Annual Update in Intensive Care and Emergency Medicine 2018

The series *Annual Update in Intensive Care and Emergency Medicine* is the continuation of the series entitled *Yearbook of Intensive Care Medicine* in Europe and *Intensive Care Medicine: Annual Update* in the United States.

Jean-Louis Vincent
Editor

Annual Update in Intensive Care and Emergency Medicine 2018

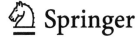 Springer

Editor

Prof. Jean-Louis Vincent
Dept. of Intensive Care
Erasme Hospital
Université libre de Bruxelles
Brussels, Belgium
jlvincent@intensive.org

The first printed copies of the book were unfortunately printed with an incorrect version of Fig. 1 in Chapter *Assessment of Fluid Responsiveness in Patients with Intraabdominal Hypertension* (page 410). An erratum sheet with the correct version was placed in the affected copies. This copy has been printed with the correct version.

ISSN 2191-5709   ISSN 2191-5717 (electronic)
Annual Update in Intensive Care and Emergency Medicine
ISBN 978-3-319-73669-3   ISBN 978-3-319-73670-9 (eBook)
https://doi.org/10.1007/978-3-319-73670-9

Cover design: WMXDesign GmbH, Heidelberg

Printed on acid-free paper

This Springer imprint is published by Springer Nature
The registered company is Springer International Publishing AG
The registred company adress is: Gewerbestrasse 11, 6330 Cham, Switzerland

Contents

Part III   Cardiovascular Concerns

Part IV   Cardiovascular Resuscitation

Part V   Respiratory Support

Part VIII   Renal Replacement Therapy

Part IX   Fluid Administration

Part X   Coagulopathy and Blood Products

Part XI   Acute Cerebral Concerns

Electronic Health Record Research in Critical Care:
S. Harris, N. MacCallum, and D. Brealey

P. R. Menon, T. D. Rabinowitz, and R. D. Stapleton

Common Abbreviations

AKI	Acute kidney injury
ARDS	Acute respiratory distress syndrome
BMI	Body mass index
CBF	Cerebral blood flow
COPD	Chronic obstructive pulmonary disease
CPB	Cardiopulmonary bypass
CPR	Cardiopulmonary resuscitation
CRRT	Continuous renal replacement therapy
CT	Computed tomography
CVP	Central venous pressure
DO_2	Oxygen delivery
ECMO	Extracorporeal membrane oxygenation
EEG	Electroencephalogram
GFR	Glomerular filtration rate
ICP	Intracranial pressure
ICU	Intensive care unit
IL	Interleukin
IVC	Inferior vena cava
LPS	Lipopolysaccharide
MAP	Mean arterial pressure
NO	Nitric oxide
OHCA	Out-of-hospital cardiac arrest
OR	Odds ratio
PEEP	Positive end-expiratory pressure
PPV	Pulse pressure variation
RAP	Right atrial pressure
RCT	Randomized controlled trial
ROS	Reactive oxygen species
RV	Right ventricular
SOFA	Sequential organ failure assessment
SVV	Stroke volume variation
TBI	Traumatic brain injury
TNF	Tumor necrosis factor

Part I
Sepsis: Underlying Mechanisms

Lipid Mediators in the Pathogenesis and Resolution of Sepsis and ARDS

B. Hamilton, L. B. Ware, and M. A. Matthay

Introduction

Recent research has demonstrated the likely importance of lipid mediators in both the pathogenesis and the resolution of sepsis and the acute respiratory distress syndrome (ARDS) [1–3]. Compared to cytokines, lipid mediators have been little studied. However, newer methods using mass spectrometry and comprehensive lipidomic analysis have facilitated more detailed investigations into lipid mediator profiles [4]. Use of broad lipid mediator profiling may uncover previously unidentified patterns in a variety of disease processes [3], including sepsis and ARDS.

The first section of this review will describe a relatively new class of lipid molecules that plays a major role in the resolution of acute inflammation and infection, termed specialized pro-resolving mediators (SPMs). The second section will review evidence that supports an important role for these endogenous lipid mediators in the resolution of localized infections as illustrated in experimental models, including viral and bacterial infections. The last section will consider the contribution of pro-inflammatory and pro-resolving lipid mediators in the resolution phase of sepsis and ARDS, including prostaglandins, leukotrienes, lipoxins, protectins and resolvins, with a focus on clinical and biological data from patients with sepsis or ARDS.

B. Hamilton
Department of Surgery, University of California
San Francisco, CA, USA

L. B. Ware
Department of Medicine and Division of Allergy, Critical Care and Pulmonary Medicine, Vanderbilt University
Nashville, TN, USA

M. A. Matthay (✉)
Cardiovascular Research Institute, University of California
San Francisco, CA, USA
e-mail: Michael.matthay@ucsf.edu

© Springer International Publishing AG 2018   3
J.-L. Vincent (ed.), *Annual Update in Intensive Care and Emergency Medicine 2018*,
Annual Update in Intensive Care and Emergency Medicine,
https://doi.org/10.1007/978-3-319-73670-9_1

Specialized Pro-Resolving Mediators and Resolution of Inflammation

The initial inflammatory responses to tissue infection have been recognized and studied for more than three decades, specifically the production of arachidonic acid metabolites, including thromboxane, prostaglandins and cysteinyl leukotrienes [1]. In the presence of infection, prostaglandin E2 (PGE2) increases local blood flow and leukotrienes C and D increase vascular permeability to augment delivery of host defense factors to the site of infection. Pro-inflammatory cytokines, such as interleukin (IL)-8, the pro-inflammatory lipid leukotriene B4 (LTB4) and activated complement factors (C3a and C5a), are key chemoattractants for neutrophils and M1-like pro-inflammatory monocytes to the site of infection [2]. Plasma factors including immunoglobulins accumulate in the extravascular site of infection.

Once the invading pathogen has been neutralized by these initial pro-inflammatory innate immune responses, the process of lipid-mediated resolution begins. This process has been termed class switching in which arachidonic acid metabolism changes from production of leukotrienes to the generation of SPMs. This new class of pro-resolving lipid mediators was initially described in studies from the laboratory of Charles Serhan [1]. These SPMs are primarily generated from essential fatty acids that include arachidonic acid, eicosapentaenoic acid (EHA) and docosahexaenoic acid (DHA). A major class of the SPMs is the lipoxins. In the circulation, lipoxins can be synthesized from leukocyte-derived 5-lipoxygenase and platelet-derived 12-lipoxygenase. In the extravascular compartments, lipoxins are produced by conversion of arachidonic acid by epithelial cell- or monocyte-derived 15-lipoxygenase and leukocyte-derived 5-lipoxygenase. In addition to the pro-resolving lipoxins, acute inflammatory and infectious exudates also include other SPMs, specifically resolvins, protectins and maresins. The receptors for some of the SPMs have been identified. The lipoxin A4 (LXA4) receptor is termed ALX in humans (and FPR2 in mice) and is a G-protein coupled receptor with high affinity. The receptor for resolvin D1 is also a G-protein receptor, termed GPR18, although resolvin D1 can also bind to ALX with high affinity [2]. Receptors for the other SPMs have not been comprehensively identified.

Several reviews have described the major features of how these SPMs function to resolve the different components of the acute inflammatory response [1, 2]. Initially, SPMs inhibit transendothelial and transepithelial migration of neutrophils. At the same time, SPMs enhance the capacity of macrophages to clear tissue debris, pathogens, and apoptotic neutrophils by a process termed efferocytosis. SPMs also induce production of the anti-inflammatory cytokine IL-10 and inhibit pro-inflammatory cytokine production in macrophages and in epithelial cells. In pulmonary studies, LXA4 has several effects that favor resolution of acute lung injury. LXA4 increases transepithelial electrical resistance by enhancing tight junctions through increased expression of zona occludens-1 and claudin-1 [5]. LXA4 also reverses the endotoxin-induced production of extracellular matrix and perivascular lung stiffening as measured by atomic force microscopy [6]. In addition, LXA4 increases Na-K-ATPase dependent alveolar fluid clearance across lung epithelium in rats in the presence of oleic acid-induced lung injury [7]. SPMs can also shift the balance to resolution by enhancing natural killer cells to accelerate neutrophil apoptosis. There is also some evidence that SPMs may activate lymphocytes to enhance resolution of acute lung injury. Resolvin E1 can decrease the production of IL-17 from T helper 17 cells, an effect that would dampen pro-inflammatory responses [2].

Specialized Pro-Resolving Mediators and Resolution of Infection

The role of pro-resolving lipid mediators in the resolution of infection needs to be assessed in the context of the contribution of both the pro-inflammatory and the pro-resolving lipids, without focusing exclusively on the SPMs. Modern methods for lipidomic profiling have made possible a more comprehensive understanding of the lipid mediators that induce and resolve inflammation in the presence of infection [4].

In the case of influenza infection, lipid chromatography and mass spectrometry were used to study 141 lipid species in mouse models of influenza (X31/H3N2 and PR8/H1N1) and also in nasopharyngeal samples from patients with influenza infection from the 2009–2011 seasons [8]. In the mouse studies, the protein levels of cytokines and chemokines indicated a straightforward positive relationship between the influenza pathogenicity and the immune response. However, the lipidomic patterns showed overlap between the pro- and anti-inflammatory pathways and more complex dynamics. On balance, the pro-resolving lipids predominated in the resolving phase of the viral infections. In the human samples, there was a general increase in both the pro-inflammatory lipids and the pro-resolving lipids in the more severely ill patients. Thus, determining the specific contributions of the endogenous pro-resolving lipids will require more complex experiments with blockade of key receptors. In one mouse study of X31/H3N2 influenza infection, supplemental therapy with substrate to enhance production of the pro-resolving lipid protectin D1 improved survival and lung pathology [9].

In a mouse model of bacterial pneumonia due to *Klebsiella pneumoniae*, early treatment with LXA4 at 1 h decreased the inflammatory response and in fact worsened the infection and decreased survival. However, treatment with LXA4 at 24 h increased survival. The results are difficult to interpret, in part, because antibiotic-treated arms were not included [10]. In another mouse study that combined hydrochloric acid-induced injury with live *Escherichia coli* instilled into one lung, resolvin E1 was administered as a pre-treatment. The treated mice had less lung injury, reduced tissue levels of pro-inflammatory cytokines, improved bacterial clearance and better survival [11]. However, resolvin E1 was not tested as a therapy after the development of acid-induced lung injury with Gram-negative pneumonia. In a cecal-ligation model of bacterial peritonitis in mice, LXA4 was given as a therapy 5 h after the initial surgery. The treated mice had enhanced 8-day survival in the absence of antibiotic therapy. The LXA4 treated mice had a reduced bacterial load, an increase in peritoneal macrophages and less systemic inflammation as reflected by lower plasma levels of IL-6 and monocyte chemotactic protein-1 [12].

Some studies have identified an important role for SPMs in promoting protection against bacterial periodontitis [2]. For example, resolvin E1 has therapeutic benefits in experimental models of aggressive periodontitis. In tuberculosis, the balance between pro-inflammatory and pro-resolving lipids is a determinant of survival. In mouse models of tuberculosis, excess production of either LTB4 or LXA4 had deleterious results with dysregulated production of tumor necrosis factor (TNF) [13].

Finally, in a recent experimental study from our research group, the beneficial effects on survival of bone marrow-derived mesenchymal stromal cells (MSCs) in endotoxin-induced lung injury in mice depended in part on the secretion of LXA4 by the MSCs [14]. In these studies, pretreatment with the LXA4 receptor inhibitor, WRW4, prevented the beneficial effects of MSCs on severity of lung injury and survival. In addition, administration of LXA4 alone increased survival from endotoxin-induced lung injury (Fig. 1).

Fig. 1 The effects of mesenchymal stromal cells (MSCs), ALX/FPR2 agonists (lipotoxin A4 [LXA4]) and antagonist (WRW4) on 48-hour survival of lipopolysaccharide (LPS)-injured mice (**a** and **b**). Four hours after LPS injury (5 mg/kg, intra-tracheal), mice received MSCs (500,000 cells), LXA4 (10 ug/kg), WRW4 (1 mg/kg) or vehicle intra-tracheally. Statistical analysis was performed using a log-rank test. Results are expressed as percentage survival (n = 25–35 per group). * p < 0.05 versus no injury, # p < 0.05 versus LPS group. Reproduced from [14] with permission

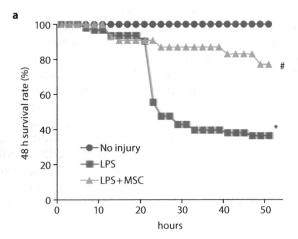

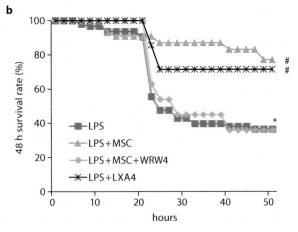

Contribution of Arachidonic Acid Metabolites in Sepsis and ARDS

In a recent clinical study of 22 patients, plasma was collected within 48 h after the onset of sepsis and follow up samples on days 3 and 7 [3]. More than 30 bioactive compounds were measured by mass spectrometry and lipid profiling. Patients were divided into survivors and non-survivors. Some interesting patterns emerged from this study. In the patients who did not survive, there were significantly higher levels of the inflammation-initiating prostaglandin F2α (PGF2α) and the pro-inflammatory LTB4, but there were also elevated levels of the pro-resolving mediators, resolvin E1, resolvin D5 and 17r-protectin D1. This pattern persisted through day 7. Thus, the higher pro-resolving lipids in the non-survivors could be interpreted as a failed endogenous attempt to resolve the infection and inflammation. However, the multiplicity of factors, including comorbidities, that determine mortality in sepsis patients makes interpretation of these results challenging. This study did not include measurements of biomarkers such as IL-6 and IL-8, or other biomarkers that have been used to profile biological responses in sepsis.

Before the availability of more comprehensive lipidomic assays, our research group used radioimmunoassay and high pressure liquid chromatography to measure selected products of arachidonic acid metabolism in the pulmonary edema fluid in the early phase of patients with ARDS, including several patients with sepsis [15]. There were 10 patients with ARDS based on bilateral chest radiographic infiltrates and severe arterial hypoxemia, a normal pulmonary arterial wedge pressure in seven patients and a normal central venous pressure in three patients. The 10 patients with ARDS had an edema fluid to plasma total protein ratio of 0.80 ± 0.16, consistent with increased protein permeability edema. There were five control patients with hydrostatic pulmonary edema, three of whom had an elevated pulmonary arterial wedge pressure (28, 30 and 33 mmHg) and the other two patients had decreased left ventricular function on echocardiography. In these five patients with hydrostatic pulmonary edema, the mean edema fluid-to-plasma total protein ratio was 0.46 ± 0.14, consistent with hydrostatic edema. Radioimmunoassay and high pressure liquid chromatography measured several products of arachidonic acid metabolism in the pulmonary edema fluid of these patients, including PGE2, thromboxane A2 (TXA2), LTB4, LTC4 and LTD4. LTD4 was significantly elevated in the edema fluid from the 10 patients with ARDS compared to in the five patients with hydrostatic edema (mean $\pm$ SD 19 ± 7 versus 4 ± 1 pmol/ml, $p < 0.001$). LTB4 levels were numerically elevated in the ARDS edema fluid samples compared to the hydrostatic edema fluid samples (11 ± 8 versus 4 ± 3 pmol/ml), although this difference did not reach statistical significance. Of the 10 patients with ARDS, five had sepsis as the primary cause of ARDS. Prior studies had focused on cyclooxygenase products of arachidonic metabolism, which had been recognized for their vasoconstrictor properties [16]. This clinical study was focused on the leukotrienes, especially LTB4 and LTD4. The elevated LTD4 was thought to be a likely contributor to the increase in lung vascular permeability. LTB4 was recognized at the time to be an important neutrophil chemoattractant that allowed large numbers of neutrophils to cross the normally tight alveolar epithelial barrier in humans without inducing a significant increase in protein permeability [17]. A follow-up study documented the presence of both LTD4 and LTE4 in the edema fluid of patients with ARDS at significantly higher concentrations than in patients with hydrostatic edema [18]. Biologically, LTE4 has similar properties to LTD4 for increasing vascular permeability. These studies were done prior to the recognition of the pro-resolution lipid pathways.

In more recent work, our research group studied 20 mechanically ventilated patients with acute pulmonary edema, 14 with ARDS and six with hydrostatic pulmonary edema [19]. The patients were categorized as ARDS or hydrostatic edema based on clinical data and the edema fluid-to-plasma protein ratio, as in prior studies. Undiluted pulmonary edema fluid was collected, centrifuged and frozen within 24 h of intensive care unit (ICU) admission from ventilated patients with pulmonary edema. The etiology of ARDS was infectious in nine of the 14 patients (pneumonia or sepsis) and is provided in Table 1. The baseline clinical data and patient characteristics are provided in Table 2. The clinical characteristics were comparable between patients with hydrostatic edema and those with ARDS except that oxygenation was significantly worse in the patients with ARDS.

To take advantage of the comprehensive lipidomic analysis using more advanced liquid chromatography and mass spectrometry and multiple reaction monitoring methods [20], seven pro-inflammatory or pro-resolving lipid mediators were measured including arachidonic acid, PGE2, PGF2α, TXB2, LTB4, LTE4 and LXA4. Levels of three of the lipid mediators were significantly higher in the ARDS edema fluid, specifically LTB4, LTE4 and LXA4 (p < 0.05) (Fig. 2). These findings provide evidence for the likely contribution of the two pro-inflammatory leukotrienes, LTB4

Table 1 Etiology and underlying medical disorders in the patients with hydrostatic pulmonary edema (HPE) and those with acute respiratory distress syndrome (ARDS)

Etiology	HPE	ARDS	Underlying disorder
Pneumonia	0	5	Community-acquired; myasthenia gravis; metastatic cancer; perioperative; fungal
Myocardial infarct	1	0	Peri-catheterization
Sepsis	0	4	S/p small bowel resection; gastroparesis & end-stage liver disease; sepsis vs. aspiration with cardiac arrest
TACO/TRALI	1	1	End-stage liver disease with TACO; transfusion s/p spinal fusion with TRALI
Idiopathic	0	2	Intracranial tumor; acute hepatic failure
Volume overload	1	0	Mitral stenosis/congestive heart failure
Drug overdose	0	1	Fulminant hepatic failure
Reperfusion injury	0	1	S/p lung transplant
Neurogenic	1	0	Subarachnoid hemorrhage
Heart failure	1	0	Hypoxic respiratory failure
Hypertension	1	0	ESRD

TACO: transfusion-associated circulatory overload; *TRALI*: transfusion-related acute lung injury; *s/p*: status post; *ESRD*: end-stage renal disease

Table 2 Baseline clinical characteristics in the patients with hydrostatic pulmonary edema (HPE) and those with acute respiratory distress syndrome (ARDS)

Characteristic	HPE	ARDS	p value
Male, *n (%)*	3 (50%)	8 (57%)	1.00
Age, years, *median (IQR)*	63 (51, 71)	46 (37, 55)	0.12
PaO_2/FiO_2 ratio, *median (IQR)*	115 (106, 137)	53 (47, 76)	0.03
Lung injury score, *median (IQR)*	3.0 (2.4, 3.0)	3.0 (2.7, 3.5)	0.19
Tidal volume per kg, *median (IQR)*	6.3 (5.9, 7.4)	6.6 (4.8, 8.4)	1.00
Use of vasopressors, *n (%)*	2 (50%)	10 (91%)	0.15
Alveolar fluid clearance, *median (IQR) (%/hour)*	4.2 (2.4, 7.8)	0.6 (0.0, 3.3)	0.17
Days ventilated, *median (IQR)*	4.5 (2.5, 5.8)	3.0 (2.0, 6.0)	0.79
Death, *n (%)*	0 (0%)	7 (43%)	0.06

Continuous data are shown as median with interquartile ranges (IQR; 25th to 75th percentile) and compared using Wilcoxon rank-sum tests because of the non-normal distribution of the data. Categorical data are shown as number and percent and compared using Fisher's exact test

and LTE4, in the pathogenesis of the increased protein permeability in ARDS. The statistically higher level of LXA4 is particularly interesting given the growing data that pro-resolving lipids play an important role in tissue repair. Elevation of LXA4 early in ARDS may indicate that the process of resolving injury has been initiated

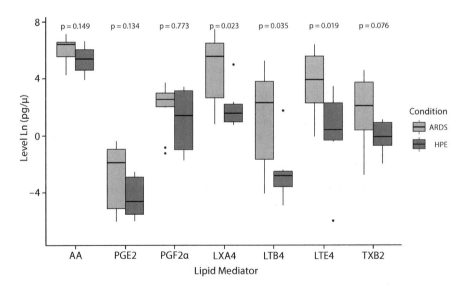

Fig. 2 Lipid mediator levels in the undiluted pulmonary edema fluid of the patients with hydrostatic pulmonary edema (HPE) and acute respiratory distress syndrome (ARDS). The levels are displayed on the y-axis in Ln (natural log transformed) as pg/µl and the data are shown as median with confidence intervals (25th to 75th intervals). The seven measured lipid mediators were arachidonic acid (AA), prostaglandin E2 (PGE2), prostaglandin F2α (PGF2α), lipoxin A4 (LXA4), leukotriene B4 (LTB4), leukotriene E4 (LTE4) and thromboxane B2 (TXB2). p < 0.05 for LTB4, LTE4 and LXA4

at an early stage, similar to some of the experimental studies cited earlier in this review. Thus, the lipid mediator levels measured in the alveolar fluid compartment demonstrate distinct patterns in patients with ARDS versus hydrostatic edema. Further studies are needed to determine the association and function of lipid mediators in the pathogenesis of ARDS.

Conclusion

The availability of comprehensive lipidomic and mass spectrometry assays has made it possible to study both pro-inflammatory and pro-resolving lipids in experimental and clinical studies of sepsis and acute lung injury. The important contribution of SPMs in the resolution of tissue injury has now been established in several clinically relevant experimental models of infection, sepsis and acute lung injury. More clinical studies are needed to characterize the pro-inflammatory and pro-resolving lipid patterns in patients with sepsis and ARDS, potentially making it possible to endotype these patients into sub-populations that have different clinical outcomes, as our group has done by combining protein biomarkers and clinical data using latent class analysis [21, 22]. Given developments in lipid mediator pharmacology, identification of specific targets could lead to novel therapeutic strategies for sepsis and ARDS.

References

1. Serhan CN (2014) Pro-resolving lipid mediators are leads for resolution physiology. Nature 510:92–101
2. Basil MC, Levy BD (2016) Specialized pro-resolving mediators: endogenous regulators of infection and inflammation. Nat Rev Immunol 16:51–67
3. Dalli J, Colas RA, Quintana C et al (2017) Human sepsis eicosanoid and proresolving lipid mediator temporal profiles: correlations with survival and clinical outcomes. Crit Care Med 45:58–68
4. Cajka T, Fiehn O (2014) Comprehensive analysis of lipids in biological systems by liquid chromatography-mass spectrometry. Trends Anal Chem 61:192–206
5. Grumbach Y, Quynh NVT, Chiron R, Urbach V (2009) LXA4 stimulates ZO-1 expression and transepithelial resistance in human airway epithelial cells. Am J Physiol Lung Cell Mol Physiol 296:L101–L108
6. Meng F, Mambetsariev I, Tian Y et al (2015) Attenuation of lipopolysaccharide-induced lung vascular stiffening by lipoxin reduces lung inflammation. Am J Respir Cell Mol Biol 52:152–161
7. Wang Q, Lian QQ, Li B et al (2013) Lipoxin A4 activates alveolar epithelial sodium channel, Na,K-ATPase, and increases alveolar fluid clearance. Am J Respir Cell Mol Biol 48:610–618
8. Tam VC, Quehenberger O, Oshansky C et al (2013) Lipidomic profiling of influenza infection identifies mediators that induce and resolve inflammation. Cell 154:213–227
9. Morita M, Kuba K, Ichikawa A et al (2013) The lipid mediator protectin D1 inhibits influenza viral replication and improves severe influenza. Cell 153:112–125
10. Sordi R, Menez-de-Lima O Jr, Horewicz V et al (2013) Dual role of lipoxin A4 in pneumosepsis pathogenesis. Int Immunopharm 17:283–292

11. Seki H, Fukunaga K, Artia M et al (2009) The anti-inflammatory and proresolving mediator resolving E1 protects mice from bacterial pneumonia and acute lung injury. J Immunol 184:836–843

12. Walker J, Dichter E, Lacorte G et al (2011) Lipoxin A4 increases survival by decreasing systemic inflammation and bacterial load in sepsis. Shock 36:410–416

13. Tobin D, Roca JF, Oh SF et al (2012) Host genotype-specific therapies can optimize the inflammatory response to mycobacterial infections. Cell 148:434–446

14. Fang X, Abbott J, Cheng L, Lee JW, Levy BD, Matthay MA (2015) Human mesenchymal stem (stromal) cells promote the resolution of acute lung injury in part through lipoxin A4. J Immunol 195:875–881

15. Matthay M, Eschenbacher WL, Goetzl EJ (1984) Elevated concentrations of leukotriene D4 in pulmonary edema fluid of patients with the adult respiratory distress syndrome. J Clin Immunol 4:479–483

16. Snapper JR, Hutchinson AA, Ogletree ML, Brigham KL (1983) Effects of cyclooxygenase inhibitors on the alterations in lung mechanics caused by endotoxemia in the unanesthetized sheep. J Clin Invest 72:63–76

17. Martin TR, Pistoresse BP, Chi EY, Goodman RB, Matthay MA (1989) Effects of leukotriene B4 in the human lung. J Clin Invest 84:1609–1619

18. Ratnoff WD, Matthay MA, Wong MY et al (1988) Sulfidopeptide-leukotriene peptidases in pulmonary edema fluid from patients with the adult respiratory distress syndrome. J Clin Immunol 8:250–258

19. Hamilton B, Gronert K, Gotts JE, Calfee CS, Ware LB, Matthay MA (2017) Integrated analysis method of soluble lipid mediators in alveolar fluid discriminates ARDS from hydrostatic pulmonary edema. Am J Respir Crit Care Med 195:A4356 (abst)

20. von Moltke J, Trinidad NJ, Moayeri M et al (2012) Rapid induction of inflammatory lipid mediators by the inflammasome in vivo. Nature 490:107–111

21. Calfee CS, Delucchi K, Parsons PE, Thompson BT, Ware LB, Matthay MA (2014) Subphenotypes in acute respiratory distress syndrome: latent class analysis of data from two randomized controlled trials. Lancet Respir Med 2:611–620

22. Famous K, Delucchi K, Ware LB et al (2017) Acute respiratory distress syndrome subphenotypes respond differently to randomized fluid management strategy. Am J Respir Crit Care Med 195:331–338

Immune Paralysis in Sepsis: Recent Insights and Future Development

B. M. Tang, V. Herwanto, and A. S. McLean

Introduction

Immune paralysis, or the inability of the immune response to recover despite clearance of pathogens by antimicrobials, is a major cause of death in patients with sepsis. Persistent immune paralysis leads to failure to eradicate the primary infection and increased susceptibility to secondary infection [1, 2]. The clinical relevance of this immunosuppressed state in sepsis patients is evidenced by the frequent occurrence of infection with opportunistic and multidrug-resistant bacterial pathogens and the reactivation of latent viruses (cytomegalovirus, Epstein-Barr virus and herpes simplex virus-1) [3–8]. Here, we review recent insights related to the cellular mechanisms of sepsis-induced immune paralysis and the development of novel therapies for treating immune paralysis.

How Does Immune Paralysis Occur?

We begin with a brief review of the established literature on the mechanisms of immune paralysis. These mechanisms have been well studied in animal models and human studies. They fall into three main categories as follows:

B. M. Tang
Department of Intensive Care Medicine, Nepean Hospital
Kingswood, NSW 274, Australia
Centre for Immunology and Allergy Research, Westmead Institute for Medical Research
Westmead, NSW 2145, Australia

V. Herwanto · A. S. McLean (✉)
Department of Intensive Care Medicine, Nepean Hospital
Kingswood, NSW 274, Australia
e-mail: anthony.mclean@sydney.edu.au

© Springer International Publishing AG 2018   13
J.-L. Vincent (ed.), *Annual Update in Intensive Care and Emergency Medicine 2018*,
Annual Update in Intensive Care and Emergency Medicine,
https://doi.org/10.1007/978-3-319-73670-9_2

Death of Immune Cells

Sepsis causes progressive, apoptosis-induced loss of cells of the immune system. Apoptosis is prominent in CD4 T$^+$-cells, CD8$^+$ T-cells, B-cells, natural killer (NK) cells and follicular dendritic cells in sepsis patients. Two pathways for apoptosis have been identified: (1) the death-receptor pathway; and (2) the mitochondrial-mediated pathway [9].

The detrimental effects of apoptosis are not only related to the severe loss of immune cells but also to the impact that apoptotic cell uptake has on the surviving immune cells. Uptake of apoptotic cells by monocytes, macrophages and dendritic cells either leads to increased anti-inflammatory cytokine production (e.g., inter-leukin [IL]-10) or results in an anergy state (see below) that further exacerbates the immune suppressive state [10, 11].

Immune Cell Exhaustion or 'Anergy'

A robust cytokine response, after stimulation by pathogens or bacterial antigens (e.g., lipopolysaccharide [LPS]), is a common characteristic of healthy, well-functioning immune cells. The progressive loss of such a response is a well-recognized condition in sepsis. This condition has been named as "immune cell exhaustion", "anergy" or "endotoxin tolerance" [12]. T-cell anergy, or an impaired response to an antigen with decreased release of cytokines in the T cells, can lead to immune dysfunction in sepsis patients. Immune cell anergy also occurs in macrophages and monocytes. Loss of their expression of surface receptor, major histocompatibility complex (MHC) class II, contributes to macrophage and monocyte dysfunction [13]. Furthermore, the decrease in monocyte CD14/human leukocyte antigen (HLA)-DR co-expression correlates with the degree of immune dysfunction and results in a poorer outcome in severe sepsis [14].

Anti-Inflammatory State

During sepsis, the anti-inflammatory cytokine, IL-10, is produced by T regulatory (Treg) and T helper (Th)2 cells and suppresses the Th1 response. This suppressive environment results in a marked decrease in monocyte production of pro-inflammatory cytokines tumor necrosis factor (TNF)-α, IL-1β, and IL-6 [13, 14].

What Are the New Insights from Recent Studies?

The above three processes, although well supported by many studies, are unlikely to be the only mechanisms that underpin sepsis-induced immune paralysis. Additional mechanisms have been discovered in more recent studies.

Immune-Metabolic Dysfunction

Immune cells rely on oxidative phosphorylation as their main energy source. However, during sepsis, immune cells shift their metabolism towards aerobic glycolysis [15, 16]. This shift is an important adaptive mechanism that helps maintain host defense. The failure of this shift may explain immune paralysis during sepsis. In a recent landmark study, investigators found that in immune cells during sepsis both oxidative phosphorylation and aerobic glycolysis were greatly diminished. The investigators also observed that the expected metabolic shift did not occur [17]. The cellular consequence of this metabolic failure is significant, as immune cells require an adequate supply of adenosine triphosphate and other metabolic intermediates (e.g., NAD^+) to maintain critical cellular functions during host defense, including activation, differentiation and proliferation [18].

Transcriptomics Changes

Changes in cellular function are controlled, in part, at a gene-expression level. Therefore, studies on gene-expression changes (i.e., transcriptomics) have revealed considerable insight into the host response in sepsis. The findings from these studies demonstrated increased gene-expressions in pro-inflammatory, anti-inflammatory, and mitochondrial dysfunction and decreased gene-expression in translational initiation, mTOR signaling, adaptive immunity and antigen presentation [19–21]. A recent landmark gene-expression study explored the correlation between gene-expression changes and patient level outcomes (e.g., mortality). The authors discovered a subgroup of sepsis patients who displayed gene-expression changes that corresponded to an immunosuppressive phenotype and termed these gene-expression changes the "sepsis response signature" 1. Genes included in this gene-expression signature indicate changes in T cell exhaustion, endotoxin tolerance, and downregulation of HLA class II. The authors showed that the presence of this immunosuppressive signature predicted poor prognosis [22].

Epigenetic Modifications

Gene-expression can be modulated at an epigenetic level. Epigenetic modification could retain unfavorable changes in gene-expression and maintain these changes beyond the acute phase of infection. This 'imprinting' process may contribute to the persistence of the immune suppressive state during the post-resuscitation period of sepsis. For example, epigenetic imprinting might occur in progenitor cells in the bone marrow and in other immune tissues, such as spleen and thymus. This effect may explain why the immune system is not completely recovered by the generation of new immune cells from the bone marrow. Similarly, epigenetic reprogramming may be retained in the progenitor cells of patients who survive sepsis, allowing them to perpetuate the epigenetic marks into well differentiated cells, which further compromises the immune response [23]. Together, these findings suggest that epigenetic changes in immune cells may be important factors contributing to the prolonged effect of post-septic complications [24].

How Do Leukocytes Contribute to Immune Paralysis?

Monocytes and Macrophages

Monocytes and macrophages play important roles in sepsis-induced immune paralysis. In sepsis, the capacity of monocytes to release pro-inflammatory cytokines in response to endotoxin (e.g., LPS) or other Toll-like receptor (TLR) agonists is diminished. This phenomenon is known as endotoxin tolerance [25]. Two major consequences of endotoxin tolerance on monocytes and macrophages are (1) an increase in the release of immunosuppressive mediators (mainly IL-10) and (2) a decrease in antigen presentation as a result of reduced expression of HLA-DR. Both consequences are associated with augmented susceptibility to secondary microbial infection and a worse outcome in sepsis [26, 27].

Neutrophils and Myeloid-Derived Suppressor Cells (MDSC)

Neutrophils contribute to immune paralysis in three ways. First, neutrophils produce large amounts of the immunosuppressive cytokine, IL-10, during sepsis. These alterations are assumed to be due to abnormalities in TLR signaling, which is analogous to endotoxin tolerance in monocytes. Second, suppressive neutrophil-like cells (i.e., MDSCs), a subtype of differentiated neutrophils that accumulate in the lymphoid organ after infection, could also contribute to immune paralysis by blocking T cell function and promoting T regulatory cells. Third, neutrophils release nuclear extracellular traps (NETs) that may be immunosuppressive. NETs are normal parts of host defense; however, an excessive release of NETs can lead to extensive tissue damage. Sepsis patients have been observed to have increased NETs in their circulation, which correlated with organ dysfunction [24, 28].

Dendritic Cells

Dendritic cells are central components for linking the innate and adaptive immunity. Sepsis causes loss of dendritic cells in various lymphoid and non-lymphoid tissues. Plasmacytoid and myeloid dendritic cells are particularly vulnerable to sepsis-induced apoptosis. Dendritic cell loss was more apparent in patients with sepsis who died than in those who survived, and it was also more marked in patients who subsequently developed nosocomial infections than in those patients who did not. Monocyte-derived dendritic cells from patients with sepsis were unable to induce a robust effector T cell response but instead induced T cell anergy. These anergic

T cells, in turn, may disrupt dendritic cell function. Collectively, these data suggest that dendritic cell death/dysfunction is an important determinant of sepsis-induced immunosuppression and mortality [11].

CD4+ Th Cell Subsets

Mature CD4+ Th cells have been characterized into Th1, Th2 and Th17 cell subsets based on the type of cytokines that they produce in response to stimulation. Th1 and Th2 cell-associated cytokine production is decreased during the initial immune response to sepsis. This could be related to the significant reductions in the expression of T-bet and GATA-binding protein 3 (GATA3), which are transcription factors that modulate the Th1 and Th2 cell response. The Th17 cell response is also reduced in sepsis, possibly as a result of decreased expression of the retinoic acid receptor-related orphan receptor-γt (RORγt), which is the transcription factor that is specific for Th17 cells. This defect in the Th17 cell phenotype in sepsis is likely to be a contributing factor to the increased susceptibility of these patients to secondary fungal infections [29].

T Regulatory Cells

The number of Treg cells increases during sepsis. One reason for this could be that they are more resistant to sepsis-induced apoptosis, presumably because of an increase expression of the anti-apoptotic protein, B-cell lymphoma (BCL)-2. Another reason is the increase in alarmins, including heat shock proteins and histones, which are strong inducers of Treg cells. In addition, Treg cells inhibit both monocyte and neutrophil function. Furthermore, Treg cells precipitate an NK cell-dependent endotoxin tolerance-like phenomenon that is characterized by decreased production of interferon (IFN)γ and granulocyte-macrophage colony-stimulating factor (GM-CSF). Based on these observations, it is clear that Treg cells play a critical role in sepsis-induced immune paralysis [10].

$\gamma\delta$ T Cells

The $\gamma\delta$ T cells are a distinct subset of lymphocytes that reside mainly in the intestinal mucosa. They recognize invading pathogens and mount a prompt, innate-like immune response by releasing IFN-γ, IL-17 and various chemokines. The number of circulating $\gamma\delta$ T cells is significantly decreased in patients with sepsis and the depletion is parallel to sepsis severity. The loss of their number in the intestinal mucosa might be detrimental because it allows invasion of intestinal pathogens into the circulation or the peritoneal cavity, thereby causing secondary infections [30].

Natural Killer Cells

In patients with sepsis, the number of circulating NK cells is markedly decreased, often for weeks, and the low numbers of NK cells are associated with increased mortality. Their cytotoxic function and cytokine productions are also reduced. In addition, decreased IFNγ production by NK cells was identified as a possible contributing factor to increased secondary infection in sepsis and reactivation of latent infection [31].

B-Lymphocytes

B cells or B-lymphocytes have a relevant immunoregulatory role in that they present antigens to T lymphocytes and differentiate into antibody producing cells. B cell exhaustion is a hallmark of sepsis; it compromises the ability of B cells to produce antibodies and the efficient eradication of pathogens [32, 33].

Future Approach in Immunotherapeutics: New Ways to Treat Sepsis?

The above review suggests that there are many potential targets for immune modulation therapy, which might help reverse or reduce the effect of sepsis-induced immune paralysis. Such therapy may include agents that inhibit apoptosis, block negative costimulatory molecules, decrease the level of anti-inflammatory cytokines, increase HLA-DR expression, and reactivate 'exhausted' or anergic T cells [34]. These agents (currently investigated in preclinical studies) are summarized in Table 1.

Table 1 Proposed therapies targeting immune cells implicated in sepsis-induced immune paralysis

Immune cells	Mechanisms implicated in sepsis	Immunotherapy
Monocytes and macrophages	Endotoxin tolerance Increase immunosuppressive mediators, esp. IL-10 Reduce expression of HLA-DR Reprogramming to M2 phenotype	IFN-γ, G-CSF, GM-CSF, anti-PD-L1-antibody, IL-15
Neutrophil and MDSC	Decrease apoptosis Increase IL-10 Increase immature cells with decreased antimicrobial function Block T cell function and promote Treg Release NET	IL-15, recombinant human IL-7, G-CSF, GM-CSF

Table 1 (Continued)

Immune cells	Mechanisms implicated in sepsis	Immunotherapy
Dendritic cell	Increase apoptosis Induce T cell anergy Induce Treg proliferation Reduce antigen presentation to T cell and B cell	IL-15
CD4+ Th cell subset	Increase apoptosis Exhaustion Th2 cell polarization	Recombinant human IL-7, anti-PD-1-antibody, anti-PD-L1-antibody, IL-15, anti-IL-10, anti-TGF-ß
Treg cell	Resistance to apoptosis Inhibit monocyte and neutrophil function Precipitate NK cell-dependent endotoxin tolerance-like phenomenon	Recombinant human IL-7, anti-IL-10, anti-TGF-ß
$\gamma\delta$ T cell	Decrease number, esp. in intestinal mucosa	Recombinant human IL-7
NK cell	Increase apoptosis Reduce cytotoxic function Decrease IFN-γ production	IL-15
B-lymphocyte	Increase apoptosis Exhaustion → compromise ability of antibody production and pathogen eradication	Recombinant human IL-3

IL: interleukin; *NK*: natural killer; *TGF*: transforming growth factor; *Th*: T helper cell; *PD*: programmed death; *PD-L*: programmed death ligand; *G-CSF*: granulocyte colony-stimulating factor; *GM-CSF*: granulocyte-macrophage colony-stimulating factor; *IFN*: interferon; *NET*: nuclear extracellular trap; *MDSC*: myeloid-derived suppressor cells

Recombinant Human IL-7

IL-7 is essential for T cell development and function. It upregulates the expression of anti-apoptotic molecule BCL-2, induces the proliferation of peripheral T cells and sustains increased numbers of circulating blood CD4+ and CD8+ T cells. In addition, IL-7 administration causes reduction in the proportion of Treg cells in the circulation, rejuvenates exhausted T cells by decreasing programmed death 1 (PD-1) expression and increases the expression of cell adhesion molecules, thereby facilitating the trafficking of T cells to sites of infection [10, 13].

IL-15

IL-15 has been targeted to reverse apoptosis and improve immune suppression in sepsis and its administration reduces apoptosis of NK cells, dendritic cells, CD8$^+$ T cells and gut epithelial cells. It also increases IFNγ levels and percentage of NK cells [35].

IFNγ

A key immunological defect in sepsis is the decreased production of IFNγ. Treatment with recombinant IFNγ has been observed to reverse monocyte dysfunction in sepsis patients whose monocytes had decreased HLA-DR expression and reduced amounts of TNF in response to LPS [36]. Thus, IFNγ might be effective in sepsis patients who have entered the immunosuppressive phase.

Granulocyte Colony-Stimulating Factor and Granulocyte-Macrophage Colony-Stimulating Factor

Administration of these agents has resulted in the restoration of HLA-DR expression, fewer days on the ventilator and in the ICU, restored TNF production, and reduced the acquisition of nosocomial infection; however, there was no clear benefit in terms of mortality [37].

Blockade of PD-1 and PD-L1 Signaling

Blockade of PD-1 and programmed death ligand 1 (PD-L1) with specific antibodies has shown improved survival in clinically relevant animal models of bacterial sepsis. These agents work by reversing several effects of PD-1 and PD-L1 proteins (apoptosis, T cell suppression and anti-inflammatory cytokine production) [34].

Mesenchymal Stem Cells

Administration of allogenic mesenchymal stem cells is a relatively new approach. Administration is associated with lower organ dysfunction and mortality in animal models via antimicrobial, anti-apoptotic, immunomodulatory and barrier-preserving effects [38].

Should We Use a Biomarker-Guided Approach?

A prerequisite for the application of immunotherapy in sepsis-induced immune paralysis is the proper selection of patients. Therefore, we advocate a precision medicine approach where biomarkers are used to select patients with abnormalities in specific immune pathways. Potential biomarkers include decreased monocyte HLA-DR expression and increased circulating IL-10 concentrations, both of which assess innate immune function and therefore can be utilized to stratify patients for IFNγ or GM-CSF treatment. Other parameters include decreased absolute CD4$^+$ T cell number and increased percentage of Treg cells, which can be used to stratify patients for IL-7 therapy. Additional parameters include PD-1 expression on CD4$^+$ and CD8$^+$ cells or PD-L1 expression on monocytes, which could help in selecting candidates for PD-1 and PD-L1-specific antibody therapy. IFNγ production by T cells and the IL-10/TNF ratio are some other biomarker options that can be used to guide immunotherapy in sepsis [10, 39, 40].

Conclusion

This review summarizes recent advances and new insights relating to the mechanisms of immune paralysis in sepsis. Current evidence clearly indicates that no single therapeutic agent can adequately treat the broad range of immunological abnormalities present in sepsis. In this regard, clinical trials recruiting a heterogeneous patient population are unlikely to succeed due to their poor discrimination in recognizing subsets of patients with specific immunological deficits. Future clinical trials should therefore adopt a precision medicine approach in which clinicians use 'omics' technology to select the right patients (i.e., those with biomarker-proven abnormalities in immune pathways) and treat these patients with the right therapeutic agents (i.e., drugs that target these pathways).

References

1. Myrianthefs PM, Karabatsos E, Baltopoulos GJ (2014) Sepsis and immunoparalysis. In: Hall JB, Schmidt GA, Kress JP (eds) Principles of Critical Care, 4th edn. McGraw-Hill, New York
2. Angus DC, van der Poll T (2013) Severe sepsis and septic shock. N Engl J Med 369:840–851
3. Zhao GJ, Li D, Zhao Q et al (2016) Incidence, risk factors and impact on outcomes of secondary infection in patients with septic shock: an 8-year retrospective study. Sci Rep 6:38361
4. Sakr Y, Lobo SM, Moreno RP et al (2012) Patterns and early evolution of organ failure in the intensive care unit and their relation to outcome. Crit Care 16:R222
5. Otto GP, Sossdorf M, Claus RA et al (2011) The late phase of sepsis is characterized by an increased microbiological burden and death rate. Crit Care 15:R183
6. Morrow LE, Kollef MH (2010) Recognition and prevention of nosocomial pneumonia in the intensive care unit and infection control in mechanical ventilation. Crit Care Med 38:S352–S362
7. Walton AH, Muenzer JT, Rasche D et al (2017) Reactivation of multiple viruses in patients with sepsis. PLoS One 9:e98819

8. Delaloye J, Calandra T (2014) Invasive candidiasis as a cause of sepsis in the critically ill patient. Virulence 5:161–169

9. Czabotar PE, Lessene G, Strasser A, Adams JM (2014) Control of apoptosis by the BCL-2 protein family – implications for physiology and therapy. Nat Rev Mol Cell Biol 15:49–63

10. Hotchkiss RS, Monneret G, Payen D (2013) Sepsis-induced immunosuppression: from cellular dysfunctions to immunotherapy. Nat Rev Immunol 13:862–867

11. Fan X, Liu Z, Jin H, Yan J, Liang HP (2015) Alterations of dendritic cells in sepsis: featured role in immunoparalysis. Biomed Res Int 2015:903720

12. Cheng SC, Scicluna BP, Arts RJW, Gresnigt MS, Lachmandas E, Giamarellos-Bourboulis EJ (2016) Broad defects in the energy metabolism of leukocytes underlie immunoparalysis in sepsis. Nat Immunol 17:406–413

13. Boomer JS, Green JM, Hotchkiss RS (2014) The changing immune system in sepsis – is individualized immuno-modulatory therapy the answer? Virulence 5:45–56

14. Sundar KM, Sires M (2013) Sepsis induced immunosuppression: Implications for secondary infections and complications. Indian J Crit Care Med 17:162–169

15. Vachharajani V, Liu T, McCall CE (2014) Epigenetic coordination of acute systemic inflammation: potential therapeutic targets. Expert Rev Clin Immunol 10:1141–1150

16. Cheng SC, Joosten LA, Netea MG (2014) The interplay between central metabolism and innate immune responses. Cytokine Growth Factor Rev 25:707–713

17. Nalos M, Parnell G, Robergs R, Booth D, McLean A, Tang B (2016) Transcriptional reprogramming of metabolic pathways in critically ill patients. Intensive Care Med Exp 4:21

18. Carre JE, Orban JC, Re L et al (2010) Survival in critical illness is associated with early activation of mitochondrial biogenesis. Am J Respir Crit Care Med 182:745–751

19. Scicluna BP, Klein Klouwenberg PM, van Vught LA et al (2015) A molecular biomarker to diagnose community-acquired pneumonia on intensive care unit admission. Am J Respir Crit Care Med 192:826–835

20. Van Vught LA, Klein Klouwenberg PMC, Spitoni C (2016) Incidence, risk factors, and attributable mortality of secondary infections in the intensive care unit after admission for sepsis. JAMA 315:1469–1479

21. Parnell G, Tang B, Nalos M et al (2013) Identifying key regulatory genes in the whole blood of septic patients to monitor underlying immune dysfunctions. Shock 40:166–174

22. Davenport EE, Burnham KL, Radhakrishnan J et al (2016) Genomic landscape of the individual host response and outcomes in sepsis: a prospective cohort study. Lancet Respir Med 4:259–271

23. Carson WF, Cavassani KA, Dou Y, Kunkel SL (2011) Epigenetic regulation of immune cell functions during post-septic immunosuppression. Epigenetics 6:273–283

24. Gimenez JLG, Carbonell NE, Mateo CR et al (2016) Epigenetics as the driving force in long-term immunosuppression. J Clin Epigenet 2:2

25. Shalova IN, Lim JY, Chittezhath M et al (2015) Human monocytes undergo functional reprogramming during sepsis mediated by hypoxia-inducible factor-1. Immunity 42:484–498

26. Chan C, Li L, McCall CE, Yoza BK (2005) Endotoxin tolerance disrupts chromatin remodeling and NF-κB transactivation at the IL-1β promoter. J Immunol 175:461–468

27. El Gazzar M, Yoza BK, Chen X, Garcia BA, Young NL, McCall CE (2009) Chromatin-specific remodeling by HMGB1and linker histone H1 silences proinflammatory genes during endotoxin tolerance. Mol Cell Biol 29:1959–1971

28. Van der Poll T, van de Veerdonk FL, Scicluna BP, Netea MG (2017) The immunopathology of sepsis and potential therapeutic targets. Nat Rev Immunol 17:407–420

29. Cabrera-Perez J, Condotta SA, Badovinac VP, Griffith TS (2014) Impact of sepsis on CD4 T cell immunity. J Leukoc Biol 96:767–777

30. Andreu-Ballester JC, Tormo-Calandín C, Garcia-Ballesteros C et al (2013) Gamma-delta T cells in septic patients: association with severity and mortality. Clin Vaccine Immunol 20:738–746

31. Souza-Fonseca-Guimaraes F, Cavaillon JM, Adib-Conquy M (2013) Bench-to-bedside review: natural killer cells in sepsis – guilty or not guilty? Crit Care 17:235
32. De Pablo R, Monserrat J, Prieto A, Alvarez-Mon M (2014) Role of circulating lymphocytes in patients with sepsis. Biomed Res Int 2014:671087
33. Griffith TC, Condotta SA, Tygrett LT, Rai D, Yang JA, Pape KA et al (2016) Sepsis compromises primary B cell-mediated responses. J Immunol 195(1 Suppl):15 (abst)
34. Hotchkiss RS, Monneret G, Payen D (2013) Immunosuppression in sepsis: a novel understanding of the disorder and a new therapeutic approach. Lancet Infect Dis 13:260–268
35. Inoue S, Unsinger J, Davis CG et al (2010) IL-15 prevents apoptosis, reverses innate and adaptive immune dysfunction, and improves survival in sepsis. J Immunol 184:1401–1409
36. Nalos M, Santner-Nanan B, Parnell G, Tang B, McLean AS, Nanan R (2012) Immune effects of interferon gamma in persistent staphylococcal sepsis. Am J Respir Crit Care Med 185:110–112
37. Bo L, Wang F, Zhu J, Li J, Deng X (2011) Granulocyte-colony stimulating factor (G-CSF) and granulocyte-macrophage colony stimulating factor (GM-CSF) for sepsis: a meta-analysis. Crit Care 15:R58
38. Kingsley SM, Bhat BV (2016) Could stem cells be the future therapy for sepsis? Blood Rev 30:439–452
39. Biron BM, Ayala A, Lomas-Neira JL (2015) Biomarkers for sepsis: what is and what might be? Biomark Insights 10:7–17
40. Trapnell B (2009) A novel biomarker-guided immunomodulatory approach for the therapy of sepsis. Am J Respir Crit Care Med 180:585–587

Persistent Inflammation, Immunosuppression and Catabolism after Severe Injury or Infection

P. A. Efron, F. A. Moore, and S. C. Brakenridge

Introduction

Starting in the 1990s, reports describing chronic critical illness emerged under a variety of descriptive terms including the "neuropathy of critical illness", "myopathy of critical illness", "intensive care unit (ICU)-acquired weakness" and most recently "post-ICU syndrome". These reports largely originated from medical ICUs that included individuals with a wide variety of admission diagnoses, most common of which was acute exacerbation of chronic disease. These patients required prolonged mechanical ventilation and were often discharged to long-term care facilities. Given the clinical heterogeneity of this patient population, the underlying pathophysiology of chronic critical illness has remained ill-defined. However, with recent improved implementation of evidence-based ICU care, the epidemiology of multiple organ failure (MOF) has evolved. Early hospital mortality has decreased substantially and the incidence of late onset MOF deaths in the ICU has largely disappeared. As a result, protracted low grade MOF has become a common cause of chronic critical illness. Based on substantial laboratory and clinical research data, the Persistent, Inflammation, Immunosuppression and Catabolism (PICS) paradigm was proposed as a mechanistic framework in which to explain the increased incidence of chronic critical illness in surgical ICUs, which we believe represents the next major challenge in surgical critical care. The purpose of this review is to provide a historic perspective of the epidemiologic evolution of MOF into PICS, discuss the long-term outcomes of chronic critical illness and PICS and review the mechanisms that can induce PICS.

P. A. Efron (✉) · F. A. Moore · S. C. Brakenridge
Departments of Surgery and the Sepsis and Critical Illness Research Center, University of Florida College of Medicine
Gainesville, FL, USA
e-mail: philip.efron@surgery.ufl.edu

© Springer International Publishing AG 2018
J.-L. Vincent (ed.), *Annual Update in Intensive Care and Emergency Medicine 2018*,
Annual Update in Intensive Care and Emergency Medicine,
https://doi.org/10.1007/978-3-319-73670-9_3

Evolving Epidemiology of MOF into PICS

MOF has plagued ICUs for over four decades and its epidemiology has evolved as advances in critical care have allowed patients to survive previously lethal insults. Over the years, different predominant clinical presentations of MOF have come and gone, all having consumed tremendous amounts of healthcare resources with associated prolonged ICU stays and prohibitive mortality [1]. The advent of ICUs in the early 1970s facilitated survival of patients with single organ failure; concurrently, MOF emerged as a highly lethal syndrome (with mortality greater than 80%). Early case series from the USA concluded that MOF occurred as the result of uncontrolled sepsis (principally intraabdominal infections) and research efforts were effectively focused on curbing this condition.

In the mid-1980s, European studies reported MOF frequently after blunt trauma with no identifiable site of infection [2]. It was then recognized that both infectious and non-infectious insults could induce a similar overwhelming destructive systemic inflammatory response syndrome (SIRS). Research thus shifted to determining the underlying mechanisms of this phenomenon (e.g., bacterial translocation, 'cytokine storm', ischemia-reperfusion). Simultaneously, through the early 1990s, tremendous advances in trauma care substantially reduced early deaths from bleeding but resulted in an epidemic of abdominal compartment syndrome (ACS) that emerged in ICUs worldwide.

While clinical interest focused on understanding ACS as a new malignant presentation of MOF, epidemiological studies revealed that MOF was a bimodal phenomenon [3]. Early MOF occurred after either an overwhelming insult (one-hit model) or sequential amplifying insults (2-hit model), whereas late MOF was precipitated by secondary nosocomial infections. SIRS, followed by a compensatory anti-inflammatory response syndrome (CARS), was proposed to explain this bimodal distribution of MOF. SIRS-induced early MOF was thought to occur because of exaggerated innate immune and inflammatory response, whereas CARS was viewed as progressive depression in adaptive immunity, resulting in secondary infections.

By the late 1990s, fundamental changes in the initial care of patients arriving with severe bleeding were widely implemented, including sonography, massive transfusion protocols, avoidance of excessive crystalloids and abandonment of pulmonary artery catheter directed resuscitation. Subsequently, the epidemic of ACS virtually disappeared [4]. Concordantly, evidence-based medicine became a health care mandate; subsequently, this has become a major driver for improved ICU care. As a result of these initiatives, there has been another striking change in the epidemiology of MOF. Early in-hospital mortality has decreased substantially, and the incidence of late-onset MOF deaths has largely disappeared [5].

However, a substantial portion of these high-risk patients with MOF survive prolonged ICU stays to progress into a new predominant MOF phenotype of chronic critical illness that we have termed "PICS" (Fig. 1; [6]). Following major insults (e.g., trauma, burns, pancreatitis and sepsis), pro-inflammation (SIRS), immune suppression and anti-inflammation (CARS) occur simultaneously. In some cases,

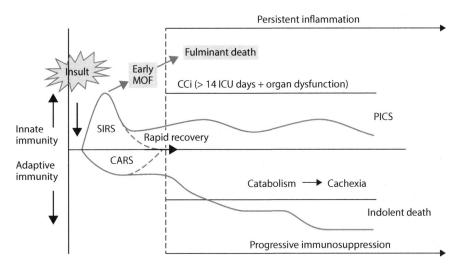

Fig. 1 Model of persistent inflammation, immunosuppression and catabolism syndrome (PICS). Following the simultaneous inflammatory and immunosuppressive responses, patients may return to a homeostatic immune state, leading to a rapid recovery, or develop chronic critical illness (CCi) and PICS, resulting from protein catabolism, cachexia, organ failure and secondary infections. A significant number of these patients fail to ever recover and suffer an indolent death. *CARS*: compensatory anti-inflammatory response syndrome; *MOF*: multi-organ failure; *SIRS*: systemic inflammatory response syndrome. Adapted from [9] with permission

SIRS becomes overwhelming, leading to early MOF and fulminant death trajectory. Fortunately, modern ICU care allows medical practitioners to detect and prevent this trajectory's fatal expression. If patients do not succumb to early MOF, they follow one of two pathways: either their aberrant immunology rapidly recovers (i.e., restores homeostasis) or its dysfunction persists and they enter a state of chronic critical illness, which we define as > 14 days in ICU with organ dysfunction.

These patients with chronic critical illness experience ongoing immunosuppression (e.g., lymphopenia) and inflammation (e.g., neutrophilia) that is associated with a persistent acute phase response (e.g., high C-reactive protein [CRP] and low pre-albumin levels) with ongoing protein catabolism. Despite aggressive nutritional intervention, there is a tremendous loss of lean body mass and proportional decrease in functional status and poor wound healing. Clinically, PICS patients suffer from recurrent nosocomial infections, poor wound healing and develop decubitus ulcers. They are commonly discharged to long-term acute care facilities where they often experience sepsis recidivism requiring re-hospitalization, failure to rehabilitate and an indolent death.

Long-Term Outcomes of Chronic Critical Illness and PICS

As stated, there has been a significant decline in inpatient mortality after critical illness secondary to severe trauma or sepsis [7–10]. While we may be tempted to celebrate these successes of inpatient survival, the incidence of chronic critical illness continues to increase and the long-term outcomes of these intensive care survivors remain unclear. The majority of published descriptions of the clinical phenotype of patients that survive critical illness come from patient cohorts with primary pulmonary failure and acute respiratory distress syndrome (ARDS).

Appropriately utilizing general descriptive terms such as post-intensive care syndrome, neuropathy of critical illness and ICU-acquired weakness, these studies describe a significant burden and persistence of functional deficits after prolonged respiratory failure and ventilator dependence [11, 12].

The definitions of chronic critical illness and PICS as described in this chapter attempt to elucidate or characterize the underlying pathophysiology driving these morbidities. We offer an operational definition of resource utilization and persistent organ injury, as well as a conceptual framework for the underlying pathophysiologic mechanisms that drive the persistent immunologic, organ and physical deficits. All of these factors contribute to poor long-term outcomes after severe pro-inflammatory insults such as trauma or sepsis.

While it is well-described that survivors of critical illness are at significant risk of death after hospital discharge, the mechanisms driving this mortality risk remain unclear. It has been demonstrated that hospital discharge dispositions that provide high levels of functional support for extended periods of time (i.e., skilled nursing facilities and long-term acute care facilities) are associated with significantly higher long-term mortality rates after trauma or surgical sepsis [8, 13]. As an example, overall patient mortality has decreased significantly over the past 15 years in conjunction with the application of evidenced-based standard operating protocols for the care of severely injured trauma patients at a cohort of Level 1 trauma centers in the USA [7]. Despite these apparent successes, a US state-population based long-term outcomes analysis of trauma patients revealed that, although inpatient mortality after severe trauma steadily decreased over a 13-year period to as low as 5%, subsequent 3-year mortality was nearly three-fold greater [13]. Additionally, advancing age and discharge to a skilled nursing facility (as compared to discharge to home or a rehabilitation facility) were the strongest predictors of long-term mortality [13]. These findings likely reflect the reality of the gentrification of the population and the associated increasing age and frailty of patients that now survive severe injury.

Post-trauma long-term outcomes are poor, but long-term outcomes associated with sepsis are dismal. In a combined analysis of two interventional randomized controlled trials after severe sepsis/septic shock, initial 28-day mortality for this critically ill cohort was approximately 20%, but 6-month mortality jumped to nearly 35% [14]. Even more striking than the discrepancy between short- and long-term mortality were the significant functional limitations and morbidity burden amongst sepsis survivors. Of sepsis survivors at 6 months, nearly half reported significant difficulties with mobility, poor quality of life and could not live independently [14].

Another more recent prospective longitudinal cohort study of 88 patients with severe sepsis/septic shock has revealed that early (within the first week) inpatient mortality from refractory shock and MOF is now less than 5%. However, 40% of this population subsequently developed chronic critical illness and had inpatient discharge dispositions (i.e., long-term acute care, skilled nursing facility) known to be associated with poor outcomes and a striking 6-month mortality of nearly 30% (Fig. 2; [10]).

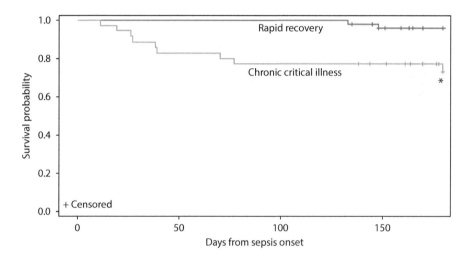

Fig. 2 Six-month mortality of sepsis patients with chronic critical illness versus rapid recovery. Eighty-eight critically ill surgical sepsis patients were enrolled in a prospective observational study and classified as chronic critical illness or rapid recovery [35]. Chronic critical illness was defined as an ICU length of stay (LOS) greater than or equal to 14 days with evidence of persistent organ dysfunction, measured using components of the Sequential Organ Failure Assessment (SOFA) score at 14 days (i.e., cardiovascular SOFA ≥ 1, or score in any other organ system ≥ 2). In addition, patients with an ICU LOS less than 14 days would also qualify for chronic critical illness if they were discharged to another hospital, a long-term acute care facility, or to hospice and demonstrated evidence of organ dysfunction at the time of discharge. Those patients experiencing death within 14 days of sepsis onset were excluded from the analysis. Rapid recovery was defined as any patient who did not meet criteria for chronic critical illness or early death. The Kaplan-Meier analysis demonstrates their cumulative survival rate over six months in chronic critical illness versus rapid recovery patients (*log-rank; $p = 0.0023$). Patients who had yet to reach six months after their initial sepsis event were censored and are denoted with tick marks. Adapted from [10] with permission

Mechanisms That Induce PICS

A vicious cycle of pathophysiological alterations is engendered in patients with chronic critical illness and PICS, which is reflected and propagated by chronic low-grade inflammation, such as elevated CRP and cytokine concentrations; immuno-suppression, such as lymphocyte dysfunction and reduced antigen-presentation; and catabolism, including defects in carbohydrate, lipid and protein metabolism ([6, 9, 15]; Fig. 3a). Organ injury, such as acute kidney injury and acute respiratory insuffi-ciency/failure, contributes to the persistence of PICS and vice-versa [16]. This also includes other organ systems not historically thought of as having systemic effects, such as muscle and intestine, but are now recognized to have significant impact on inflammation and immune suppression [16].

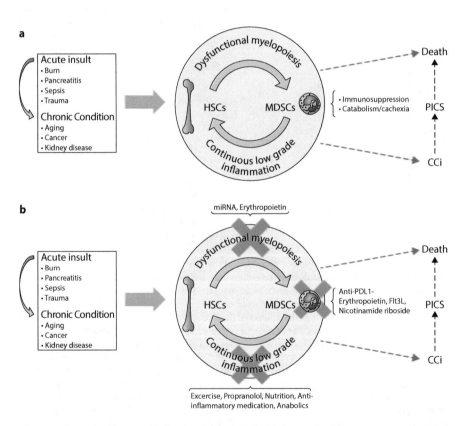

Fig. 3 Depiction of the myelodysplasia of persistent inflammation, immunosuppression and catabolism syndrome (PICS). **a** The vicious cycle and immune dyscrasia of PICS and its subse-quent outcomes. Chronic critical illness (CCi) and PICS are more likely to occur when combined with certain chronic conditions or aging. **b** Interventions that have the potential to be investigated to determine whether they can disrupt the vicious cycle of CCi and PICS. *HSC*: hematopoietic stem cells; *MDSCs*: myeloid-derived suppressor cells; *PD-L1*: programmed death ligand-1

Most hematopoietic stem cells (HSCs) are relatively quiescent, participating in maintaining immune and hematologic homeostasis in the host. The upregulation of the HSC activity in response to stress, however, is an integral function of innate immunity [17, 18]. After injury or infection, host HSCs become active, entering the cell cycle as well as differentiating. This process, known as 'emergency myelopoiesis', aims to repopulate innate immune effector cells after host stressors stimulate the release of mature populations and the creation of bone marrow niches [18, 19]. The increased and preferential generation of these myelopoietic cells occurs at the expense of lymphopoiesis and erythropoiesis [18].

This emergency activation occurs through multiple, redundant pathways and mechanisms, including ligands such as growth factors (e.g., granulocyte/granulocyte-macrophage colony stimulating factor [G/GM-CSF], FltL) and cytokines (e.g., interleukin [IL]-6 and IL-17), as well as through mesenchymal or immune cells [6, 20, 21]. One result of this HSC response is the creation of immature myeloid populations including myeloid-derived suppressor cells (MDSCs), which are a wide range of myeloid cells in various stages of differentiation [18]. Although the exact roles of MDSCs are still being elicited, they are *acutely* believed to be part of a physiologic response to sepsis and trauma in order to help reduce inflammation through immunosuppression, while not eliminating all protective innate immunity [18, 22]. This includes the toxicity that can occur due to excessive T-cell proliferation and cytokine production [23]. It is clear, however, that their *chronic persistence* is associated with poor outcomes in sepsis patients, as initially demonstrated by Mathias et al. and then confirmed by Uhel et al. [9, 18, 24, 25].

Chronic critical illness is associated with several stimuli and mechanisms. In chronic critical illness, there is a persistent presence of damage-associated molecular pattern (DAMP) and/or pathogen-associated molecular pattern (PAMP) molecules [23]. This is physiologic in the acute phase of an insult, as the host is programmed to recognize specific 'danger signals' or 'alarmins' with microbial invasion or tissue damage [26]. These PAMPs and DAMPs can bind to multiple receptors, including Toll-like receptors (TLRs), NOD-like receptors (NLRs), complement, retinoic acid-inducible gene (RIG)-like receptors and mannose-binding lectin/scavenger receptors [23, 26]. This leads to the activation of common and redundant signaling pathways of immunity in various cell types, including immune, epithelial and endothelial cells [23, 26]. In turn, pro- and anti-inflammatory cytokine, reactive oxygen and reactive nitrogen species production increases, as well as there being increased tissue wasting and apoptosis [23]. There is an accompanying recruitment of myeloid (e.g., neutrophils, macrophages) and lymphoid cells and there are direct and indirect effects of infection and injury on endothelium and parenchymal tissue as well as the neurologic and coagulation systems [23, 26]. Altogether, this leads the host to suffer from common immunosuppressive mechanisms, such as: the expansion of MDSCs, T-regulatory cells (Treg), and M2 macrophages; T-cell exhaustion; immunosuppressive mediator (e.g., IL-10, transforming growth factor [TGF]-β) release; and inhibitory ligand expression on parenchymal cells [23].

As mentioned previously, the immediate and simultaneous SIRS/CARS response, or "cytokine storm", is an appropriate mammalian reaction to an insult with the intent of addressing injury or infection and subsequently restoring the host to homeostasis [27]. However, the perseverance of inflammation, immunosuppression and catabolism in the host is highly dysfunctional. The medical practitioner's capacity to compensate for organ dysfunction in critically ill patients creates a host environment in which damaged organs and tissues maintain a low grade continuous pro-inflammatory state [26]. This is presumed to be through DAMPs and alarmins, many of which are well described in the literature: hyaluronan products, ATP, adenosine, protein S100A, high-mobility group protein B1 (HMGB1), histones, nucleosides and mitochondrial/nuclear DNA. The downstream effects of this chronic inflammation make the host susceptible to opportunistic infections and viral reactivations, alters the host microbiota, and often requires the continuation of intensive care interventions such as mechanical ventilation and catheters. This, in turn, perpetuates a vicious cycle by preventing the return of the host to homeostasis regarding immune, organ and metabolic function [26].

The downstream effects of persistent inflammation are numerous. Interestingly, it engenders a host immune environment similar to that of an elderly individual at baseline – i.e., "inflammaging" (constant low-grade inflammation in the aged) contributing to immunosenescence (the dysfunction of the innate and adaptive immune systems of the aged) [28, 29]. Lymphopenia occurs due to both acute apoptosis of effector T and B lymphocytes during sepsis, as well as the HSC shift to myelopoiesis [9, 26]. Lymphocytes also undergo Th2 polarization as well as expansion of Treg cells. Neutrophilia occurs, but these effector immature myeloid cells are suboptimal, as they have a decreased capacity for antigen presentation, expression of adhesion molecules and formation of extracellular traps, as well as an altered cytokine and chemokine expression pattern [26]. In addition, there is a shift in macrophages to the M2 phenotype as well as dendritic cell apoptosis [26, 30]. Finally, there is an increase in the number of and suppressive capacity in circulating MDSCs [24].

Although research regarding the classification of MDSCs is ongoing, they are generally divided into two forms, monocytic and granulocytic [24]. The *sine quo none* of these immature myeloid cells is their ability to suppress T cell function. The immunosuppression of MDSCs is carried out in several ways, which may be dependent on their subtype [9]. First, MDSCs secrete the anti-inflammatory cytokines IL-10 and TGF-β. Two of the many effects of these cytokines are to polarize macrophages to a type II phenotype and upregulate Treg cells. Second, MDSCs deplete L-arginine via arginase 1 (ARG1) and inducible nitric oxide (NO) synthase (iNOS), which alters the function, impairs the intracellular signaling and induces apoptosis of T cells. Third, MDSCs produce increased reactive oxygen species (ROS), which with NO (the byproduct of iNOS), produce peroxynitrites. These peroxynitrites then nitrosylate several lymphocyte cell surface proteins and cysteine residents, resulting in decreased T-cell responsiveness and altered IL-2 signaling. Additionally, NO can impede the stability of IL-2 mRNA and ROS can suppress natural killer (NK) cell function. Finally, direct MDSC cell contact via CD40 receptors results in induction of Treg cells, and upregulation of programmed death ligand-1 (PD-L1) and other checkpoint inhibitors in MDSCs cause T-cell apoptosis [9]. In addition, although its association with MDSCs has not been established, chronic exposure to these factors involved in PICS can induce HSC defects, including, but not limited to, their ability to repopulate and differentiate [31–33].

MDSCs have been associated with poor clinical outcomes, specifically after sepsis. Mathias et al. demonstrated that MDSCs are persistently elevated in the circulation, predominantly granulocytic, transcriptomically unique and immunosuppressive to T lymphocytes after severe sepsis or septic shock in the surgical ICU [24]. Persistent increased percentages of blood MDSCs in this study were associated with increased nosocomial infections, prolonged ICU stays, increased mortality and poor functional status at discharge [24]. Uhel et al. verified these findings in the medical ICU population. Although both monocytic and granulocytic MDSCs were expanded in their medical ICU population and both of these cell populations inhibited T-cell proliferation, granulocytic MDSCs were more specifically increased in patients with sepsis [25]. The granulocytic MDSCs, which demonstrated a high level of ARG1 activity, displayed high levels of degranulation markers, and most importantly, their early expansion predicted the development of nosocomial infections in these patients [25].

Conclusion

PICS describes the underlying pathophysiology, or immune dyscrasia, that results after an inciting inflammatory response. After severe inflammation, which can also include burns and pancreatitis, patients with chronic critical illness fail to achieve immune and organ homeostasis [6, 15, 19, 34]. Due to the complexity and redundancy of pathways after a severe inflammatory insult to humans, it is unlikely that a 'silver bullet' therapy will be identified to improve the outcomes of patients with chronic critical illness or PICS. However, PICS is, in part, a myelodysplastic disease, and this aspect of the syndrome, possibly through immunomodulation, will need to be addressed as part of a multi-phased approach to optimize post-trauma and post-sepsis morbidity and mortality – both acute and chronic (Fig. 3b). Further discovery of the underlying mechanisms will undoubtedly require more studies, including additional genomic and proteomic analyses, as well as the creation of improved animal models of PICS. Hopefully, ongoing clinical trials testing of approved therapies for other diseases (e.g., PD-L1 inhibitors) will provide further direction. Ideally, these therapies will directly influence dysregulated host immunity and prevent the perpetual cycle of PICS (Fig. 3b).

Acknowledgement

PAE was supported by the National Institutes of Health (NIH) National Institute of General Medical Sciences (NIGMS) grant 1 R01 GM113945-01, and PAE and

SCB were supported by P30 AG028740 from the National Institute on Aging (NIA). PAE, FAM and SCB were all supported by P50 GM111152-01 (NIGMS).

References

1. Moore FA, Moore EE (1995) Evolving concepts in the pathogenesis of postinjury multiple organ failure. Surg Clin North Am 75:257–277
2. Faist E, Baue AE, Dittmer H, Heberer G (1983) Multiple organ failure in polytrauma patients. J Trauma 23:775–787
3. Moore FA, Sauaia A, Moore EE et al (1996) Postinjury multiple organ failure: a bimodal phenomenon. J Trauma 40:501–510
4. Balogh Z, McKinley BA, Cox CS Jr et al (2003) Abdominal compartment syndrome: the cause or effect of postinjury multiple organ failure. Shock 20:483–492
5. Sauaia A, Moore EE, Johnson JL et al (2014) Temporal trends of postinjury multiple-organ failure: still resource intensive, morbid, and lethal. J Trauma Acute Care Surg 76:582–592
6. Gentile LF, Cuenca AG, Efron PA et al (2012) Persistent inflammation and immunosuppression: a common syndrome and new horizon for surgical intensive care. J Trauma Acute Care Surg 72:1491–1501
7. Cuschieri J, Johnson JL, Sperry J et al (2012) Benchmarking outcomes in the critically injured trauma patient and the effect of implementing standard operating procedures. Ann Surg 2555:993–999
8. Mira JC, Cuschieri J, Ozrazgat-Baslanti T et al (2017) The epidemiology of chronic critical illness after severe traumatic injury at two-level one trauma centers. Crit Care Med 45:1989–1996
9. Mira JC, Gentile LF, Mathias BJ et al (2017) Sepsis pathophysiology, chronic critical illness, and persistent inflammation-immunosuppression and catabolism syndrome. Crit Care Med 452:253–262
10. Stortz JA, Murphy TJ, Raymond SL et al (2017) Evidence for persistent immune suppression in patients who develop chronic critical illness after sepsis. Shock. https://doi.org/10.1097/SHK.0000000000000981 (epub ahead of print)
11. Herridge MS, Cheung AM, Tansey CM et al (2003) One-year outcomes in survivors of the acute respiratory distress syndrome. N Engl J Med 348:683–693
12. Cheung AM, Tansey CM, Tomlinson G et al (2006) Two-year outcomes, health care use, and costs of survivors of acute respiratory distress syndrome. Am J Respir Crit Care Med 174:538–544
13. Davidson GH, Hamlat CA, Rivara FP, Koepsell TD, Jurkovich GJ, Arbabi S (2011) Long-term survival of adult trauma patients. JAMA 305:1001–1007
14. Yende S, Austin S, Rhodes A et al (2016) Long-term quality of life among survivors of severe sepsis: analyses of two international trials. Crit Care Med 44:1461–1467
15. Rosenthal MD, Moore FA (2015) Persistent inflammatory, immunosuppressed, catabolic syndrome (PICS): a new phenotype of multiple organ failure. J Adv Nutr Hum Metab 1:e784
16. Rosenthal MD, Moore FA (2016) Persistent inflammation, immunosuppression, and catabolism: evolution of multiple organ dysfunction. Surg Infect (larchmt) 17:167–172
17. Pietras EM, Warr MR, Passegue E (2011) Cell cycle regulation in hematopoietic stem cells. J Cell Biol 195:709–720
18. Goldszmid RS, Dzutsev A, Trinchieri G (2014) Host immune response to infection and cancer: unexpected commonalities. Cell Host Microbe 15:295–305
19. Mira JC, Brakenridge SC, Moldawer LL, Moore FA (2017) Persistent inflammation, immunosuppression and catabolism syndrome. Crit Care Clin 33:245–258
20. Boettcher S, Ziegler P, Schmid MA et al (2012) Cutting edge: LPS-induced emergency myelopoiesis depends on TLR4-expressing nonhematopoietic cells. J Immunol 188:5824–5828

21. Boiko JR, Borghesi L (2012) Hematopoiesis sculpted by pathogens: toll-like receptors and inflammatory mediators directly activate stem cells. Cytokine 57:1–8
22. Cuenca AG, Delano MJ, Kelly-Scumpia KM et al (2011) A paradoxical role for myeloid-derived suppressor cells in sepsis and trauma. Mol Med 17:281–292
23. Hotchkiss RS, Moldawer LL (2014) Parallels between cancer and infectious disease. N Engl J Med 371:380–383
24. Mathias B, Delmas AL, Ozrazgat-Baslanti T et al (2017) Human myeloid-derived suppressor cells are associated with chronic immune suppression after severe sepsis/septic shock. Ann Surg 265:827–834
25. Uhel F, Azzaoui I, Gregoire M et al (2017) Early expansion of circulating granulocytic myeloid-derived suppressor cells predicts development of nosocomial infections in patients with sepsis. Am J Respir Crit Care Med 196:315–327
26. Hotchkiss RS, Moldawer LL, Opal SM et al (2016) Sepsis and septic shock. Nat Rev Dis Primers 2:16045
27. Xiao W, Mindrinos MN, Seok J et al (2011) A genomic storm in critically injured humans. J Exp Med 208:2581–2590
28. Nacionales DC, Gentile LF, Vanzant E et al (2014) Aged mice are unable to mount an effective myeloid response to sepsis. J Immunol 192:612–622
29. Nacionales DC, Szpila B, Ungaro R et al (2015) A detailed characterization of the dysfunctional immunity and abnormal myelopoiesis induced by severe shock and trauma in the aged. J Immunol 195:2396–2407
30. Efron PA, Martins A, Minnich D et al (2004) Characterization of the systemic loss of dendritic cells in murine lymph nodes during polymicrobial sepsis. J Immunol 173:3035–3043
31. Baldridge MT, King KY, Goodell MA (2011) Inflammatory signals regulate hematopoietic stem cells. Trends Immunol 32:57–65
32. Skirecki T, Kawiak J, Machaj E et al (2015) Early severe impairment of hematopoietic stem and progenitor cells from the bone marrow caused by CLP sepsis and endotoxemia in a humanized mice model. Stem Cell Res Ther 6:142
33. Zhang H, Rodriguez S, Wang L et al (2016) Sepsis Induces hematopoietic stem cell exhaustion and myelosuppression through distinct contributions of TRIF and MYD88. Stem Cell Reports 6:940–956
34. Yang N, Li B, Ye B et al (2017) The long-term quality of life in patients with persistent inflammation-immunosuppression and catabolism syndrome after severe acute pancreatitis: A retrospective cohort study. J Crit Care 42:101–106
35. Loftus TJ, Mira JC, Ozrazgat-Baslanti T et al (2017) Sepsis and Critical Illness Research Center investigators: protocols and standard operating procedures for a prospective cohort study of sepsis in critically ill surgical patients. BMJ Open 7:e15136

Current Trends in Epidemiology and Antimicrobial Resistance in Neonatal Sepsis

S. Chavez-Bueno and R. J. McCulloh

Introduction

Invasive infections are the cause of approximately 25% of deaths in newborns worldwide. In 2015, 336,300 neonatal deaths globally were attributed to sepsis and other neonatal infections [1]. Rates of neonatal sepsis are highest in African countries and lowest in North American and developed European countries. In addition to the different incidence of neonatal invasive disease, the pathogens causing neonatal sepsis and their antibiotic resistance patterns also vary in different regions of the world. This manuscript focuses on the epidemiological characteristics of sepsis in infants younger than 30 days of age in the developed world, and on recent antibiotic resistance trends observed in the pathogens that cause neonatal sepsis in the USA.

Rates of sepsis in newborns are inversely related to gestational age. Neonates rely on innate immune responses as the first line of defense against infections. These mechanisms are impaired in preterm newborns compared to term infants. Likewise, the normal maturation of T and B cell responses to infection is interrupted in preterm newborns, resulting in a higher risk for infection in this group. Preterm newborns, particularly those born < 34 weeks' gestational age, are more likely to require hospitalization for interventions such as mechanical ventilation, intravas-

S. Chavez-Bueno
Children's Mercy Kansas City
Kansas City, MO, USA
University of Missouri
Kansas City, MO, USA

R. J. McCulloh (✉)
Children's Mercy Kansas City
Kansas City, MO, USA
University of Missouri
Kansas City, MO, USA
University of Kansas Medical Center
Kansas City, KS, USA
e-mail: rmcculloh@cmh.edu

© Springer International Publishing AG 2018
J.-L. Vincent (ed.), *Annual Update in Intensive Care and Emergency Medicine 2018*,
Annual Update in Intensive Care and Emergency Medicine,
https://doi.org/10.1007/978-3-319-73670-9_4

Table 1 Microorganisms that commonly cause early- and/or late-onset neonatal sepsis

Organism	Transmission	Usual onset
Bacteria		
Escherichia coli	Intrapartum/postpartum	Early-onset, late-onset
Streptococcus agalactiae (GBS)	Intrapartum/postpartum	Early-onset, late-onset
Other GNRs	Intrapartum/postpartum	Late-onset
Staphylococcus aureus	Postpartum	Late-onset
CoNS	Postpartum	Late-onset
Viruses		
HSV	Intrapartum/postpartum	Early-onset, late-onset
Enteroviruses	Postpartum	Late-onset
Influenza	Postpartum	Late-onset
VZV	Transplacental	Late-onset
Fungi		
Candida spp.	Postpartum	Late-onset

GNRs: Gram-negative rods; *GBS*: group B streptococci; *CoNS*: coagulase-negative staphylococci; *HSV*: herpes simplex virus; *VZV*: varicella zoster virus

cular catheterization, parenteral nutrition, and treatment for underlying respiratory and cardiovascular diseases, which further increase their risk for invasive infections. In addition to host and environmental factors as determinants for the susceptibility to infection in newborns, the mechanisms of transmission of the various neonatal pathogens also affect the timing and the incidence of the different infections found in this population.

Based on the age of presentation, neonatal sepsis is classified into early-onset and late-onset. The US Centers for Disease Control and Prevention (CDC) use the designation of early-onset disease for infants diagnosed within the first week of life, and late-onset sepsis for cases occurring between 7 and 89 days of age. The Neonatal Research Network (NRN) from the Eunice Kennedy Shriver National Institute of Child Health and Human Development (NICHD), and the Vermont Oxford Network designate early-onset sepsis as those cases presenting within the first 72 h of life. Common pathogens responsible for early- and late-onset sepsis are listed in Table 1.

Early-Onset Sepsis

Early-onset sepsis is caused by organisms vertically transmitted from a colonized mother to her newborn in the perinatal period. The rate of early-onset sepsis reported to the CDC's Active Bacterial Core surveillance (ABCs) from 2005 to 2008 was 0.77 per 1,000 live births [2]. Data from 2006 to 2009 obtained from participating centers of the NRN showed an overall early-onset sepsis rate of 0.98 cases per 1,000 live births [3]. The incidence of early-onset sepsis correlates inversely with gestational age, and consequently, with birth weight. The overall rate of early-onset sepsis in infants born with weight > 2,500 g has been reported at 0.57 cases per 1,000 live births, and as high as 10.96 cases per 1,000 live births in very low birth weight (VLBW) newborns (i.e., birth weight 401–1,500 g) [3]. In addition to gestational age, race is another factor affecting the incidence of early-onset sepsis. Rates of early-onset sepsis in black newborns are two- to several-fold greater when compared to non-black infants [2, 4].

Bacterial Pathogens in Early-Onset Sepsis

In the US and Europe, Group B streptococcus (GBS) has been the leading cause of early-onset sepsis since the 1970s [5]. Although the incidence of GBS early-onset sepsis has decreased by > 80% since the introduction of maternal intrapartum antibiotic prophylaxis, GBS continues to be the most frequent pathogen causing early-onset sepsis in newborns overall [6, 7], although in recent years *Escherichia coli* has surpassed GBS as a cause of early-onset sepsis in some parts of the US [4]. In the US, GBS early-onset sepsis rates have decreased from approximately 1.7 cases per 1,000 live births in the 1990s to 0.23 per 1,000 live births in 2015, which is below the target goal of 0.25 cases per 1,000 live births set by the CDC's Healthy People 2020 [8].

GBS has a predominant role as a cause of early-onset sepsis in term newborns. However, this is not the case in preterm neonates. *E. coli* is now the most frequent pathogen causing early-onset sepsis in preterm newborns. With the marked decrease in the incidence of GBS early-onset sepsis due to the implementation of intrapartum antibiotic prophylaxis, concerns have arisen for the possibility of concurrent increasing rates of Gram-negative early-onset sepsis, and possibly increasing rates of ampicillin resistance in early-onset sepsis pathogens. In the US, data from studies published between 1994 and 2002 showed that all-cause early-onset sepsis rates decreased in some centers. However, some centers reported increasing rates of *E. coli* specifically, and only in preterm newborns [9]. Subsequent reports confirmed *E. coli* as the predominant causative agent in early-onset sepsis in preterm newborns, and that resistance to ampicillin in this pathogen is now prevalent [2, 3, 10].

In addition to GBS and *E. coli*, other bacterial pathogens that cause early-onset sepsis in term and preterm newborns include other Gram-negative bacteria, such as *Haemophilus influenzae*, *Citrobacter* spp., and *Enterobacter* spp., each in < 5% of early-onset sepsis cases. Among Gram-positive bacteria, viridans streptococci were involved in 4 and 12% of cases of early-onset sepsis in term and preterm infants, respectively [2, 10]. Coagulase-negative staphylococci (CoNS) was found in 14.7% cases of early-onset sepsis in VLBW newborns, while *Listeria monocytogenes* was the cause in 2% [10].

Overall mortality due to early-onset sepsis is 16%, with a range from 54% in infants born at 22–24 weeks' gestational age to 3% in term infants [3]. Mortality due to Gram-negative early-onset sepsis is greater than in early-onset sepsis caused by Gram-positive bacteria. Overall mortality in early-onset sepsis due to *E. coli* ranges from 23.1% to 33% and due to GBS is 4–9% [2–4, 6]. The highest mortality rates reported for early-onset sepsis are approximately 40% and occur in black preterm newborns infected with *E. coli* [2, 4]. Most deaths in early-onset sepsis occur in the first 72 h of life [3].

Late-Onset Sepsis

Late-onset sepsis occurs after the first week of life and is considered to be a community-acquired infection in otherwise healthy infants, or a hospital-acquired infection in the case of newborns that remain hospitalized after birth. The incidence of late-onset serious bacterial infections in healthy infants born at term is approximately 0.57 per 1,000 births [11]. Not surprisingly, the incidence of late-onset sepsis is greater in preterm newborns, particularly in those that remain hospitalized, and ranges from 0.78 cases per 1,000 hospital days in late-preterm infants to 5.15 cases per 1,000 hospital days in those born < 25 weeks' gestational age [12]. In the latter group, NRN data have shown a decreased incidence of overall late-onset sepsis in recent years [13].

Bacterial Pathogens in Late-Onset Sepsis

The epidemiology of late-onset sepsis in term newborns is changing. GBS late-onset sepsis rates have remained stable after the introduction of maternal intrapartum antibiotic prophylaxis because this measure is effective only for decreasing the incidence of GBS early-onset sepsis as discussed earlier. The incidence of GBS late-onset sepsis in 2015 was 0.32 cases per 1,000 live births, similar to the 0.34 per 1,000 live births in 1996 when the first recommendations for intrapartum antibiotic prophylaxis were issued [14]. While the incidence of GBS late-onset sepsis has not changed, the rates of late-onset sepsis caused by other pathogens show relevant differences in recent years.

In previously healthy term newborns between ages 7–28 days, late-onset sepsis is currently caused predominantly by *E. coli*. Bacteremia in newborns in this age group was caused by *E. coli* in 49% of cases in a large population of infants at Kaiser Permanente Northern California [11]. The second and third most common pathogens associated with late-onset sepsis in that study were GBS (31%) and *Staphylococcus aureus* (8%). The remaining cases were caused by *Klebsiella* spp., *Citrobacter* spp., *Salmonella* spp., and viridans streptococci. No cases of *L. monocytogenes*, *Streptococcus pneumoniae* or enteroccal infections were found in this age group in this population. This study also found that previously healthy term newborns age 7–28 days diagnosed with late-onset sepsis bacteremia had an additional focus of infection (i.e., meningitis and/or urinary tract infection) significantly more frequently compared to infants 30–90 days old [11]. Another recent study in infants up to 30 days old with bacteremia, confirmed *E. coli* as the most frequent causative pathogen (46% of cases), followed by GBS (23%), *Klebsiella* spp. (5%), *S. aureus* (4%), and *S. pneumoniae* (2%). *L. monocytogenes* was not isolated from any of these bacteremic newborns [15].

In preterm newborns, Gram-positive bacteria are the main cause of late-onset sepsis, and among them, CoNS predominates. CoNS causes 22–55% of late-onset sepsis episodes in VLBW infants. Overall, *S. aureus* is the cause of late-onset sepsis in 4–8% of cases, followed by *Enterococcus* spp. (3%) and GBS (2%). Gram-negative organisms are responsible for approximately 18% of late-onset sepsis cases in VLBW newborns. In VLBW the frequency of *E. coli* has significantly increased in recent years [16]. In late-preterm newborns, late-onset sepsis is caused most frequently by CoNS (16%), followed by *S. aureus* in 13%, enterococci in 8%, and GBS in 3%. Gram-negative bacteria that cause late-onset sepsis in preterm infants include *E. coli* in 10% of cases, *Klebsiella* spp. in 7%, *Enterobacter* spp. in 4%, *Serratia* spp. in 2% and *Pseudomonas* spp. in 1% [17].

Overall, the mortality rate due to late-onset sepsis in term infants is ≤ 5% [11]. In late preterm newborns, the overall mortality rate is 7%, and highest when associated with Gram-negative bacteremia, such as that caused by *Pseudomonas* spp. (40% mortality) [17]. Late-onset sepsis caused by Gram-positive bacteria in late-preterm newborns carries a mortality rate of 8.3%. *Candida* spp. late-onset sepsis in this subgroup of preterm infants has a mortality rate of 6.4% [17]. Preterm newborns born < 25 weeks' gestational age have the highest mortality rates secondary to late-onset sepsis compared to newborns of other gestational ages. Although the incidence of late-onset sepsis has decreased recently in these extremely VLBW (EVLBW) infants, mortality rates have not. Overall, mortality in EVLBW newborns with late-onset sepsis is 26%. In this group of infants, Gram-positive infections have a mortality rate of 22%, Gram-negative late-onset sepsis has a mortality rate of 39%, and in fungal late-onset sepsis the mortality rate is also 39% [13].

Antimicrobial Resistance in Bacterial Pathogens Causing Neonatal Sepsis

Despite the widespread use of intrapartum antibiotic prophylaxis in pregnant women, GBS has remained susceptible to penicillin, ampicillin and first generation cephalosporins. GBS isolates with increased minimum inhibitory concentrations (MICs) to penicillin, ampicillin and cefazolin have been reported rarely in the US [6]. However, the clinical significance of the increased MIC values to these antibiotics in GBS remains unclear. All GBS isolates are considered to be susceptible to vancomycin. Resistance to clindamycin is approximately 15–20% [3, 18].

In contrast to GBS, antibiotic resistance in Gram-negative pathogens causing neonatal sepsis continues to increase. Most reports available in the US regarding antibiotic resistance in Gram-negative neonatal infections focus on *E. coli*. Resistance of *E. coli* to ampicillin reported in the US is as high as 85% in VLBW with early-onset sepsis, and at least 44% in other groups of neonates with *E. coli* sepsis. The proportion of ampicillin-resistant *E. coli* in newborns with early-onset sepsis bacteremia is significantly greater in those whose mothers received intrapartum antibiotic prophylaxis than in those without this exposure [4]. Resistance to gentamicin and third-generation cephalosporin in *E. coli* has not surpassed 10% yet (see

Table 2 Resistance rates to common antibiotics used for treating *E. coli* neonatal bacteremia

Antibiotic	Early-onset sepsis	Late-onset sepsis	References
Ampicillin	49–78% (85% in VLBW neonates)	44–47%	[2–4, 16, 20, 46]
3rd generation cephalosporins	3–4%	6%	[3, 11, 16]
Gentamicin	4–10%	2%	[3, 4, 11]

VLBW: very-low birth weight

Table 2). A concerning recent finding is the simultaneous resistance to ampicillin and gentamicin in neonatal *E. coli* isolates [4, 11, 19]. *E. coli* extended-spectrum beta-lactamase (ESBL) producers are reported in up to 3% of cases [3, 20]. Data on resistance in neonatal *E. coli* isolates to other antibiotics, such as tobramycin, amikacin or beta-lactam/lactamase inhibitors, are not commonly included in most reports.

Other Potential Microbial Etiologies of Neonatal Sepsis

Although bacterial infections are responsible for the majority of neonatal sepsis and sepsis-related deaths in developed countries, fungal and viral infections can cause severe disease. As in bacterial neonatal sepsis, the risk of neonatal sepsis due to fungi and viruses depends largely on perinatal factors and gestational age.

Invasive Candidiasis

Fungal infections are the cause in up to 12% of cases of late-onset sepsis and account for 2.5% of bloodstream infections in preterm infants [12, 21, 22]. Fungal infections due to *Candida* spp. (invasive candidiasis) comprise the vast majority of these cases. Common infecting species are those that typically colonize neonates and most often include *C. albicans* or *C. parapsilosis*, but can also include *C. tropicalis*, *C. krusei*, *C. lusitaniae*, or *C. glabrata* [23]. Risk factors for developing invasive candidiasis include exposure to a combination of predisposing factors, particularly long-term antibiotic use, corticosteroid exposure and indwelling central vascular catheters (CVCs) [24, 25]. Additionally, infants born premature and those born at low birth weight (particularly those < 1,500 g) are at increased risk of infection; up to 10% of these infants who become colonized with *Candida* spp. may develop invasive disease [26].

Neonates can experience several unique infection syndromes due to *Candida* spp. that can result in invasive candidiasis and sepsis. Congenital candidiasis is due to ascending infection of the uterus prior to birth. Affected infants will have a diffuse erythematous rash at birth that can progress to a vesicular and desquamating dermatitis. Although usually benign in infants > 1,500 g, smaller and/or more preterm infants can develop extensive dermatitis and disseminated infection; prompt and

Table 3 Empirical antimicrobial therapy for bacterial, viral, and fungal infections. Adapted in part from [47]

Organism	Antimicrobial (s) (dose/kg, i.v.[a])	Frequency (h)	Usual duration (days)
Early-onset sepsis (no meningitis)	Ampicillin (50 mg) PLUS gentamicin (2.5 mg)	q 8–12[b]	10
Late-onset sepsis (no meningitis)	Ampicillin (50 mg) PLUS gentamicin (2.5 mg)	q 8–12[b]	7–10
Nosocomial	Vancomycin PLUS gentamicin (2.5 mg) OR amikacin (10 mg)[c,d]	q 12[b,c]	10–14
Early-onset sepsis (meningitis)	Ampicillin (100 mg) PLUS gentamicin (2.5 mg) PLUS cefotaxime (50 mg)	q 8[b] q 12	14–21
Late-onset sepsis (meningitis)	Ampicillin (75 mg) PLUS gentamicin (2.5 mg) OR amikacin (15 mg) PLUS cefotaxime (50 mg)	q 6 q 8[c,d]	14–21
Suspected gastrointestinal source	Add clindamycin (10 mg) OR piperacillin-tazobactam (50 mg) PLUS aminoglycoside	q 6–8 q 8	10–14 unless complications
Influenza	Oseltamivir (3 mg)[e,f,g]	q 12	5
Enteroviruses	IGIV[h]	–	–
HSV	Acyclovir (20 mg)	q 8	21
Candidiasis	Amphotericin B (AmB) deoxycholate (1 mg)[i] OR Fluconazole (12 mg)[j]	q 24	Minimum 14[k]

[a]Except for oseltamivir (oral)

[b]Dosing for postconteptual age < 30 weeks, gentamicin should be 3 mg/kg with dosing per serum levels (goal peak 5/12 mcg/ml, trough < 2.0 mcg/ml). Postconteptual age 30–37 weeks, 3 mg/kg for day-of-life ≤ 7, then 2.5 mg/kg thereafter

[c]Dosing for postconteptual age < 30 weeks, vancomycin should be 20 mg/kg with frequency depending on serum levels (goal peak 24–40 mcg/ml, trough 5–15 mcg/ml). Postconteptual age 30–37 weeks, vancomycin dosing should be 20 mg/kg day-of-life 1–7, then 15 mg/kg thereafter. For postconteptual age > 37 weeks, vancomycin dosing should be 15 mg/kg

[d]Goal serum levels for amikacin: 20–35 mcg/ml (peak), < 10 mcg/ml (trough)

[e]For term infants 14 days old to 1 year old

[f]Limited data on dosing in preterm infants. The US National Institute of Allergy and Infectious Diseases Collaborative Antiviral Study Group provides the following recommended dosing based on postmenstrual (PM) age (gestational age + chronological age): < 38 weeks PM age, 1.0 mg/kg/dose twice daily; 38–40 weeks PM age, 1.5 mg/kg/dose twice daily; > 40 weeks PM age, 3.0 mg/kg/dose twice daily

[g]Recommended dosing not established for zanamavir and peramivir in neonates

[h]Efficacy not well-established. Dosing varies by report; many experts use up to 2 g/kg total dose

[i]Lipid formulation AmB, 3–5 mg/kg daily (5 mg/kg daily for central nervous system (CNS) disease), is an alternative, but AmB deoxycholate is preferred in neonates

[j]For infants not previously exposed to fluconazole

[k]For CNS disease, therapy should continue until cerebrospinal fluid, radiology, and symptoms normalize

i. v.: intravenous; *HSV*: herpes simplex virus; *IGIV*: Immune globulin, i. v.

early treatment is associated with improved outcomes [27]. Invasive fungal dermatitis develops later after birth, usually within the first two weeks of life. Extremely premature infants, particularly those exposed to corticosteroids and who experience significant hyperglycemia, are at increased risk. Invasive fungal dermatitis can rapidly progress to severe erosions and crusting, with many infants developing candidemia.

Sepsis due to invasive candidiasis is clinically quite similar to sepsis due to other etiologies, making recognition of risk factors critically important [28]. The combination of thrombocytopenia and hyperglycemia during symptom onset, particularly in an infant born at < 28 weeks, with a history of VLBW (< 1,500 g), and prior antibiotic exposure should prompt the clinician to consider evaluation and empirical treatment for fungal infection. Unfortunately fungal cultures are poorly sensitive and require significant blood volumes (relative to the patient's total blood volume) to achieve sensitivity of > 50% [29]. Positive urine culture for *Candida* spp. should prompt further assessment for concomitant invasive candidiasis. Biomarkers typically considered for use in adults and older children lack established criteria for interpretation in neonates, including serum $(1-3)$-β-d-glucan, mannan and anti-mannan antibodies. Empirical treatment for suspected sepsis due to invasive candidiasis is outlined in Table 3. Even with prompt treatment, mortality from invasive candidiasis can exceed 10%, with up to 60% of extremely low birth weight (< 1,000 g) infants suffering permanent neurodevelopmental impairment [30].

Viruses

Viral infections are one of the most common causes of fever in otherwise healthy neonates [31], and respiratory viral pathogens were identified as the only pathogen in infants evaluated for late-onset sepsis in a neonatal intensive care unit (ICU) [32]. Although viral infections in children are commonly considered self-limiting, neonatal viral infections more often can result in a dysregulated inflammatory response that progresses to sepsis and septic shock, due to differences in innate and adaptive immune responses in early infancy [33]. Common viral pathogens responsible for neonatal sepsis are detailed in Table 1. Some viral pathogens (e.g., enteroviruses, varicella zoster virus [VZV]), when acquired transplacentally late in pregnancy can result in devastating illness. Most other viral pathogens are acquired intrapartum or post-natally. Congenital viral infections that can result in neonatal sepsis are beyond the scope of this chapter.

Enteroviruses
Neonatal enteroviral infection can result in devastating sepsis in neonates. Infants are at greatest risk in the first 10 days of life, which may be due in part to host immune immaturity, particularly macrophage function, in the first weeks of postnatal life [34]. Lack of maternal neutralizing antibody is also a major factor in disease severity, which is why eliciting a careful history of maternal fever, abdominal pain and other potential symptoms of enterovirus infection in the weeks before delivery

of an infant who develops enterovirus-mediated sepsis is important. Neonatal infection can result in hepatitis, coagulopathy, myocarditis with cardiovascular collapse and meningoencephalitis. Despite the devastating potential of neonatal enterovirus infection, available treatments are limited due to the relative rarity of neonatal infection. Neutralizing antibodies to multiple enterovirus subtypes can be found in human immune globulin preparations, and limited published reports support some potential benefit if given early. Limited data have also been published on the use of antiviral agents including pleconaril [35] and pocapavir [36], but access to these medications is extremely limited, and efficacy is not established.

Herpes Simplex Virus

Neonatal HSV infection can result in a variety of infection syndromes, all of which can progress to sepsis. About half of infants born to mothers who have active genital lesions due to primary HSV infection will contract HSV as compared to < 5% of those exposed to recurrent genital outbreaks during delivery [37]. Neonates can manifest HSV infection in one of three general presentations [38]. Disseminated infection typically occurs in the first week of life as severe shock with multiorgan dysfunction, particularly coagulopathy, hepatitis and respiratory distress. Skin/eye/mucous membrane infection occurs most commonly in the second week of life, and can present as keratoconjunctivitis, oral vesicles/ulcers or vesicular lesions at skin sites of trauma (e.g., fetal scalp electrode site). Central nervous system infection occurs usually after day 14 of life and presents as irritability, seizures and/or fever. The mortality from each infection syndrome after appropriate antiviral treatment varies widely, from 0% for treated skin/eye/mucous membrane disease to > 50% for disseminated infection. The treatment of choice for neonatal HSV infection is acyclovir (Table 3). Risk-based screening and empiric treatment recommendations can help guide the management of infants born to mothers suspected of HSV infection near the time of delivery (Table 4).

Varicella-Zoster Virus

VZV is a member of the herpesvirus family that can cause severe congenital or neonatal infection. When maternal infection occurs during the final few days of gestation, 1 in 5 infants may be infected, although infants born at > 1 week of life are not at high risk of severe disease [39]. Neonatal VZV is most severe if maternal infection occurs within 5 days before delivery, due to the fact that transplacental transfer of maternal neutralizing IgG antibody has not occurred. In the infants of mothers who develop symptoms of varicella between 5 days before and 2 days after delivery, the untreated mortality of neonatal varicella can exceed 30%. Post-exposure passive immunoprophylaxis is recommended for infants at high risk of neonatal varicella disease (Table 4). Antiviral therapy with acyclovir is recommended for symptomatic infants, although its efficacy in these patients is uncertain.

Influenza

Respiratory viral infections are the cause of fever in up to 8% of infants evaluated for late-onset sepsis in neonatal ICUs [31] and are responsible for 40–70% of fevers

Table 4 Current recommendations for preventing neonatal sepsis due to specific pathogens

Organism	Recommended prophylaxis	Eligibility
S. agalactiae (GBS)	Maternal chemoprophylaxis[a]	Mothers with: 1) known GBS rectal-vaginal colonization; 2) GBS bacteriuria during pregnancy; or 3) history of previous child with invasive GBS infection OR Unknown maternal GBS status and: 1) preterm delivery; 2) amniotic membrane rupture ≥ 18 h; 3) intrapartum fever; or 4) intrapartum GBS testing positive
HSV	Infant pre-emptive therapy[b] Cesarean delivery	Infants born to mothers with active genital lesions and suspected primary or first non-primary infection, positive infant HSV testing at ≥ 24 h of life, or signs/symptoms of neonatal HSV infection Maternal active genital lesions or prodromal symptoms at delivery
Influenza	Maternal vaccination[c]	All pregnant mothers
VZV	Infant post-exposure prophylaxis[d,e]	1. Mother had onset of varicella infection (chickenpox) within 5 days before or 48 h after delivery, OR 2. Hospitalized preterm infant ≥ 28 weeks gestation born to mother lacking evidence of VZV immunity, OR 3. Hospitalized preterm infant < 28 weeks gestation or birth weight $< 1,000$ g regardless of maternal VZV immunity
Candida spp.	Infant chemoprophylaxis[f]	Admission to a NICU with $> 10\%$ prevalence of invasive candidiasis

[a]Penicillin G, 5 million units i. v. initial dose, then 2.5–3.0 million units q4h until delivery, OR ampicillin 2 g i. v. initial dose, then 1 g i. v. q4h until delivery. Alternatives: cefazolin 2 g i. v. q8H, clindamycin 900 mg i. v. q8h (if isolate susceptible), or vancomycin 1 g q12h until delivery
[b]Acyclovir, 60 mg/kg, divided three times daily
[c]Antiviral chemoprophylaxis not recommended for infants < 3 months of age
[d]Immune globulin, i. v. (IGIV), 400 mg/kg, OR VariZIG, intramuscularly, 125 units/10 kg body weight (62.5 units if ≤ 2 kg), up to maximum of 625 units (5 vials)
[e]Must be given within 10 days of exposure
[f]Infants $< 1,000$ g: Fluconazole, 3–6 mg/kg 2x/wk × 6 weeks; OR Infants $< 1,500$ g: nystatin orally 100,000 units 3 × daily × 6 weeks
NICU: neonatal intensive care unit; *GBS*: group B streptococci; *HSV*: herpes simplex virus; *RSV*: respiratory syncytial virus; *VZV*: varicella zoster virus

in term neonates [40]. Influenza in particular places mother and fetus at increased risk of severe illness, with rates of hospitalization approaching that of nonpregnant women with high-risk medical conditions [41]. Infants born to vaccinated mothers experience a 48% decreased risk of developing influenza [42]. Although data for neonates is scant, data on infants < 6 months old who are hospitalized for influenza have found this age group at highest risk for ICU admission and death. Treatment options for influenza infection are limited and are outlined in Table 3.

Prophylaxis for Specific Pathogens Causing Neonatal Sepsis

Recommended prophylaxis measures for select pathogens are detailed in Table 4. Of these measures, GBS prophylaxis has proven to have the greatest effect on risk of bacterial early-onset sepsis. Ongoing research on potential vaccine targets for GBS may one day provide an antibiotic-free alternative for reducing the risk of invasive infection due to this organism [43]. Prophylaxis of at-risk preterm infants in neonatal ICUs against invasive candidiasis is of questionable benefit, and depends in part on the institutional prevalence of invasive candidiasis in the neonatal ICU [44, 45].

Conclusion

Neonates are at increased risk of sepsis from a broad range of microorganisms due to immune immaturity and a variety of potential adverse exposures. Continued monitoring of the epidemiology and antimicrobial resistance of pathogens that cause neonatal sepsis is imperative for designing the most appropriate empiric and definitive therapeutic approaches in this population. Morbidity and mortality from Gram-negative sepsis in newborns is significant, and antimicrobial resistance is increasing in this group of pathogens. The use of improved diagnostic approaches for early detection of serious bacterial infections in newborns will result in a decrease in antibiotic use and more targeted antimicrobial regimens. Currently there is no prevention strategy for *E. coli* neonatal sepsis, but future antibiotic-sparing prophylactic regimens for neonatal GBS disease may reduce maternal and neonatal antibiotic exposure and slow the spread of antimicrobial resistance in this at-risk population. Sepsis due to fungal or viral pathogens requires careful attention to maternal and infant exposure history and a high index of suspicion, given the much lower prevalence of these pathogens in neonatal sepsis.

References

1. GBD 2015 Mortality and Causes of Death Collaborators (2016) Global, regional, and national life expectancy, all-cause mortality, and cause-specific mortality for 249 causes of death, 1980–2015: a systematic analysis for the Global Burden of Disease Study 2015. Lancet 388:1459–1544
2. Weston EJ, Pondo T, Lewis MM et al (2011) The burden of invasive early-onset neonatal sepsis in the United States, 2005–2008. Pediatr Infect Dis J 30:937–941
3. Stoll BJ, Hansen NI, Sanchez PJ et al (2011) Early onset neonatal sepsis: the burden of group B Streptococcal and E. coli disease continues. Pediatrics 127:817–826
4. Schrag SJ, Farley MM, Petit S et al (2016) Epidemiology of Invasive early-onset neonatal sepsis, 2005 to 2014. Pediatrics 138:e20162013
5. Le Doare K, Heath PT (2013) An overview of global GBS epidemiology. Vaccine 31(Suppl 4):D7–D12
6. Verani JR, McGee L, Schrag SJ, Division of Bacterial Diseases, National Center for Immunization and Respiratory Diseases, Centers for Disease Control and Prevention (CDC) (2010)

Prevention of perinatal group B streptococcal disease—revised guidelines from CDC, 2010. MMWR Recomm Rep 59:1–36

7. Edmond KM, Kortsalioudaki C, Scott S et al (2012) Group B streptococcal disease in infants aged younger than 3 months: systematic review and meta-analysis. Lancet 379:547–556

8. CDC: Centers for Disease Control and Prevention (2015) Active bacterial core surveillance report, emerging infections program network, group B streptococcus, 2015. Available at www.cdc.gov/abcs/reports-findings/survreports/gbs15.pdf. Accessed 27 December 2017

9. Moore MR, Schrag SJ, Schuchat A (2003) Effects of intrapartum antimicrobial prophylaxis for prevention of group-B-streptococcal disease on the incidence and ecology of early-onset neonatal sepsis. Lancet Infect Dis 3:201–213

10. Stoll BJ, Hansen NI, Higgins RD et al (2005) Very low birth weight preterm infants with early onset neonatal sepsis: the predominance of gram-negative infections continues in the National Institute of Child Health and Human Development Neonatal Research Network, 2002–2003. Pediatr Infect Dis J 24:635–639

11. Greenhow TL, Hung YY, Herz AM (2012) Changing epidemiology of bacteremia in infants aged 1 week to 3 months. Pediatrics 129:e590–e596

12. Stoll BJ, Hansen N, Fanaroff AA et al (2002) Late-onset sepsis in very low birth weight neonates: the experience of the NICHD Neonatal Research Network. Pediatrics 110:285–291

13. Greenberg RG, Kandefer S, Do BT et al (2017) Late-onset sepsis in extremely premature infants: 2000–2011. Pediatr Infect Dis J 36:774–779

14. Jordan HT, Farley MM, Craig A et al (2008) Revisiting the need for vaccine prevention of late-onset neonatal group B streptococcal disease: a multistate, population-based analysis. Pediatr Infect Dis J 27:1057–1064

15. Biondi E, Evans R, Mischler M et al (2013) Epidemiology of bacteremia in febrile infants in the United States. Pediatrics 132:990–996

16. Bizzarro MJ, Dembry LM, Baltimore RS, Gallagher PG (2008) Changing patterns in neonatal Escherichia coli sepsis and ampicillin resistance in the era of intrapartum antibiotic prophylaxis. Pediatrics 121:689–696

17. Cohen-Wolkowiez M, Moran C, Benjamin DK et al (2009) Early and late onset sepsis in late preterm infants. Pediatr Infect Dis J 28:1052–1056

18. Phares CR, Lynfield R, Farley MM et al (2008) Epidemiology of invasive group B streptococcal disease in the United States, 1999–2005. JAMA 299:2056–2065

19. Shakir SM, Goldbeck JM, Robison D, Eckerd AM, Chavez-Bueno S (2014) Genotypic and phenotypic characterization of invasive neonatal Escherichia coli clinical isolates. Am J Perinatol 31:975–982

20. Bergin SP, Thaden JT, Ericson JE et al (2015) Neonatal Escherichia coli bloodstream infections: clinical outcomes and impact of initial antibiotic therapy. Pediatr Infect Dis J 34:933–936

21. Shane AL, Stoll BJ (2013) Recent developments and current issues in the epidemiology, diagnosis, and management of bacterial and fungal neonatal sepsis. Am J Perinatol 30:131–141

22. Camacho-Gonzalez A, Spearman PW, Stoll BJ (2013) Neonatal infectious diseases: evaluation of neonatal sepsis. Pediatr Clin North Am 60:367–389

23. Kelly MS, Benjamin DK Jr., Smith PB (2015) The epidemiology and diagnosis of invasive candidiasis among premature infants. Clin Perinatol 42:105–117 (viii–ix)

24. Singhi S, Rao DS, Chakrabarti A (2008) Candida colonization and candidemia in a pediatric intensive care unit. Pediatr Crit Care Med 9:91–95

25. Garzillo C, Bagattini M, Bogdanovic L et al (2017) Risk factors for Candida parapsilosis bloodstream infection in a neonatal intensive care unit: a case-control study. Ital J Pediatr 43:10

26. Kaufman D, Boyle R, Hazen KC, Patrie JT, Robinson M, Donowitz LG (2001) Fluconazole prophylaxis against fungal colonization and infection in preterm infants. N Engl J Med 345:1660–1666

27. Kaufman DA, Coggins SA, Zanelli SA, Weitkamp JH (2017) Congenital cutaneous candidiasis: prompt systemic treatment is associated with improved outcomes in neonates. Clin Infect Dis 64:1387–1395

28. Calley JL, Warris A (2017) Recognition and diagnosis of invasive fungal infections in neonates. J Infect 74(Suppl 1):S108–S113

29. Cuenca-Estrella M, Verweij PE, Arendrup MC et al (2012) ESCMID guideline for the diagnosis and management of Candida diseases 2012: diagnostic procedures. Clin Microbiol Infect 18(Suppl 7):9–18

30. Benjamin DK Jr., Stoll BJ, Fanaroff AA et al (2006) Neonatal candidiasis among extremely low birth weight infants: risk factors, mortality rates, and neurodevelopmental outcomes at 18 to 22 months. Pediatrics 117:84–92

31. Cioffredi LA, Jhaveri R (2016) Evaluation and management of febrile children: a review. JAMA Pediatr 170:794–800

32. Cerone JB, Santos RP, Tristram D et al (2017) Incidence of respiratory viral infection in infants with respiratory symptoms evaluated for late-onset sepsis. J Perinatol 37:922–926

33. van Well GTJ, Daalderop LA, Wolfs T, Kramer BW (2017) Human perinatal immunity in physiological conditions and during infection. Mol Cell Pediatr 4:4

34. Zhu K, Yang J, Luo K et al (2015) TLR3 signaling in macrophages is indispensable for the protective immunity of invariant natural killer T cells against enterovirus 71 infection. Plos Pathog 11:e1004613

35. Abzug MJ, Michaels MG, Wald E et al (2016) A randomized, double-blind, placebo-controlled trial of pleconaril for the treatment of neonates with Enterovirus sepsis. J Pediatric Infect Dis Soc 5:53–62

36. Torres-Torres S, Myers AL, Klatte JM et al (2015) First use of investigational antiviral drug pocapavir (v-073) for treating neonatal enteroviral sepsis. Pediatr Infect Dis J 34:52–54

37. Kimberlin DW, Baley J, Committee on Infectious Diseases, Committee on Fetus and Newborn (2013) Guidance on management of asymptomatic neonates born to women with active genital herpes lesions. Pediatrics 131:383–386

38. James SH, Kimberlin DW (2015) Neonatal herpes simplex virus infection. Infect Dis Clin North Am 29:391–400

39. Smith CK, Arvin AM (2009) Varicella in the fetus and newborn. Semin Fetal Neonatal Med 14:209–217

40. Dagan R, Powell KR, Hall CB, Menegus MA (1985) Identification of infants unlikely to have serious bacterial infection although hospitalized for suspected sepsis. J Pediatr 107:855–860

41. Rasmussen SA, Jamieson DJ, Uyeki TM (2012) Effects of influenza on pregnant women and infants. Am J Obstet Gynecol 207(3 Suppl):S3–S8

42. Nunes MC, Madhi SA (2017) Influenza vaccination during pregnancy for prevention of influenza confirmed illness in the infants: a systematic review and meta-analysis. Hum Vaccin Immunother 14:1–9

43. Chen VL, Avci FY, Kasper DL (2013) A maternal vaccine against group B Streptococcus: past, present, and future. Vaccine 31(Suppl 4):D13–D19

44. Manzoni P, Stolfi I, Pugni L et al (2007) A multicenter, randomized trial of prophylactic fluconazole in preterm neonates. N Engl J Med 356:2483–2495

45. Lee J, Kim HS, Shin SH et al (2016) Efficacy and safety of fluconazole prophylaxis in extremely low birth weight infants: multicenter pre-post cohort study. BMC Pediatr 16:67

46. Fanaroff AA, Stoll BJ, Wright LL et al (2007) Trends in neonatal morbidity and mortality for very low birthweight infants. Am J Obstet Gynecol 196:147.e1–147.e8

47. Edwards MS, Baker CJ (2008) Bacterial infections in the neonate. In: Long SS, Pickering LK, Prober CG (eds) Principles and Practice of Pediatric Infectious Diseases, 3rd edn. Churchill Livingstone, Philadelphia, p 537

Prolonged Infusion of Beta-lactam Antibiotics in Critically Ill Patients: Revisiting the Evidence

S. A. M. Dhaese, V. Stove, and J. J. De Waele

Introduction

Infection in critically ill patients remains a highly challenging issue. Mortality attributed to sepsis in the intensive care unit (ICU) is estimated to be as high as 30% [1]. Appropriate antibiotic therapy is well recognized as the cornerstone of sepsis management, but increasing resistance rates and a paucity of new antimicrobials in the pipeline continue to pose a serious threat for the clinical utility of antimicrobial drugs [2, 3]. Health care institutions are increasingly adopting antimicrobial stewardship (AMS) programs to help preserve our antimicrobial armamentarium [4]. AMS initiatives have been shown to reduce antimicrobial resistance, antimicrobial costs and the consumption of broad-spectrum antimicrobials [3]. Dose-optimization of antimicrobial therapy is an example of an AMS initiative undertaken after the prescription of initial antibiotic therapy [4]. Scientific advances in the field of dose-optimization are mainly driven by antimicrobial pharmacokinetic (PK) and pharmacodynamic (PD) principles, the science relating drug exposure to an outcome measurement [3].

Beta-lactam antibiotics, amongst the antimicrobials most commonly prescribed in the ICU [4], are a present-day example of how PK/PD considerations led to the adoption of alternative dosing regimens to optimize their use [5]. These PK/PD-optimized dosing regimens are based on the time-dependent killing properties of beta-lactam antibiotics. For optimal antibacterial activity, beta-lactam antibiotic concentrations need to be maintained above the minimum inhibitory concentration (MIC)

S. A. M. Dhaese · J. J. De Waele (✉)
Dept of Intensive Care Medicine, Ghent University Hospital
Ghent, Belgium
e-mail: jan.dewaele@ugent.be

V. Stove
Dept of Clinical Chemistry, Microbiology and Immunology, Ghent University
Ghent, Belgium
Dept of Laboratory Medicine, Ghent University Hospital
Ghent, Belgium

© Springer International Publishing AG 2018   53
J.-L. Vincent (ed.), *Annual Update in Intensive Care and Emergency Medicine 2018*,
Annual Update in Intensive Care and Emergency Medicine,
https://doi.org/10.1007/978-3-319-73670-9_5

for extended periods [6]. In critically ill patients however, the time beta-lactam concentrations remain above the MIC may be shortened due to specific PK alterations often encountered in these patients [7].

To maintain antibiotic concentrations at therapeutic levels, extending the duration of infusion, i.e. prolonged infusion, has been introduced [8, 9]. In clinical practice, prolonged infusion strategies encompass both extended infusion with infusion duration of at least 50% of the dosing interval and continuous infusion with a steady infusion rate throughout the entire dosing interval [11]. Intermittent infusion with an infusion duration ranging from bolus administration to 30 min infusion is package insert dosing and is regarded as standard practice in the ICU. However, several institutions are moving towards the adoption of prolonged infusion dosing regimens [10, 11]. In recent years, the amount of research assessing the anticipated advantage of prolonged infusion in terms of mortality and clinical cure has increased dramatically but a definitive benefit of prolonged infusion has not yet been demonstrated [9].

In this chapter, we review and unravel preclinical comparative experiments and the available clinical evidence for prolonged infusion of beta-lactam antibiotics in the ICU. Some suggestions for future research are listed as well.

Beta-Lactam Pharmacokinetics/Pharmacodynamics

Beta-Lactam Pharmacodynamics

For antibiotics, three major patterns of antimicrobial killing have been defined. Each of these killing patterns is described by a PK/PD index. The PK/PD index best describing beta-lactam killing properties is $\%fT_{>MIC}$, or the time (T) the free (f) fraction of the drug exceeds the MIC of the causative pathogen. The MIC is defined as the lowest concentration of an antimicrobial agent that prevents visible growth of a microorganism in an agar or broth dilution susceptibility test, usually after 18–24 h of incubation. By convention, the exact magnitude of the PK/PD index necessary to achieve a certain outcome (for example a 3 $\log_{10}$ reduction of colony forming units (CFU/ml) is called the PK/PD target [12]).

Beta-lactam antibiotics typically do not require concentrations greater than the MIC throughout the entire dosing interval to exert their bactericidal effect and PK/PD targets of 40–70% $fT_{>MIC}$ are frequently cited [13–15]. However, the optimal PK/PD target remains highly controversial. For example, targets of 100% $fT_{>4\times MIC}$ and higher have been deemed necessary [16]. In contrast to the number of preclinical experiments assessing beta-lactam killing efficacy, far fewer experiments have focused on the PK/PD index and target necessary for the suppression of antimicrobial resistance. Recently, Tam et al. [17] reported that C_{min}/MIC (trough concentration/MIC) ratios ≥ 3.8 were necessary to suppress the emergence of *Pseudomonas aeruginosa* and *Klebsiella pneumoniae* resistance, whereas others report C_{min}/MIC ratios as high as 10.4 with extended infusion of piperacillin [18].

As of today, only a limited number of clinical studies, with a limited number of patients and a limited set of infection foci have defined an optimal PK/PD target [16].

Pharmacokinetic/Pharmacodynamic Considerations in Critically Ill Patients

Dose and dosing regimens of beta-lactam antibiotics in ICU patients were traditionally developed using healthy volunteer PK studies. However, it is well known that severe illness may profoundly alter the PK of antimicrobials in critically ill patients [7].

In the case of time-dependent antibiotics such as beta-lactam antibiotics, altered PK raises questions regarding target attainment and tissue penetration. Because of their hydrophilic nature, beta-lactam PK is strongly influenced by altered renal clearance and changes in volume of distribution. Renal clearance in sepsis patients may be increased due to increased renal perfusion associated with an increased cardiac output and decreased systemic vascular resistance. Hypoalbuminemia is also frequently encountered in critically ill patients and can increase the renal clearance of highly protein-bound substances, such as ceftriaxone. A rise in interstitial fluid volume following third spacing and fluid resuscitation may significantly increase the volume of distribution, especially for hydrophilic drugs. Additionally, decreased end-organ perfusion in patients with septic shock and severe sepsis can lead to decreased tissue perfusion and decreased levels of free drug at the site of infection [7, 19, 20].

Although there is no conclusive evidence, it has been suggested that higher PK/PD targets may be necessary within the subgroup of critically ill patients. For example, 100% $fT_{>MIC}$, based on little clinical PK/PD data [21, 22], and 100% $fT_{>4\times MIC}$, based on preclinical data [16], have both been recommended.

With these PK/PD targets in mind, the probability of PK/PD target attainment in ICU patients has been studied. In 2013, a landmark study by Roberts et al. [22] demonstrated that approximately 16% of the patients treated for infection with an intermittent dosing regimen did not achieve the PK/PD target of 50% $fT_{>MIC}$. In a more recent review by Delattre et al. [16], the probability of achieving recommended PK/PD targets at first dose in critically ill patients was assessed. They conclude that reaching 100% $fT_{>MIC}$ for piperacillin (4 g), ceftazidime (2 g), cefepime (2 g) or meropenem (1 g) via intermittent infusion (30 min) was only achieved in 56, 87, 63 and 59% of the patients for each beta-lactam antibiotic, respectively. The PK/PD target of 100% $fT_{>4\times MIC}$ (or C_{min}/MIC of 4) was attained in less than 20% of the patients. Aardema et al. [23] recently evaluated target attainment of a PK/PD target of 100% $fT_{>4\times MIC}$ with continuous infusion piperacillin in a population of critically ill patients. All patients received a loading dose of 4 g/0.5 g piperacillin/tazobactam followed by a 12/1.5 g piperacillin/tazobactam continuous infusion. Overall, less than one third of their patients achieved piperacillin concentrations $\geq 100\% fT_{>4\times MIC}$ within one hour after administration and throughout the entire treatment period.

Tissue Penetration in Critically Ill Patients

Proof-of-concept studies comparing antibiotic concentrations were performed as an initial step to assess whether or not prolonged infusion could increase target site antibiotic concentrations. Although serum concentrations are often used as a surrogate parameter, data evaluating tissue concentrations in infected patients are available and likely to provide more accurate information [24]. Achieving adequate antibiotic concentrations at the focus of infection is a necessity but potentially challenging in ICU patients because sepsis and septic shock may result in decreased tissue perfusion [25].

Studies comparing tissue concentrations of beta-lactam antibiotics between intermittent and continuous infusion dosing regimens have consistently shown higher tissue steady state concentrations (C_{ss}) with continuous infusions. However, it is worth mentioning that many of these experiments used tissue concentrations in patients who were either not infected (e.g., during elective surgery) or, if patients were infected, concentrations were not measured at the actual site of infection (e.g., subcutaneous tissue concentrations in sepsis patients) [26].

Cousson et al. [27] measured ceftazidime epithelial lining fluid concentrations in patients with pneumonia. Equal ceftazidime serum AUC_{0-48} (area under the curve) values were reported in both the intermittent and continuous infusion groups. A significantly higher epithelial lining fluid C_{ss} was achieved in the continuous infusion arm versus the intermittent infusion arm. As mentioned by the authors, additional epithelial lining fluid samples would have been useful to calculate and compare serum/tissue AUC_{0-48} for intermittent versus continuous infusion. Indeed, when comparing tissue antibiotic exposure between intermittent and prolonged infusion in infectious patients, one could focus on tissue AUC rather than tissue C_{ss} or C_{min} to get a more complete picture. Buijk et al. [28] compared abdominal fluid concentrations in patients with severe abdominal infections when ceftazidime was administered intermittently (1.5 g q8h) or continuously (1 g loading dose plus 4.5 g/24 h infusion). Comparable serum AUCs were achieved. The authors had sufficient data to also provide tissue AUC values. In their experiment, AUC_{tissue}/AUC_{serum} ratios on days 2 and 4 were not significantly different in the continuous infusion arm versus the intermittent infusion arm. Unfortunately, no AUC_{tissue}/AUC_{serum} values are provided for the first few hours of therapy. It is possible that, because of the higher first dose with intermittent infusion compared to the loading dose with continuous infusion, target concentrations were reached faster with intermittently infused ceftazidime. However, by day 2, this effect may already have leveled out.

Based on these data, it appears that continuous infusion ensures higher trough concentrations at the target site, whereas total tissue antibiotic exposure may be comparable with the two modes of infusion if equal first doses and equal total daily doses are used.

Preclinical Experiments Comparing Intermittent and Prolonged Infusion in Terms of Bacterial Cell Kill

Few comparative *in vitro* or animal experiments have been undertaken to confirm the theoretical advantage of prolonged infusion of beta-lactam antibiotics in terms of bacterial cell kill. The little research that is available in this field has been almost exclusively limited to *P. aeruginosa* and *in vitro* infection models.

Extended Infusion

Zelenitsky et al. [29] simulated piperacillin/tazobactam intermittent infusion (3.375 g q6h) and extended infusion (3.375 g q6h for 3-hour infusions and 3.375 g q8h for 4-hour infusions) to compare the killing characteristics of intermittent and extended infusions in an *in vitro P. aeruginosa* infection model. Piperacillin MICs were 8, 16 and 32 mg/l. The authors reported that the final bacterial kill at the end of every dosing interval was significantly greater for prolonged infusion against isolates with an MIC of 32 mg/l. The overall antibacterial effect (calculated as the $\log_{10}$ of the area under the growth control curve divided by the area under the piperacillin/tazobactam kill curve) was similar for both intermittent and extended infusion dosing regimens. Kim et al. [30] reported doripenem intermittent infusion (1 h) and extended infusion (4 h) experiments with comparable AUC in a *P. aeruginosa in vitro* infection model. For *P. aeruginosa* with doripenem MICs from 2 to 16 mg/l, the authors reported change in $\log_{10}$ CFU/ml and their corresponding $\%fT_{>MIC}$ for both intermittent and extended infusion dosing regimens. For strains with an MIC of 2 mg/l, the intermittent and extended infusion dosing regimen provided approximately equal killing. For 2 out of the 4 isolates with an MIC of 4 mg/l, extended infusion showed regrowth while intermittent infusion showed (moderate) bacterial kill, despite higher $\%fT_{>MIC}$ for extended compared to intermittent infusion (30% vs 52.5%$fT_{>MIC}$). For MICs greater than 8 mg/l, the extended infusion regimen did not achieve concentrations greater than the MIC (0% $fT_{>MIC}$). Felton et al. [18] published an *in vitro P. aeruginosa* hollow fiber infection model for piperacillin in 2013. Dosing of 3, 9 and 17 g either via intermittent infusion (0.5 h) or extended infusion (4 h) was simulated. Targets (in C_{min}/MIC ratios) reported for stasis, 1, 2 and 3 $\log_{10}$ kill and suppression of resistance for extended infusion were consistently higher compared to targets documented for intermittent infusion.

Continuous Infusion

Cappelletty et al. [31] compared the *in vitro* bactericidal activity of ceftazidime in continuous versus intermittent infusion against susceptible and resistant *P. aeruginosa* with and without amikacin. Simulated dosing regimens for ceftazidime monotherapy were 2 g q8h, 2 g q12h and continuous infusion with C_{ss} of 20 µg/ml, 10 µg/ml and 5 µg/ml. The susceptible *P. aeruginosa* strain had a ceftazidime MIC value of 1.56 µg/ml and the resistant strain had a ceftazidime MIC of 50 µg/ml. Time kill curves for the susceptible strain showed that only the continuous infusion of 5 µg/ml (C_{ss}/MIC ratio of 3.2) led to regrowth after 48 h of exposure (despite providing 100% $fT_{>MIC}$). None of the intermittent infusion experiments showed regrowth at 48 h. Importantly, AUCs of the central compartment for the intermittent and continuous infusions were far from equal in their experiment, which makes it difficult to compare the two regimens. Indeed, the continuous infusion regimen inducing regrowth (C_{ss} of 5 µg/ml) had an AUC_{24-48} of only 137.1 µg/h/l, whereas the 2 g q12h dosing regimen had an AUC_{24-48} of 875.3 µg/h/l and the 2 g q8h dosing regimen had an AUC_{24-48} of 1,780.7 µg/h/l. Not unexpectedly, none of the ceftazidime monotherapy regimens achieved a 3 $\log_{10}$ reduction in CFU in the time kill curves with the resistant *P. aeruginosa* strain (MIC 50 µg/l). Robaux et al. [32] conducted a very similar *in vivo* animal experiment. In a *P. aeruginosa* rabbit endo-carditis model, intermittent and continuous infusions of ceftazidime were studied with or without amikacin. Continuous infusions of 4, 6 and 8 g over 24 h and an intermittent infusion of 2 g q8h were simulated. Ceftazidime MICs of the *P. aerug-inosa* strains used in the experiment were 1, 4 and 8 mg/l. For the susceptible strain (PA3) with a MIC of 4 mg/l, the intermittent 2 g q8h infusion did not produce a significant decrease in CFU compared to controls, whereas an equal daily dose as a continuous infusion (C_{ss}/MIC ratio of 8.7) provided a significant decrease in CFU compared to controls. AUC_{0-8} for the 2 g q8h intermittent infusion was 369 mg/h/l and AUC_{0-8} for the 6 g continuous infusion (34.8×8) was 278.4 mg/h/l, indicating that despite lower total exposure, continuous infusion appeared to be more efficient in bacterial killing.

Three experiments compared bacterial killing with continuous versus intermit-tent infusion for comparable AUCs. In 1994, Mouton et al. [33] published an *in vitro* PD experiment comparing intermittent and continuous infusion of ceftazidime against three *P. aeruginosa* strains with different susceptibilities (MIC of 1, 4 and 16 mg/l). The same dose of 300 mg/kg was used in both treatment arms. In their time-kill experiment, initial killing (the first 8 h) was comparable between intermit-tent and continuous infusion for all strains. After 8 h, the intermittent infusion arm showed a gradual increase in CFU for the strains with low MICs (MIC 1 and 4 mg/l) whereas during continuous infusion, growth for these strains increased a little until 16 h and then remained constant for the rest of the experiment. When less suscepti-ble strains were used (MIC = 16 mg/l), regrowth appeared in both regimens and, at 32 h, the numbers of CFU for both regimens were equal. In conclusion, continuous infusion for the strains with low MICs (MIC 1 and 4 mg/l) was more efficacious in killing off bacteria compared to intermittent infusion but for strains with higher MICs, regrowth occurred in both regimens. In 1997, Mouton et al. [34] used the data from their 1994 [33] experiment for the assessment of *in vitro* bacterial killing rates of ceftazidime concentrations over time. To account for the regrowth seen in the time-kill curves, the adaptation rate during intermittent and continuous infusion was modeled. Remarkably, for the P16 strain (MIC = 16 mg/l), the adaptation rate was twice as high for continuous infusion compared to intermittent infusion despite the fact that the continuous infusion provided 100% $fT_{>1.25 \times MIC}$, while intermittent infusion concentrations fell below the MIC for at least a proportion of the dosing interval (trough concentrations were 1–2 mg/l, the target reached was approximately 50% $fT_{>MIC}$) (Fig. 1).

In an *in vitro* PD model, Alou et al. [35] exposed three *P. aeruginosa* strains with different susceptibilities (MIC = 8, 16 and 32 mg/l) to either intermittent (simulation of 2 g every 8 h) or continuous (simulation 6 g over 24 h) infusion of ceftazidime. In their experimental design, AUC_{0-24} for both intermittent and continuous infusion was comparable. The steady state concentration for the continuous infusion regimen was 40.38 mg/l. As such, 100% $fT_{>MIC}$ was achieved against all strains with the continuous infusion regimen. The PK/PD targets in this experiment were a C_{ss}/MIC ratio of 5, 2.5 and 1.25 (continuous infusion) and 99.8, 69 and 47.6% $fT_{>MIC}$ (intermittent infusion) for the three strains involved. When the reduction in initial inoculum was assessed, both continuous and intermittent infusion provided at least a 3 $\log_{10}$ reduction in CFU/ml for strains with an MIC up till 16 mg/l. However, for the more resistant strain (MIC = 32 mg/l), regrowth was seen with both modes of infusion at 30 and 32 h after antibiotic exposure with significantly more regrowth in the intermittent infusion compared to the continuous infusion arm.

Tessier et al. [36] compared intermittent and continuous infusions of cefepime in an *in vitro P. aeruginosa* PD model. Cefepime doses simulated were 1 g q12h and a continuous infusion of 2 g after a loading dose of 1 g. The tested strains had MICs of 2 and 8 μg/ml. AUC_{0-24} was 317.3 and 344.3 μg/h/ml and AUC_{24-48} was 303.4 and 275 μg/h/ml for intermittent and continuous infusions, respectively. When added up, intermittent infusion (620.7 μg/h/ml) and continuous infusion

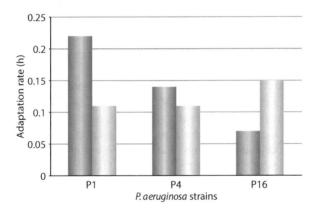

Fig. 1 Adaptation rate for three *P. aeruginosa* strains (P1 with minimum inhibitory concentration [MIC] = 1 mg/l, P4 with MIC = 4 mg/l and P16 with MIC = 16 mg/l). A dose of 300 mg/kg ceftazidime was infused either intermittently (*dark blue*) or continuously (*light blue*). Comparable AUCs were achieved. For strain P16 with MIC 16 mg/l, targets achieved were 100% $fT_{>1.25\times MIC}$ (continuous infusion) and approximately 50% $fT_{>MIC}$ (intermittent infusion). At comparable AUCs (28.575 mg/h/l for continuous infusion and 31.8 mg/h/l for intermittent infusion), the continuous infusion group showed a greater tendency towards resistance development for strain P16. Data from [34]

(619.3 µg/h/ml) had comparable AUC_{0-48} values. For continuous infusion cefepime, C_{ss} was 11.48 µg/ml. For intermittent infusion cefepime, C_{max} (peak concentration) was 106.6 µg/ml after a 30 min infusion and the half-life was 1.93 h. With intermittent infusion cefepime, trough concentrations approximately equal to the MIC of the most susceptible strain (MIC 2 µg/ml) were achieved (C_{min}/MIC equals 1) but trough concentrations dropped below the MIC of the less susceptible strain (MIC 8 µg/ml). With continuous infusion cefepime, C_{ss} remained above the MIC during the entire dosing interval (C_{ss}/MIC of 5.74 and 1.4 for the susceptible and less susceptible strain respectively). The authors found a significant difference in decrease in CFU at 24, 36 and 48 h in favor of continuous infusion of cefepime; however, both the intermittent and continuous infusion regimen for the strain with MIC 8 mg/l led to resistance after 36–48 h of antibiotic exposure.

Update on Clinical Evidence for Prolonged Infusion in Critically Ill Patients

Clinical Trials, Systematic Reviews and Meta-Analyses

Several clinical trials have been published in recent years to assess the anticipated clinical benefit of prolonged infusion compared with intermittent infusion. The majority of these clinical trials mainly focused on outcomes in terms of mortality and clinical cure and little attention has been paid to possible adverse events of prolonged infusion such as toxicity or the emergence of resistance. In the late seventies and early eighties, the first randomized clinical trials (RCT) were conducted [8] but it was not until the early 2000s that the first clinical trials focusing on ICU patients were published [37, 38]. Not surprisingly, research in this field was especially boosted when the finding of altered PK was acknowledged in ICU patients [39].

Many of the published RCTs yielded inconsistent results [5] and meta-analyses were undertaken, aiming to provide consensus on the highly controversial topic. A 2013 Cochrane review by Shiu et al. [37] reported no difference in all-cause mortality, infection reoccurrence, clinical cure or super-infection post therapy between intermittent and continuous infusion. The authors concluded that evidence was insufficient to recommend the widespread adoption of continuous infusion antibiotics. Shortly thereafter, in 2014, Teo et al. [40] published a meta-analysis combining the results of 18 RCTs and 11 observational studies. Primary outcomes evaluated were mortality and clinical success. Compared with intermittent infusion, the authors concluded that prolonged infusion was associated with a significant reduction in mortality and improvement in clinical success. However, the mortality benefit was only associated with prolonged infusion in observational studies and not in RCTs. When the statistical analysis was performed on studies using equivalent daily doses, no difference in mortality was noted. However, mortality was lower with prolonged infusion when a subset of critically ill patients with APACHE II scores ≥ 15 was evaluated. In terms of clinical success, a significant difference in favor of prolonged infusion was again only detected in observational studies. Analysis of studies with equivalent total daily doses and studies with patients with APACHE II scores ≥ 15 were both in favor of prolonged infusion.

In 2013, the Beta-Lactam Infusion Group (BLING), an Australian-based initiative, compared continuous infusion versus intermittent infusion of beta-lactam antibiotics in ICU patients [41]. The primary outcome was C_{min}/MIC ratios ≥ 1 on days 3 and 4 of therapy. Clinical outcomes were clinical response 7–14 days after drug cessation, ICU-free days at day 28 and ICU and hospital survival. Sixty ICU patients were included and equal doses were administered. In the continuous infusion group, significantly more patients achieved concentrations above the MIC compared to the intermittent infusion treatment arm. A significant difference in clinical cure rate in favor of continuous infusion versus intermittent infusion was reported for the beta-lactam antibiotics under study (meropenem, piperacillin-tazobactam and ticarcillin-clavulanate). ICU-free days at day 28, hospital- and ICU-mortality were not significantly different between the two treatment arms. In 2015, Dulhunty et al. [42] reported the results of the BLING II study, a multicenter randomized trial of continuous versus intermittent infusion of piperacillin/tazobactam, ticarcillin/clavulanic acid and meropenem in severe sepsis. Equal total daily doses were administered and the primary outcome was alive ICU-free days at day 28 after randomization. No difference was found between treatment groups for alive ICU-free days at day 28, 90-day survival, clinical cure, organ failure-free days at day 14 and duration of bacteremia. Of note, in BLING II, 26% of the patients included received renal replacement therapy. The lack of evidence in favor of prolonged infusion was, according to the authors, at least partly explained by the high rate of renal impairment. Also in 2015, Yang et al. [43] documented a significant benefit in favor of piperacillin prolonged infusion compared to intermittent infusion in terms of mortality and clinical cure. Bacterial cure was not significantly different. The meta-analysis included 14 studies of which 2 were prospective studies, 7 were retrospective and 5 were RCTs. ICU patients (5 studies) and non-ICU patients (9 studies) were included for analysis. Studies with non-equal daily dosing were included. In 2016, Yang et al. [44] published a more up-to-date systematic review and meta-analysis. Two of their previously included RCTs were excluded from the meta-analysis, and three retrospective observational studies were added. By contrast with their earlier findings, prolonged infusion of piperacillin no longer demonstrated a significant benefit in terms of mortality or clinical cure.

Roberts et al. [45] published an individual patient data meta-analysis in 2016 solely focusing on severe sepsis patients. The idea behind it was the expectation that in critically patients, based on their altered PK, lower PK/PD targets would be achieved and the benefit of prolonged infusion was more likely to rise to the surface. The authors concluded that compared with intermittent infusion, administration of beta-lactam antibiotics by continuous infusion in critically ill patients with severe sepsis was associated with decreased hospital mortality. Clinical cure was not statistically different between the two groups [45]. In 2017, Fan et al. [46] published a prospective clinical trial comparing intermittent infusion and extended infusion in ICU patients with bacterial infections or neutropenic fever. Equal daily doses were used. The extended infusion group had a mean creatinine clearance of 42 ml/min and the intermittent infusion group had a creatinine clearance of 36 ml/min. There was no significant difference in mortality, as the primary outcome, between the two groups. In their post-hoc subgroup analysis, there was a significant decrease in mortality rate in favor of the extended infusion group when performing analysis for patients with respiratory tract infections. When stratified on higher (≥ 29.5) or lower (< 29.5) APACHE II scores, there was no significant difference between the groups. However, it is worth mentioning that the high mean creatinine clearance rates in both groups may have distorted the relationship between mode of infusion and primary and secondary outcomes.

Finally, a clinical trial protocol for BLING III, a large phase III RCT powered for survival has been registered on clinicaltrials.gov. Meropenem and piperacillin-tazobactam are the antibiotic drugs under study and the aim is to enroll 7,000 ICU patients. The primary outcome is comparing all-cause mortality censored at day 90 after randomization for intermittent infusion versus continuous infusion. Amongst others, new acquisition, colonization and infection with a multidrug resistant organism and *C. difficile* diarrhea are listed as secondary outcomes.

Interpreting the Available Data: What Can We Expect from Prolonged Infusion?

Preclinical Data

Preclinical data suggest that extended infusion and continuous infusion have different killing properties. Although both extended and continuous infusion have demonstrated their ability to achieve higher target attainment rates, only continuous infusion has been shown to be superior in terms of actual bacterial cell kill. This has been demonstrated in preclinical experiments using comparable drug exposure (AUC/MIC). Fig. 2 shows the concentration-time curve of intermittent infusion and continuous infusion of ceftazidime at comparable AUC/MIC. Killing with continuous infusion, despite equal AUC/MIC, was significantly better at 32 h.

The same conclusion however cannot be drawn for extended infusion versus intermittent infusion. Kim et al. [30] reported regrowth with their extended regimen for 2 out of 4 strains with an MIC of 4 mg/l whereas intermittent infusion at comparable AUC/MIC for these strains showed (moderate) killing. In the experiment by Felton et al. [18], the C_{min}/MIC ratios corresponding to an equal outcome (log_{10} kill or resistance suppression) for either intermittent or extended infusion corresponded with (slightly) higher AUC/MIC ratios for the extended dosing regimens compared to the intermittent dosing regimens.

The benefit of continuous infusion is therefore rather demonstrated by its ability to kill more efficaciously for the same exposure (comparable AUC/MIC) than by its ability to achieve equal or higher PK/PD targets. Indeed, preclinical experiments demonstrate that attaining an equal PK/PD target does not necessarily lead to equal bacterial cell kill (Fig. 3). For example, Cappelletty et al. [31] showed in their

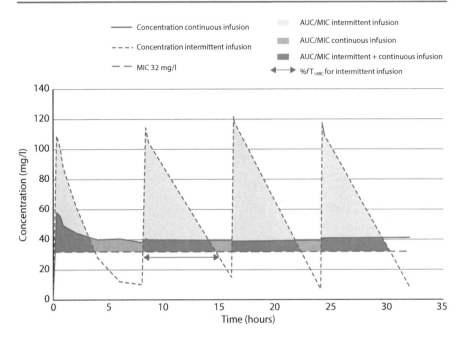

Fig. 2 Concentration-time curve of continuous and intermittent ceftazidime infusion for compara-ble area under the curve/minimal inhibitory concentration (AUC/MIC). Concentration-time curve of continuous infusion (6 g/24 h, *solid line*) and intermittent infusion (2 g q8h, *dashed line*) of ceftazidime. An MIC of 32 mg/l is depicted. Shaded areas are AUC/MIC ratios for intermittent and continuous infusion (30.21 and 29.52 mg/h/l, respectively). The AUC/MIC ratios for the two modes of infusion were comparable. The steady state concentration (C_{ss})/MIC ratio for the con-tinuous infusion regimen was 100% $fT_{>1.2\times MIC}$, while the intermittent infusion regimen achieved a pharmacokinetic/pharmacodynamics (PK/PD) target of 47.6% $fT_{>MIC}$. Killing at 32 h was sig-nificantly better for the continuous infusion dosing regimen. Adapted from [35]

experiment that 'higher' PK/PD targets might be associated with a less favorable outcome when different modes of infusion are used. Regrowth in their experiment was seen at a C_{ss}/MIC ratio of 3.2 (which is equal to 100% $fT_{>3.2\times MIC}$), whereas for intermittent infusion of 2 g q12h, killing at 48 h was seen for a PK/PD target of approximately 100% $fT_{>1.7\times MIC}$ (trough concentration was 2.6–2.8 µg/ml). *Vice versa*, as demonstrated by Felton et al. [18], equal bacterial cell kill with different modes of infusion may require different PK/PD targets.

There are no preclinical experiments available comparing PK/PD targets for maximal bacterial cell kill between intermittent and continuous infusion under the exact same circumstances for the exact same causative pathogen. The above-de-scribed comparative preclinical experiments have used a limited set of different doses and usually a fixed dosing interval. These experiments were designed to com-pare bacterial cell kill between different modes of infusion and were not intended as true dose-ranging and dose-fractionating studies. However, it is worth consider-ing that, when targets for efficacy are considered, the conventional PK/PD target

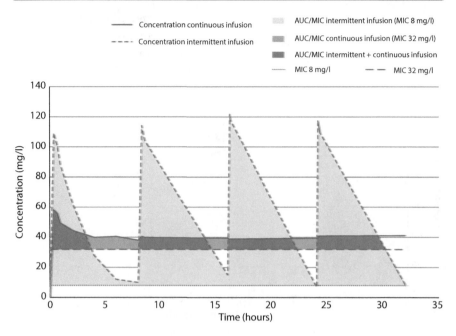

Fig. 3 Concentration-time curve of continuous and intermittent ceftazidime infusion for comparable % $fT_{>MIC}$. Concentration-time curve of continuous infusion (6 g/24 h, *solid line*) and intermittent infusion (2 g q8h, *dashed line*) of ceftazidime. A mean inhibitory concentration (MIC) of 8 mg/l (*dotted line*) and 32 mg/l are depicted. Shaded areas are area under the curve (AUC)/MIC ratios for intermittent (MIC 8 mg/l) and continuous (MIC 32 mg/l) infusion (120.83 and 29.52 mg/h/l respectively). PK/PD targets were comparable, i.e., 100% $fT_{>1.2\times MIC}$ for continuous infusion and 99.8% $fT_{>MIC}$ for intermittent infusion. Despite attaining comparable PK/PD targets, the intermittent regimen achieved ≥ 3 $\log_{10}$ kill at 32 h while the continuous infusion regimen showed regrowth at 32 h. Adapted from [35]

(40–70% $fT_{>MIC}$) is a PK/PD target derived from actual dose-ranging and dose-fractionating studies whereas the PK/PD target of $4 \times MIC$, generally considered as a more stringent or 'higher' PK/PD target, is in fact derived from time-kill experiments where bacteria were exposed to constant, or continuous, concentrations of several MIC multiples for 24 h. As follows, different modes of infusion requiring seemingly different PK/PD targets may explain, at least partly, why it is difficult to demonstrate a benefit in favor of prolonged infusion. Essentially, prolonged infusion is subject to the same PK alterations as is intermittent infusion and may therefore face the same difficulties to achieve therapeutic levels or the respective PK/PD target. Hence, target attainment may be equally difficult to achieve. For example, Aardema et al. [23] demonstrated recently that more than 70% of their patients did not achieve a C_{ss}/MIC ratio of 4 for continuous infusion piperacillin, whereas in the Defining Antibiotic Levels in Intensive Care (DALI) study, approximately 16% of the patients did not achieve 50% $fT_{>MIC}$ [22].

Clinical Data

Limitations of previous clinical studies may have clouded the anticipated difference between intermittent and prolonged infusion in terms of clinical cure and mortality. Examples are limitations in study design, delayed start of the intervention beyond the first 24 h of antibiotic therapy, inclusion of a heterogeneous patient population, inclusion of patients receiving antimicrobials for noninfectious diseases, co-administration of other antimicrobials, differences in total daily doses, unequal or absent loading doses before initiating therapy and limited evaluation of possible adverse effects such as toxicity or antimicrobial resistance.

Limitations in study design are mainly small samples sizes, especially when ICU patients are concerned. In the meta-analysis by Roberts et al. [45], a total of 632 patients with severe sepsis were included. However, in the near future, BLING III may provide data on a much larger and more representative sample of up to 7,000 ICU patients. Clinical trials in which the intervention, i.e., prolonged infusion, could be delayed until 24 h after initiation of standard antimicrobial therapy, lack the ability to evaluate the first 'golden' hours in sepsis management.

Although previous clinical trials and meta-analyses did not demonstrate a convincing benefit in favor of prolonged infusion in a heterogeneous patient population, these trials are of value to detect sub-groups of patients in whom prolonged infusion of beta-lactam antibiotics could still optimize clinical outcomes. Patients with high disease severity, patients infected with less susceptible bacteria and patients suffering from respiratory disease have all been suggested as niche populations likely to benefit from prolonged infusion [47]. In patients with a high disease severity, we expect more profound PK alterations leading to more variable and possibly lower antibiotic concentrations. Prolonging the duration of infusion may lead to higher trough concentrations. As such, intermittent dosing regimens are more likely to result in sub-MIC trough concentrations compared to prolonged infusion regimens. Therefore, demonstrating the advantage of prolonged over intermittent infusion is considered to have a higher probability of success in clinical trials focusing on patients who are most at risk for low trough concentrations. By contrast, including patients in whom mean beta-lactam antibiotic concentrations and concentration/MIC ratios are likely to be higher may cloud the anticipated benefit of prolonged infusion. Examples are patients with renal impairment and patients infected with very susceptible bacteria. Patients infected with very susceptible bacteria are expected to achieve high C_{min}/MIC ratios because the MIC is small. Therefore, trials including patients with a low disease severity, patients with renal dysfunction and patients infected with very susceptible causative organisms are likely to have included patients with high trough concentrations (beyond 100% $fT_{>MIC}$), even with intermittent infusions. Beta-lactam antibiotics exert no further killing beyond a certain antibiotic concentration/MIC ratio, hence we do not expect to easily detect between-group differences if the mean C_{min}/MIC or C_{ss}/MIC in both treatment arms is very high [6].

The observed benefit of prolonged infusion in respiratory infections has been attributed to better penetration of beta-lactam antibiotics into pulmonary tissue when infused continuously compared to intermittently [47]. Although research in this area is very scarce, it is worth pursuing the idea that the type or focus of infection may play a role.

Inclusion of patients with noninfectious diagnoses and co-administration of other antimicrobials may further cloud between-group differences. In patients suffering from inflammation but not infection, clinical outcome may still be suboptimal despite optimal antibiotic dosing. When other antimicrobials are co-administered, e.g., aminoglycosides for additional Gram-negative coverage, it is difficult to delineate the exclusive contribution of beta-lactam antibiotics to improved cure rates or decreased mortality.

Another issue is the use of unequal total daily doses and/or unequal or absent loading doses before the start of the therapy. Local antibiotic prescribing practices may imply the use of different total daily doses in intermittent versus prolonged infusion. Although Teo et al. [40] could not demonstrate a mortality benefit of prolonged infusion when equal daily doses were applied, it seems reasonable to assume that the use of a higher total daily dose in one infusion arm could bias results in favor of this mode of infusion. Administering a loading dose prior to initiating beta-lactam antibiotic therapy is paramount to achieve early target concentrations [48]. In clinical trials, however, the loading dose may differ across different modes of infusion [40]. Higher loading doses (with a higher C_{max}) may allow a more rapid diffusion into peripheral tissue and may therefore influence outcome. So, when dosing is concerned, it is preferable to use both an equal loading dose and an equal total daily dose in comparative clinical trials.

Finally, very few clinical data are available evaluating differences in terms of toxicity or antimicrobial resistance between intermittent and prolonged infusion. Beta-lactam toxicity has been linked to C_{min}/MIC ratios and not dose [49]. Therefore, it seems reasonable to assume that strategies increasing C_{min}, such as prolonged infusion, may increase toxicity. Although a theoretical advantage of prolonged infusion is also expected when antimicrobial resistance is concerned, a recently published retrospective study did not demonstrate a lower risk of emergence of antimicrobial resistance in *P. aeruginosa* with extended infusion meropenem compared to intermittent infusion meropenem [50]. Despite the fact that data on this topic are far from adequate to draw any firm conclusions, one should remain vigilant when resistance is concerned.

Conclusion

Prolonged infusion of beta-lactam antibiotics has consistently been shown to increase target attainment in ICU patients. Nevertheless, clinical trials failed to demonstrate a definitive mortality benefit. Methodological limitations of clinical trials may have masked the clinical superiority of prolonged infusion but, on the other hand, we may have incompletely understood preclinical data as well. Distinguishing extended and continuous infusion as two separate infusion modalities and using equal first and total daily doses to achieve comparable AUC/MIC ratios in all patients are important aspects in the design of clinical trials. Additionally, monitoring toxicity and antimicrobial resistance in comparative clinical trials is indispensable to complete the global picture. Overall, considering the high level of uncertainty, there is an important need to further pursue large and methodologically strong clinical trials in order to definitively demonstrate or refute the advantage of prolonged infusion of beta-lactam antibiotics in the ICU.

References

1. Levy M, Artigas A, Phillips GS et al (2012) Outcomes of the Surviving Sepsis Campaign in intensive care units in the USA and Europe: a prospective cohort study. Lancet Infect Dis 12:919–924
2. Rhodes A, Evans L, Alhazzani W et al (2017) Surviving sepsis campaign: international guidelines for management of sepsis and septic shock: 2016. Intensive Care Med 43:304–377
3. Kollef M, Bassetti M, Francois B et al (2017) The intensive care medicine research agenda on multidrug-resistant bacteria, antibiotics, and stewardship. Intensive Care Med 43:1187–1197
4. Cotta M, Roberts J, Tabah A, Lipman J, Vogelaers D, Blot S (2014) Antimicrobial stewardship of β-lactams in intensive care units. Expert Rev Anti Infect Ther 12:581–595
5. Roberts J, Lipman J, Blot S, Rello J (2008) Better outcomes through continuous infusion of time-dependent antibiotics to critically ill patients? Curr Opin Crit Care 14:390–396
6. Craig (1995) Interrelationship between pharmacokinetics and pharmacodynamics in determining dosage regimens for broad-spectrum cephalosporins. Diagn Microbiol Infect Dis 22:89–96
7. Gonçalves-Pereira J, Póvoa P (2011) Antibiotics in critically ill patients: a systematic review of the pharmacokinetics of β-lactams. Crit Care 15:R206
8. Craig WA, Ebert SC (1992) Continuous infusion of beta-lactam antibiotics. Antimicrob Agents Chemother 36:2577–2583
9. Osthoff M, Siegemund M, Balestra G, Abdul-Aziz M, Roberts J (2016) Prolonged administration of β-lactam antibiotics – a comprehensive review and critical appraisal. Swiss Med Wkly 146:w14368
10. Charmillon A, Novy E, Agrinier N et al (2016) The ANTIBIOPERF study: a nationwide cross-sectional survey about practices for β-lactam administration and therapeutic drug monitoring among critically ill patients in France. Clin Microbiol Infect 22:625–631
11. Buyle FM, Decruyenaere J, De Waele J et al (2013) A survey of beta-lactam antibiotics and vancomycin dosing strategies in intensive care units and general wards in Belgian hospitals. Eur J Clin Microbiol Infect Dis 32:763–768
12. Mouton J (2016) General concepts of pharmacodynamics for anti-infective agents. In: Rotschafer JC, Andes DR, Rodvold KA (eds) Antibiotic pharmacodynamics. Springer, New York, pp 3–27
13. Drusano G (2004) Antimicrobial pharmacodynamics: critical interactions of 'bug and drug'. Nat Rev Microbiol 2:289–300
14. Levison M, Levison J (2009) Pharmacokinetics and pharmacodynamics of antibacterial agents. Infect Dis Clin North Am 23:791–815
15. Craig WA (1998) Pharmacokinetic/pharmacodynamic parameters: rationale for antibacterial dosing of mice and men. Clin Infect Dis 26:1–10
16. Delattre I, Taccone F, Jacobs F et al (2017) Optimizing β-lactams treatment in critically-ill patients using pharmacokinetics/pharmacodynamics targets: are first conventional doses effective? Exp Rev Anti Infect Ther 15:677–688
17. Tam V, Chang KT, Zhou J et al (2017) Determining beta-lactam exposure threshold to suppress resistance development in Gram-negative bacteria. J Antimicrob Chemother 72:1421–1428
18. Felton TW, Goodwin J, O'Connor L et al (2013) Impact of bolus dosing versus continuous infusion of piperacillin and tazobactam on the development of antimicrobial resistance in Pseudomonas aeruginosa. Antimicrob Agents Chemother 57:5811–5819

19. Roberts J, Abdul-Aziz M, Lipman J et al (2014) Individualised antibiotic dosing for patients who are critically ill: challenges and potential solutions. Lancet Infect Dis 14:498–509
20. Felton T, Roberts J, Lodise TP et al (2014) Individualization of piperacillin dosing for critically ill patients: dosing software to optimize antimicrobial therapy. Antimicrob Agents Chemother 58:4094–4102
21. McKinnon P, Paladino J, Schentag J (2008) Evaluation of area under the inhibitory curve (AUIC) and time above the minimum inhibitory concentration (T)MIC) as predictors of outcome for cefepime and ceftazidime in serious bacterial infections. Int J Antimicrob Agents 31:345–351
22. Roberts J, Paul S, Akova M et al (2014) DALI: defining antibiotic levels in intensive care unit patients: are current β-lactam antibiotic doses sufficient for critically ill patients? Clin Infect Dis 58:1072–1083
23. Aardema H, Panday P, Wessels M et al (2017) Target attainment with continuous dosing of piperacillin/tazobactam in critical illness: a prospective observational study. Int J Antimicrob Agents 50:68–73
24. Felton T, Hope WW, Roberts JA (2014) How severe is antibiotic pharmacokinetic variability in critically ill patients and what can be done about it? Diagn Microbiol Infect Dis 79:441–447
25. Joukhadar C, Frossard M, Mayer BX et al (2001) Impaired target site penetration of beta-lactams may account for therapeutic failure in patients with septic shock. Crit Care Med 29:385–391
26. Roberts J, Lipman J (2009) Tissue distribution of beta-lactam antibiotics: continuous versus bolus dosing. J Pharm Pract Res 39:219–222
27. Cousson J, Floch T, Guillard T et al (2015) Lung concentrations of ceftazidime administered by continuous versus intermittent infusion in patients with ventilator-associated pneumonia. Antimicrob Agents Chemother 59:1905–1909
28. Buijk SL, Gyssens IC, Mouton JW, Van Vliet A, Verbrugh HA, Bruining HA (2002) Pharmacokinetics of ceftazidime in serum and peritoneal exudate during continuous versus intermittent administration to patients with severe intra-abdominal infections. J Antimicrob Chemother 49:121–128
29. Zelenitsky S, Nash J, Weber Z, Iacovides H, Ariano R (2016) Targeted benefits of prolonged-infusion piperacillin-tazobactam in an in vitro infection model of Pseudomonas aeruginosa. J Chemother 28:390–394
30. Kim A, Banevicius M, Nicolau D (2008) In vivo pharmacodynamic profiling of doripenem against pseudomonas aeruginosa by simulating human exposures. Antimicrob Agents Chemother 52:2497–2502
31. Cappelletty DM, Kang SL, Palmer SM, Rybak MJ (1995) Pharmacodynamics of ceftazidime administered as continuous infusion or intermittent bolus alone and in combination with single daily-dose amikacin against Pseudomonas aeruginosa in an in vitro infection model. Antimicrob Agents Chemother 39:1797–1801
32. Robaux MA, Dube L, Caillon J et al (2001) In vivo efficacy of continuous infusion versus intermittent dosing of ceftazidime alone or in combination with amikacin relative to human kinetic profiles in a Pseudomonas aeruginosa rabbit endocarditis model. J Antimicrob Chemother 47:617–622
33. Mouton J, den Hollander JG (1994) Killing of Pseudomonas aeruginosa during continuous and intermittent infusion of ceftazidime in an in vitro pharmacokinetic model. Antimicrob Agents Chemother 38:931–936
34. Mouton J, Vinks A, Punt N (1997) Pharmacokinetic-pharmacodynamic modeling of activity of ceftazidime during continuous and intermittent infusion. Antimicrob Agents Chemother 41:733–738
35. Alou L, Aguilar L, Sevillano D et al (2005) Is there a pharmacodynamic need for the use of continuous versus intermittent infusion with ceftazidime against Pseudomonas aeruginosa? An in vitro pharmacodynamic model. J Antimicrob Chemother 55:209–213
36. Tessier PR, Nicolau DP, Onyeji CO, Nightingale CH (1999) Pharmacodynamics of intermittent- and continuous-infusion cefepime alone and in combination with once-daily

tobramycin against Pseudomonas aeruginosa in an in vitro infection model. Chemotherapy 45:284–295

37. Shiu J, Wang E, Tejani A, Wasdell M (2013) Continuous versus intermittent infusions of antibiotics for the treatment of severe acute infections. Cochrane Database Syst Rev CD008481

38. Nicolau DP, McNabb J, Lacy MK, Quintiliani R, Nightingale CH (2001) Continuous versus intermittent administration of ceftazidime in intensive care unit patients with nosocomial pneumonia. Int J Antimicrob Agents 17:497–504

39. Lipman J (2000) Towards better ICU antibiotic dosing. Crit Care Resusc 2:282–289

40. Teo J, Liew Y, Lee W, Kwa A (2014) Prolonged infusion versus intermittent boluses of β-lactam antibiotics for treatment of acute infections: a meta-analysis. Int J Antimicrob Agents 43:403–411

41. Dulhunty J, Roberts J, Davis J et al (2013) Continuous infusion of beta-lactam antibiotics in severe sepsis: a multicenter double-blind, randomized controlled trial. Clin Infect Dis 56:236–244

42. Dulhunty J, Roberts J, Davis J et al (2015) A multicenter randomized trial of continuous versus intermittent β-lactam infusion in severe sepsis. Am J Respir Crit Care Med 192:1298–1305

43. Yang H, Zhang C, Zhou Q, Wang Y, Chen L (2015) Clinical outcomes with alternative dosing strategies for piperacillin/tazobactam: a systematic review and meta-analysis. PLoS One 10:e116769

44. Yang H, Cui X, Ma Z, Liu L (2016) Evaluation outcomes associated with alternative dosing strategies for piperacillin/tazobactam: a systematic review and meta-analysis. J Pharm Pharm Sci 19:274–289

45. Roberts J, Abdul-Aziz MH, Davis J et al (2016) Continuous versus Intermittent β-lactam infusion in severe sepsis. a meta-analysis of individual patient data from randomized trials. Am J Respir Crit Care Med 194:681–691

46. Fan SY, Shum HP, Cheng WY, Chan YH, Leung SY, Yan WW (2017) Clinical outcomes of extended versus intermittent infusion of piperacillin/tazobactam in critically ill patients: a prospective clinical trial. Pharmacotherapy 37:109–119

47. Taccone F, Laupland K, Montravers P (2016) Continuous infusion of β-lactam antibiotics for all critically ill patients? Intensive Care Med 42:1604–1606

48. Waele J, Lipman J, Carlier M, Roberts J (2015) Subtleties in practical application of prolonged infusion of β-lactam antibiotics. Int J Antimicrob Agents 45:461–463

49. Beumier M, Casu GS, Hites M et al (2015) Elevated β-lactam concentrations associated with neurological deterioration in ICU septic patients. Minerva Anestesiol 81:497–506

50. Yusuf E, Herendael B, Verbrugghe W et al (2017) Emergence of antimicrobial resistance to Pseudomonas aeruginosa in the intensive care unit: association with the duration of antibiotic exposure and mode of administration. Ann Intensive Care 7:72

Colistin Dosing in Continuous Renal Replacement Therapy

P. M. Honore, M. L. N. G. Malbrain, and H. D. Spapen

Introduction

Colistin is a multicomponent polypeptide antibiotic produced by strains of the *Paenibacillus polymyxa* bacteria [1]. It was abandoned from clinical use in the 1970s because of significant renal and neurological toxicity. Currently, colistin is increasingly proposed as a last resort treatment for severe multidrug-resistant (MDR) Gram-negative bacterial infections, particularly in the intensive care unit (ICU). Colistin has a relatively narrow spectrum but is very effective against Enterobacteriaceae (*Escherichia coli, Klebsiella* spp., *Enterobacter* spp., *Citrobacter* spp., *Salmonella* spp. and *Shigella* spp., including extended spectrum beta-lactamase [ESBL], *Klebsiella pneumoniae* carbapenemase [KPC], verona integron-encoded metallo-β-lactamase [VIM] and New Delhi metallo [NDM]-1 producers), and MDR *Pseudomonas aeruginosa, Acinetobacter baumannii, Stenotrophomonas maltophilia and Aeromonas* spp. [2]. Resistance is rare and mediated by plasmid transfer between bacterial strains. The plasmid-borne MCR-1 gene was first detected in 2011 and is now widespread throughout South East Asia, several European countries and the United States of America [3].

Colistin is commercially available as colistin sulfate and colistimethate sodium (CMS). CMS is an inactive prodrug that is hydrolyzed to a series of sulfomethylated derivatives and to colistin that exhibits antibacterial activity. CMS is predominantly (~ 70%) cleared by the kidneys. Colistin undergoes extensive renal tubular reabsorption and mainly has a non-renal route of elimination [4]. CMS is mostly administered intravenously but can be nebulized in pneumonia and injected intrathecally or intraventricularly [5]. Colistin sulfate is used to treat intestinal infections and is also available in creams, powders and eardrops.

P. M. Honore (✉) · M. L. N. G. Malbrain · H. D. Spapen
Department of Intensive Care, Universitair Ziekenhuis Brussel, Vrije Universiteit Brussel (VUB)
Brussels, Belgium
e-mail: Patrick.Honore@az.vub.ac.be

© Springer International Publishing AG 2018   71
J.-L. Vincent (ed.), *Annual Update in Intensive Care and Emergency Medicine 2018*,
Annual Update in Intensive Care and Emergency Medicine,
https://doi.org/10.1007/978-3-319-73670-9_6

Pharmacological Insights

The 'resurgence' of colistin in the critical care arena invokes questions with regard to optimal dosing regimens aimed at maximal efficacy with minimal toxicity and minimal development of resistance [6]. From a pharmacodynamic/pharmacokinetic (PK/PD) viewpoint, colistin possesses rapid concentration-dependent bacterial killing against susceptible strains but the unbound area under the concentration time curve above the minimum inhibitory concentration (AUC/MIC) ratio is the PK/PD parameter that correlates best with the antibacterial effect [7]. Colistin is bactericidal when a steady-state plasma concentration of at least 2 mg/l is achieved.

For decades, colistin treatment consisted of a 'standard' CMS dose of 3 million international units (MIU) every 8 h. Plachouras et al. first reported the PK effects of this dosing regimen in a cohort of critically ill patients with normal renal function [8]. Predicted maximum concentrations of colistin in plasma were 0.60 mg/l for the first CMS dose of 3 MIU and 2.3 mg/l at steady state. These observations implied that plasma colistin levels were largely insufficient before and probably not always therapeutic during steady state and suggested that administration of a loading dose should be considered and, at least in severely ill patients, a higher maintenance dose. Another challenging issue is the large interpatient PK/PD variability of colistin resulting in plasma concentrations that may either fail to achieve an antibacterial effect or be too high, thus causing nephrotoxicity.

Current understanding of colistin PK/PD relationships in different populations, including patients receiving renal replacement therapy (RRT), has yielded user-friendly algorithms for individualized dosing to achieve effective plasma steady-state colistin concentrations [9]. Of note, however, is the paucity of colistin PK/PD data in subjects receiving continuous RRT (CRRT). This is problematic because CRRT is increasingly used in critically ill patients. Compared with intermittent dialysis, CRRT indeed is better hemodynamically tolerated, offers rapid correction of life-threatening metabolic alterations, allows more adequate control of fluid balance and may even lower the incidence of post-ICU need for chronic dialysis.

CRRT Elimination of Colistin

Molecular weight, protein binding, hydro- or lipophilicity and the membrane sieving coefficient all determine CRRT-related drug elimination [10–13]. Colistin is bound to albumin and alpha-1 acid glycoprotein (AAG). AAG is an acute phase reactant protein produced by the liver [1]. Plasma AAG concentrations (~ 0.75 g/l) are much lower than those of human serum albumin (~ 45 g/l) but may increase 15 to 30 fold in stressful conditions [14–16]. During inflammation or in infectious disease, AAG drug binding capacity may increase up to 95% [17]. As such, AAG-bound colistin is not likely to be eliminated by convection alone, because convection allows drug removal only at a binding level less than 80% [18]. Moreover, AAG production not only shows significant infection-related variability between patients but also depends on liver function, which may result in unpredictable colistin protein binding over time.

Mariano et al. evaluated colistin removal in a small cohort of septic patients treated with continuous veno-venous hemodiafiltration (CVVHDF) using non-adsorptive polysulfone membranes, coupled plasma filtration adsorption with hemofiltration (CPFA-HF), or hemoperfusion [19]. Significant convective elimination of colistin was observed during CVVHDF. However, extracorporeal clearance of colistin during CVVHDF exceeded values reported so far suggesting some adsorptive activity of the polysulfone membrane. CPFA-HF most efficiently removed colistin, probably because colistin was partly adsorbed on the sorbent cartridge [19].

We measured colistin concentrations in plasma and ultrafiltration (UF) fluid in a patient undergoing continuous venovenous hemofiltration (CVVH) [20] using a highly adsorptive membrane [21]. Different elimination over time curves of CMS and colistin were observed. A decrease in CMS elimination from plasma was seen after each dose, which is typical of elimination through convection. In contrast, colistin removal followed an asymptotic curve representing slow elimination and accumulation as seen with adsorption. This supports the concept that the prodrug CMS is eliminated by convection whereas colistin removal is determined by the adsorptive capacity of the CRRT membrane [20].

Colistin Dosing in CRRT

PK/PD analysis in nine critically ill patients (seven receiving continuous venovenous hemodialysis and two undergoing hemofiltration) in whom CRRT dialysate clearance of CMS and colistin was determined, suggested a maximum loading dose of 9 MIU CMS followed 12 h later by a daily CMS dose of approximately 13 MIU [9]. Plasma levels between 1.5 and 2 mg/l were obtained in 8 patients. One patient had a concentration > 4 mg/l [9]. Karaiskos et al. confirmed rapid achievement of target colistin concentrations in critically ill patients under CVVHDF after administering a loading dose of 9 MIU CMS. However, following implementation of a predicted pharmacokinetic model on plasma CMS/colistin concentrations, a loading dose of 12 MIU CMS appeared more appropriate, and a CMS maintenance dosage of at least 6.5 to 7.5 MIU every 12 h was suggested [22].

We recently performed a retrospective observational study in 16 critically ill patients infected with Gram-negative infections only susceptible to colistin [23]. Causative pathogens were *P. aeruginosa*, *K. pneumoniae* and *Enterobacter* spp. All patients were receiving CVVH using a 1.5 m^2 highly adsorptive acrylonitrile 69 surface-treated filter. CVVH was performed at a dose of 35 ml/kg/h under regional citrate anticoagulation. A loading dose of 9 MIU CMS was administered followed by 4.5 MIU/8 h. To reconcile dose- and time-dependent PK/PD properties of colistin, we chose to divide the maintenance dose into three. Clinical and microbiological efficacy were assessed at end of therapy. Serum creatinine was evaluated before and at the end of therapy and at hospital discharge in survivors. MIC values for colistin ranged from 0.03 to 3 mg/l. CVVH was provided for 13 (6–27) days. A favorable clinical response was obtained in 14 (88%) patients. Microbiological eradication was complete in 10, presumed in four and absent in two subjects. Seven

Table 1 Clinical studies on high-dose colistin treatment in patients receiving continuous renal replacement therapy (CRRT)

Author [ref]	Number of patients	Loading dose	Maintenance dose	CRRT modality	Anticoagulation	CRRT membrane	TDM	Hospital mortality (%)	Renal function at discharge
Mariano [19]	12	None	4.5 MIU bid	CVVHDF CPFA-HF HMP	RCA	Polysulfone (less adsorptive)	In plasma and UF	33%	Not reported
Karaiskos [22]	8	9 MIU (12 MIU suggested)	4.5 MIU bid (6.5–7.5 MIU bid suggested)	CVVHDF	Not reported	AN68	In plasma	Not reported	Not reported
Verdoodt [23]	16	9 MIU	4.5 MIU tid	CVVH	RCA	AN69 ST (highly adsorptive)	No	45%	Normal renal function in 6/7 survivors

TDM: therapeutic drug monitoring; *CVVHDF*: continuous venovenous hemodiafiltration; *CPFA-HF*: coupled plasma filtration adsorption with hemofiltration; *HMP*: hemoperfusion; *CVVH*: continuous venovenous hemofiltration; *RCA*: regional citrate anticoagulation; *MIU*: million international units; *AN69 ST*: acrylonitrile 69 surface treated; *bid*: twice daily; *tid*: three times daily; *UF*: ultrafiltrate

(45%) patients left the hospital alive. Renal function was preserved in six patients. One patient required intermittent dialysis at ICU discharge.

Clinical studies evaluating high-dose colistin treatment in CRRT are summarized in Table 1.

Monitoring Colistin Therapy During CRRT

Therapeutic drug monitoring of colistin in plasma and ultrafiltration fluid during CRRT is recommended [24]. Apart from its variable PK/PD behavior, adjustments of maintenance colistin dosing may also be required because of changes in porosity and adsorptive capacity of the dialysis membrane. Given their different elimination profiles, colistin and not CMS must be measured. Any colistin therapeutic drug monitoring study in patients undergoing CRRT should provide detailed information about the method of CRRT used (with or without adsorptive column), the type of membrane (not, partly, or highly adsorptive), and the anticoagulation protocol (regional citrate anticoagulation may improve membrane adsorptive capacity!).

Conclusion

Colistin at a loading dose of 9 MIU, followed by a divided maintenance dose of 13 to 15 MIU daily, guarantees adequate and safe treatment in patients undergoing CRRT. We suggest that CRRT should be equipped with highly adsorptive filters to avoid colistin accumulation and performed under regional citrate anticoagulation to preserve functional membrane capacity [25]. Ideally therapeutic drug monitoring should be performed, especially in patients with increased clearance.

References

1. Falagas ME, Rafailidis PI (2008) Re-emergence of colistin in today's world of multidrug-resistant organisms: personal perspectives. Expert Opin Investig Drugs 17:973–981
2. Karaiskos I, Giamarellou H (2014) Multidrug-resistant and extensively drug-resistant Gram-negative pathogens: current and emerging therapeutic approaches. Expert Opin Pharmacother 15:1351–1370
3. Kumarasamy KK, Toleman MA, Walsh TR et al (2010) Emergence of a new antibiotic resistance mechanism in India, Pakistan, and the UK: a molecular, biological, and epidemiological study. Lancet Infect Dis 10:597–602
4. Bergen PJ, Landersdorfer CB, Zhang J et al (2012) Pharmacokinetics and pharmacodynamics of 'old' polymyxins: what is new? Diagn Microbiol Infect Dis 74:213–223
5. Gilbert B, Morrison C (2017) Evaluation of intraventricular colistin utilization: a case series. J Crit Care 40:161–163
6. Landersdorfer CB, Nation RL (2015) Colistin: how should it be dosed for the critically ill? Semin Respir Crit Care Med 36:126–135
7. Grégoire N, Aranzana-Climent V, Magréault S, Marchand S, Couet W (2017) Clinical pharmacokinetics and pharmacodynamics of colistin. Clin Pharmacokinet 56:1441–1460

8. Plachouras D, Karvanen M, Friberg LE et al (2009) Population pharmacokinetic analysis of colistin methanesulfonate and colistin after intravenous administration in critically ill patients with infections caused by gram-negative bacteria. Antimicrob Agents Chemother 53:3430–3436

9. Nation RL, Garonzik SM, Thamlikitkul V et al (2017) Dosing guidance for intravenous colistin in critically-ill patients. Clin Infect Dis 64:565–571

10. Leypoldt JK, Jaber BL, Lysaght MJ, McCarthy JT, Moran J (2003) Kinetics and dosing predictions for daily haemofiltration. Nephrol Dial Transplant 18:769–776

11. Jeffrey RF, Khan AA, Prabhu P et al (1994) A comparison of molecular clearance rates during continuous hemofiltration and hemodialysis with a novel volumetric continuous renal replacement system. Artif Organs 18:425–428

12. Elbers PW, Girbes A, Malbrain ML, Bosman R (2015) Right dose, right now: using big data to optimize antibiotic dosing in the critically ill. Anaesthesiol Intensive Ther 47:457–463

13. Martinkova J, Malbrain ML, Havel E, Šafránek P, Bezouška J, Kaška M (2016) A pilot study on pharmacokinetic/pharmacodynamic target attainment in critically ill patients receiving piperacillin/tazobactam. Anaesthesiol Intensive Ther 48:23–28

14. Azad MA, Huang JX, Cooper MA et al (2012) Structure-activity relationships for the binding of polymyxins with human α-1-acid glycoprotein. Biochem Pharmacol 84:278–291

15. Dudhani RV, Li J, Nation RL (2009) Plasma binding of colistin involves multiple proteins and is concentration dependent: potential clinical implications. Abstracts of the forty-ninth Interscience Conference on Antimicrobial Agents and Chemotherapy. American Society for Microbiology, Washington, p 41

16. Herve F, Gomas E, Duche JC, Tillement JP (1993) Evidence for differences in the binding of drugs to the two main genetic variants of human alpha 1-acid glycoprotein. Br J Clin Pharmacol 36:241–249

17. Israili ZH, Dayton PG (2001) Human alpha-1-glycoprotein and its interactions with drugs. Drug Metab Rev 33:161–235

18. Pea F, Viale P, Pavan F, Furlanut M (2007) Pharmacokinetic considerations for antimicrobial therapy in patients receiving renal replacement therapy. Clin Pharmacokinet 46:997–1038

19. Mariano F, Leporati M, Carignano P, Stella M, Vincenti M, Biancone L (2015) Efficient removal of colistin A and B in critically ill patients undergoing CVVHDF and sorbent technologies. J Nephrol 28:623–631

20. Honore PM, Jacobs R, Lochy S et al (2013) Acute respiratory muscle weakness and apnea in a critically ill patient induced by colistin neurotoxicity: key potential role of hemoadsorption elimination during continuous venovenous hemofiltration. Int J Nephrol Renovasc Dis 6:107–111

21. Honore PM, Jacobs R, Joannes-Boyau O et al (2013) Newly designed CRRT membranes for sepsis and SIRS—a pragmatic approach for bedside intensivists summarizing the more recent advances: a systematic structured review. ASAIO J 59:99–106

22. Karaiskos I, Friberg LE, Galani L et al (2016) Challenge for higher colistin dosage in critically ill patients receiving continuous venovenous haemodiafiltration. Int J Antimicrob Agents 48:337–341

23. Verdoodt A, Honore PM, Jacobs R, Van Gorp V, Hubloue I, Spapen HD (2017) High-dose colistin combined with continuous veno-venous haemofiltration for treatment of multidrug-resistant Gram-negative infection in critically ill patients. Intensive Care Med Exp 5(Suppl 2):44-0986 (abst)

24. Gobin P, Lemaître F, Marchand S, Couet W, Olivier JC (2010) Assay of colistin and colistin methanesulfonate in plasma and urine by liquid chromatography-tandem mass spectrometry. Antimicrob Agents Chemother 54:1941–1948

25. Honore PM, Jacobs R, Hendrickx I, De Waele E, Van Gorp V, Spapen HD (2015) Higher colistin dose during continuous renal replacement therapy: look before leaping! Crit Care 19:235

Part III
Cardiovascular Concerns

Left Ventricular Diastolic Dysfunction in the Critically Ill

F. Guarracino, P. Bertini, and M. R. Pinsky

Introduction

Intrinsic left ventricular (LV) cardiac pump function plays a major role in defining cardiovascular reserve and the ability of the host to respond to circulatory stress. The three major processes defining myocardial contractile reserve relate to processes directly altering systolic pump function, contraction synchrony and diastolic relaxation. The most common process limiting intrinsic cardiac performance worldwide is diastolic dysfunction. Diastolic dysfunction increases perioperative risk and hemodynamic derangement in the intensive care unit (ICU). In the unstressed state, diastolic dysfunction often exists at a subclinical level, becoming overtly manifest only during stress states as seen with acute hypovolemic or distributive shock and in the management of acute respiratory failure. Preoperative diagnosis often requires exercise testing because patients are usually asymptomatic at rest. Diastolic dysfunction often becomes manifest by cardiovascular stressors commonly seen in the critically ill and postoperative state, namely systemic hypertension, fluid overload or atrial fibrillation.

Myocardial relaxation after end-systole is the energy-dependent process of the cardiac cycle; thus, coronary artery disease-induced regional ischemia causes immediate diastolic stiffening of the involved area, which presents as an S3 gallop and regional wall motion abnormalities. Furthermore, diastolic relaxation is not only energy dependent, the rate of relaxation is greater than if the myocardium relaxed passively. Such active relaxation can be quantified during cardiac catheterization

F. Guarracino (✉) · P. Bertini
Department of Anesthesia and Critical Care Medicine, Azienda Ospedaliero Universitaria Pisana
Pisa, Italy
e-mail: fabiodoc64@hotmail.com

M. R. Pinsky
Department of Critical Care Medicine, University of Pittsburgh
Pittsburgh, PA, USA

© Springer International Publishing AG 2018
J.-L. Vincent (ed.), *Annual Update in Intensive Care and Emergency Medicine 2018*,
Annual Update in Intensive Care and Emergency Medicine,
https://doi.org/10.1007/978-3-319-73670-9_7

as the negative LV dP/dt, which if extrapolated to complete relaxation would give a negative LV diastolic pressure.

Normal LV diastolic function can be defined as the ability of the left ventricle to first relax enough to allow filling and then to fill up to an end-diastolic volume without significant increase in left atrial pressure (LAP) [1]. Thus, LAP or its surrogate, pulmonary artery occlusion pressure (PAOP), have been used to diagnose diastolic dysfunction, though this screening approach is not without limitations. Relevant to the practice of intensive care medicine, LV failure with subsequent increases in LAP can occur without impaired LV systolic function. Thus, a LV ejection fraction (LVEF), e.g., >0.5 does not exclude diastolic dysfunction. Indeed, the presence of diastolic dysfunction is often unexpected and occasionally misdiagnosed because of its lack of presence at rest and, with resuscitation, a low cardiac output and high LV filling pressure but a preserved LVEF. The extent that diastolic dysfunction can proceed to cardiogenic shock is a function of the underlying etiologies. But heart failure can occur due to isolated diseased diastolic physiology or in combination with mild systolic dysfunction [2].

Physiology of the Cardiac Cycle

The LV cardiac cycle can be represented as a sequence of transvascular pressure, volume and electrocardiographic events on the timeline known as Wiggers' diagram (Fig. 1). Most clinicians concentrate their attention on the systolic period, although, as seen on the diagram, the left ventricle spends most of the time in diastole, a time needed for both diastolic relaxation and LV filling. The diastolic phase of LV pump function is underappreciated in critical care medicine and anesthesia probably because common hemodynamic monitoring systems can only measure systemic arterial pressure, thus focusing only on systolic performance. However, both stroke volume and cardiac output are intimately related to diastolic function. Clearly, the left ventricle can only eject an amount of volume slightly less than LV end-diastolic volume. Thus, if diastolic filling is impaired, LV stroke volume will be equally restricted, independent of LV systolic function.

Diastole can be separated into four phases: isovolumic relaxation, rapid filling, diastasis and atrial systole. Isovolumic relaxation occurs after the aortic valve closes and the mitral valve is still closed. This is the major energy-dependent aspect of diastole and, in ischemic states, delayed diastolic relaxation limits the time necessary for the other four phases of diastole. The second phase is rapid LV filling; as the left ventricle relaxes enough, left atrial pressure exceeds LV pressure causing the mitral valve to open and pulmonary venous blood to fill the LV cavity. This is the phase in which the largest amount of blood volume is introduced into the left ventricle. However, filling is limited by the passive pressure gradients between the pulmonary veins and the left ventricle. That these pressures are low and diastolic compliance high means that filling occurs both rapidly and under low pressure, allowing coronary blood flow to perfuse the subendocardium. Diastasis occurs as LV pressures approach LAP and is responsible for 5% or less of diastolic volume as some LV in-

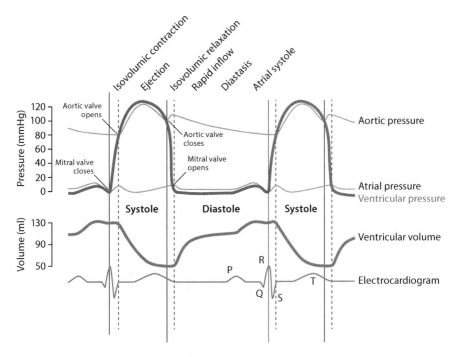

Fig. 1 The Wiggers' diagram

flow occurs owing to inertia. The last phase occurs as the atria contract, increasing LAP and increasing LV volume to end-diastole, but at a much higher pressure than seen during diastasis. At rest, left atrial contraction adds an additional 15% to end-diastolic-volume. During exercise, when diastolic time is shortened, atrial contraction adds progressively more volume. Thus, atrial fibrillation, by abolishing atrial contraction markedly decreases LV end-diastolic volume during exercise and also when LV diastolic compliance is reduced. Regrettably, none of these phases of the cardiac cycle are routinely explored using routine bedside hemodynamic monitoring tools! So the intensivist is usually blind to the diastolic physiology and often surprised at stroke volume limitation during volume loading in a patient without impaired contractility.

Epidemiology of Diastolic Dysfunction in the Critical Care Population

Approximately half of all patients with a diagnosis of heart failure have diastolic dysfunction. It is more common in women, the aged and those with co-morbidities of diabetes, hypertension, coronary artery disease and LV hypertrophy [3–6]. Relevant to this review, recent studies suggest also that diastolic dysfunction might negatively impact on the prognosis of the critically ill [7].

Diagnosis of Altered Diastolic Physiology

Invasive catheter based measurement of LV pressures is considered the most reliable method to assess elevated LV filling pressures and, by definition to grade diastolic dysfunction. Unfortunately, this method is difficult to perform in the critically ill [8]. The most recent European Cardiology recommendations [9] report that diastolic dysfunction is not only common but presents as heart failure with preserved ejection fraction. Echocardiography is the most used and convenient diagnostic test to identify and stratify diastolic dysfunction based on etiology. In patients with normal LVEF, diastolic dysfunction can be diagnosed by four altered echocardiographic parameters: $E/e' > 14$, e' velocity < 7 cm/s (septal) or < 10 cm/s (lateral), tricuspid regurgitation velocity > 2.8 m/s and left atrial volume index > 34 ml/m^2. The presence of less than 50% of these parameters indicates normal LV diastolic function, if 50% are positive, diagnosis of diastolic dysfunction is indeterminate, and if more than 50% are positive, diastolic dysfunction is diagnosed. Relevant to this echocardiographic diagnosis, in subjects with reduced LVEF, mitral inflow $E/A < 0.8$ with $E < 50$ cm/s are indexes of normal LAP and therefore diastolic dysfunction is considered as grade I; if $E/A < 0.8$ and $E > 50$ cm/s or E/A is between 0.8 and 2, diastolic dysfunction is considered grade II; finally, when E/A is > 2, grade III diastolic dysfunction is diagnosed. However, transmitral flow analysis as well as E wave deceleration time may be difficult to obtain in the critically ill and the results are usually difficult to interpret by the non-cardiologist. Therefore, echocardiographic tissue Doppler imaging (TDI), if available is a reasonable and less time consuming method of processing the echocardiographic mages to make the diagnosis of diastolic dysfunction. A recent study in a critically ill population of patients with septic shock documented that measures of e' and E/e' alone could be used to diagnose diastolic dysfunction with reasonable accuracy [10].

It is important to underline the difference between diastolic dysfunction and diastolic heart failure. Diastolic dysfunction consists of altered physiology of LV relaxation or/and compliance, whereas diastolic heart failure consists of signs and symptoms of reduced ventricular compliance and abnormal relaxation with preserved or mildly reduced systolic function. This difference is crucial to appreciate, as many factors commonly occurring in the critical care setting can turn diastolic dysfunction into diastolic heart failure.

Factors Triggering Diastolic Heart Failure

In the setting of diastolic dysfunction, decreased preload (e.g., hypovolemia, positive-pressure breathing), tachycardia, loss of atrial pump filling, afterload increase and myocardial ischemia (Fig. 2) can all induce diastolic heart failure. Importantly, diastolic failure is rarely responsive to fluid therapy or isolated inotropic drug infusion. Specifically, impaired LV filling may be exacerbated by fluid loading because right ventricular (RV) dilation will only decrease further LV diastolic compliance. Thus, conditions common to critically ill patients, such as rapid fluid administra-

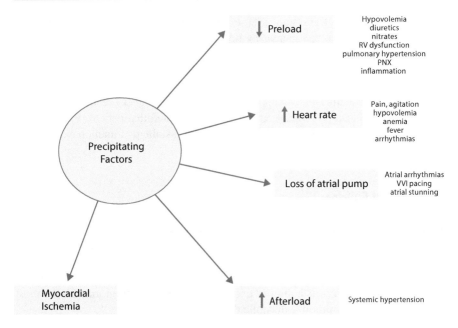

Fig. 2 Factors that can trigger diastolic dysfunction or turn diastolic dysfunction into diastolic heart failure. *RV*: right ventricular; *VVI*: V = ventricle paced, V = ventricle sensed, I = pacing inhibited if ventricular beat is sensed; *PNX*: pneumothorax

tion, RV dysfunction, elevated positive end-expiratory pressure (PEEP; increasing pulmonary vascular resistance and decreasing venous return) and pneumothorax can all precipitate diastolic failure. Tachycardia limits diastolic filling and may also cause myocardial ischemia, decreasing diastolic compliance further. Arterial hypertension and coronary artery disease may cause non-heart rate dependent myocardial ischemia [11]. Myocardial ischemia deserves a further comment. Ischemia can precipitate diastolic dysfunction due to primary pump failure decreasing coronary blood flow making it important to keep mean arterial pressure (MAP) above some minimal value to maintain coronary perfusion. Finally, stress as may occur associated with pain, agitation, invasive maneuvers and surgery can also trigger diastolic heart failure.

Impact of Diastolic Dysfunction on Major Critical Care Scenarios

The Weaning Process from the Ventilator

Weaning from mechanical ventilation is a form of cardiovascular exercise [12]. Several studies have investigated the relationship between diastolic dysfunction and the weaning process [13–17]. When a patient is changed to spontaneous ventilation, several things occur simultaneously: intrathoracic pressure decreases leading to an increase in LV transmural systolic pressure, which increases LV afterload decreasing LV ejection and increasing myocardial O_2 demand (MVO_2); and an increase in LV preload increasing LAP. Collectively, these processes cause weaning-induced pulmonary edema. Weaning-induced pulmonary edema is exacerbated by diastolic dysfunction. Indeed, Liu et al. [18] demonstrated that 59% of ICU patients who developed weaning-induced pulmonary edema had higher E/e' than those without weaning-induced pulmonary edema. They suggested that patients who develop weaning-induced pulmonary edema need to have diastolic dysfunction excluded or treated if present treated [19].

Right Heart Failure

Right heart failure is a common co-traveler with diastolic dysfunction. Whether the cause of diastolic dysfunction or induced by it, LV diastolic stiffening is commonly seen. The mechanisms are multiple and include reactive pulmonary hypertension and RV dilation with septal shift into the left ventricle. Mechanical ventilatory support without lung over-distention or excessive fluid resuscitation may be the most effective strategy to minimize diastolic dysfunction.

Septic Shock

In a recent meta-analysis, Sanfilippo et al. [20] demonstrated that diastolic dysfunction was associated with mortality in a septic shock population, whereas systolic dysfunction did not show the same association. The etiology of septic diastolic dysfunction is not well understood. Several studies have documented both systolic and diastolic dysfunction in septic shock patients [21]. Clearly, in sepsis, diastolic dysfunction should alert the clinician to be more cautious in fluid resuscitation. Since early and aggressive fluid resuscitation are part of the Surviving Sepsis Guidelines, caution needs to be exercised in this approach in patients with known chronic hypertension, diabetes or right heart failure as such fluid resuscitation might make cardiac function worse.

Hemodynamic Monitoring

Conventional hemodynamic monitoring of the critically ill patient using central venous pressure (CVP) monitoring and an arterial pressure monitor will reveal most of the hallmarks of diastolic dysfunction. Static pressures (CVP and PAOP) most of the time fail to provide adequate information on filling conditions due to altered LV compliance, but their increase in response to fluid loading should trigger stopping of the infusion and assessment for evidence of right heart failure [22, 23]. Regrettably, even applying functional hemodynamic monitoring principles of assessing dynamic indices of preload responsiveness [24] (stroke volume variation [SVV], pulse pressure variation [PPV] and dynamic elastances) will not detect diastolic dysfunction at an early stage, only once diastolic failure has developed. At the present time, the only reliable bedside monitoring tool capable of assessing diastolic dysfunction is echocardiography. Echocardiography identifies RV dilation, septal shift and impaired mitral flow. Moreover, echocardiography provides a comprehensive evaluation of cardiovascular function, thus putting the intensivist in the best position to reflect on the patient's pathophysiology and decide on the hemodynamic treatment [25].

Management of the Critically Ill Patient with Diastolic Dysfunction

Based on the above discussion, it should be clear that the critical care patient can suffer from chronic diastolic dysfunction due to pre-existing cardiovascular or systemic disease, or develop an acute diastolic dysfunction due to an acute illness impacting on diastolic function.

No treatment is available that can acutely revert chronic diastolic dysfunction. Each causal etiology has different treatments. Diastolic dysfunction caused by LV hypertrophy is made worse by tachycardia, thus keeping heart rate low enough to allow LV filling (e.g., < 90/min) should maintain end-diastolic volume. Since impaired contractility is not the major problem causing diastolic dysfunction, beta-adrenergic blocking agents are beneficial. The only therapies known to treat LV diastolic dysfunction are those able to reverse myocardial remodeling, and they take time and are not a realistic option for most patients in circulatory shock with diastolic dysfunction. For example, aortic valve replacement to treat aortic stenosis and blood pressure control to treat systemic arterial hypertension will minimize diastolic dysfunction over months. The only rapidly reversible causes of diastolic dysfunction are acute cor pulmonale and tamponade-like physiology. In the patient with chronic obstructive pulmonary disease (COPD), minimizing hyperinflation and alveolar hypoxia will reduce pulmonary artery pressures allowing the right ventricle to become smaller, thus minimizing ventricular interdependence.

Since intensivists cannot treat diastolic dysfunction, all they can do is minimize the inciting processes that exacerbate it to prevent diastolic dysfunction from deteriorating into diastolic heart failure. Fig. 2 lists the various triggers that may move diastolic dysfunction towards diastolic heart failure. These need to be considered on a case-by-case basis. As listed above for LV hypertrophy, wherein LV isometric relaxation is impaired, one of the most important measures is to avoid tachycardia. By balancing a fixed stroke volume and lower heart rate with its associated limit of O_2 delivery, efforts to minimize O_2 demand become adjuvant treatments. Thus, providing mechanical ventilatory support, stopping seizures and tremors and preventing fever will all minimize O_2 demands. By slowing the heart rate, diastole is prolonged, allowing adequate LV filling time and coronary perfusion, which will secondarily benefit both LV output and contractility. In this setting, continuing beta-blocker therapy becomes a central line of therapy. Avoiding myocardial ischemia also plays a major role, the diastolic phase being very dependent on myocardial perfusion [26]. This implies use of normal cardiovascular practice in the management of patients with coronary insufficiency, namely maintaining an adequate diastolic arterial pressure, low heart rate and low global O_2 demand. Unlike hypovolemic shock, in which fluid resuscitation is the primary treatment, maintaining an appropriate circulating blood volume becomes paramount to defining circulatory reserve. Too little filling and tachycardia and low stroke volumes develop, too much filling and pulmonary edema and hypoxemia ensue. Thus, these patients may not tolerate vasodilator therapy, fluid boluses or mechanical ventilatory settings that limit venous return or increase pulmonary vascular resistance. Furthermore, if some mild systolic dysfunction co-exists, slight increases in arterial pressure may greatly impair LV ejection worsening diastolic dysfunction. Loss of atrial kick, as occurs with the sudden onset of atrial fibrillation, can change asymptomatic diastolic dysfunction into diastolic heart failure then circulatory shock. Avoiding drugs that induce atrial fibrillation, keeping serum potassium levels > 4.5 mEg/dl and avoiding acidosis represent smart strategies. If atrial fibrillation occurs, pharmacologic or electric cardioversion should be attempted. Once stable, if atrial contraction is shown to be central to cardiovascular stability, inserting an atrio-ventricular sequential pacemaker may be indicated. The value of atrial contraction in maintaining an adequate stroke volume in patients with diastolic dysfunction cannot be over emphasized. Finally, a patient with diastolic dysfunction requiring inotropic support represents one of the more challenging critical care situations. In fact, beta-agonists tend to worsen diastolic function by increasing intracellular calcium (delaying isovolemic relaxation) and increasing MVO_2, thus leading to increased wall tension and reduced LV compliance. In this scenario, the choice should be a drug that can increase the contractile state without causing detrimental effects on diastole. Currently the only class of drugs with such a pharmacodynamic profile is the calcium sensitizers, whose effect on long term outcomes is, however, still under debate. For all these reasons, fluid management, vasoactive drugs and beta-blockers must be titrated in a very precise and patient-specific manner as no two patients will require the same circulating blood volume, heart rate or arterial pressure combination.

Conclusion

In the management of patients with circulatory shock, attention usually focuses on fluid resuscitation and LV systolic function. However, the literature strongly supports that clinicians focus more on diastolic dysfunction as a leading cause of cardiovascular limitation. This requires recognition of diastolic dysfunction in the ICU patient, and management aimed at sustaining filling times, minimizing RV dilation and sustaining coronary blood flow. This approach should include the bedside evaluation of diastolic function in order to assess diastolic physiology at baseline and monitor it following intensive care treatments. As a consequence, intensive care medicine physicians should include echocardiography analysis as part of their ongoing cardiovascular assessment.

References

1. Vignon P (2013) Ventricular diastolic abnormalities in the critically ill. Curr Opin Crit Care 19:242–249
2. Ponikowski P, Voors AA, Anker SD et al (2016) 2016 ESC guidelines for the diagnosis and treatment of acute and chronic heart failure. Eur J Heart Fail 18:891–975
3. Jeong EM, Dudley SC Jr (2015) Diastolic dysfunction. Circ J 79:470–477
4. Masoudi FA, Havranek EP, Smith G et al (2003) Gender, age, and heart failure with preserved left ventricular systolic function. J Am Coll Cardiol 41:217–223
5. Nishimura RA, Tajik AJ (1997) Evaluation of diastolic filling of left ventricle in health and disease: doppler echocardiography is the clinician's Rosetta stone. J Am Coll Cardiol 30:8–18
6. Phillip B, Pastor D, Bellows W, Leung JM (2003) The prevalence of preoperative diastolic filling abnormalities in geriatric surgical patients. Anesth Analg 97:1214–1221
7. Gonzalez C, Begot E, Dalmay F et al (2016) Prognostic impact of left ventricular diastolic function in patients with septic shock. Ann Intensive Care 6:36
8. Pirracchio R, Cholley B, De Hert S, Solal AC, Mebazaa A (2007) Diastolic heart failure in anaesthesia and critical care. Br J Anaesth 98:707–721
9. Nagueh SF, Smiseth OA, Appleton CP et al (2016) Recommendations for the evaluation of left ventricular diastolic function by Echocardiography: an update from the American Society of Echocardiography and the European association of cardiovascular imaging. Eur Heart J Cardiovasc Imaging 17:1321–1360
10. Lanspa MJ, Gutsche AR, Wilson EL et al (2016) Application of a simplified definition of diastolic function in severe sepsis and septic shock. Crit Care 20:243
11. Kawaguchi M, Hay I, Fetics B, Kass DA (2003) Combined ventricular systolic and arterial stiffening in patients with heart failure and preserved ejection fraction: implications for systolic and diastolic reserve limitations. Circulation 107:714–720
12. Pinsky MR (2000) Breathing as exercise: the cardiovascular response to weaning from mechanical ventilation. Intensive Care Med 26:1164–1166
13. Caille V, Amiel JB, Charron C, Belliard G, Vieillard-Baron A, Vignon P (2010) Echocardiography: a help in the weaning process. Crit Care 14:R120
14. Lamia B, Maizel J, Ochagavia A et al (2009) Echocardiographic diagnosis of pulmonary artery occlusion pressure elevation during weaning from mechanical ventilation. Crit Care Med 37:1696–1701
15. Moschietto S, Doyen D, Grech L, Dellamonica J, Hyvernat H, Bernardin G (2012) Transthoracic Echocardiography with Doppler Tissue Imaging predicts weaning failure from mechanical ventilation: evolution of the left ventricle relaxation rate during a spontaneous breathing trial is the key factor in weaning outcome. Crit Care 16:R81
16. Papanikolaou J, Makris D, Saranteas T et al (2011) New insights into weaning from mechanical ventilation: left ventricular diastolic dysfunction is a key player. Intensive Care Med 37:1976–1985
17. Voga G (2012) Early and simple detection of diastolic dysfunction during weaning from mechanical ventilation. Crit Care 16:137
18. Liu J, Shen F, Teboul JL et al (2016) Cardiac dysfunction induced by weaning from mechanical ventilation: incidence, risk factors, and effects of fluid removal. Crit Care 20:369
19. de Meirelles Almeida CA, Nedel WL, Morais VD, Boniatti MM, de Almeida-Filho OC (2016) Diastolic dysfunction as a predictor of weaning failure: a systematic review and meta-analysis. J Crit Care 34:135–141
20. Sanfilippo F, Corredor C, Fletcher N et al (2015) Diastolic dysfunction and mortality in septic patients: a systematic review and meta-analysis. Intensive Care Med 41:1004–1013
21. Landesberg G, Gilon D, Meroz Y et al (2012) Diastolic dysfunction and mortality in severe sepsis and septic shock. Eur Heart J 33:895–903

22. Cecconi M, De Backer D, Antonelli M et al (2014) Consensus on circulatory shock and hemo-dynamic monitoring. Task force of the European Society of Intensive Care Medicine. Intensive Care Med 40:1795–1815
23. Monnet X, Marik PE, Teboul JL (2016) Prediction of fluid responsiveness: an update. Ann Intensive Care 6:111
24. Pinsky MR (2015) Functional hemodynamic monitoring. Crit Care Clin 31:89–111
25. Guarracino F, Bertini P (2014) Perioperative haemodynamic management: is echocardiography the right tool? Curr Opin Crit Care 20:431–437
26. Vanhecke TE, Kim R, Raheem SZ, McCullough PA (2010) Myocardial ischemia in patients with diastolic dysfunction and heart failure. Curr Cardiol Rep 12:216–222

Management of Intraoperative Hypotension: Prediction, Prevention and Personalization

T. W. L. Scheeren and B. Saugel

Introduction

The human cardiovascular system is pressure regulated with relatively high arterial pressures to guarantee organ perfusion. Arterial blood pressure is kept fairly constant, at least in healthy individuals. The system can be compared to a water tower providing a constant pressure head, with changes in local resistance (like opening the water tap), allowing a distribution of flow to the different organs, according to their need. Some organ systems (e.g., the brain and kidneys) regulate blood flow – within certain limits – independently of blood pressure. This phenomenon is called 'autoregulation of blood flow' and aims at protecting these organs from hypoperfusion. Below the lower limits of this autoregulation, organ perfusion becomes linearly dependent on blood pressure. Even in some circulatory shock states (hypovolemic shock and cardiogenic shock), blood pressure is kept constant for a long time due to stimulation of the sympathetic nervous system, and arterial hypotension is a rather late physiological response. Nevertheless, arterial hypotension occurs frequently in patients undergoing surgery under general anesthesia. This intraoperative hypotension has been demonstrated to jeopardize organ perfusion and to be associated with postoperative morbidity and mortality.

In this chapter, we will discuss the pathophysiology and relevance of intraoperative hypotension with a special focus on recent publications and innovative concepts for the management of intraoperative hypotension based on the three mainstays: prediction, prevention and personalization.

T. W. L. Scheeren (✉)
Department of Anesthesiology, University of Groningen, University Medical Center Groningen
Groningen, Netherlands
e-mail: t.w.l.scheeren@umcg.nl

B. Saugel
Department of Anesthesiology, Center of Anesthesiology and Intensive Care Medicine,
University Medical Center Hamburg-Eppendorf
Hamburg, Germany

© Springer International Publishing AG 2018   89
J.-L. Vincent (ed.), *Annual Update in Intensive Care and Emergency Medicine 2018*,
Annual Update in Intensive Care and Emergency Medicine,
https://doi.org/10.1007/978-3-319-73670-9_8

Intraoperative Hypotension: Definition and Epidemiology

Despite its relevance for postoperative patient outcome, intraoperative hypotension is poorly defined. In a literature review, 140 different definitions of intraoperative hypotension were found in 130 articles [1]. Definitions are based on absolute thresholds for mean arterial pressure (MAP) or systolic blood pressure, relative declines from baseline blood pressure, or combine absolute and relative cut-off values. Because of the lack of an unambiguous definition of intraoperative hypotension, the incidence of intraoperative hypotension varies between 5 and 99%, depending on the definition used [1].

One problem related to finding a physiologically sound and clinically applicable definition of intraoperative hypotension is the definition of 'baseline' blood pressure. The question of which blood pressure to consider as the baseline value has recently been addressed in a study including 4,408 patients ≥ 60 years old undergoing non-cardiac surgery. Of note, the average pre-induction blood pressure was higher than the preoperative blood pressure obtained outside the operating room, with a huge variability both within and among patients [2].

Retrospective data analysis from 15,509 patients undergoing anesthesia for non-cardiac surgery revealed that intraoperative hypotension frequently occurred when the most common definition of intraoperative hypotension (MAP < 65 mmHg) was used; the incidence was 65% for 1 min below this threshold, 49% for 5 min and 31% for 10 min [1].

Etiology of Intraoperative Hypotension

Multiple patient-related and procedural factors can contribute to the development of intraoperative hypotension during the induction and maintenance of anesthesia and during surgery (e.g., age, comorbidities, cardio-depressant and vasodilatory effects of anesthetics or neuraxial blockade, hemorrhage, patient positioning).

Risk factors for intraoperative hypotension include advanced age (≥ 50 years), lower baseline MAP, use of propofol and fentanyl for induction of anesthesia, and higher American Society of Anesthesiologists (ASA) physiological status [3].

In a recent retrospective study in more than 2,000 patients undergoing general anesthesia for non-cardiac surgery, the authors differentiated between post-induction hypotension (i.e., arterial hypotension occurring during the first 20 min after anesthesia induction) and early intraoperative hypotension (i.e., arterial hypotension during the first 30 min of surgery) [4]. Independent variables significantly related to post-induction hypotension were a low pre-induction systolic blood pressure (odds ratio 0.97), advanced age (odds ratio 1.03), and emergency surgery (odds ratio 1.75). For early intraoperative hypotension, pre-induction systolic blood pressure (odds ratio 0.99), age (odds ratio 1.02), emergency surgery (odds ratio 1.83), supplementary administration of spinal or epidural anesthetic techniques (odds ratio 3.57), male sex (odds ratio 1.41) and ASA physical status IV (odds ratio 2.18) were identified as significant predictors [4].

In general, because blood pressure is mathematically and physiologically coupled with cardiac output and systemic vascular resistance, intraoperative hypotension can be caused by decreased cardiac preload, decreased cardiac afterload, decreased cardiac contractility, or any combination of these factors. Intraoperative hypotension should be diagnosed and managed based on these physiological principles.

Intraoperative Hypotension and Outcome

There is increasing evidence that (even a short period of) intraoperative hypotension is associated with postoperative mortality [5–7], myocardial injury [8–11], acute kidney injury (AKI) [8, 9, 12–14] and postoperative stroke [15] in patients undergoing non-cardiac surgery under general anesthesia. One study showed that the negative effect of intraoperative hypotension on mortality might even be persistent for as long as one year after surgery [16].

A low intraoperative MAP as part of a "triple low" state, meaning a combination of low arterial pressure, low bispectral index and low minimum alveolar concentration of volatile anesthetics in non-cardiac surgical patients was associated with significantly increased 30-day mortality (odds ratio 3.96) in a large retrospective cohort analysis [17].

Regarding postoperative complications, large database studies suggest that the risk for both kidney and myocardial injury gradually increases with the duration and severity of hypotension [8, 9].

Management of Intraoperative Hypotension

Prediction

Considering the association of intraoperative hypotension and adverse patient outcome and the pathophysiology of intraoperative hypotension, it would be an intriguing and promising approach to establish prediction models that enable the development of intraoperative hypotension to be identified before the blood pressure drops to a critical level. Prediction of hypotension before it occurs would allow the clinician to apply preemptive treatment strategies to prevent hypotension and thus potentially improve outcome.

Clinical signs of hypotension that are routinely available to the clinician in the operating room occur late in the process of hemodynamic instability, i.e., when cardiovascular dynamics are already markedly altered [18, 19]. Currently, standard hemodynamic monitoring is aimed at detecting ongoing hemodynamic instability, but these means of hemodynamic monitoring are not good at predicting instability before its development or at detecting instability at a very early stage.

Fig. 1 shows an exemplary time progression of a hemodynamic instability event. Standard clinical signs of the event that are obtained during routine monitoring ap-

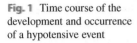 Time course of the
development and occurrence
of a hypotensive event

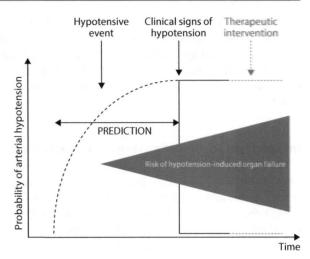

pear late when the event has already occurred. Resuscitation possibly starts even later, after a time delay. This may result in the patient spending a significant amount of time in hemodynamic instability, potentially resulting in hypoperfusion and organ failure as discussed previously.

From a physiologic point of view, hypotensive events do not start with the appearance of the clinical signs of hypotension. In fact, such events start earlier, long before the patient exhibits clinical signs of instability. Early stages of instability are typically characterized by subtle and complex changes in the dynamics of physiological waveforms and the physiological association between them as a result of altered compensatory mechanisms [18, 19]. An example of this complex interplay is heart rate variability which has been shown to decrease before a hypotensive event [20]. Similar to heart rate variability, spontaneous variability exists in all continuously measured clinical variables and physiological waveforms [21, 22]. The spontaneous variability is caused by various compensatory mechanisms in the cardiovascular system that try to maintain hemodynamics stable. Measuring early alterations in the compensatory mechanisms reflected by changes in the spontaneous variability of hemodynamic variables during early stages of instability might enable an upcoming hypotensive event to be detected early, even before it occurs.

The compensatory mechanisms also create complex physiological associations and dynamic links between different hemodynamic variables and physiological waveforms. One example of such an interactive physiological link is the baroreflex sensitivity [23, 24] that is based on the feedback loop between MAP and heart rate (with any decrease in MAP, heart rate increases and *vice versa*). A correlation between these two variables indicates high baroreflex sensitivity and thus strong compensatory activity, whereas a lack of correlation indicates weak compensatory activity.

From a technical point of view, it is complex to assess and monitor the changes in the physiologic signals that might serve as early indicators for upcoming hypotensive events. The dynamic changes in the variability and complexity of physiological signals and their physiological associations are not easily discernible to the human eye or detectable with simple signal processing algorithms [19]. Machine learning methods are powerful mathematical tools that allow very accurate quantification of these dynamic multivariate interconnections and can be used to construct reliable mathematical models for predicting hemodynamic instability or hypotension [25, 26].

The physiological principles discussed above can be used to develop algorithms for real-time prediction of hypotension based on the continuous analysis of a large number of hemodynamic features extracted from the arterial pressure waveform and machine learning models. Within each cardiac cycle, several cardiac sub-phases of the arterial pressure waveform can be analyzed and related to specific physiological effects (Fig. 2). For each phase, several features can be calculated and analyzed, such as the times (or durations), amplitudes, areas under each phase (measuring its energy power), the standard deviation (measuring its pulsatility/variability), slopes and frequency components. Information about additional hemodynamic features, such as pulse rate, cardiac output, stroke volume variation, systemic vascular resistance, and arterial tone can also be derived from the arterial waveform. The huge set of data including various hemodynamic variables and features of the arterial pressure waveform can be further processed and analyzed. Thus, certain features or combination of features of the arterial waveform can be statistically assessed for their predictive capabilities for hypotension and machine learning techniques can be used to finally generate a prediction model for hypotension.

An algorithm for prediction of hypotension recently became commercially available as a feature of the EV1000 clinical monitoring platform (Edwards Lifesciences, Irvine, CA, USA) and was named the "Hypotension Probability Indicator" (HPI). The HPI provides the clinician with information regarding the probability of a patient trending towards a hypotensive event, defined as MAP < 65 mmHg for at least one minute, and is displayed as a percentage, ranging from 0–100%. In a secondary screen, which pops up automatically when the HPI exceeds 85%, more hemody-

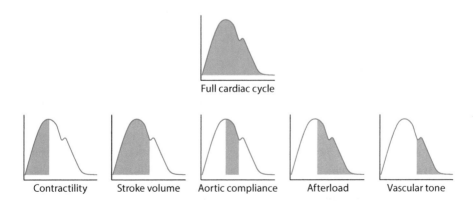

Full cardiac cycle

Contractility   Stroke volume   Aortic compliance   Afterload   Vascular tone

Fig. 2 Sub-phases of the arterial pressure waveform

namic information about the patient is provided in order to help clinicians gain insight into probable causes of the hypotensive event, and take respective measures to prevent or treat hypotension. Before any recommendations regarding the clinical use of the HPI software can be given, clinical validation and outcome studies are needed. These studies are required to show whether use of this system will change hemodynamic management and if this will have an impact on patient outcome.

Prevention

Early identification of intraoperative hypotension or prediction before its clinical occurrence would enable preemptive treatment strategies to be applied in order to minimize the time spent in intraoperative hypotension. However, because the prediction of intraoperative hypotension is not yet established in clinical practice, data on prevention or preemptive treatment of intraoperative hypotension are scarce.

As a first step, the preoperative clinical assessment (history and physical examination) of a patient scheduled for surgery might allow the patient's risk of intraoperative hypotension to be identified and perioperative hemodynamic management to be adapted accordingly. To avoid the development of intraoperative hypotension or to provide a specific causative treatment for intraoperative hypotension early during its development it is necessary to evaluate the underlying pathophysiologic cause of intraoperative hypotension in an individual patient and a specific clinical setting. This remains highly complex because intraoperative hypotension can be caused by a variety of different factors (and a combination of these) including (but not limited to) a decrease in systemic vascular resistance, a decrease in cardiac preload, or an impairment of myocardial contractility. Therefore, therapeutic concepts for the prevention or treatment of intraoperative hypotension include the intravenous administration of fluids (crystalloids and colloids, blood products) to optimize the intravascular volume status and cardiac preload and the administration of vasoactive and inotropic agents to optimize vasomotor tone and cardiac contractility. In addition to these established therapeutic concepts, peristaltic pneumatic compression of the patients' legs has been suggested in patients undergoing minor surgery under general anesthesia to prevent and treat intraoperative hypotension [27].

Personalization

The underlying pathophysiology of intraoperative hypotension calls for personalized approaches to the management of intraoperative hypotension [28]. Depending on a patient's blood pressure profile (e.g., presence or history of chronic arterial hypertension, circadian blood pressure changes), the blood flow/perfusion pressure autoregulation curve has specific properties that determine the upper and lower limits of blood flow autoregulation and thus the critical blood pressure thresholds that define clinically relevant intraoperative hypotension in the individual patient. The great variability in the lower pressure limit of blood flow autoregulation implies that a fixed general blood pressure threshold to define intraoperative hypotension cannot match the value that represents the critical blood pressure in each individual patient.

This fact is illustrated by a study in 152,445 adult patients undergoing non-cardiac surgery, the results of which showed that the lower the MAP, the greater was the increase in 30-day mortality and that for each hypotensive MAP threshold, less time needed to be accumulated in patients with a history of hypertension (in comparison to patients without a history of hypertension) to incur the same relative increase in the odds ratio for 30-day mortality [29].

So far, there are very limited data on circadian blood pressure profiles and their relation to perioperatively obtained blood pressure values [30, 31].

More and larger clinical studies are needed to establish the concept of personalized blood pressure management in the perioperative phase [28]. This might include the preoperative assessment of a patient's baseline blood pressure or circadian blood pressure profile in patients scheduled for surgery, the individual estimation of lower limits of blood flow autoregulation, and the definition of intraoperative hypotension (and thus blood pressure target values) for each individual patient.

Conclusions

Hypotension is frequently observed in the perioperative period and is associated with postoperative morbidity and mortality. Yet, despite its relevance for postoperative patient outcome, intraoperative hypotension is poorly defined and an unambiguous definition of intraoperative hypotension is urgently needed. Multiple patient-related and procedural factors can contribute to the development of intraoperative hypotension during the induction and maintenance of anesthesia and during surgery.

Future concepts for the management of intraoperative hypotension might be based on the early identification or even prediction of intraoperative hypotension. This approach may enable treatment for intraoperative hypotension to be applied very early – or even in a preemptive way – to prevent intraoperative hypotension. Personalized treatment strategies may help enable fluids and vasoactive agents to be titrated to individual targets for each patient based on baseline blood pressure or individual circadian blood pressure profiles.

References

1. Bijker JB, van Klei WA, Kappen TH, van Wolfswinkel L, Moons KG, Kalkman CJ (2007) Incidence of intraoperative hypotension as a function of the chosen definition: literature definitions applied to a retrospective cohort using automated data collection. Anesthesiology 107:213–220
2. van Klei WA, van Waes JA, Pasma W et al (2017) Relationship between preoperative evaluation blood pressure and preinduction blood pressure: a cohort study in patients undergoing general anesthesia. Anesth Analg 124:431–437

3. Reich DL, Hossain S, Krol M et al (2005) Predictors of hypotension after induction of general anesthesia. Anesth Analg 101:622–628
4. Südfeld S, Brechnitz S, Wagner JY et al (2017) Post-induction hypotension and early intraoperative hypotension associated with general anaesthesia. Br J Anaesth 119:57–64
5. Monk TG, Bronsert MR, Henderson WG et al (2015) Association between intraoperative hypotension and hypertension and 30-day postoperative mortality in noncardiac surgery. Anesthesiology 123:307–319
6. Mascha EJ, Yang D, Weiss S, Sessler DI (2015) Intraoperative mean arterial pressure variability and 30-day mortality in patients having noncardiac surgery. Anesthesiology 123:79–91
7. Devereaux PJ, Yang H, Yusuf S et al (2008) Effects of extended-release metoprolol succinate in patients undergoing non-cardiac surgery (POISE trial): a randomised controlled trial. Lancet 371:1839–1847
8. Walsh M, Devereaux PJ, Garg AX et al (2013) Relationship between intraoperative mean arterial pressure and clinical outcomes after noncardiac surgery: toward an empirical definition of hypotension. Anesthesiology 119:507–515
9. Salmasi V, Maheshwari K, Yang D et al (2017) Relationship between intraoperative hypotension, defined by either reduction from baseline or absolute thresholds, and acute kidney and myocardial injury after noncardiac surgery: a retrospective cohort analysis. Anesthesiology 126:47–65
10. Alcock RF, Kouzios D, Naoum C, Hillis GS, Brieger DB (2012) Perioperative myocardial necrosis in patients at high cardiovascular risk undergoing elective non-cardiac surgery. Heart 98:792–798
11. van Waes JA, van Klei WA, Wijeysundera DN, van Wolfswinkel L, Lindsay TF, Beattie WS (2016) Association between intraoperative hypotension and myocardial injury after vascular surgery. Anesthesiology 124:35–44
12. Sun LY, Wijeysundera DN, Tait GA, Beattie WS (2015) Association of intraoperative hypotension with acute kidney injury after elective noncardiac surgery. Anesthesiology 123:515–523
13. Mizota T, Hamada M, Matsukawa S, Seo H, Tanaka T, Segawa H (2017) Relationship between intraoperative hypotension and acute kidney injury after living donor liver transplantation: a retrospective analysis. J Cardiothorac Vasc Anesth 31:582–589
14. Heringlake M, Nowak Y, Schon J et al (2014) Postoperative intubation time is associated with acute kidney injury in cardiac surgical patients. Crit Care 18:547
15. Bijker JB, Persoon S, Peelen LM et al (2012) Intraoperative hypotension and perioperative ischemic stroke after general surgery: a nested case-control study. Anesthesiology 116:658–664
16. Bijker JB, van Klei WA, Vergouwe Y et al (2009) Intraoperative hypotension and 1-year mortality after noncardiac surgery. Anesthesiology 111:1217–1226
17. Sessler DI, Sigl JC, Kelley SD et al (2012) Hospital stay and mortality are increased in patients having a "triple low" of low blood pressure, low bispectral index, and low minimum alveolar concentration of volatile anesthesia. Anesthesiology 116:1195–1203
18. Pinsky MR (2010) Complexity modeling: identify instability early. Crit Care Med 38:S649–S655
19. Pinsky MR, Dubrawski A (2014) Gleaning knowledge from data in the intensive care unit. Am J Respir Crit Care Med 190:606–610
20. Padley JR, Ben-Menachem E (2017) Low pre-operative heart rate variability and complexity are associated with hypotension after anesthesia induction in major abdominal surgery. J Clin Monit Comput. https://doi.org/10.1007/s10877-017-0012-4 (epub ahead of print)
21. Pagani M, Somers V, Furlan R et al (1988) Changes in autonomic regulation induced by physical training in mild hypertension. Hypertension 12:600–610
22. de Boer RW, Karemaker JM, Strackee J (1986) On the spectral analysis of blood pressure variability. Am J Physiol 251:H685–H687

23. Westerhof BE, Gisolf J, Stok WJ, Wesseling KH, Karemaker JM (2004) Time-domain cross-correlation baroreflex sensitivity: performance on the EUROBAVAR data set. J Hypertens 22:1371–1380

24. Zavodna E, Honzikova N, Hrstkova H et al (2006) Can we detect the development of barore-flex sensitivity in humans between 11 and 20 years of age? Can J Physiol Pharmacol 84:1275–1283

25. Convertino VA, Moulton SL, Grudic GZ et al (2011) Use of advanced machine-learning techniques for noninvasive monitoring of hemorrhage. J Trauma 71:S25–S32

26. Convertino VA, Grudic G, Mulligan J, Moulton S (2013) Estimation of individual-specific progression to impending cardiovascular instability using arterial waveforms. J Appl Physiol 115:1196–1202

27. Kiefer N, Theis J, Putensen-Himmer G, Hoeft A, Zenker S (2011) Peristaltic pneumatic compression of the legs reduces fluid demand and improves hemodynamic stability during surgery: a randomized, prospective study. Anesthesiology 114:536–544

28. Saugel B, Vincent J-L, Wagner JY (2017) Personalized hemodynamic management. Curr Opin Crit Care 23:334–341

29. Stapelfeldt WH, Yuan H, Dryden JK et al (2017) The SLUScore: a novel method for detecting hazardous hypotension in adult patients undergoing noncardiac surgical procedures. Anesth Analg 124:1135–1152

30. Berger JJ, Donchin M, Morgan LS, van der Aa J, Gravenstein JS (1984) Perioperative changes in blood pressure and heart rate. Anesth Analg 63:647–652

31. Soo JC, Lacey S, Kluger R, Silbert BS (2011) Defining intra-operative hypotension—a pilot comparison of blood pressure during sleep and general anaesthesia. Anaesthesia 66:354–360

Vasodilatory Shock in the ICU: Perils, Pitfalls and Therapeutic Options

S. Vallabhajosyula, J. C. Jentzer, and A. K. Khanna

Introduction

Circulatory failure is commonly seen in the intensive care unit (ICU) and manifests as cardiovascular instability. Shock is defined as hypotension leading to decreased organ perfusion and inadequate cellular oxygen utilization [1, 2]. Even brief periods of hypotension in the intraoperative period can lead to renal and myocardial injury [3]. The degree of hypotension leading to end organ dysfunction has been defined as a mean arterial pressure (MAP) of < 65 mmHg in the operating room [3]. The threshold MAP associated with adverse outcomes is as yet unclear in critically ill patients admitted to the ICU, and likely depends on the baseline blood pressure and other patient characteristics [4]. The most recent Surviving Sepsis Campaign Guidelines define this threshold using a MAP of < 65 mmHg [5]. Hypotension in critically ill patients is often multifactorial in etiology and is a consequence of pathological vasodilation, impaired cardiac performance, hypovolemia, sedation, processes of care and worsening morbidity due to underlying pathology. Distributive shock due to vasodilation remains the most commonly seen shock state in the ICU and is a consequence of medical or surgical conditions that cause vasoplegia and vascular dysfunction. Vasodilatory shock that requires escalating doses of vasopressors and remains unresponsive to these interventions is associated with significant mortality and morbidity due to a multitude of factors [1, 6]. The optimal combination and dosing of vasoactive medications, thresholds for defining severe or refractory

S. Vallabhajosyula · J. C. Jentzer
Department of Cardiovascular Medicine, Mayo Clinic
Rochester, MN, USA
Division of Pulmonary and Critical Care Medicine, Mayo Clinic
Rochester, MN, USA

A. K. Khanna (✉)
Center for Critical Care, Anesthesiology Institute and Department of Outcomes Research, Cleveland Clinic
Cleveland, OH, USA
e-mail: khannaa@ccf.org

© Springer International Publishing AG 2018
J.-L. Vincent (ed.), *Annual Update in Intensive Care and Emergency Medicine 2018*,
Annual Update in Intensive Care and Emergency Medicine,
https://doi.org/10.1007/978-3-319-73670-9_9

shock and role of rescue therapies remains to be determined [6]. In this chapter, we seek to highlight the pathophysiology, risk factors, evaluation and management of refractory vasodilatory shock in the ICU.

Etiology and Pathogenesis

The etiology of vasodilatory shock is multifactorial and results from multiple in-ter-related pathophysiological mechanisms. Sepsis is a leading etiology of refrac-tory shock (81%) in the ICU [7]. Prior randomized and observational data have noted 50–80% of cases of refractory vasodilatory shock to be due to sepsis [1, 8]. Vasoplegia is frequently seen in post-surgical patients, especially after cardiac surgery with the use of cardiopulmonary bypass (CPB) [9]. Preoperative and in-traoperative factors contribute to the development of vasoplegia and low-cardiac output syndrome in the postoperative population leading to refractory shock in a minority [10]. In the Angiotensin II for the Treatment of High-Output Shock (ATHOS-3) trial, postoperative patients with vasoplegic shock formed 6% of the to-tal population [1]. Other less common etiologies include pancreatitis, anaphylaxis, severe metabolic acidosis, post-cardiac arrest syndrome and multifactorial shock states.

In septic patients, dysregulation of the immune system and pathological va-sodilatation are associated with coagulation abnormalities, immunodeficiency and activation or dysfunction of the endothelium. This pathological process can be ag-gravated by delayed administration of antibiotics, use of unbalanced crystalloids and concomitant renal failure [11]. Additionally, sepsis is associated with tachy-cardia due to autonomic dysreflexia that contributes to impaired diastolic filling, worsening arrhythmias and decreased cardiac output. In cardiac surgery patients, the use of CPB is associated with the release of inflammatory vasodilators and impairment of the arginine-vasopressin system that results in a decreased sensi-tivity to catecholamines and a hemodynamic state mimicking sepsis [9]. Preop-erative left ventricular dysfunction and the use of renin-angiotensin-aldosterone system (RAAS) inhibitors can be associated with a higher incidence of postopera-tive vasoplegia in post-surgical patients [10]. Patients with shock often have relative adrenal insufficiency, hyperglycemia and hypocalcemia, all of which predispose to decreased efficacy of catecholamine vasopressors. In critically ill patients, this can be further complicated by cardiomyopathy due to stress, sepsis and/or cate-cholamine vasopressors used to counteract the shock state [12, 13]. Left and/or right ventricular systolic and diastolic dysfunction may impact preload, fluid responsive-ness and response to vasoactive medications [14].

Regardless of the etiology, the pathogenesis of vasodilatory shock follows a com-mon pathway as detailed in Fig. 1 [8]. At the cellular and molecular level, alterations in pathways related to nitric oxide (NO), prostaglandins and reactive oxygen species (ROS) result in inappropriate vasodilatation [8]. Activation of adenosine triphos-phate (ATP)-sensitive potassium channels in vascular smooth muscle cells prevents calcium entry required for vasoconstriction, representing a final common pathway

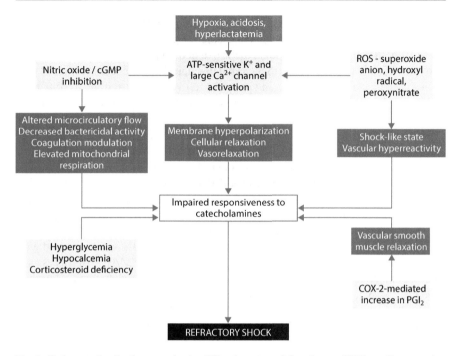

Fig. 1 Pathogenesis of refractory shock. *ATP*: adenosine triphosphate; *cGMP*: cyclic guanosine monophosphate; *COX*: cyclooxygenase; *PGI₂*: prostaglandin I₂; *ROS*: reactive oxygen species. Adapted from [8] with permission

linking metabolic derangements (i.e., tissue hypoxia and acidosis) and inflammation (including NO production) with vasoplegia [8].

Defining Hypotension and Associated Complications

Myocardial Injury

As a result of physiologic blood flow autoregulation, end-organ perfusion pressure remains stable over a normal MAP range, typically above 60 mmHg [15]. Below this MAP threshold, organ perfusion decreases in proportion to a further decrease in MAP and organ failure can ensue. Chronic end-organ damage from hypertension or acute organ dysfunction due to sepsis can alter the autoregulatory threshold, allowing organ hypoperfusion to occur at higher MAP thresholds. The myocardium is exquisitely sensitive to changes in hemodynamics and coronary blood flow impairment during shock. Increased tachycardia and tachyarrhythmia in shock is associated with decreased diastolic time leading to coronary hypoperfusion [14]. Bradycardia, either spontaneously or by the use of beta-blockers, may confer a survival advantage in critically ill septic patients [16, 17]. In patients with critically low diastolic blood pressure, the use of norepinephrine can improve cardiac hemodynamics and systemic perfusion pressure [18]. Elevation in cardiac troponins in critically ill patients is proportional to the extent of hypotension, suggesting a role of hypotension in causing occult myocardial damage [14]. Often, restoration of vascular tone and adequate fluid loading unmasks left ventricular systolic dysfunction, which may be an adaptive mechanism and is not associated with adverse outcomes in septic patients [12, 19].

Critically ill patients, especially those with sepsis, face dysregulation of the inflammatory and coagulation cascades that are associated with end-organ damage in the heart, kidneys and the brain independent of the hemodynamic status [11, 20]. A direct implication of this 'double insult' (hypotension and sepsis) may be that thresholds for blood pressure targets of safety may be higher in the ICU patient population as noted by Khanna et al. [21]. Therefore, septic critically ill patients may need a higher perfusion pressure to maintain vital organ integrity. In a clinical trial of septic patients, resuscitation to a MAP goal of 65 mmHg was associated with similar mortality to a MAP goal of 85 mmHg [4]. The higher MAP goal was associated with more catecholamine-related adverse effects such as arrhythmias, but may have been associated with reduced rates of acute kidney injury (AKI), particularly in patients with chronic hypertension [4]. These results emphasize the delicate balance between adverse events related to hypotension and those related to vasoactive drug therapy.

Hypotension, even transiently, in the operating room is associated with worse outcomes [3, 22, 23]. This relationship is clearly defined in terms of time duration and MAP thresholds in the operating room [3, 22, 23]. A recent post-hoc analysis of the Perioperative Ischemic Evaluation 2 (POISE-2) trial demonstrated a substantial increase in the risk of myocardial infarction and mortality in patients with clinically important hypotension on postoperative days 1–4, after adjustment for relevant confounders [24]. In the ICU, data from septic and non-septic patients with vasodilatory shock have shown that both the duration and extent of hypotension are associated with progression of renal injury [25]. In another large retrospective cohort, mean MAP < 65 mmHg in patients with septic shock was the strongest predictor of mortality after serum lactate levels [26]. Data from a cohort of critically ill non-cardiac surgery patients in the ICU during the initial 7 postoperative days showed that a MAP of < 75 mmHg was associated with a composite of myocardial injury after non-cardiac surgery and mortality. In addition, the threshold appeared to be higher and the relationship nearly linear for AKI [21]. Among patients with sepsis, those with a history of hypertension appear to be at increased risk of significant AKI when treated to a lower MAP goal of 65 mmHg versus 85 mmHg [4].

Renal and Cerebral Injury

In the kidney, alterations in renal hemodynamics resulting from hypotension can be associated with AKI [11]. In a meta-analysis of 160 studies on septic patients, normal or increased renal blood flow was noted in nearly 30% of the patients [27].

The diversion of renal blood flow towards the renal cortex resulting in relative renal medullary hypoxia has been stated to be responsible for renal ischemia and acute tubular necrosis [28]. In critically ill patients, AKI has been associated with longer lengths of stay and increased mortality in post-surgical and septic populations [3, 11]. In addition to the heart and the kidney, hypotension also compromises the cerebral circulation. In the cerebral circulation, the cerebral perfusion pressure is tightly controlled in a given MAP range. However, rapid shifts in hemodynamics result in hypoperfusion contributing to impaired autoregulation [29]. Hypotension in combination with inflammation, use of sedative-hypnotics and neurotransmitter imbalance is associated with encephalopathy and delirium in critically ill patients, which are associated with worse short and long-term outcomes [20, 30].

Refractory Shock

The inability to achieve target MAPs despite escalating vasopressor therapy, need for rescue vasopressor therapy or the need for high-dose vasopressors are all methods to define refractory shock in this population [1, 6]. The incidence and outcomes of refractory shock vary with differences in definition and vasoactive medication cut-offs, however it is consistently associated with poor outcomes [31]. Reversible etiologies that contribute to worsening shock include untreated infection, severe metabolic acidosis, hypocalcemia, sedative overdose and hypovolemia [11, 31]. The pathophysiology, diagnosis and management of refractory shock have been previously described elegantly by Jentzer et al. [8].

Clinical Features and Diagnostic Evaluation

End-organ hypoperfusion in shock manifests with changes in mental status, decreased urine output, decreased capillary refill and mottling over the extremities. Patients with shock will be hypotensive, often tachycardic, and typically require vasopressor therapy; tachypnea and hypoxemia are common, especially from concomitant acute respiratory distress syndrome (ARDS) [5]. End-organ hypoperfusion may occur in chronically hypertensive patients at higher MAP values defining a subgroup that might benefit from maintenance of higher MAP targets during resuscitation [4]. In addition, critically ill patients with sepsis may have higher thresholds of sufficient blood pressure, though the data are preliminary and based on associative relationships only. The diagnosis, evaluation and management of shock in critical illness often happen simultaneously [2].

The primary step is to evaluate the hemodynamic picture to discern the type of shock and likely etiology. Bedside point-of-care ultrasonography is frequently used in current clinical practice to diagnose and manage shock. Invasive hemodynamic measures, such as pulmonary artery wedge pressure and central venous pressures, are used less commonly in modern practice to evaluate the hemodynamic status [32]. Cardiac surgery patients often have an in-dwelling pulmonary artery catheter from the operating room that can be used to evaluate hemodynamic parameters. Modern practice has moved away from static variables of hemodynamic status such as filling pressures to more reliable measures of dynamic fluid assessment [5]. Vasodilatory shock typically presents as a hyperdynamic circulation with decreased systemic vascular resistance, high cardiac output and preserved ventricular function; central or mixed venous saturation is typically normal or elevated. A complete review of hemodynamic monitoring and fluid responsiveness is beyond the scope of this review.

Laboratory parameters typically reflect anion-gap metabolic acidosis with elevated lactic acid in these patients, often with respiratory alkalosis that may occur prior to development of metabolic acidosis. Mixed respiratory and metabolic acidosis or mixed anion-gap and non-gap acidosis warrant evaluation for alternate etiologies, such as AKI, ARDS, mesenteric ischemia and tumor lysis syndrome [33]. Rapid identification and correction of metabolic and electrolyte derangements, such as extreme acidosis (pH < 7.15), hypocalcemia, or hyperglycemia, is an important adjunct measure in restoring vascular tone.

Vasodilatory shock is often complicated by deranged hepatic metabolism and coagulopathy due to ischemic hepatitis and/or disseminated intravascular coagulation. Early evaluation for source of infection, timely source control and prompt initiation of antimicrobial therapy remain the cornerstones of sepsis management and have been shown to decrease mortality independent of other aspects of bundled sepsis care [5, 34].

Management

The management of vasodilatory shock requires timely fluid resuscitation and vasopressor therapy that form the cornerstone of therapy. Prompt recognition of reversible factors of refractory shock, such as metabolic and electrolyte derangements, source control for septic shock and lung-protective mechanical ventilation for respiratory failure are important therapeutic adjuncts. Use of invasive, non-invasive and minimally invasive devices for hemodynamic monitoring is recommended based on the clinical setting and individual patient variables [32]. Numerous methods for assessment of fluid-responsiveness are available to guide rational fluid resuscitation, and should be employed to avoid volume overload from excessive fluid administration [32]. Most patients requiring vasopressor therapy require invasive central venous and arterial catheters for safe administration and monitoring of therapy. A summary of the proposed treatment algorithm is presented in Fig. 2 [8].

Vasopressors

Pathologic vasodilation of arterioles impairs systemic perfusion pressure, while vasodilation within the venous circulation triggers mesenteric venous pooling reducing stressed blood volume. Initiation of vasopressors such as norepinephrine

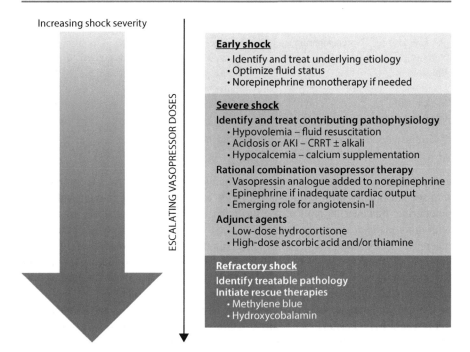

Increasing shock severity

ESCALATING VASOPRESSOR DOSES

Early shock
- Identify and treat underlying etiology
- Optimize fluid status
- Norepinephrine monotherapy if needed

Severe shock
Identify and treat contributing pathophysiology
- Hypovolemia – fluid resuscitation
- Acidosis or AKI – CRRT ± alkali
- Hypocalcemia – calcium supplementation

Rational combination vasopressor therapy
- Vasopressin analogue added to norepinephrine
- Epinephrine if inadequate cardiac output
- Emerging role for angiotensin-II

Adjunct agents
- Low-dose hydrocortisone
- High-dose ascorbic acid and/or thiamine

Refractory shock
Identify treatable pathology
Initiate rescue therapies
- Methylene blue
- Hydroxycobalamin

Fig. 2 Treatment algorithm for vasodilatory shock. *AKI*: acute kidney injury; *CRRT*: continuous renal replacement therapy. Adapted from [8] with permission

will restore arteriolar tone while facilitating venous return by reversing venous pooling and increasing stressed blood volume. This can facilitate the clinical response to fluid resuscitation, supporting early initiation of vasopressors in severe shock. Vasopressors are the mainstay of therapy for maintaining adequate MAP in shock to ensure adequate end-organ perfusion (Table 1; [5, 35]). Norepinephrine is the first line vasopressor in vasodilatory shock, including septic shock, and causes pure vasoconstriction via alpha-adrenergic receptors with modest cardiac beta-receptor agonism [5, 7, 35]. Current guidelines recommend and endorse the utility of norepinephrine as the primary pressor in septic vasodilatory shock (Grade 1C evidence) [5]. Dopamine was historically used based on the theory that its favorable renal hemodynamic effects could be reno-protective, but randomized clinical trials failed to demonstrate any beneficial effects of dopamine on renal or clinical outcomes [36]. On the contrary, dopamine is associated with increased risk of arrhythmias and mortality when used as a primary vasopressor in critically ill patients with sepsis or cardiogenic shock [7, 36]. The Sepsis Occurrence in Acutely Ill Patients (SOAP) study comparing dopamine versus norepinephrine as the initial vasopressor in unselected patients showed a trend to lower mortality with norepinephrine and an increased incidence of arrhythmias with dopamine [7]. Current guidelines recommend adding vasopressin or epinephrine as a second line agent to norepinephrine to allow for dose reduction, offset adverse effects and contribute to

Table 1 Hemodynamic effects and equipotent doses of vasoactive medications [6, 35]

Vasopressor	Norepinephrine equivalence	Receptor of action	CI	SVR	HR
Norepinephrine	1	$\alpha_1 > \beta_1 > \beta_2$	↑↓	↑↑	↑
Epinephrine	1	$\beta_1 > \alpha_1 > \beta_2$	↑↑	↑	↑↑
Dopamine	0.01	$\alpha_1 \approx \beta_1 > \beta_2$	↑	↑	↑↑
Vasopressin	5	$V_1 (\approx \alpha_1)$	↓	↑	↓↔
Phenylephrine	0.45	α_1	↓	↑	↓↔

CI: cardiac index; *HR*: heart rate; *SVR*: systemic vascular resistance

vasoconstriction via alternate receptor mechanisms [5]. Epinephrine, recommended as a second line agent in septic shock, has been considered equipotent with norepinephrine; however its clinical use has been in disfavor owing to its association with more lactic acidosis, tachycardia and arrhythmia compared to norepinephrine when used as a primary vasopressor [37]. Due to the potential toxicity of high-dose epinephrine, many experts prefer vasopressin for refractory vasodilatory shock with adequate or increased cardiac output. Epinephrine is preferred when the cardiac output is marginal or inadequate contributing to worsening hypotension.

Critically ill patients may develop a relative vasopressin deficiency contributing to persistent hypotension and impaired vasopressor response, leading to exploration of the use of physiologic vasopressin doses in septic shock [38]. In the Vasopressin and Septic Shock Trial, use of low-dose vasopressin (up to 0.03 units/min) did not reduce mortality significantly compared to norepinephrine when used as a norepinephrine-sparing vasopressor, although there may have been a reduced rate of AKI [39, 40]. The Vasopressin vs Norepinephrine as Initial Therapy in Septic Shock (VANISH) study tested the hypothesis that early initiation of vasopressin in septic shock would be beneficial when compared to norepinephrine, and also tested the hypothesis that there would be synergy between vasopressin and low-dose hydrocortisone [41]. However, no evidence of improved mortality was seen with either vasopressin or hydrocortisone, and the evidence of a renal-protective effect was conflicting. The 2016 Surviving Sepsis Campaign Guidelines suggest adding vasopressin (≤ 0.03 units/min) to norepinephrine to help achieve MAP target or decrease norepinephrine dosage [5]. Vasopressin analogs have been investigated as alternatives. Of these terlipressin is a long-acting, non-selective synthetic analogue that showed a catecholamine sparing effect in early pilot studies [42]. However, this came at the cost of decreased cardiac output, oxygen delivery and consumption. This agent continues to be used in most of Europe, and parts of Australia and New Zealand, but has not received United States Food and Drug Administration Agency approval. Meta-analyses have been conflicting about whether addition of vasopressin or terlipressin reduced mortality in septic shock when compared to catecholamines alone [43]. Selepressin, a selective V_1A analogue, promises an effect profile similar to vasopressin while reducing the non-selective effects such as fluid overload and microvascular thrombosis. While selepressin safety has been established in phase IIa trials, a phase IIb/IIIa trial was recently stopped for futility [44]. This agent is also unavailable in the United States currently. Phenylephrine is a pure alpha-1 adrenergic receptor agonist that causes vasoconstriction without any change to cardiac output. It can be safely administered at a lower concentration peripherally while awaiting central access for other vasopressors. The current Surviving Sepsis Campaign guidelines do not recommend the use of phenylephrine in septic shock except when norepinephrine is associated with severe arrhythmias or as salvage therapy when other vasopressors have failed [5].

Recent literature has shown angiotensin-II to be an effective vasopressor in patients with refractory shock [1, 45]. Recruitment of the RAAS pathway can decrease the requirement and tachyphylaxis from the use of catecholamine vasopressors [45]. The recent Angiotensin II for the Treatment of High-Output Shock 3 (ATHOS-3) trial demonstrated the efficacy and potency of human, synthetic stable angiotensin II with a significantly higher proportion of patients achieving the primary outcome of a target MAP of 75 mmHg or 10 mmHg greater than baseline compared with placebo in patients with catecholamine resistant hypotension [1]. There was a concomitant improvement in cardiovascular illness severity scores at 48 h. This phase 3 trial with > 300 patients did not demonstrate a significant mortality benefit in patients with refractory shock, although there was a trend to improved survival [1]. Importantly, overall adverse events were similar across groups underlining safety of the drug in question.

Inotropes

Inotropes have a limited role in vasodilatory shock and are reserved for patients with low cardiac output. The current guidelines do not recommend using inotropes in patients with adequate cardiac output [5]. Low doses of epinephrine, dopamine and dobutamine can be used to increase cardiac output in patients with myocardial dysfunction or cardiogenic shock under careful hemodynamic monitoring. All of these agents can produce significant toxicity related to excessive beta-adrenergic stimulation including tachycardia, arrhythmias and myocardial ischemia. These effects may be particularly harmful in patients with cardiogenic shock due to myocardial infarction.

With the vasopressor toolbox adding new tools as described above, an obvious message for the clinician at the bedside is clearly focused on the use of moderate doses of multiple vasopressors with complementary and synergistic mechanisms of action. This will help achieve and maintain a vital perfusion pressure and may avoid toxicity associated with high doses of a single agent. We advocate for earlier initiation of combination vasopressor therapy utilizing a rational combination to achieve best outcomes in severe vasodilatory shock.

Rescue Therapies

A complete discussion of rescue therapies and their mechanisms of action are beyond the scope of this review [31]. Glucocorticoids, calcium, vitamin C, hydoxycobalamin, sodium bicarbonate and renal replacement therapy (RRT) can all improve MAP in selected patients with refractory shock on high-dose vasopressors. Relative or functional adrenal insufficiency in critical illness is offset by the use of low dose hydrocortisone, which can decrease the dose and duration of vasopressors without a consistent effect on mortality [46]. Bicarbonate and non-bicarbonate based buffers have been used to correct severe acidemia and are recommended for pH < 7.15 despite lack of data demonstrating consistent clinical benefits [5]. However, the use of bicarbonate has to be balanced against the risks of intracellular acidosis and increased carbon dioxide production that can paradoxically worsen the acidosis. Currently, there is uncertainty amongst intensivists regarding the optimal timing of initiation of RRT; however more recent literature has favored early initiation, especially in post-surgical patients [47]. In an observational study of patients with septic shock, institution of a protocol combining hydrocortisone, high-dose vitamin C and thiamine was associated with improved shock reversal and decreased organ failure severity [48]. These results however need further verification in carefully designed prospective studies to evaluate the utility of vitamin C supplementation in septic shock.

Mechanical Circulatory Support

There are limited data on the use mechanical circulatory support in vasodilatory shock [49, 50]. Extracorporeal life support (ECLS) is primarily used for management of severe cardiopulmonary compromise, such as cardiogenic shock or ARDS, and is less hemodynamically effective in patients with vasodilatory shock and inadequate vascular tome. Despite careful patient selection, survival in septic shock patients with ECLS is ~ 20% and it offers uncertain benefit in patients with myocardial dysfunction [49]. The use of other percutaneous mechanical support is restricted to vasodilatory shock with a primary cardiac insult – cardiogenic shock, acute coronary syndrome and cardiac surgery. Because mechanical circulatory support devices function by augmenting cardiac output, they are only expected to be effective for improving hypotension in patients with low cardiac output; efficacy for improving MAP will be limited in vasoplegic patients.

Conclusions

In conclusion, vasodilatory shock remains a significant challenge in the ICU. Prompt assessment and diagnosis of vasodilatory shock is associated with improved clinical outcomes. Hypotension, even transiently, is associated with significant cardiac, renal and neurological injury and dysfunction that is associated with worse short and long-term outcomes. Fluid, vasopressors and antimicrobials form the cornerstone of therapy for this population. Careful selection of vasopressors and inotropes and the use of moderate doses of combination vasoactive medications appear to confer the most benefit while decreasing adverse effects. There are limited data for adjunct and rescue therapies in patients with pure vasodilatory shock.

References

1. Khanna A, English SW, Wang XS et al (2017) Angiotensin II for the treatment of vasodilatory shock. N Engl J Med 377:419–430
2. Vincent J-L, De Backer D (2013) Circulatory shock. N Engl J Med 369:1726–1734
3. Walsh M, Devereaux PJ, Garg AX et al (2013) Relationship between intraoperative mean arterial pressure and clinical outcomes after noncardiac surgery: toward an empirical definition of hypotension. Anesthesiology 119:507–515
4. Asfar P, Meziani F, Hamel JF et al (2014) High versus low blood-pressure target in patients with septic shock. N Engl J Med 370:1583–1593
5. Rhodes A, Evans LE, Alhazzani W et al (2017) Surviving Sepsis Campaign: international guidelines for management of sepsis and septic shock: 2016. Intensive Care Med 43:304–377
6. Brown SM, Lanspa MJ, Jones JP et al (2013) Survival after shock requiring high-dose vasopressor therapy. Chest 143:664–671
7. De Backer D, Biston P, Devriendt J et al (2010) Comparison of dopamine and norepinephrine in the treatment of shock. N Engl J Med 362:779–789
8. Jentzer JC, Vallabhajosyula S, Khanna AK, Chawla LS, Busse LW, Kashani KB (2018) Management of refractory vasodilatory shock. Chest. https://doi.org/10.1016/j.chest.2017.12.021 (Jan 9, Epub ahead of print)
9. Mekontso-Dessap A, Houel R, Soustelle C, Kirsch M, Thebert D, Loisance DY (2001) Risk factors for post-cardiopulmonary bypass vasoplegia in patients with preserved left ventricular function. Ann Thorac Surg 71:1428–1432
10. Algarni KD, Maganti M, Yau TM (2011) Predictors of low cardiac output syndrome after isolated coronary artery bypass surgery: trends over 20 years. Ann Thorac Surg 92:1678–1684
11. Kotecha A, Vallabhajosyula S, Coville HH, Kashani K (2017) Cardiorenal syndrome in sepsis: a narrative review. J Crit Care 43:122–127
12. Vallabhajosyula S, Jentzer JC, Geske JB et al (2017) New-onset heart failure and mortality in hospital survivors of sepsis-related left ventricular dysfunction. Shock. https://doi.org/10.1097/SHK.0000000000000952 (Jul 19, Epub ahead of print)
13. Champion S, Belcour D, Vandroux D et al (2015) Stress (Tako-tsubo) cardiomyopathy in critically-ill patients. Eur Heart J Acute Cardiovasc Care 4:189–196
14. Landesberg G, Jaffe AS, Gilon D et al (2014) Troponin elevation in severe sepsis and septic shock: the role of left ventricular diastolic dysfunction and right ventricular dilatation. Crit Care Med 42:790–800
15. Leone M, Asfar P, Radermacher P, Vincent J-L, Martin C (2015) Optimizing mean arterial pressure in septic shock: a critical reappraisal of the literature. Crit Care 19:101
16. Beesley SJ, Wilson EL, Lanspa MJ et al (2017) Relative bradycardia in patients with septic shock requiring vasopressor therapy. Crit Care Med 45:225–233
17. Morelli A, Ertmer C, Westphal M et al (2013) Effect of heart rate control with esmolol on hemodynamic and clinical outcomes in patients with septic shock: a randomized clinical trial. JAMA 310:1683–1691
18. Hamzaoui O, Georger JF, Monnet X et al (2010) Early administration of norepinephrine increases cardiac preload and cardiac output in septic patients with life-threatening hypotension. Crit Care 14:R142
19. Boissier F, Razazi K, Seemann A et al (2017) Left ventricular systolic dysfunction during septic shock: the role of loading conditions. Intensive Care Med 43:633–642
20. Kress JP (2010) The complex interplay between delirium, sepsis and sedation. Crit Care 14:164
21. Khanna A, Mao G, Liu L et al (2018) Hypotension increases acute kidney injury, myocardial injury and mortality in surgical critical care. Crit Care Med 46:71 (abst)
22. Mascha EJ, Yang D, Weiss S, Sessler DI (2015) Intraoperative mean arterial pressure variability and 30-day mortality in patients having noncardiac surgery. Anesthesiology 123:79–91

23. Salmasi V, Maheshwari K, Yang D et al (2017) Relationship between intraoperative hypotension, defined by either reduction from baseline or absolute thresholds, and acute kidney and myocardial injury after noncardiac surgery: a retrospective cohort analysis. Anesthesiology 126:47–65

24. Sessler DI, Meyhoff CS, Zimmerman NM et al (2017) Period-dependent associations between hypotension during and for 4 days after noncardiac surgery and a composite of myocardial infarction and death: A sub-study of the POISE-2 trial. Anesthesiology https://doi.org/10.1097/ALN.0000000000001985 (Nov 21, Epub ahead of print)

25. Janssen van Doorn K, Verbrugghe W, Wouters K, Jansens H, Jorens PG (2014) The duration of hypotension determines the evolution of bacteremia-induced acute kidney injury in the intensive care unit. PLoS One 9:e114312

26. Houwink AP, Rijkenberg S, Bosman RJ, van der Voort PH (2016) The association between lactate, mean arterial pressure, central venous oxygen saturation and peripheral temperature and mortality in severe sepsis: a retrospective cohort analysis. Crit Care 20:56

27. Langenberg C, Wan L, Egi M, May CN, Bellomo R (2006) Renal blood flow in experimental septic acute renal failure. Kidney Int 69:1996–2002

28. Wan L, Bagshaw SM, Langenberg C, Saotome T, May C, Bellomo R (2008) Pathophysiology of septic acute kidney injury: what do we really know? Crit Care Med 36(4 Suppl):S198–S203

29. Donnelly J, Budohoski KP, Smielewski P, Czosnyka M (2016) Regulation of the cerebral circulation: bedside assessment and clinical implications. Crit Care 20:129

30. Singh TD, O'Horo JC, Gajic O et al (2017) Risk factors and outcomes of critically ill patients with acute brain failure: a novel end point. J Crit Care 43:42–47

31. Bassi E, Park M, Azevedo LC (2013) Therapeutic strategies for high-dose vasopressor-dependent shock. Crit Care Res Pract 2013:654708

32. Cecconi M, De Backer D, Antonelli M et al (2014) Consensus on circulatory shock and hemodynamic monitoring. Task force of the European Society of Intensive Care Medicine. Intensive Care Med 40:1795–1815

33. Kimmoun A, Novy E, Auchet T, Ducrocq N, Levy B (2015) Hemodynamic consequences of severe lactic acidosis in shock states: from bench to bedside. Crit Care 19:175

34. Seymour CW, Gesten F, Prescott HC et al (2017) Time to treatment and mortality during mandated emergency care for sepsis. N Engl J Med 376:2235–2244

35. Jentzer JC, Coons JC, Link CB, Schmidhofer M (2015) Pharmacotherapy update on the use of vasopressors and inotropes in the intensive care unit. J Cardiovasc Pharmacol Ther 20:249–260

36. De Backer D, Aldecoa C, Njimi H, Vincent J-L (2012) Dopamine versus norepinephrine in the treatment of septic shock: a meta-analysis. Crit Care Med 40:725–730

37. Levy B, Perez P, Perny J, Thivilier C, Gerard A (2011) Comparison of norepinephrine-dobutamine to epinephrine for hemodynamics, lactate metabolism, and organ function variables in cardiogenic shock. A prospective, randomized pilot study. Crit Care Med 39:450–455

38. Russell JA (2011) Bench-to-bedside review: vasopressin in the management of septic shock. Crit Care 15:226

39. Russell JA, Walley KR, Singer J et al (2008) Vasopressin versus norepinephrine infusion in patients with septic shock. N Engl J Med 358:877–887

40. Gordon AC, Russell JA, Walley KR et al (2010) The effects of vasopressin on acute kidney injury in septic shock. Intensive Care Med 36:83–91

41. Gordon AC, Mason AJ, Thirunavukkarasu N et al (2016) Effect of early vasopressin vs norepinephrine on kidney failure in patients with septic shock: The VANISH randomized clinical trial. JAMA 316:509–518

42. Leone M, Albanese J, Delmas A, Chaabane W, Garnier F, Martin C (2004) Terlipressin in catecholamine-resistant septic shock patients. Shock 22:314–319

43. Avni T, Lador A, Lev S, Leibovici L, Paul M, Grossman A (2015) Vasopressors for the treatment of septic shock: systematic review and meta-analysis. PLoS One 10:e129305

44. Russell JA, Vincent J-L, Kjolbye AL et al (2017) Selepressin, a novel selective vasopressin V1A agonist, is an effective substitute for norepinephrine in a phase IIa randomized, placebo-controlled trial in septic shock patients. Crit Care 21:213
45. Chawla LS, Busse L, Brasha-Mitchell E et al (2014) Intravenous angiotensin II for the treatment of high-output shock (ATHOS trial): a pilot study. Crit Care 18:534
46. Annane D, Sebille V, Charpentier C et al (2002) Effect of treatment with low doses of hydrocortisone and fludrocortisone on mortality in patients with septic shock. JAMA 288:862–871
47. Park JY, An JN, Jhee JH et al (2016) Early initiation of continuous renal replacement therapy improves survival of elderly patients with acute kidney injury: a multicenter prospective cohort study. Crit Care 20:260
48. Marik PE, Khangoora V, Rivera R, Hooper MH, Catravas J (2017) Hydrocortisone, vitamin C, and thiamine for the treatment of severe sepsis and septic shock: a retrospective before-after study. Chest 151:1229–1238
49. Park TK, Yang JH, Jeon K et al (2015) Extracorporeal membrane oxygenation for refractory septic shock in adults. Eur J Cardiothorac Surg 47:e68–e74
50. Cheng A, Sun HY, Lee CW et al (2013) Survival of septic adults compared with non-septic adults receiving extracorporeal membrane oxygenation for cardiopulmonary failure: a propensity-matched analysis. J Crit Care 28:532.e1–532.e10

Angiotensin in Critical Care

A. Hall, L. W. Busse, and M. Ostermann

Introduction

Hypotension is a key feature of shock and strongly correlated with the development of multisystem organ failure. Multiple studies have highlighted that even short durations of hypotension are harmful [1, 2]. In a retrospective analysis of 33,000 non-cardiac surgical patients, Walsh et al. showed that short periods of intraoperative hypotension were associated with a significant increase in the risk of acute kidney injury (AKI), myocardial injury or cardiac complications and mortality [1]. The risk of renal and cardiac injury increased with duration of hypotension and was significant for periods as short as 1–5 min. Similarly, using data from over 57,000 patients undergoing non-cardiac surgery, Salmasi et al. showed that patients with a mean arterial pressure (MAP) less than 65 mmHg during the intraoperative period had a significantly higher risk of myocardial injury and AKI, confirming that hypotension does not need to be severe to affect organ function [2]. On the basis of these and other studies, European and international guidelines for the treatment of shock recommend that a minimum MAP should be maintained at all times and that the target should be at least 65 mmHg [3, 4]. Heretofore, the restoration and maintenance of MAP has been accomplished through the judicious use of fluids as well as vasopressors, namely catecholamines and vasopressin analogs. However, patients with sepsis in particular often show marked hyporeactivity to traditionally administered

A. Hall
Department of Critical Care, Guy's & St Thomas' NHS Foundation Hospital
London, UK

L. W. Busse
Emory University School of Medicine, Department of Medicine, Emory Saint Joseph's Hospital
Atlanta, GA, USA

M. Ostermann (✉)
Department of Critical Care, King's College London, Guy's & St Thomas' NHS Foundation Hospital
London, UK
e-mail: Marlies.Ostermann@gstt.nhs.uk

© Springer International Publishing AG 2018   113
J.-L. Vincent (ed.), *Annual Update in Intensive Care and Emergency Medicine 2018*,
Annual Update in Intensive Care and Emergency Medicine,
https://doi.org/10.1007/978-3-319-73670-9_10

therapies. To date, no vasopressor has consistently been proven to be superior to the others in terms of clinical outcomes [5–7]. In 2015, a meta-analysis concluded that in terms of survival, with the exception of noted superiority of norepinephrine over dobutamine, there was insufficient evidence to recommend any vasopressor agent or combination over another [8].

Angiotensin II (Ang II) has emerged as an effective therapy to raise blood pressure in patients with vasodilatory shock [9]. The first reports of Ang II administration in patients with shock date back 50 years, but interest was re-ignited following several small studies and a recent larger randomized controlled trial (RCT) confirming that Ang II was effective at maintaining MAP at target and reducing norepinephrine requirements without an increase in adverse effects [9–11]. The following review provides an overview of the physiological effects of angiotensin and summarizes existing data in the literature.

Role of Renin-Angiotensin System

After the discovery of renin in 1898, angiotensinogen and angiotensin-converting enzyme (ACE) were later identified as additional key components of the classical circulating renin-angiotensin system (RAS) [12, 13]. Angiotensinogen, the precursor of angiotensin, is an α-glycoprotein produced primarily by the liver and released into the systemic circulation where it is converted to angiotensin I (Ang I) under activity by renin (Fig. 1). Ang I is cleaved into Ang II, predominantly by endothelial-bound ACE in the lungs but also in plasma and the vascular bed of kidneys, heart and brain, and to some extent by chymases stored in secretory granules in mast cells [13, 14].

Renin is an enzyme produced by pericytes in the vicinity of the afferent arterioles and cells of the juxtaglomerular apparatus. It is stored in intracellular vesicles and rapidly secreted in response to three stimuli: a decrease in blood pressure as detected by baropressors, a decrease in the sodium concentration delivered to the distal tubules, and activation of the sympathetic nervous system (through β_1 adrenergic receptors). Renin itself has no peripheral receptors and no direct hemodynamic effects [14].

Ang II, an octapeptide, has strong vasopressor properties but its action is terminated by rapid degradation to angiotensin III by angiotensinases located in red blood cells and the vascular beds of most tissues. Ang II is also hydrolized into Ang (1–7) through the actions of ACE 2. It has a half-life in circulation of around 30 s, whereas, in tissue, this may be as long as 15–30 min [15].

In addition to the 'classic' systemic RAS, which regulates blood pressure, fluid and electrolyte homeostasis and preserves volume status and vascular tone, most organs contain a tissue RAS and an intracellular RAS. The tissue RAS is predominantly involved in local cardiovascular regulation and inflammatory processes, including vascular permeability, apoptosis, cellular growth, migration and cell differentiation, and the intracellular RAS participates in intracellular signaling pathways [16].

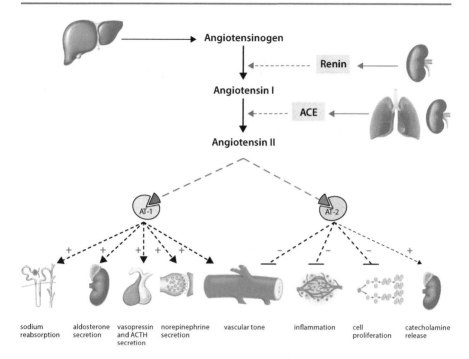

sodium   aldosterone   vasopressin   norepinephrine   vascular tone   inflammation   cell   catecholamine
reabsorption   secretion   and ACTH   secretion   proliferation   release
                              secretion

Fig. 1 The renin-angiotensin system. *ACE*: angiotensin-converting enzyme; *ACTH*: adrenocorti-cotropin hormone; *AT*: angiotensin receptor

Physiologic Effects of Angiotensin II

Ang II exerts its effects by binding to specific angiotensin (AT) receptors based on the cell membrane of various cell types: AT-1, AT-2, AT-4 and Mas receptors. In humans, the major physiological effects are mediated by AT-1 receptors located in the kidneys, vascular smooth muscle, lung, heart, brain, adrenals, pituitary gland and liver, and relate to maintenance of hemodynamic stability and fluid and electrolyte regulation ([14, 16]; Fig. 1 and Table 1).

In the healthy adult, the AT-2 receptor is expressed in certain cell types and tissues, such as vascular endothelial cells, distinct areas of the brain, adrenal glands, myometrium and ovaries and selected cutaneous, renal and cardiac structures [17, 18]. Although their expression level is often much lower than that of AT-1 receptors, AT-2 receptors have an important role in injury and repair mechanisms and, under conditions such as mechanical injury or ischemia, expression may be increased. There is also good evidence that AT-2 receptors are involved in the regulation of Ang II mediated adrenal catecholamine secretion, for example during sepsis [18]. The main biological effects of the AT-2 receptor are often opposite to the AT-1 receptors with focus on anti-proliferation, vasodilation and anti-inflammation. Stimulation of AT-2 receptors confers protection against an overstimulation of AT-1 receptors: for example, vasoconstriction mediated by the AT-1 receptors can

Table 1 Main physiological effects of angiotensin (Ang) II

Organ system	Physiological effects
Vascular	Vasoconstriction of venous and arterial vessels Increased vascular permeability by inducing VEGF
Renal	Stimulation of Na reabsorption and H^+ excretion in the proximal tubule via the Na/H^+ exchanger Stimulation of the release of aldosterone, which stimulates the distal tubule and collecting ducts of the kidneys to re-absorb sodium and water Variable effects on glomerular filtration and renal blood flow depending on the physiological and pharmacological setting: i) Constriction of the afferent and efferent glomerular arterioles; although this will tend to restrict renal blood flow, the effect on the efferent arteriole is markedly greater, and as a result, this tends to increase or maintain GFR ii) Constriction of the glomerular mesangium, thereby reducing the area for glomerular filtration iii) Enhanced sensitivity to tubuloglomerular feedback and thereby prevention of excessive rise in GFR iv) Stimulation of local release of prostaglandins, which oppose the effect of Ang II and antagonize renal vasoconstriction
Endocrine	Stimulation of the secretion of vasopressin from the posterior pituitary gland Secretion of ACTH in the anterior pituitary gland Enhancement of release of norepinephrine by direct action on postganglionic sympathetic fibers
Nervous	Enhancement of norepinephrine secretion
Cardiac	Mediation of cardiac remodeling through activated tissue RAS in cardiac myocytes
Coagulation	Prothrombotic potential through adhesion and aggregation of platelets and stimulation of PAI-1 and PAI-2
Immune	Promotion of cell growth and inflammation Increased expression of endothelium-derived adhesion molecules Synthesis of pro-inflammatory cytokines and chemokines Generation of reactive oxygen species

ACTH: adrenocorticotropin hormone; *GFR*: glomerular filtration rate; *RAS*: renin-angiotensin system; *PAI*: plasminogen activator inhibitor; *VEGF*: vascular endothelial growth factor

be opposed by the vasodilatory effects of Ang II linked to the AT-2 receptor ([19]; Fig. 1). AT-2 receptors also play a role in pressure natriuresis, opposing the anti-natriuretic effects of AT-1 receptor activation, and in cardiovascular remodeling following myocardial infarction and hypertension, heart failure and stroke. Finally, in the fetus and neonate, AT-2 receptors are involved in fetal tissue development, neuronal regeneration and cellular differentiation.

The AT-4 receptor is activated by the Ang II metabolite Ang IV, and appears to contribute to the regulation of the extracellular matrix in the central nervous system, as well as modulation of oxytocin release.

Sepsis-Induced Dysregulation of the Renin-Angiotensin System

The natural role of the RAS is to preserve volume status and arterial blood pressure, thereby maintaining the systemic circulation and also the microcirculation. In sepsis, both over- and under-stimulation of the RAS have been reported in patients [20–25]. The capacity of ACE and the functionality of angiotensin receptors are key factors that determine whether hemodynamic stability can be achieved and maintained.

ACE is an ectoenzyme that is distributed primarily on the pulmonary capillary endothelium but can also be found in endothelial and renal epithelial cells. ACE molecules are uniformly distributed along the luminal pulmonary endothelial surface including the membrane caveolae [26]. As a result, ACE is directly accessible to blood-borne substrates and able to convert Ang I to Ang II rapidly, but also very susceptible to disease processes that affect the pulmonary vasculature [27].

Effects of Sepsis on Ang II Levels

During sepsis, renin, Ang I and Ang II are usually activated. However, variable and even low plasma levels of Ang II have been reported [20, 21]. The reasons are multifactorial. Pre-morbid treatment with an ACE-inhibitor will prevent conversion of Ang I to Ang II. There is also evidence that endotoxin associated with Gram-negative sepsis has potential to deactivate ACE [22]. Additionally, in diseases that affect the pulmonary capillary endothelium, such as acute respiratory distress syndrome (ARDS) and pneumonia, ACE activity is altered at an early stage, resulting in reduced capacity to convert Ang I to Ang II [23, 28–30].

Low levels of Ang II and ACE have clinical implications. Zhang et al. measured serial Ang II and ACE concentrations in 58 patients with severe sepsis and showed that the cohort with low levels exhibited more complications and had a greater risk of dying [20].

Sepsis-Induced Downregulation of Ang II Receptors

Ang II is antagonized by the endogenous vasodilator, nitric oxide (NO), and each has a role in influencing the production and functioning of the other. Several studies have shown that sepsis is associated with downregulation of AT-1 receptors, likely mediated by pro-inflammatory cytokines and NO [31, 32]. In addition, reduced activity of the AT-1 receptor associated protein 1 (Arap 1) has been reported [33]. The physiological role of Arap 1 is to support the trafficking of the AT-1 receptor to the cell membrane. As such, reduced activity of Arap 1 is associated with decreased sensitivity of the AT-1 receptor.

Downregulation of AT-2 receptors may also occur during septic shock [18]. The consequences of this process are reduced catecholamine release by the adrenal medulla and attenuation of the responsiveness of blood pressure and aldosterone formation.

Clinical Studies with Angiotensin

Ang II was discovered in the 1930s and has been used in clinical studies since the early 1960s. To date, over 31,000 subjects have been exposed to Ang II either as monotherapy or in combination with catecholamines and non-catecholamine vasopressors in various clinical settings [34].

Prevention of Hypotension During Obstetric Anesthesia

Hypotension is a frequently occurring adverse effect during spinal anesthesia. In the obstetric population where utero-placentary blood flow depends directly on maternal blood pressure and where moderate maternal hypotension is associated with fetal hypoxemia and neurological morbidity, every attempt is made to prevent hypotension [35]. Phenylephrine and ephedrine are often used in clinical practice. Ephedrine was the vasoconstrictor agent of choice in obstetric anesthesia for many years because of its marked increase in utero-placentary blood flow [36]. However, it has fallen out of favor because of its association with lower umbilical artery pH values, likely due to increased fetal metabolic activity [37].

Phenylephrine is a synthetic sympathicomimetic agent that is regarded to be safe in the treatment of regional anesthesia-induced maternal hypotension [35].

Ang II has been shown to cause less vasoconstriction of the utero-placental vascular bed compared with uterine or other systemic vessels [38, 39]. In 1994, Ramin et al. randomized 30 healthy pregnant women undergoing elective Cesarean section either to a control group or prophylactic Ang II infusion versus prophylactic ephedrine infusion in order to maintain a diastolic blood pressure 0–10 mmHg above the baseline [40]. In women randomized to Ang II infusion, the maternal Ang II levels were increased nearly fourfold but Ang II levels in the umbilical artery and vein were unchanged. Of note, no one in the Ang II cohort had a recorded umbilical artery blood pH < 7.20 in contrast to 40% of the ephedrine group. Vincent et al. reported similar results in 54 women randomized to Ang II versus ephedrine during spinal anesthesia for elective Cesarean delivery [41]. The umbilical arterial and venous pH and base excess were higher in the angiotensin group compared to women who had received ephedrine, and maternal heart rate was higher in the ephedrine group. The authors concluded that Ang II maintained systolic blood pressure during anesthesia without causing fetal acidosis or increasing maternal heart rate.

Treatment of Hypotension Following ACE Inhibitor Overdose

ACE-inhibitor overdose may result in severe refractory hypotension. Several case reports have highlighted successful treatment with Ang II [42–44]. Although in all cases, Ang II was administered in combination with other therapies, including gut decontamination, intravenous fluids, vasopressors and naloxone, there was a profound effect on blood pressure immediately after starting Ang II infusion. Physiologically, it is logical to regard Ang II as a rational treatment for ACE-inhibitor induced hypotension.

Treatment of Vasodilatory Shock

The most immediate and critical need of patients with vasodilatory shock is the achievement of hemodynamic stability to prevent multiorgan dysfunction whilst allowing time to treat the underlying etiology. Multiple vasopressors and catecholamines are often needed [45]. Studies using Ang II as a vasopressor for management of shock were originally conducted in the 1960s. Ang II was compared to catecholamines in non-randomized designs and was shown to have comparable effects to norepinephrine [46, 47].

In the first RCT, Chawla et al. reported a catecholamine-sparing effect in patients with high output shock treated with Ang II administration [10]. The subsequent Angiotensin for the Treatment of High Output Shock (ATHOS)-3 trial was a phase 3, placebo-controlled, double-blind, multicenter RCT including 321 patients with refractory vasodilatory shock who were randomized to Ang II infusion or placebo [9]. Analysis of the primary efficacy endpoint (defined as the percentage of patients achieving the pre-specified target blood pressure response) was statistically significant ($p < 0.0001$). Twenty-three percent of the 158 placebo-treated patients had a desired blood pressure response compared to 70% of the 163 patients treated with Ang II. Treatment with Ang II also resulted in a significant decrease in the standard of care vasopressor use, as measured by a change in the cardiovascular Sequential Organ Failure Assessment (SOFA) score at 48 h (-1.75 versus -1.28, $p = 0.01$). No difference in mortality was noted but there were fewer adverse events with Ang II. In a recent systematic review including data from $> 31,000$ patients, Busse et al. also confirmed that Ang II was safe to be used in humans [34].

Conclusion

The RAS plays a key role in maintaining hemodynamic stability, vascular tone and electrolyte homeostasis. Studies suggest that its physiological regulation is disturbed in sepsis and critical illness, which results in altered ACE functionality, reduced generation of Ang II and downregulation of Ang II receptors. Recent RCTs stipulate that Ang II is an effective and safe treatment for hypotension in patients with refractory vasodilatory shock, allowing for sparing of catecholamines. It may also have a role in cardiogenic, distributive and unclassified shock [48].

Innate to the human body are three molecules (catecholamines, vasopressin and angiotensin) that maintain and regulate BP. The addition of Ang II as a potential tool in the armamentarium against shock offers clinicians the opportunity to provide a 'balanced' approach to vasopressor therapy. The combination of different vasoactive drugs that mimic the natural response to severe vasodilatation and hypotension makes physiological sense [49]. With this approach, the likelihood of hemodynamic recovery is enhanced and toxicity from large doses of monotherapy can be minimized.

References

1. Walsh M, Devereaux PJ, Garg AX et al (2013) Relationship between intraoperative mean arterial pressure and clinical outcomes after noncardiac surgery: toward an empirical definition of hypotension. Anesthesiology 119:507–515
2. Salmasi V, Maheshwari K, Yang D et al (2017) Relationship between intraoperative hypotension, defined by either reduction from baseline or absolute thresholds, and acute kidney and myocardial injury after noncardiac surgery. Anesthesiology 126:47–65
3. Cecconi M, De Backer D, Antonelli M et al (2014) Consensus on circulatory shock and hemodynamic monitoring. Task force of the European Society of Intensive Care Medicine. Intensive Care Med 40:1795–1815
4. Rhodes A, Evans LE, Alhazzani W et al (2017) Surviving sepsis campaign: international guidelines for management of sepsis and septic shock: 2016. Intensive Care Med 43:304–377
5. Sakr Y, Reinhart K, Vincent J-L et al (2006) Does dopamine administration in shock influence outcome? Results of the Sepsis Occurrence in Acutely Ill Patients (SOAP) Study. Crit Care Med 34:589–597
6. Myburgh JA, Higgins A, Jovanovska A et al (2008) A comparison of epinephrine and norepinephrine in critically ill patients. Intensive Care Med 34:2226–2234
7. Russell JA, Walley KR, Singer J et al (2008) Vasopressin versus norepinephrine infusion in patients with septic shock. N Engl J Med 358:877–887
8. Zhou F, Mao Z, Zeng X et al (2015) Vasopressors in septic shock: a systematic review and network meta-analysis. Ther Clin Risk Manag 11:1047–1059
9. Khanna A, English SW, Wang XS et al (2017) Angiotensin II for the treatment of vasodilatory shock. N Engl J Med 377:419–430
10. Chawla LS, Busse L, Brasha-Mitchell E et al (2014) Intravenous angiotensin II for the treatment of high-output shock (ATHOS trial): a pilot study. Crit Care 18:534
11. Correa TD, Takala J, Jakob SM (2015) Angiotensin II in septic shock. Crit Care 19:98
12. Tigerstedt R, Bergman P (1898) Niere und Kreislauf. Scand Arch Physiol 8:223–271
13. Correa TD, Takala J, Jakob S (2015) Angiotensin II in septic shock. Crit Care 19:98
14. Paul M, Mehr A, Kreutz R (2006) Physiology of local renin-angiotensin systems. Physiol Rev 86:747–803
15. Kopf P, Campbell W (2013) Endothelial metabolism of angiotensin II to angiotensin III, not angiotensin (1–7), augments the vasorelaxation response in adrenal cortical arteries. Endocrinology 154:4768–4776
16. Fyhrquist F, Saijonmaa O (2008) Renin-angiotensin system revisited. J Intern Med 264:224–236
17. Steckelings UM, Kaschina E, Unger T (2005) The AT2 receptor – a matter of love and hate. Peptides 26:1401–1419
18. Bucher M, Hobbhahn J, Kurtz A (2001) Nitric oxide-dependent down-regulation of angiotensin II type 2 receptors during experimental sepsis. Crit Care Med 29:1750–1755
19. Carey RM, Wang ZQ, Siragy HM (2000) Role of the angiotensin type 2 receptor in the regulation of blood pressure and renal function. Hypertension 35:155–163
20. Zhang W, Chen X, Huang L et al (2014) Severe sepsis: Low expression of the renin-angiotensin system is associated with poor prognosis. Exp Ther Med 7:1342–1348
21. Dong LW, Chang YZ, Tong LJ, Tang J, Su JY, Tang CS (1994) Role of regulatory peptide in pathogenesis of shock. Sci China B 37:162–169

22. Dunn CW, Horton JW (1993) Role of angiotensin II in neonatal sepsis. Circ Shock 40:144–150

23. Chawla LS, Busse LW, Brasha-Mitchell E, Alotaibi Z (2016) The use of angiotensin II in distributive shock. Crit Care 20:13

24. Wray GM, Coakley JH (1995) Severe septic shock unresponsive to noradrenaline. Lancet 346:1604

25. Salgado DR, Rocco JR, Silva E, Vincent J-L (2010) Modulation of the renin-angiotensin-aldosterone system in sepsis: a new therapeutic approach? Expert Opin Ther Targets 14:11–20

26. Orfanos SE, Langleben D, Khoury J et al (1999) Pulmonary capillary endothelium-bound angiotensin-converting enzyme activity in humans. Circulation 99:1593–1599

27. Orfanos SE, Armaganidis A, Glynos C et al (2000) Pulmonary capillary endothelium-bound angiotensin-converting enzyme activity in acute lung injury. Circulation 102:2011–2018

28. Casey L, Krieger B, Kohler J, Rice C, Oparil S, Szidon P (1981) Decreased serum angiotensin converting enzyme in adult respiratory distress syndrome associated with sepsis: a preliminary report. Crit Care Med 9:651–654

29. Johnson AR, Coalson JJ, Ashton J, Larumbide M, Erdös EG (1985) Neutral endopeptidase in serum samples from patients with adult respiratory distress syndrome. Comparison with angiotensin-converting enzyme. Am Rev Respir Dis 132:1262–1267

30. Kuba K, Imai Y, Penninger JM (2006) Angiotensin-converting enzyme 2 in lung disease. Curr Opin Pharmacol 6:271–276

31. Bucher M, Ittner KP, Hobbhahn J, Taeger K, Kurtz A (2001) Downregulation of angiotensin II type 1 receptors during sepsis. Hypertension 38:177–182

32. Schmidt C, Höcherl K, Kurt B, Moritz S, Kurtz A, Bucher M (2010) Blockade of multiple but not single cytokines abrogates downregulation of angiotensin II type-I receptors and anticipates septic shock. Cytokine 49:30–38

33. Mederle K, Schweda F, Kattler V et al (2013) The angiotensin II AT1 receptor-associated protein Arap1 is involved in sepsis-induced hypotension. Crit Care 17:R130

34. Busse LW, Wang XS, Chalikonda DM et al (2017) Clinical experience with IV angiotensin ii administration: a systematic review of safety. Crit Care Med 45:1285–1294

35. Chooi C, Cox JJ, Lumb RS et al (2017) Techniques for preventing hypotension during spinal anaesthesia for caesarean section. Cochrane Database Sys Rev CD002251

36. McGrath J, Chestnut D, Vincent R et al (1994) Ephedrine remains the vasopressor of choice for treatment of hypotension during ritodrine infusion and epidural anesthesia. Anesthesiology 80:1073–1081

37. Shearer VE, Ramin SM, Wallace DH, Dax JS, Gilstrap LC 3rd (1996) Fetal effects of prophylactic ephedrine and maternal hypotension during regional anesthesia for cesarean section. J Matern Fetal Med 5:79–84

38. Naden RP, Rosenfeld CR (1981) Effect of angiotensin II on uterine and systemic vasculature in pregnant sheep. J Clin Invest 68:468–474

39. Rosenfeld CR, Naden RP (1989) Uterine and nonuterine vascular responses to angiotensin II in ovine pregnancy. Am J Physiol 257:H17–H24

40. Ramin SM, Ramin KD, Cox K, Magness RR, Shearer VE, Gant NF (1994) Comparison of prophylactic angiotensin II versus ephedrine infusion for prevention of maternal hypotension during spinal anesthesia. Am J Obstet Gynecol 171:734–739

41. Vincent RD Jr, Werhan CF, Norman PF et al (1998) Prophylactic angiotensin II infusion during spinal anesthesia for elective cesarean delivery. Anesthesiology 88:1475–1479

42. Jackson T, Corke C, Agar J (1993) Enalapril overdose treated with angiotensin infusion. Lancet 341:703

43. Newby DE, Lee MR, Gray AJ, Boon NA (1995) Enalapril overdose and the corrective effect of intravenous angiotensin II. Br J Clin Pharmacol 40:103–104

44. Trilli LE, Johnson KA (1994) Lisinopril overdose and management with intravenous angiotensin II. Ann Pharmacother 28:1165–1167

45. Brand DA, Patrick PA, Berger JT et al (2017) Intensity of vasopressor therapy for septic shock and the risk of in-hospital death. J Pain Symptom Manag 53:938–943

46. John JN, Luria MH (1965) Studies in clinical shock and hypotension. II. Hemodynamic effects of norepinephrine and angiotensin. J Clin Invest 44:1494–1504

47. Belle MS, Jaffee RJ (1965) The use of large doses of angiotensin in acute myocardial infarction with shock. J Lancet 85:193–194

48. Busse LW, McCurdy MT, Osman A, Hall A, Chen H, Ostermann M (2017) The effect of angiotensin II on blood pressure in patients with circulatory shock: a structured review of the literature. Crit Care 21:34

49. Bellomo R, Hilton A (2017) The ATHOS-3 trial, angiotensin II and The Three Musketeers. Crit Care Resusc 19:3–4

Part IV
Cardiovascular Resuscitation

Making Sense of Early High-dose Intravenous Vitamin C in Ischemia/Reperfusion Injury

A. M. E. Spoelstra-de Man, P. W. G. Elbers, and H. M. Oudemans-van Straaten

Introduction

In Europe, each day over 1,000 patients have a cardiac arrest [1]. Only half of these patients arrive at the hospital alive. Of these survivors, 50% will still die or remain severely disabled due to the post-cardiac arrest syndrome [2]. Apart from targeted temperature management, there is no effective therapy to improve prognosis. Crucial to the post-cardiac arrest syndrome is the overwhelming oxidative stress caused by systemic ischemia/reperfusion injury and leading to endothelial dysfunction with cardiovascular failure, brain damage and death. These effects provide a strong rationale for targeting this overwhelming oxidative stress with antioxidant therapy.

Recently, early high-dose intravenous (i. v.) vitamin C for the treatment of sepsis has attracted a lot of attention in the critical care community as well as in the lay press. The potential benefit of vitamin C, the main circulating antioxidant, has indeed recently been shown in this population. High-dose i. v. vitamin C was associated with earlier recovery from organ failure in a small randomized controlled trial (RCT) with the most pronounced effect in the highest dose group [3], and with earlier shock reversal and improved survival in a small RCT in a surgical sepsis population [4]. Most impressively, high-dose i. v. vitamin C combined with i. v. thiamine and stress dose steroids substantially accelerated shock reversal and improved survival in a before and after study [5]. Of course, these results require confirmation, but are nonetheless thought-provoking.

Sepsis and ischemia/reperfusion injury have a common pathophysiological pathway comprising overwhelming amounts of reactive oxygen species (ROS) causing endothelial dysfunction, cellular injury and multiple organ failure. This massive production of ROS has been demonstrated *in vitro*. Plasma derived from cardiac arrest patients induced an acute pro-oxidant state in endothelial cells with impair-

A. M. E. Spoelstra-de Man (✉) · P. W. G. Elbers · H. M. Oudemans-van Straaten
Department of Intensive Care Medicine, Amsterdam Cardiovascular Sciences, Amsterdam
Infection and Immunity Institute, VU University Medical Center Amsterdam
Amsterdam, Netherlands
e-mail: am.spoelstra@vumc.nl

© Springer International Publishing AG 2018
J.-L. Vincent (ed.), *Annual Update in Intensive Care and Emergency Medicine 2018*,
Annual Update in Intensive Care and Emergency Medicine,
https://doi.org/10.1007/978-3-319-73670-9_11

ment of the mitochondrial respiratory chain activity, resulting in major endothelial toxicity [6]. Therefore, high-dose i. v. vitamin C could be beneficial in the setting of ischemia/reperfusion as well. In particular, it could be a promising novel therapeutic intervention to improve clinical outcome post-cardiac arrest.

That vitamin C may protect against ischemia/reperfusion injury is also supported by the finding that pond turtles, which have a remarkable tolerance for oxygen depletion during hours of diving under water, have extremely high vitamin C concentrations in their brain. The high levels of vitamin C in the central nervous system are possibly an evolutionary adaptation to protect the brain from oxidative damage during re-oxygenation after a long hypoxic dive [7]. Humans have lost the capacity to make vitamin C.

An increasing number of preclinical and clinical studies have investigated the role of vitamin C in ischemia/reperfusion injury. In this narrative review, we will discuss the rationale of the use of vitamin C for post-cardiac arrest syndrome and summarize the results of the relevant (pre)clinical studies focusing on high-dose i. v. vitamin C for post-cardiac arrest, myocardial and cerebral ischemia/reperfusion injury.

Pathophysiology of Ischemia/Reperfusion Injury and the Post-Cardiac Arrest Syndrome

The pathophysiology of the post-cardiac arrest syndrome is complex. During cardiac arrest, systemic ischemia causes cellular and tissue damage by depletion of energy and oxygen stores. Despite the low oxygen tension, ROS are generated, mainly by the mitochondria due to uncoupling of oxidative phosphorylation. After successful resuscitation, reperfusion of blood to ischemic organs can paradoxically exacerbate organ damage. Being highly metabolic organs, the brain and heart are particularly vulnerable to these deleterious effects. Upon reperfusion, huge amounts of ROS are produced within minutes from different sources, including mitochondrial electron-transport chain reactions; upregulation of the enzymes NADPH oxidase, xanthine oxidase, lipoxygenase, cyclooxygenase and inducible nitric oxide synthase (iNOS); and oxidation of catecholamines. This massive release of ROS, especially when unopposed by antioxidants such as vitamin C, can damage proteins, membrane lipids and DNA, trigger necrotic and apoptotic cell death and induce cellular and organ dysfunction. Endothelial dysfunction results in heterogeneity of the microcirculation and a diminished response to endothelial-dependent vasodilators and vasoconstrictors causing hypotension. In addition, loss of the endothelial barrier leads to leakage of plasma fluid from the vasculature inducing hypovolemia, hypotension and edema. Organ edema further impedes gas exchange in the lungs and oxygenation in other organs. Multiple organ dysfunction necessitates intensive care support.

Acute Vitamin C Depletion

The overpowering oxidative stress during the post-cardiac arrest syndrome can quickly exhaust body stores of vitamin C due to massive cellular consumption. Already on the first day after cardiac arrest, vitamin C plasma concentrations are reduced by more than 50% compared to healthy volunteers and after 3 days more than half the patients are deficient [8]. Plasma vitamin C levels are decreased not only after cardiac arrest, but also in many other critically ill patients (with sepsis, hemorrhage, myocardial infarction or traumatic brain injury). That low plasma levels reflect real deficiency is supported by the finding that they are accompanied by a significant decrease in intracellular leukocyte ascorbic acid concentrations to scorbutic levels, and that muscle vitamin C content follows plasma concentrations. Vitamin C is the primary circulatory antioxidant used and depleted during oxidative stress, thereby sparing other endogenous antioxidants. This unique function of vitamin C as a first-line "ROS sink" is supported by *in vitro* studies on plasma vitamin C, in which various kinds of ROS primarily cause a fast depletion of vitamin C. Vitamin E and glutathione are oxidized only after exhaustion of vitamin C. Decreased recycling of dehydroascorbate (DHA, the oxidized form of vitamin C) to vitamin C may further contribute to low plasma vitamin C levels post-cardiac arrest due to the altered redox state.

We found that low vitamin C levels in intensive care unit (ICU) patients were associated with vasopressor requirements, kidney injury, multiple organ dysfunction (higher SOFA scores) and increased mortality (Figs. 1 and 2; [8]). Vitamin C deficient patients had an 8-point higher SOFA score, corresponding to two fully fail-

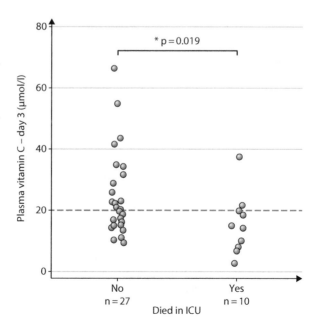

Fig. 1 Plasma vitamin C concentration on day 3 categorized by subsequent mortality. Vitamin C concentrations are markedly lower in patients dying in the ICU. *Dashed line* is deficiency plasma concentration in non-ICU patients. From [8] with permission

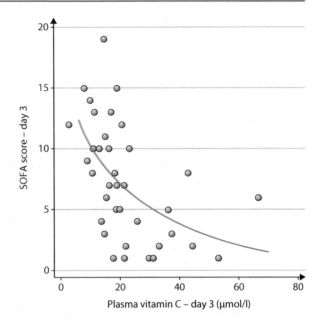

Fig. 2 Vitamin C concentration on day 3 versus sequential organ failure assessment (SOFA) score on day 3. *Blue line* is an ordinary least squares (OLS) regression fit: SOFA = 20.3 − 3.08 * $\log_2$ (Vit-C), $p_{coef} < 0.001$, $R^2 = 0.31$. From [8] with permission

ing organs and 6.9 times higher odds of dying. The association between vitamin C levels and multiple organ failure has also been demonstrated in septic patients [9].

Vitamin C deficiency in ICU patients will often go unnoticed. Because of the complexity and cost of its laboratory measurement, plasma levels of vitamin C are not routinely available in hospitals. Furthermore, in clinical practice the vitamin C content of standard nutrition is assumed to be sufficient to normalize the vitamin C levels. However, even after 700 mg vitamin C via enteral nutrition for one week, plasma concentrations remained deficient in the majority of patients [10].

Rationale of High-dose Intravenous Vitamin C

The administration of high-dose vitamin C is often considered as unnecessary or even alternative medicine. This does not do justice to the strong scientific base of the pleiotropic beneficial effects of high i. v. doses (not enteral!) as demonstrated in multiple preclinical and clinical studies [11]. Beyond simply preventing scurvy by the correction of vitamin C deficiency, supraphysiological vitamin C levels can exert very strong multifaceted effects. With enteral supplementation, maximally tolerated dosages (3–4 g/day) cannot achieve plasma levels of > 250 μmol/l because of saturable absorption [12]. Intravenous vitamin C administration can generate much higher plasma levels, thus yielding more potent antioxidative effects. The underlying pathophysiological mechanisms have now been well elucidated (Fig. 3).

High plasma levels of vitamin C not only limit the generation of ROS, repair other oxidized scavengers such as glutathione, urate and vitamin E, and modulate

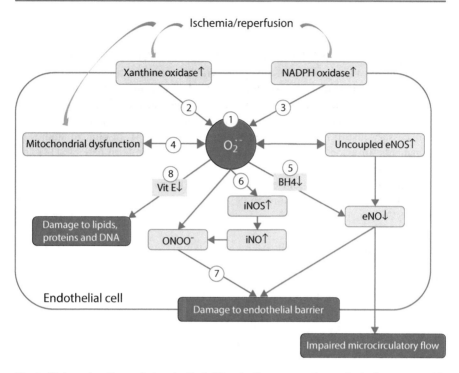

Fig. 3 Pleiotropic effects of vitamin C. *1*. Vitamin C scavenges free radicals from superoxide ($O_2^{·-}$). *2*. Vitamin C inhibits activation of xanthine oxidase and of *3*, NADPH oxidase. *4*. Vitamin C protects the mitochondria from oxidative stress caused by increased leakage of electrons from the dysfunctional electron transport chain. *5*. Vitamin C recovers tetrahydrobiopterin (BH_4) from dihydrobiopterin (BH_2), restoring endothelial nitric oxide synthase (eNOS) activity and increasing eNO bioavailability. *6*. Vitamin C inhibits inducible NOS (iNOS) activation, preventing profuse iNO production and peroxynitrite ($ONOO^-$) generation. *7*. Vitamin C scavenges $ONOO^-$, preventing loosening of the tight junctions of the endothelium. *8*. Vitamin C recovers α-tocopherol, which protects against lipid peroxidation

numerous enzyme reactions, but can also act as a direct radical scavenger. The low electron reduction potential of both vitamin C (282 mV) and its one-electron oxidation product, the ascorbyl radical (−174 mV), enable them to reduce virtually all clinically important radicals and oxidants. In addition, vitamin C maintains NO-mediated endothelial integrity and vasomotor control. Furthermore, as a necessary cofactor, vitamin C supplementation can also recover endogenous vasopressor synthesis. In addition, and very relevant for post-cardiac arrest patients, vitamin C may protect the brain. Neurons in the brain have high rates of oxidative metabolism and contain some of the highest concentrations of vitamin C. Intracerebral vitamin C provides protection against oxidative stress and glutamate toxicity and supports peptide amidation, myelin formation, synaptic potentiation and catecholamine synthesis.

Pharmacokinetics of Vitamin C

Normal plasma vitamin C levels are around 60 μmol/l (deficiency < 20 μmol/l, severe deficiency < 11 μmol/l). Enteral uptake via the vitamin C transporter (SVCT1) is saturable and intestinal uptake during critical illness may be even more limited. Without supplementation, baseline low plasma concentrations (6–20 μmol/l) in critically ill patients further declined and a minimum of 3 g vitamin C i. v./day was necessary just to normalize plasma concentrations [13]. In clinical studies in ICU patients, infusion of 66 mg/kg/h vitamin C for 24 h in burn patients [14] and 200 mg/kg/day for 4 days in septic patients [3] attained plasma vitamin C concentrations of up to 600 μmol/l on day 1 and 5,700 μmol/l on day 4, respectively. Vitamin C is filtered by the glomerulus, and actively reabsorbed in the proximal tubule (SVCT1). Urinary excretion is low in deficient patients and increases at higher plasma levels.

Uptake from plasma into cells occurs via vitamin C transporters (SVCT2) or as dehydroascorbate across the blood-brain barrier via glucose transporters. As a result of active transport, cerebrospinal fluid concentrations are about 4-fold and intracellular concentrations are up to 25- to 80-fold higher than in plasma, especially in leukocytes and neurons, protecting them against oxidative injury. High plasma concentrations facilitate cellular entry and the vitamin C content of granulocytes, erythrocytes and platelets is significantly related to plasma concentration and oxidative stress-induced transporter expression.

Safety of High-dose Vitamin C

Significant adverse events from high-dose vitamin C have not yet been reported [11]. In critically ill patients with sepsis, 200 mg/kg/day was well tolerated [3] as were megadoses up to 1,500 mg/kg i. v. vitamin C three times weekly in cancer patients [15]. Risks comprise a paradoxical pro-oxidative effect in case of iron overload and oxalate kidney stones. However, these risks are limited to susceptible patients and only reported as cases. Vitamin C can reduce catalytic metals such as Fe^{3+} (to Fe^{2+}) facilitating generation of ROS by subsequent Fenton cycles and cause pro-oxidative effects in patients with hemochromatosis. Patients with hemochromatosis have been excluded in most studies. High-dose vitamin C increases urinary oxalate excretion. However, oxalate nephrocalcinosis and calcium oxalate stones take months to years to develop and none of the studies with short-term vitamin C administration reported kidney stone formation [3–5, 14].

High-dose Vitamin C Post-Cardiac Arrest

The effect of high-dose i. v. vitamin C on the systemic ischemia/reperfusion injury post-cardiac arrest has only been investigated in three preclinical studies and not in a clinical setting. All studies used a rat model of ventricular fibrillation and electrical shock. During cardiac arrest, the myocardium is harmed not only by the underlying ischemic heart disease and ischemia/reperfusion injury, but also by ventricular fibrillation and electrical shocks. The resulting myocardial injury is an important cause of in-hospital mortality post-cardiac arrest. Of note, the electrical shock doses used in the rat cardiac arrest models are large when converting to humans on a weight basis.

In two rat studies, vitamin C (50 and 100 mg/kg i. v.) decreased myocardial damage and improved survival rate and neurological outcome [16, 17]. Oxidative stress of the myocardium, estimated by malonaldehyde concentrations, was significantly reduced. These beneficial effects were not only observed when vitamin C was administered at the start of cardiopulmonary resuscitation (CPR), but also when given after return of spontaneous circulation. In contrast, another study using both vitamin C and DHA, the oxidized form of vitamin C, in a much higher dose of 250 mg/kg i. v. showed compromised resuscitability [18].

High-dose Vitamin C and Myocardial Ischemia/Reperfusion Injury

Acute myocardial ischemia followed by reperfusion therapies, such as thrombolysis, percutaneous coronary intervention (PCI) or coronary bypass surgery, can also cause substantial myocardial ischemia/reperfusion injury.

Preclinical Studies

Myocardial ischemia/reperfusion injury can induce four types of major cardiac dysfunction: lethal reperfusion injury (infarction), reperfusion arrhythmias, microvascular damage (no-reflow phenomenon) and contractile dysfunction (myocardial stunning).

Reperfusion injury accounts for up to 50% of the final myocardial infarction. In animal studies, high-dose i. v. vitamin C mostly reduced infarct size [19–22]. However, some studies showed no reduction [23–25], or only reduction in diabetic hearts [19] or when vitamin C was administered in the oxidized form, DHA [26], or when combined with glutathione [27]. Ischemia/reperfusion arrhythmias contribute to many episodes of sudden death in humans [28]. The burst of ROS caused by reperfusion leads to peroxidation of lipids in the cell membrane, which can result in an influx of calcium through the damaged sarcolemma. Furthermore, ROS inhibit calcium uptake in the sarcoplasmatic reticulum. These factors increase intracellular free calcium which can lead to abnormal impulse formation/conduction and initiation of arrhythmias. High-dose i. v. vitamin C reduced reperfusion arrhythmias, such as ventricular fibrillation, ventricular tachycardia and premature ventricular complexes [27–31], although not all changes were significant [28]. In some studies a significant reduction was only present when vitamin C was combined with deferoxamine [29] or glutathione [27]. Post-ischemic reperfusion induces endothelial cell swelling and luminal membrane blebbing in the myocardial microcirculation. These factors contribute to decreased microcirculatory flow (the 'no-reflow' phenomenon). In addition, swollen myocytes compress neighboring capillaries. Vitamin C prevented endothelial cell and myocyte swelling and reduced membrane blebbing [32].

Even when damage is not irreversible and coronary flow is completely restored after myocardial ischemia, contractile dysfunction can persist after reperfusion (myocardial stunning). This can lead to systolic and diastolic failure and even cardiogenic shock. Vitamin C improved left ventricular function in many [19–21], although not all studies [23].

Clinical Studies

Few clinical studies have investigated i. v. vitamin C during PCI for myocardial ischemia. Periprocedural myocardial injury occurs in about 15–35% of PCI procedures and ranges from obvious clinical myocardial infarction to a mild increase in cardiac enzymes [33]. It is associated with increased long-term mortality, recurrent infarction and revascularization at follow-up. Periprocedural myocardial injury can take place as a result of side branch occlusion near the intervention site or because of structural and functional microvascular dysfunction in the downstream territory of the treated artery with persistent no-reflow. Two studies with vitamin C have been performed in patients undergoing elective PCI for stable angina pectoris. Infusion of vitamin C before elective PCI reduced oxidative stress in both studies [34, 35] and periprocedural myocardial injury in the larger study (n = 532) [35]. Vitamin C administered before PCI strongly improved microcirculatory reperfusion, with 79% of the patients reaching TIMI myocardial perfusion grade III versus 39% in controls [34]. The potential mechanism for better microcirculatory perfusion due to vitamin C is increased bioavailability of NO. Vitamin C prevents the oxidation of tetrahydrobiopterin (BH_4), a cofactor of NOS that is highly sensitive to oxidation. When BH_4 is oxidized, endothelial NOS activity becomes uncoupled, resulting in the production of superoxide instead of NO, thus enhancing the oxidative damage.

Only one very small study (n = 21) estimated the effect of vitamin C administered just before PCI for acute myocardial infarction on oxidative stress (estimated as 8-epi prostaglandin F2α in urine) and showed no effect. However, this may have been a type II error [36].

Cardiac Surgery with Cardiopulmonary Bypass

During cardiac surgery with cardiopulmonary bypass (CPB), myocardial ischemia is induced during cross-clamping of the aorta. Re-exposure to oxygen produces ischemia/reperfusion injury in the myocardium, but also a whole-body inflammatory reaction to the CPB itself. The generation of ROS was associated with decreased vitamin C levels after cardiac surgery [37], which had not returned to preoperative concentrations in most patients at hospital discharge. This suggests massive vitamin C consumption and depletion of body stores likely including the myocardium. Vitamin C may be consumed by direct reaction with ROS, by regeneration of other antioxidants (vitamin E, glutathione) or by massive synthesis of catecholamines during CPB.

Oxidative stress after cardiac surgery contributes to myocardial stunning and arrhythmias. High-dose i. v. vitamin C administered before CPB and after aortic declamping decreased oxidative stress and myocardial injury [38]. Preoperative ingestion of vitamin E and C supplements attenuated markers of oxidative stress and inhibited ischemic electrocardiographic alterations [39]. The most frequent type of heart rhythm disturbance after cardiac surgery is atrial fibrillation with an incidence of 10% to 65% and an increased risk of morbidity and mortality. In a recent meta-analysis, vitamin C therapy significantly decreased the incidence of paroxysmal atrial fibrillation with an OR of 0.47 (95% CI: 0.36–0.62; $p < 0.00001$) [40].

High-dose Vitamin C and Cerebral Ischemia/Reperfusion Injury

Ischemia/reperfusion injury of the brain results in blood-brain barrier disruption with inflammatory and oxidative damage, brain edema and necrosis. Brain tissue is highly sensitive to oxidative damage because of its high need for oxygen and its high content of polysaturated fatty acids. Stored at millimolar concentrations in brain cells, vitamin C is the most important antioxidant in the brain. During ischemia, large amounts of vitamin C are released into the extracellular compartment in the ischemic area and brain vitamin C levels decline markedly and rapidly in the intracellular compartment [41].

Vitamin C (= ascorbate) crosses the blood-brain barrier via the glucose receptor GLUT1 in the oxidized form, DHA. In the brain, DHA is converted back to vitamin C by glutathione and other intracellular thiols (Fig. 4). Intravenous administration of DHA, but not of vitamin C, generates supraphysiological concentrations of vitamin C in the brain, due to the more efficient uptake of DHA compared to vitamin C. Therefore, most studies in cerebral ischemia have focused on the effects of DHA. When DHA is converted back to vitamin C, it has a potential polymechanistic neuroprotective effect. Glutamate uptake into astrocytes is blocked by ROS and vitamin C can prevent this. Furthermore, vitamin C can prevent the formation of catechol-protein conjugates from oxidized dopamine (which is notoriously neurotoxic) and may block dopamine receptors.

Preclinical Studies

Most preclinical studies investigated the effect of DHA on cerebral ischemia/reperfusion injury. In preclinical cerebral ischemia models in mice, rats and monkeys, DHA decreased mortality [42] and, in multiple studies, infarct size [42–47]. DHA administered 15 min, but also as late as 3 h post-ischemia produced a 6- to 9-fold reduction in infarct size, improved post-ischemic cerebral blood flow and decreased

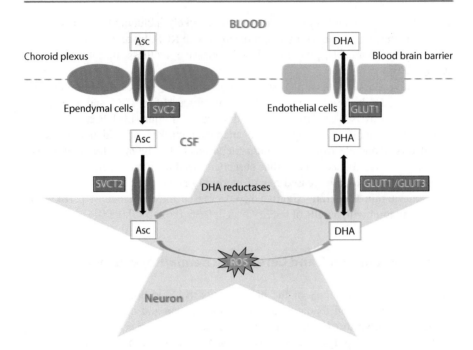

Fig. 4 Ascorbate (Asc) can enter the cerebrospinal fluid (CSF) directly through the choroid plexus via the sodium-dependent vitamin C transporter (SVCT)2. Ascorbate enters the neuron also via SVCT2. This route is a slow, saturable, controlled process. Dehydroascorbate (DHA) is transported directly and fast into the brain via the abundant glucose transporter (GLUT)1 transporters on the endothelial cells of the blood brain-barrier and via the GLUT1 or GLUT3 on the neurons. Inside the neurons, DHA can be reduced back to ascorbate

neurological impairment [42]. DHA 100 mg/kg (intra-peritoneally [i. p.]) given 10 min after occlusion decreased infarct size by 50% after 24 h. In addition, i. v. DHA rapidly replenished the significantly declined vitamin C levels in the brain after ischemic stroke, and reduced cerebral oxidative injury and edema [43, 44].

A few studies have investigated the effect of vitamin C on cerebral ischemia/reperfusion injury. In monkeys pretreated with 2 g i. v. vitamin C just before occlusion, infarct size decreased from 22% to 7%, and in gerbils vitamin C protected the striatum [48]. The cerebral cortex, hippocampus and corpus striatum are the most vulnerable regions of the brain to ischemic insult. Vitamin C slowed the rate of dopamine release in the striatum in a concentration-dependent fashion. However, in contrast to the uniform results with DHA, vitamin C did not exert beneficial effects in two other studies [42, 49].

Clinical Studies

Only a few clinical studies have been performed investigating the effects of i. v. vitamin C or DHA on cerebral ischemia. A placebo-controlled trial in patients with stroke showed no benefit of vitamin C 500 mg/day i. v. for 10 days. There was no effect on neurological status after 10 days or 3 months [50]. A possible explanation could be the relatively low dose used and the start of vitamin C one day after stroke when irreversible damage was already done.

Variability in the Results of the Effects of High-dose i. v. Vitamin C on Ischemia/Reperfusion Injury

Although many studies investigating the effect of high-dose i. v. vitamin C in ischemia/reperfusion showed a positive effect, not all did so. Several factors could have influenced this controversy.

First, the specific experimental conditions can have a major impact on the effects of vitamin C on ischemia/reperfusion injury. The dosage, the route, duration and timing of administration were highly variable among studies. The dosage varied widely from a bolus of 500 mg vitamin C to a dose of 1 g vitamin C per kg bodyweight. The route of administration could be i. v., i. p., oral or intracoronary. Vitamin C was applied as a single bolus or as a continuous infusion, sometimes preceded by a bolus. The half-life of parenteral vitamin C is short, so bolus vitamin C will attain higher plasma levels for only a short period. All these aforementioned factors affect the achieved plasma concentrations and antioxidative capacity. The direct scavenger activity of vitamin C is only reached with plasma concentrations of 1 to 10 mmol/l or higher. Furthermore, timing of the administration of vitamin C in the studies is crucial. The huge burst of ROS is generated within minutes after the start of reperfusion. Therefore, a late start of vitamin C infusion may lead to negative results [50].

Second, there is a delicate balance between protective oxidant signaling and the detrimental effects of ROS. Vitamin C can, in the presence of metallic ions such as iron, act as a pro-oxidant (Fenton reaction). Free iron (Fe^{3+}) is an abundant ion in myocardial and endothelial cells. During ischemia, a large number of iron ions may be released during ischemia, over-saturating the serum's iron-binding capacity, especially in patients with hemochromatosis.

Third, vitamin C could potentially interfere with the beneficial signaling of adaptive responses by lowering ROS levels. Redox signaling is useful for cell survival, but excessively high ROS is one of the most critical triggers for necrotic and apoptotic cell death. Therefore, it is essential to stop the administration of high-dose i. v. vitamin C after the massive burst of ROS has subsided.

Fourth, the drug combinations used can affect the results. A negative interaction between antioxidants can occur [25]. It is possible that some antioxidant combinations interfere with this balance and abolish not only the detrimental effects, but also some protective effects of oxidant signaling.

Future Trials

Given the preclinical and clinical signals of a beneficial effect of high-dose i. v. vitamin C in ischemia/reperfusion injury and sepsis, the extensive clinical safety data in ICU patients and the convincing mechanistic understanding, it is time for a clinical RCT in post-cardiac arrest patients. There are several prerequisites to maximize the chances of revealing potential beneficial effects of vitamin C in such a trial.

To accomplish maximal pleiotropic beneficial effects of vitamin C, supraphysiological plasma levels have to be attained. This is only possible when vitamin C is administered i. v. at a dose of at least 3 g/day ($\geq$ 3 g/day is necessary to correct deficiency in ICU patients). Furthermore, although vitamin C enters the brain mainly as DHA, which is converted to vitamin C in the neurons, for cardiac arrest we believe the more stable reduced form of vitamin C is preferable. The overwhelming oxidative stress post-cardiac arrest will convert a substantial amount of the administered vitamin C to DHA, thereby ensuring sufficient vitamin C in the brain.

In addition, it is essential that infusion with vitamin C is started as early as possible. Huge amounts of ROS are created within minutes after reperfusion, and the oxidative damage of patient plasma to cultured endothelial cells is highest early after resuscitation [6]. ICU admission likely indicates the moment at which where the pro/antioxidant balance is lost and the oxidative stress response becomes uncontrolled. Starting the infusion before this point seems crucial. Finally, we suggest administering high-dose vitamin C for a short course of four days only, e.g., during the overwhelming oxidative stress when organ damage occurs. After four days, plasma concentrations will be supranormal and vitamin C can be continued in a low (nutritional) dose to allow generation of low concentrations of ROS, which are essential for physiological signaling and repair.

Conclusion

An increasing number of preclinical and clinical studies show that high-dose i. v. vitamin C can mitigate systemic, cerebral and myocardial ischemia/reperfusion injury. Vitamin C administration has been associated with reduced oxidative stress, myocardial injury and arrhythmias and improved microcirculation, neurological outcome and survival, although not all studies showed benefit. Because of the common pathophysiological pathway of sepsis and ischemia/reperfusion injury, the potential role of vitamin C for ischemia/reperfusion injury is further supported by the results of preliminary sepsis studies, showing earlier recovery from organ failure and higher survival rates. Therefore, early, high-dose i. v. vitamin C is a promising therapeutic intervention after cardiac arrest to diminish the systemic ischemia/reperfusion injury due to overwhelming oxidative stress. The supportive evidence from preclinical and clinical studies is too large to continue considering early high-dose i. v. vitamin C as alternative medicine. An RCT is urgently required to provide definitive proof as to whether this cheap and safe therapy does indeed improve outcome.

References

1. Grasner JT, Bottiger BW, Bossaert L (2014) EuReCa ONE – ONE month – ONE Europe – ONE goal. Resuscitation 85:1307–1308
2. Beesems JA, Stieglis R, Koster RW (2012) Reanimatie buiten het ziekenhuis in Noord-Holland en twente: resultaten ARREST-onderzoek. In: Koopman C, van Dis I, Visseren FLJ, Vaartjes I, Bots ML (eds) Hart- en vaatziekten in Nederland 2012, cijfers over risicofactoren, ziekte en sterfte. Hartstichting, Den Haag, pp 2006–2011
3. Fowler AA III, Syed AA, Knowlson S et al (2014) Phase I safety trial of intravenous ascorbic acid in patients with severe sepsis. J Transl Med 12:32
4. Zabet MH, Mohammadi M, Ramezani M, Khalili H (2016) Effect of high-dose ascorbic acid on vasopressor's requirement in septic shock. J Res Pharm Pract 5:94–100
5. Marik PE, Khangoora V, Rivera R, Hooper MH, Catravas J (2016) Hydrocortisone, vitamin C and thiamine for the treatment of severe sepsis and septic shock: a retrospective before-after study. Chest 151:1229–1238
6. Huet O, Dupic L, Batteux F et al (2011) Postresuscitation syndrome: potential role of hydroxyl radical-induced endothelial cell damage. Crit Care Med 39:1712–1720
7. Rice ME, Lee EJ, Choy Y (1995) High levels of ascorbic acid, not glutathione, in the CNS of anoxia-tolerant reptiles contrasted with levels in anoxia-intolerant species. J Neurochem 64:1790–1799
8. Grooth HJ, Spoelstra-de Man AME, Oudemans-van Straaten HM (2014) Early plasma Vitamin C concentration, organ dysfunction and ICU mortality. Intensive Care Med 40(Suppl 1):S199 (abst)
9. Borrelli E, Roux-Lombard P, Grau GE et al (1996) Plasma concentrations of cytokines, their soluble receptors, and antioxidant vitamins can predict the development of multiple organ failure in patients at risk. Crit Care Med 24:392–397
10. van Zanten AR, Sztark F, Kaisers UX et al (2014) High-protein enteral nutrition enriched with immune-modulating nutrients vs standard high-protein enteral nutrition and nosocomial infections in the ICU: a randomized clinical trial. JAMA 312:514–524
11. Oudemans-van Straaten HM, Spoelstra-de Man AM, de Waard MC (2014) Vitamin C revisited. Crit Care 18:460
12. Levine M, Padayatty SJ, Espey MG (2011) Vitamin C: a concentration-function approach yields pharmacology and therapeutic discoveries. Adv Nutr 2:78–88
13. Long CL, Maull KI, Krishnan RS et al (2003) Ascorbic acid dynamics in the seriously ill and injured. J Surg Res 109:144–148
14. Tanaka H, Matsuda T, Miyagantani Y et al (2000) Reduction of resuscitation fluid volumes in severely burned patients using ascorbic acid administration: a randomized, prospective study. Arch Surg 135:326–331
15. Hoffer LJ, Levine M, Assouline S et al (2008) Phase I clinical trial of i. v. ascorbic acid in advanced malignancy. Ann Oncol 19:1969–1974
16. Tsai MS, Huang CH, Tsai CY et al (2011) Ascorbic acid mitigates the myocardial injury after cardiac arrest and electrical shock. Intensive Care Med 37:2033–2040
17. Tsai MS, Huang CH, Tsai CY et al (2014) Combination of intravenous ascorbic acid administration and hypothermia after resuscitation improves myocardial function and survival in a ventricular fibrillation cardiac arrest model in the rat. Acad Emerg Med 21:257–265
18. Motl J, Radhakrishnan J, Ayoub IM, Grmec S, Gazmuri RJ (2014) Vitamin C compromises cardiac resuscitability in a rat model of ventricular fibrillation. Am J Ther 21:352–357
19. Okazaki T, Otani H, Shimazu T et al (2011) Ascorbic acid and N-acetyl cysteine prevent uncoupling of nitric oxide synthase and increase tolerance to ischemia/reperfusion injury in diabetic rat heart. Free Radic Res 45:1173–1183
20. Klein HH, Pich S, Lindert S et al (1989) Combined treatment with vitamins E and C in experimental myocardial infarction in pigs. Am Heart J 118:667–673

21. Doppelfeld IS, Parnham MJ (1992) Experimental conditions determine effects of ascorbic acid on reperfusion injury: comparison of tissue damage with hemodynamic parameters in rat isolated hearts. Methods Find Exp Clin Pharmacol 14:419–430

22. Mickle DA, Li RK, Weisel RD et al (1989) Myocardial salvage with trolox and ascorbic acid for an acute evolving infarction. Ann Thorac Surg 47:553–557

23. Chatziathanasiou GN, Nikas DN, Katsouras CS et al (2012) Combined intravenous treatment with ascorbic acid and desferrioxamine to reduce myocardial reperfusion injury in an experimental model resembling the clinical setting of primary PCI. Hellenic J Cardiol 53:195–204

24. Skyschally A, Schulz R, Gres P, Korth HG, Heusch G (2003) Attenuation of ischemic preconditioning in pigs by scavenging of free oxyradicals with ascorbic acid. Am J Physiol Heart Circ Physiol 284:H698–H703

25. Nikas DN, Chatziathanasiou G, Kotsia A et al (2008) Effect of intravenous administration of antioxidants alone and in combination on myocardial reperfusion injury in an experimental pig model. Curr Ther Res Clin Exp 69:423–439

26. Guaiquil VH, Golde DW, Beckles DL, Mascareno EJ, Siddiqui MA (2004) Vitamin C inhibits hypoxia-induced damage and apoptotic signaling pathways in cardiomyocytes and ischemic hearts. Free Radic Biol Med 37:1419–1429

27. Gao F, Yao CL, Gao E et al (2002) Enhancement of glutathione cardioprotection by ascorbic acid in myocardial reperfusion injury. J Pharmacol Exp Ther 301:543–550

28. Tan DX, Manchester LC, Reiter RJ et al (1998) Ischemia/reperfusion-induced arrhythmias in the isolated rat heart: prevention by melatonin. J Pineal Res 25:184–191

29. Karahaliou A, Katsouras C, Koulouras V et al (2008) Ventricular arrhythmias and antioxidative medication: experimental study. Hellenic J Cardiol 49:320–328

30. Woodward B, Zakaria MN (1985) Effect of some free radical scavengers on reperfusion induced arrhythmias in the isolated rat heart. J Mol Cell Cardiol 17:485–493

31. Nishinaka Y, Sugiyama S, Yokota M, Saito H, Ozawa T (1992) The effects of a high dose of ascorbate on ischemia-reperfusion-induced mitochondrial dysfunction in canine hearts. Heart Vessel 7:18–23

32. Molyneux CA, Glyn MC, Ward BJ (2002) Oxidative stress and cardiac microvascular structure in ischemia and reperfusion: the protective effect of antioxidant vitamins. Microvasc Res 64:265–277

33. Delafontaine P, Anwar A (2010) Vitamin C and percutaneous coronary intervention. Jacc Cardiovasc Interv 3:230–232

34. Basili S, Tanzilli G, Mangieri E et al (2010) Intravenous ascorbic acid infusion improves myocardial perfusion grade during elective percutaneous coronary intervention: relationship with oxidative stress markers. Jacc Cardiovasc Interv 3:221–229

35. Wang ZJ, Hu WK, Liu YY et al (2014) The effect of intravenous vitamin C infusion on periprocedural myocardial injury for patients undergoing elective percutaneous coronary intervention. Can J Cardiol 30:96–101

36. Guan W, Osanai T, Kamada T et al (1999) Time course of free radical production after primary coronary angioplasty for acute myocardial infarction and the effect of vitamin C. Jpn Circ J 63:924–928

37. Lassnigg A, Punz A, Barker R et al (2003) Influence of intravenous vitamin E supplementation in cardiac surgery on oxidative stress: a double-blinded, randomized, controlled study. Br J Anaesth 90:148–154

38. Dingchao H, Zhiduan Q, Liye H, Xiaodong F (1994) The protective effects of high-dose ascorbic acid on myocardium against reperfusion injury during and after cardiopulmonary bypass. Thorac Cardiovasc Surg 42:276–278

39. Sisto T, Paajanen H, Metsa-Ketela T et al (1995) Pretreatment with antioxidants and allopurinol diminishes cardiac onset events in coronary artery bypass grafting. Ann Thorac Surg 59:1519–1523

40. Hu X, Yuan L, Wang H et al (2017) Efficacy and safety of vitamin C for atrial fibrillation after cardiac surgery: a meta-analysis with trial sequential analysis of randomized controlled trials. Int J Surg 37:58–64

41. Flamm ES, Demopoulos HB, Seligman ML, Poser RG, Ransohoff J (1978) Free radicals in cerebral ischemia. Stroke 9:445–447
42. Huang J, Agus DB, Winfree CJ et al (2001) Dehydroascorbic acid, a blood-brain barrier transportable form of vitamin C, mediates potent cerebroprotection in experimental stroke. Proc Natl Acad Sci Usa 98:11720–11724
43. Mack WJ, Mocco J, Ducruet AF et al (2006) A cerebroprotective dose of intravenous citrate/sorbitol-stabilized dehydroascorbic acid is correlated with increased cerebral ascorbic acid and inhibited lipid peroxidation after murine reperfused stroke. Neurosurgery 59:383–388
44. Song J, Park J, Kim JH et al (2015) Dehydroascorbic acid attenuates ischemic brain edema and neurotoxicity in cerebral ischemia: an in vivo study. Exp Neurobiol 24:41–54
45. Bemeur C, Ste-Marie L, Desjardins P et al (2004) Expression of superoxide dismutase in hyperglycemic focal cerebral ischemia in the rat. Neurochem Int 45:1167–1174
46. Henry PT, Chandy MJ (1998) Effect of ascorbic acid on infarct size in experimental focal cerebral ischaemia and reperfusion in a primate model. Acta Neurochir (Wien) 140:977–980
47. Ranjan A, Theodore D, Haran RP, Chandy MJ (1993) Ascorbic acid and focal cerebral ischaemia in a primate model. Acta Neurochir (Wien) 123:87–91
48. Stamford JA, Isaac D, Hicks CA et al (1999) Ascorbic acid is neuroprotective against global ischaemia in striatum but not hippocampus: histological and voltammetric data. Brain Res 835:229–240
49. Kim EJ, Park YG, Baik EJ et al (2005) Dehydroascorbic acid prevents oxidative cell death through a glutathione pathway in primary astrocytes. J Neurosci Res 79:670–679
50. Lagowska-Lenard M, Stelmasiak Z, Bartosik-Psujek H (2010) Influence of vitamin C on markers of oxidative stress in the earliest period of ischemic stroke. Pharmacol Rep 62:751–756

Optimal Oxygen and Carbon Dioxide Targets During and after Resuscitated Cardiac Arrest

M. B. Skrifvars, G. M. Eastwood, and R. Bellomo

Introduction and Epidemiology

Cardiac arrest is major health problem with around 350,000 cases each year in Europe [1, 2]. Factors determining outcome after a sudden cardiac arrest are included in the Chain of Survival concept and include early recognition, early basic life support, early advanced life support and early post-resuscitation care and rehabilitation [3, 4].

During cardiac arrest there is an abrupt cessation of blood flow to the brain, heart and other vital organs. It has been estimated that the chances of irreversible brain injury increase by 10% every 10 min [5]. Prompt initiation of cardiopulmonary resuscitation (CPR) is therefore one of the most important determinants for both short and long-term survival [6]. Nonetheless, in patients with return of spontaneous circulation (ROSC), hypoxic brain injury remains a major problem, and most patients dying in the intensive care unit (ICU) after a cardiac arrest do so because of hypoxic brain injury [7]. For those who survive, the neurological impact may range from mild neurological deficits to severely impaired consciousness and coma. The injury can be described as a 'two-hit' model with the primary injury occurring during cardiac standstill and the secondary injury occurring during reperfusion and the following 48–72 h [8]. There are limited therapeutic interventions to alleviate this secondary injury, apart from temperature control targeting 33 to 36 degrees for a pe-

M. B. Skrifvars (✉)
Division of Intensive Care, Department of Anesthesiology, Intensive Care and Pain Medicine,
Helsinki University and Helsinki University Hospital
Helsinki, Finland
e-mail: markus.skrifvars@hus.fi

G. M. Eastwood · R. Bellomo
Department of Intensive Care, Austin Hospital
Melbourne, Australia
Australian and New Zealand Intensive Care Research Centre, School of Public Health and
Preventive Medicine, Monash University
Melbourne, Australia

© Springer International Publishing AG 2018
J.-L. Vincent (ed.), *Annual Update in Intensive Care and Emergency Medicine 2018*,
Annual Update in Intensive Care and Emergency Medicine,
https://doi.org/10.1007/978-3-319-73670-9_12

riod of at least 24 h [9]. Despite the fact that mechanical ventilation is ubiquitous during CA and after ROSC and allows for the control of both PaO_2 and $PaCO_2$ and despite the fact that optimal cerebral oxygenation is considered a major target and CO_2 a major regulator of cerebral blood flow, we still know very little about optimal oxygen and carbon dioxide targets after ROSC [10]. As optimization of oxygen and carbon dioxide levels could increase coronary artery blood flow, cerebral blood flow and cerebral oxygen delivery, in the current chapter, we describe the literature regarding both oxygen and carbon dioxide management during CPR and over the early post-resuscitation period (Table 1).

Table 1 Impact and outcomes associated with oxygen and carbon dioxide management in the pre-hospital and early in-hospital setting following cardiac arrest

	Pre-hospital and during CPR	In-hospital following ROSC
Oxygen therapy	• Existing data do not indicate that oxygen administration during CPR is harmful. • Evidence exists to show that high FiO_2 during CPR does not appear to expose brain tissue to intra-arrest hyperoxic injury. • High pre-hospital FiO_2 exposure during resuscitation period was associated with greater evidence of brain injury on histological examination. • Uncertainty exists as to whether pre-hospital titrated oxygen delivery and avoidance of arterial hyperoxemia can be achieved and whether this influences patient-centered or clinical outcomes.	• Based on a series of retrospective studies, there are limited data to support avoidance of hyperoxia in the hospital setting, though available animal data suggest potential harm associated with hyperoxia. • In-hospital increased PaO_2 values may be marker of illness severity post ROSC. Emerging evidence is indicating that increasing maximum PaO_2 vales during the first 24 h of ICU admission is associated with increased hospital mortality and poor neurological outcomes at hospital discharge.
Carbon dioxide	• Current data regarding the relationship between the $PaCO_2$ and outcome in cardiac arrest patients have focused on $etCO_2$ values drawn from observational or retrospective studies. • Current evidence supports the use of $etCO_2$ to evaluate correct endotracheal tube placement, CPR quality, usefulness of $etCO_2$ as a predictor of ROSC. • Data indicate that $etCO_2$ plays a useful role in guiding ventilation strategies to avoid hypocapnia. • Hypocapnia appears rare during cardiac arrest.	• Investigations are being performed to evaluate the relationship between targeting different $PaCO_2$ vales and patient-centered outcomes following ROSC. • Limited available evidence, based on a series of retrospective studies and phase II feasibility safety studies, supports the avoidance of hypocapnia. • Data related to the early and targeted management of $PaCO_2$ should be viewed as hypothesis generating and future large multicenter trials are warranted to assess the association between mild hypercapnia and neurological outcomes in cardiac arrest survivors.

CPR: cardiopulmonary resuscitation; *etCO_2*: end-tidal carbon dioxide; *FiO_2*: fraction of inspired oxygen; *PaO_2*: arterial oxygen tension; *PaCO_2*: arterial carbon dioxide tension; *ROSC*: return of spontaneous circulation

The Impact of Cerebral Hypoxia on Brain Injury in Cardiac Arrest

The physiological process of the primary hypoxic injury is complex and includes cerebral edema related to the cessation of important transcellular ion pumps [8]. Oxygen levels in brain tissue have been shown to be of prognostic importance in many types of neurological injuries including traumatic brain injury (TBI), and thus, by analogy, they may also be crucial during and after cardiac arrest. However, due to the invasiveness of monitoring equipment necessary to monitor tissue oxygenation, the evidence stems from animal studies and very few clinical studies have invasively measured changes in cerebral oxygen values that occur during and immediately after cardiac arrest [10]. One exception is a case report from 2003 in which a patient with a tissue oxygen probe in situ for neuromonitoring experienced a cardiac arrest following the accidental administration of potassium chloride [11]. Investigators were able to analyze the association between cerebral perfusion pressure (CPP) and PaO_2 with brain tissue oxygen (PbO_2) during and immediately after CPR. With the immediate asystole, there was a rapid and complete decline in cerebral tissue oxygen levels (Fig. 1).

One observational study in ICU patients in whom vasopressor support was withdrawn, showed that during the gradual decrease in blood pressure, near-infrared spectroscopy (NIRS) demonstrated a concomitant slow decrease in oxygen content [12]. It is likely that arterial oxygen content prior to the arrest is of importance for the development of brain injury, but few studies have addressed this in cardiac arrest patients [10]. Studies have shown that resuscitation is less likely to succeed in patients with systemic hypoxia and shock present prior to the arrest compared to those with normal physiology, but whether that is related to differences in etiology of the arrest or systemic or brain hypoxia *per se* is currently unknown [13].

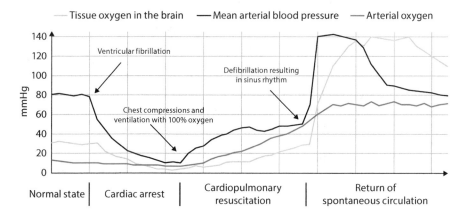

Fig. 1 Schematic presentation of mean arterial blood pressure and oxygen levels in the blood and brain tissue before, during and after cardiac arrest. Based on animal data [14] and data from one case report [11]

Brain Oxygen Levels and Means to Improve Them During Cardiac Arrest

The limited animal data currently available indicate that, with the start of CPR, even though there is an increase in oxygen content in the blood, there is only a very slow increase in invasively measured brain oxygen (Fig. 1; [14, 15]). Yeh and colleagues used a rodent model and ventilation with either 0%, 21% or 100% oxygen during CPR. They found that none of the animals survived in the group ventilated without oxygen, but there was no difference in the 21% and 100% groups [16]. However, the main determinant of the increase in PbO_2 appeared to be the increase in perfusion pressure, which is the result of chest compressions rather than the FiO_2 or achieved PaO_2 [11]. Any interruption in chest compressions will decrease both the achieved perfusion pressure, coronary perfusion and cerebral tissue oxygen values [17]. How much supplemental oxygen is needed is unclear, but one animal study comparing ventilation with 100% and 50% oxygen showed a difference in blood oxygen content but not in PbO_2 [14]. This may be one explanation as to why studies have shown similar outcomes with bystander-initiated life support with compression only compared to compression with mouth-to-mouth ventilation [18]. During advanced life support, one may argue that beyond an arterial saturation of 90–95%, oxygen delivery to the brain will not improve with increasing PaO_2. There are no data in CPR models but studies in TBI patients monitored with parenchymal oxygen catheters have shown that by increasing the FiO_2 to 100% in patients with a saturation of 100%, the oxygen levels in the brain will increase [19]. This suggests the diffusion of soluble oxygen might be of importance in increasing cerebral O_2 tension.

There are to date two clinical studies in which arterial blood oxygen tension was measured during CPR, both by Spindelboeck and colleagues [20, 21]. These two studies showed an association between high arterial oxygen tension measured during the time of arrest and higher likelihood of ROSC and hospital survival. Patients with higher oxygen were more likely to survive neurologically intact but this difference was not significant (p = 0.062). However, all patients in that study were ventilated with 100% oxygen and therefore the low PaO_2 may have been a marker of a different etiology of the arrest (suffocation, drowning, hypoxic respiratory failure) or due to lung pathology. More broadly it seems probable that the use of 100% oxygen would be more efficacious in cases of prolonged duration until start of CPR and with a hypoxic cardiac arrest than in, for example, cases with witnessed cardiac arrest with a cardiac etiology. The limited evidence available is from one patient with immediate initiation of advanced life support, and animal models without hypoxia and treated with very effective mechanical chest compressions. Thus, it is possible that the use of high FiO_2 may be of more importance especially in clinical practice when resuscitating patients with a hypoxic arrest (suffocation, drowning or pulmonary embolism) or in cases where chest compression quality cannot be adequately maintained (e.g., during the transport/movement of patients).

Intra-arrest Monitoring of Oxygenation with NIRS

NIRS is a technology used to monitor oxygenation during CPR. It uses an algorithm to display a regional oxygen saturation value (rSO_2), which appears to correspond well to cerebral venous oxygen saturation. The reported normal reference range for cerebrally-derived NIRS values is between 60 and 80% and when oxygen demand exceeds supply, cerebral venous oxygen saturation falls [22]. Low NIRS values that are identified and then sustained throughout CPR have been shown to be predictive of failure to achieve ROSC [22]. Among resuscitated out-of-hospital cardiac arrest (OHCA) patients admitted to an emergency department in Western Japan with CPR ongoing, increasing rSO_2 levels were identified as being correlated with an increased likelihood of ROSC and good neurological outcome at 90 days [23]. Of note from this study, despite the use of airway adjuncts and high concentration oxygen, no patient had rSO_2 levels above the normal reference range. Such findings may demonstrate that during cardiac arrest, even with effective CPR, it seems likely that tissue oxygen demand exceeds supply due to poor tissue perfusion [5]. Currently, it is unknown which and to what extent resuscitation factors, such as chest compression quality and ventilation, use of 100% FiO_2 or arterial PaO_2 and $PaCO_2$, influence NIRS levels during CPR. One clinical study addressed the relationship between the use of epinephrine and rSO_2 measured with NIRS and found that despite increasing perfusion pressure, epinephrine failed to increase rSO_2.

Carbon Dioxide Levels and Monitoring During CPR

Regarding carbon dioxide the situation is equally complex. Monitoring end-tidal carbon dioxide ($etCO_2$) during CPR is important for confirming correct endotracheal tube placement, for monitoring CPR quality, and may be useful as a predictor of ROSC and patient outcome [24]. However, the usefulness of continued $etCO_2$ monitoring to guide ventilation strategies is less clear. During cardiac arrest, carbon dioxide accumulates resulting in a decrease in pH, indeed carbon dioxide appears to be one of the main determinant of intra-arrest acidosis [21]. Based on animal data, $PaCO_2$ tension appears to decrease since it remains within the tissue, but following CPR initiation, $PaCO_2$ levels rise and are commonly between 8–10 kPa [14]. Hyperventilation occurs frequently both during in-hospital cardiac arrest (IHCA) and OHCA. Hyperventilation has been shown to be detrimental, but this effect has mainly been linked to an increase in intrathoracic pressure leading to decreased venous return and decreased coronary perfusion. Interestingly clinical studies do appear to suggest that intra-arrest hypocarbia is not very common [20, 21]. Indeed, it remains unclear to what extent intra-arrest carbon dioxide levels can be influenced by ventilation. Moderate hypercarbia could also have positive effects. As a vasodilator, it might increase blood flow in vasoconstricted areas. Thus far, studies have failed to show any association between intra-arrest carbon dioxide levels and outcome. The only clinical studies available did not show any difference in outcome depending on intra-arrest carbon dioxide levels [20, 21].

Changes in Oxygen Immediately After ROSC

Animal studies and the one case report available show that immediately after ROSC there is a great increase in tissue oxygen of the brain compared to both the intra- and pre-arrest situation [11, 14]. This is mainly related to a high arterial oxygen content resulting from intra-arrest ventilation with an FiO_2 of 100% and the return of pulsatile flow. This reperfusion with oxygen enriched blood may be harmful. This notion seems supported by animal studies for up to an hour after ROSC. Oxygen free radicals play an important role in the evolving reperfusion injury. However, even though it seems logical that a higher oxygen content leads to more oxygen radical generation, this has not been proven. Limiting oxygen use already during CPR would likely decrease the incidence of immediate post-ROSC extreme hyperoxia, but this is only supported by experimental evidence at present [14].

It is however unclear how common immediate post-arrest hyperoxia is in clinical practice. In a study by Spindelboeck and colleagues, arterial samples obtained immediately after ROSC found a mean PaO_2 of around 110 mmHg [20]. There were no clear differences in the peri-arrest factors between those with hyperoxia compared to those with normoxia or hypoxia. One would assume that hyperoxia is more common with short delays to initiation of CPR, such as after in-hospital cardiac arrest but the data are limited.

One other factor contributing to oxygen levels in the brain is the CPP [11]. The CPP can be elevated early after ROSC due to the intra-arrest use of epinephrine, given the elevated MAP and high CPP [11]. However, given the short half-life of epinephrine, patients commonly become hypotensive during transport and ICU admission [25].

Optimal Oxygen Tension in the Prehospital Phase and in the ICU

After ROSC, the FiO_2 needs to be adjusted to avoid hyperoxia, since prolonged use of 100% FiO_2 is likely the most common cause of extreme hyperoxia. Strict titration of the amount of oxygen administered in the pre-hospital setting seems appealing, but is very challenging to do, at least using peripheral oxygen saturation. The 'Hot or Not' study failed to show the feasibility of titration of oxygen administration by monitoring peripheral oxygen saturation, due to a high incidence of hypoxia [26]. Indeed, hyperoxia exposure most commonly occurs prior to ICU admission [27]. Obtaining arterial blood gas samples also in the pre-hospital setting may be the only option to avoid hyperoxia exposure prior to hospital admission [20, 21, 28].

There are multiple studies exploring the associations between oxygen levels and outcome in the ICU, however most of these studies are retrospective. The evidence is conflicting. Two studies on the same cohort of patients found an association between hyperoxia, based on a single arterial blood gas measurement after ICU admission, and in-hospital mortality [29, 30]. In contrast, the third study of the 'worst arterial blood gas' measurement in the first 24 h in cardiac arrest patients admitted to Australian and New Zealand ICUs, did not demonstrate this association after adjustment for potential confounding factors including illness severity and inspired oxygen concentration [31]. Collectively, these initial studies have a number of limitations. First, they did not include important predictors of clinical outcome such as initial rhythm, time to ROSC, and whether bystander CPR was provided. Second, in the case of the North American dataset, mild therapeutic hypothermia was not generally applied. Given that mild therapeutic hypothermia appears to alter the ischemia/reperfusion pathways and reduce apoptotic cell death, this is an important consideration [32].

A single-center study of 173 consecutive comatose cardiac arrest patients examined the impact of therapeutic hypothermia on oxygen exposure [33]. Using a multivariate logistic regression model adjusting for age, time to ROSC, presence of shock, bystander CPR and initial rhythm, the investigators demonstrated that higher PaO_2 levels were significantly associated with an increased risk of in-hospital mortality (OR 1.439; 95% CI 1.028–2.015; p = 0.034) and poor neurological outcome at hospital discharge (OR 1.485; 95% CI 1.032–2.136; p = 0.033). It is important to note that recognition of the association in this instance was linked with pulse oximetry assessments and as such may be inaccurate in the setting of poor peripheral perfusion, which may lead clinicians to increase oxygen delivery, thus making PaO_2 high. In an attempt to account for this, the presence of shock defined by the requirement for a vasoactive infusion was included in the multivariate analysis. However, vasopressor support requirement in itself is not necessarily predictive of a state of poor peripheral perfusion. Thereby, a high PaO_2 is likely to be a marker of illness severity rather than a mediator of adverse outcome. Data from a Dutch database including more than 5,000 mechanically ventilated cardiac arrest patients studied associations between the worst PaO_2 measured during the first 24 h (APACHE II definition) and hospital mortality [34]. They defined hypoxia as a PaO_2 less than 60 mmHg and hyperoxia as a PaO_2 greater than 300 mmHg. They found a decreased survival with hypoxia, but no clear detrimental effect with hyperoxia [34]. However, the incidence of hyperoxia was low (3%) and this may have contributed to the findings.

All retrospective studies are limited because of the potential for unmeasured confounders that might affect outcome. With this in mind, one group attempted to identify factors associated with hyperoxia in cardiac arrest patients [24]. In an Australian single center retrospective study involving resuscitated cardiac arrest patients treated in a tertiary hospital [24], patients exposed to hyperoxia were more likely to have had an OHCA than an IHCA. Moreover, the safety and efficacy of titrated oxygen therapy following cardiac arrest should be evaluated in prospective randomized clinical trials. Therefore a phase III multicenter, randomized controlled trial, the EXACT trial (NCT03138005), has started with the aim of determining whether reducing oxygen administration to target a normal level as soon as possible following successful resuscitation from OHCA, compared to current practice of maintaining 100% oxygen, improves outcome to hospital discharge.

Carbon Dioxide Levels and Cerebral Perfusion Following ROSC

During ICU care and during the first 48 h after ROSC there is a state of persistent cerebral hypoperfusion and increased oxygen extraction. In this regard, multiple studies, using positron emission tomography [35], middle cerebral artery blood flow assessment via Doppler ultrasound [36], jugular bulb oxygen saturation [37] and cerebral oximetry [38], have all confirmed the existence of cerebral vasoconstriction, cerebral hypoperfusion and cerebral hypoxia during the early post-resuscitation period.

A likely physiological mechanism for this finding is related to sustained cerebral hypoperfusion/hypoxia secondary to impaired cerebrovascular auto-regulation [7, 39]. Such impairment may make even a normal $PaCO_2$ insufficient to achieve and sustain adequate cerebral perfusion and cerebral oxygenation. However, in humans, $PaCO_2$ is the major determinant of cerebral blood flow [40, 41] and under normal physiological conditions hypercapnia markedly increases cerebral blood flow [40]. Additionally, elevated $PaCO_2$ levels are known to have anti-convulsive, anti-inflammatory and anti-oxidant properties, which may lessen the inflammatory component of reperfusion injury [42, 43]. In contrast, hypocapnia exposure is known to increase neuronal excitability, increase cerebral oxygen consumption and reduce cerebral blood flow and therein may potentially worsen reperfusion injury if experienced.

Until recently, there was no direct evidence of the effect of targeted hypercapnia on cerebral oxygenation in resuscitated cardiac arrest patients. Recently, however, a double crossover physiological study provided insight into the impact of mild hypercapnia ($PaCO_2$ 50–55 mmHg) compared to targeted normocapnia ($PaCO_2$ 35–45 mmHg) on NIRS-derived rSO_2 [44]. Investigators studied seven resuscitated adult cardiac arrest patients at a median of 24 h and 30 min after cardiac arrest, and a median ROSC of 28 min. During normocapnia, the median $PaCO_2$ was 37 mmHg with the rSO_2 in the low or lower normal range. However, during targeted hypercapnia, with a median $PaCO_2$ of 52 mmHg, the median rSO_2 increased to normal or slightly supra-normal levels. Thus, there is controlled evidence of the potential role of mild hypercapnia to safely improve cerebral oxygenation during the early post-resuscitation period.

Immediately after ROSC, carbon dioxide levels are typically elevated but rapidly decrease with the initiation of ventilation. Currently, the International Liaison Committee on Resuscitation (ILCOR) recommend targeting normocapnia ($PaCO_2$ 40–45 mmHg) for resuscitated mechanically ventilated cardiac arrest patients [9]. Recently a group of American-based investigators performed a retrospective analysis of cardiac arrest registry data to evaluate the association between post-resuscitation $PaCO_2$ and neurological outcome [45]. Their findings revealed that 27% of patients experienced hypocapnia ($PaCO_2 \leq 30$ mmHg) only, 33% had experienced hypercapnia ($PaCO_2 \geq 50$ mmHg) only, 9% had both hypocapnia and hypercapnia exposure. Overall, 74% of cardiac arrest patients (142/193 patients) were assessed at hospital discharge and had a poor neurological outcome – a Cerebral Performance Category (CPC) score ≥ 3. While unsure of the physiological mechanism, these investigators acknowledge that cerebral blood flow was not directly measured and that hypercapnia may be reflective of lung involvement and thus dyscarbia may remain a marker of illness severity.

In a larger retrospective observational study by a team of Australian-based investigators, the association of early $PaCO_2$ values with clinical outcomes for resuscitated cardiac arrest patients was also evaluated [46]. A total of 16,542 resuscitated cardiac arrest patients admitted to 125 Australian and New Zealand ICUs between 2000 and 2011 were reviewed. However, in multivariate analysis, hypocapnic patients ($PaCO_2 < 35$ mmHg) had worse outcomes when compared with either normocapnic ($PaCO_2$ 35–45 mmHg) or hypercapnic ($PaCO_2 > 45$ mmHg) patients in terms of mortality or failure to be discharged home. Importantly, their analysis revealed that hypocapnia was independently associated with worse clinical outcomes and hypercapnia with a greater likelihood of discharge home for survivors when compared with normocapnia patients. These investigators acknowledged that 'discharged home' fails to represent a full assessment of neurological recovery; it does however represent a patient-centered end point that is likely to be bias-free and may indicate a state of sufficient neurological recovery.

The association between mean $PaCO_2$ during the early resuscitation period and in-hospital mortality and neurological outcome after cardiac arrest was addressed in a single center retrospective study of 213 patients treated with therapeutic hypothermia [47]. Of 1,704 $PaCO_2$ values obtained between ROSC and end of therapeutic hypothermia, 557 (32.7%) were hypocarbic and 321 (18.8%) were hypercarbic. Following a multivariate analysis, hypocarbia was no longer associated with poor neurological outcome. Overall, this study [47], together with previous studies [45, 46] indicate that hypocarbia has a more robust relationship with mortality and may lead to poorer neurological outcomes in survivors, though larger multicenter studies are required to explicitly demonstrate any such relationships.

More recently, the Carbon Control and Cardiac Arrest (CCC) trial (ACTRN12612000690853), a prospective phase II multicenter randomized trial showed that targeting therapeutic mild hypercapnia ($PaCO_2$ 50–55 mmHg), compared to targeting normocapnia ($PaCO_2$ 35–45 mmHg) was feasible, appeared safe and resulted in attenuation of neuron specific enolase (NSE) release (a biomarker of brain injury) in resuscitated cardiac arrest patients [48]. Of note, these findings together with existing studies, suggest that mild hypercapnia could have neuroprotective properties when applied in the immediate post-resuscitation phase.

Ongoing and Planned Studies

The Carbon Dioxide, Oxygen and Mean Arterial Pressure After Cardiac Arrest and Resuscitation (COMACARE, NCT02698917) study is a multicenter Scandinavian randomized pilot trial with a factorial design comparing high or low normal levels of oxygen (75–110 mmHg vs 150–190 mmHg), carbon dioxide (34–35 mmHg compared to 44–45 mmHg) and mean arterial blood pressure (60–70 mmHg compared to 80–100 mmHg) for a period of 36 h after ICU admission [49]. The study completed in 2017, inlcuding 120 OHCA patients with witnessed ventricular fibrillation. The endpoints include feasibility, serum NSE at 48 h, rSO_2 with NIRS and epileptic activity over the first 48 h. The study will provide pilot data on three different components regulating both cerebral blood flow and oxygen content. Results are awaited in 2018.

The Targeted Therapeutic Mild Hypercapnia After Resuscitated Cardiac Arrest (TAME, NCT03114033) trial, on the other hand, is a definitive phase III multicenter randomized controlled trial to determine whether targeted therapeutic mild hypercapnia improves neurological outcome at 6 months compared to standard care (targeted normocapnia) in resuscitated cardiac arrest patients admitted to the ICU. The study treatment period is for 24 h following enrolment (< 180 min from the time of the cardiac arrest) and patients will be followed up during the ICU stay, at hospital discharge and at 6 months and 2 years. Recruiting 1,700 patients, this will be the largest trial ever of ventilation-guided therapy conducted involving resuscitated cardiac arrest patients admitted to the ICU. If the TAME Cardiac Arrest trial confirms that targeted therapeutic mild hypercapnia is effective, the induction of mild hypercapnia would be an easy intervention for most cardiac arrest patients at minimal cost that, in turn, will improve the lives of many cardiac arrest survivors and transform clinical practice.

Conclusion

The most important determinant of limiting brain hypoxia during CPR seems to be the performance of uninterrupted and high quality chest compressions. Guidelines recommend using 100% oxygen during CPR even though it seems to be supported by limited evidence. After ROSC, the best available evidence for oxygen and carbon dioxide management suggests that extreme hyperoxia and hypocapnia may cause harm and should be avoided. Apart from such considerations, there remains uncertainty as to which levels of oxygen and carbon dioxide should be targeted. Importantly, with the findings of the COMACARE trial due to be released in early 2018 and the initiation of the TAME cardiac arrest trial, evidence to support clinical decisions related to oxygen and carbon dioxide management for adult cardiac arrest patients admitted to the ICU will soon increase.

References

1. Grasner JT, Lefering R, Koster RW et al (2016) Eureca ONE-27 nations, ONE europe, ONE registry: a prospective one month analysis of out-of-hospital cardiac arrest outcomes in 27 countries in europe. Resuscitation 105:188–195
2. Bottiger BW, Grasner JT, Castren M (2014) Sudden cardiac death: good perspectives with this major health care issue. Intensive Care Med 40:907–909
3. Lund-Kordahl I, Olasveengen TM, Lorem T, Samdal M, Wik L, Sunde K (2010) Improving outcome after out-of-hospital cardiac arrest by strengthening weak links of the local Chain of

Survival; quality of advanced life support and post-resuscitation care. Resuscitation 81:422–426

4. Lopez-Herce J, Carrillo A (2012) How can we improve the results of cardiopulmonary resuscitation in out-of-hospital cardiac arrest in children? Dispatcher-assisted cardiopulmonary resuscitation is a link in the chain of survival. Crit Care Med 40:1646–1647

5. Larsen MP, Eisenberg MS, Cummins RO, Hallstrom AP (1993) Predicting survival from out-of-hospital cardiac arrest: a graphic model. Ann Emerg Med 22:1652–1658

6. Soar J, Nolan JP, Bottiger BW et al (2015) European resuscitation council guidelines for resuscitation 2015: section 3. adult advanced life support. Resuscitation 95:100–147

7. Lemiale V, Dumas F, Mongardon N et al (2013) Intensive care unit mortality after cardiac arrest: the relative contribution of shock and brain injury in a large cohort. Intensive Care Med 39:1972–1980

8. Sekhon MS, Ainslie PN, Griesdale DE (2017) Clinical pathophysiology of hypoxic ischemic brain injury after cardiac arrest: a "two-hit" model. Crit Care 21:90

9. Nolan JP, Soar J, Cariou A et al (2015) European Resuscitation Council and European Society of Intensive Care Medicine 2015 guidelines for post-resuscitation care. Intensive Care Med 41:2039–2056

10. Neumar RW (2011) Optimal oxygenation during and after cardiopulmonary resuscitation. Curr Opin Crit Care 17:236–240

11. Imberti R, Bellinzona G, Riccardi F, Pagani M, Langer M (2003) Cerebral perfusion pressure and cerebral tissue oxygen tension in a patient during cardiopulmonary resuscitation. Intensive Care Med 29:1016–1019

12. Genbrugge C, Eertmans W, Jans F, Boer W, Dens J, De Deyne C (2017) Regional cerebral saturation monitoring during withdrawal of life support until death. Resuscitation 121:147–150

13. Skrifvars MB, Nurmi J, Ikola K, Saarinen K, Castren M (2006) Reduced survival following resuscitation in patients with documented clinically abnormal observations prior to in-hospital cardiac arrest. Resuscitation 70:215–222

14. Nelskyla A, Nurmi J, Jousi M et al (2017) The effect of 50% compared to 100% inspired oxygen fraction on brain oxygenation and post cardiac arrest mitochondrial function in experimental cardiac arrest. Resuscitation 116:1–7

15. Yu J, Ramadeen A, Tsui AK et al (2013) Quantitative assessment of brain microvascular and tissue oxygenation during cardiac arrest and resuscitation in pigs. Anaesthesia 68:723–735

16. Yeh ST, Cawley RJ, Aune SE, Angelos MG (2009) Oxygen requirement during cardiopulmonary resuscitation (CPR) to effect return of spontaneous circulation. Resuscitation 80:951–955

17. Steen S, Liao Q, Pierre L, Paskevicius A, Sjoberg T (2003) The critical importance of minimal delay between chest compressions and subsequent defibrillation: a haemodynamic explanation. Resuscitation 58:249–258

18. Svensson L, Bohm K, Castren M et al (2010) Compression-only CPR or standard CPR in out-of-hospital cardiac arrest. N Engl J Med 363:434–442

19. Rosenthal G, Hemphill JC 3rd, Sorani M et al (2008) Brain tissue oxygen tension is more indicative of oxygen diffusion than oxygen delivery and metabolism in patients with traumatic brain injury. Crit Care Med 36:1917–1924

20. Spindelboeck W, Schindler O, Moser A et al (2013) Increasing arterial oxygen partial pressure during cardiopulmonary resuscitation is associated with improved rates of hospital admission. Resuscitation 84:770–775

21. Spindelboeck W, Gemes G, Strasser C et al (2016) Arterial blood gases during and their dynamic changes after cardiopulmonary resuscitation: a prospective clinical study. Resuscitation 106:24–29

22. Cournoyer A, Iseppon M, Chauny JM, Denault A, Cossette S, Notebaert E (2016) Near-infrared spectroscopy monitoring during cardiac arrest: a systematic review and meta-analysis. Acad Emerg Med 23:851–862

23. Ito N, Nishiyama K, Callaway CW et al (2014) Noninvasive regional cerebral oxygen saturation for neurological prognostication of patients with out-of-hospital cardiac arrest: a prospective multicenter observational study. Resuscitation 85:778–784

24. Touma O, Davies M (2013) The prognostic value of end tidal carbon dioxide during cardiac arrest: a systematic review. Resuscitation 84:1470–1479

25. Trzeciak S, Jones AE, Kilgannon JH et al (2009) Significance of arterial hypotension after resuscitation from cardiac arrest. Crit Care Med 37:2895–2903

26. Young P, Bailey M, Bellomo R et al (2014) HyperOxic Therapy OR NormOxic Therapy after out-of-hospital cardiac arrest (HOT OR NOT): a randomised controlled feasibility trial. Resuscitation 85:1686–1691

27. Nelskyla A, Parr MJ, Skrifvars MB (2013) Prevalence and factors correlating with hyperoxia exposure following cardiac arrest – an observational single centre study. Scand J Trauma Resusc Emerg Med 21:35

28. Kuisma M, Boyd J, Voipio V, Alaspaa A, Roine RO, Rosenberg P (2006) Comparison of 30 and the 100% inspired oxygen concentrations during early post-resuscitation period: a randomised controlled pilot study. Resuscitation 69:199–206

29. Kilgannon JH, Jones AE, Shapiro NI et al (2010) Association between arterial hyperoxia following resuscitation from cardiac arrest and in-hospital mortality. JAMA 303:2165–2171

30. Kilgannon JH, Jones AE, Parrillo JE et al (2011) Relationship between supranormal oxygen tension and outcome after resuscitation from cardiac arrest. Circulation 123:2717–2722

31. Bellomo R, Bailey M, Eastwood GM et al (2011) Arterial hyperoxia and in-hospital mortality after resuscitation from cardiac arrest. Crit Care 15:R90

32. Yenari MA, Han HS (2012) Neuroprotective mechanisms of hypothermia in brain ischaemia. Nat Rev Neurosci 13:267–278

33. Janz DR, Hollenbeck RD, Pollock JS, McPherson JA, Rice TW (2012) Hyperoxia is associated with increased mortality in patients treated with mild therapeutic hypothermia after sudden cardiac arrest. Crit Care Med 40:3135–3139

34. Helmerhorst HJ, Roos-Blom MJ, van Westerloo DJ, Abu-Hanna A, de Keizer NF, de Jonge E (2015) Associations of arterial carbon dioxide and arterial oxygen concentrations with hospital mortality after resuscitation from cardiac arrest. Crit Care 19:348

35. Edgren E, Enblad P, Grenvik A et al (2003) Cerebral blood flow and metabolism after cardiopulmonary resuscitation. Resuscitation 57:161–170

36. Buunk G, van der Hoeven JG, Meinders AE (1999) Prognostic significance of the difference between mixed venous and jugular bulb oxygen saturation. Resuscitation 41:257–262

37. Beckstead JE, Tweed WA, Lee J, MacKeen WL (1978) Cerebral blood flow and metabolism in man following cardiac arrest. Stroke 9:569–573

38. Storm C, Leithner C, Krannich A et al (2014) Regional cerebral oxygen saturation after cardiac arrest in 60 patients – a prospective outcome study. Resuscitation 85:1037–1041

39. Wiklund L, Martijn C, Miclescu A, Semenas E, Rubertsson S, Sharma HS (2012) Central nervous tissue damage after hypoxia and reperfusion in conjunction with cardiac arrest and cardiopulmonary resuscitation: mechanisms of action and possibilities for mitigation. Int Rev Neurobiol 102:173–187

40. O'Croinin D, Ni Chonghaile M, Higgins B, Laffey JG (2005) Bench-to-bedside review: permissive hypercapnia. Crit Care 9:51–59

41. Curley G, Laffey JG, Kavanagh BP (2010) Bench-to-bedside review: carbon dioxide. Crit Care 14:220

42. Gyarfas K, Pollock GH, Stein SN (1949) Central inhibitory effects of carbon dioxide; convulsive phenomena. Proc Soc Exp Biol Med 70:292

43. Shoja MM, Tubbs RS, Shokouhi G, Loukas M, Ghabili K, Ansarin K (2008) The potential role of carbon dioxide in the neuroimmunoendocrine changes following cerebral ischemia. Life Sci 83:381–387

44. Eastwood GM, Tanaka A, Bellomo R (2016) Cerebral oxygenation in mechanically ventilated early cardiac arrest survivors: the impact of hypercapnia. Resuscitation 102:11–16

45. Roberts BW, Kilgannon JH, Chansky ME, Mittal N, Wooden J, Trzeciak S (2013) Association between postresuscitation partial pressure of arterial carbon dioxide and neurological outcome in patients with post-cardiac arrest syndrome. Circulation 127:2107–2113

46. Schneider AG, Eastwood GM, Bellomo R et al (2013) Arterial carbon dioxide tension and outcome in patients admitted to the intensive care unit after cardiac arrest. Resuscitation 84:927–934

47. Lee BK, Jeung KW, Lee HY et al (2014) Association between mean arterial blood gas tension and outcome in cardiac arrest patients treated with therapeutic hypothermia. Am J Emerg Med 32:55–60

48. Eastwood GM, Schneider AG, Suzuki S et al (2016) Targeted therapeutic mild hypercapnia after cardiac arrest: a phase II multi-centre randomised controlled trial (the CCC trial). Resuscitation 104:83–90

49. Jakkula P, Reinikainen M, Hästbacka J et al (2017) Targeting low- or high-normal Carbon dioxide, Oxygen, and Mean arterial pressure After Cardiac Arrest and Resuscitation: study protocol for a randomized pilot trial. Trials 18:507

Outcome after Cardiopulmonary Resuscitation

C. J. R. Gough and J. P. Nolan

Introduction

Cardiac arrest is an absolute medical emergency. Unless effective cardiopulmonary resuscitation (CPR) is commenced within minutes, death or permanent brain injury will follow. Almost all critical care clinicians will treat cardiac arrest patients. This chapter summarizes the incidence, trends, and short- and long-term survival from both out-of-hospital (OHCA) and in-hospital (IHCA) cardiac arrest.

Out-of-Hospital Cardiac Arrest

Incidence

The incidence of emergency medical services (EMS)-treated OHCA varies significantly around the world (Table 1). A large review of 67 prospective studies, of over 100 million patients, identified wide variation in incidence of cardiac arrest across the globe, but the overall incidence for adults was 62 cases per 100,000 person-years, with the highest rates in North America (71 per 100,000 person-years) and the lowest rates in Asia (50 per 100,000 person-years) [1]. Roughly three quarters of cardiac arrests had a cardiac cause.

There is substantial variation in cardiac arrest incidence and survival even within contained regions such as North America. A study by the Resuscitation Outcomes

C. J. R. Gough
Department of Anaesthesia and Intensive Care Medicine, Royal United Hospital
Bath, UK

J. P. Nolan (✉)
Department of Anaesthesia and Intensive Care Medicine, Royal United Hospital
Bath, UK
School of Clinical Sciences, University of Bristol
Bristol, UK
e-mail: jerry.nolan@nhs.net

© Springer International Publishing AG 2018   155
J.-L. Vincent (ed.), *Annual Update in Intensive Care and Emergency Medicine 2018*,
Annual Update in Intensive Care and Emergency Medicine,
https://doi.org/10.1007/978-3-319-73670-9_13

Table 1 International survival rates for out-of-hospital cardiac arrest (OHCA). The Netherlands study included only OHCA of a cardiac cause. The Japanese survival data were for neurologically favorable survival (Cerebral Performance Category 1–2). The data cited are taken from the most recent year cited in each publication

Country	First author [ref]	Year	Treated cardiac arrests	Bystander CPR (%)	Survival all rhythms (%)	Survival VF/pVT (%)	Survival PEA/ asystole (%)
United States (CARES)	Chan [6]	2012	16,614	36.3	9.8	27.9	4.4
United States (ROC)	Daya [7]	2010	11,215	40.1	10.4	29.3	4.3
Denmark (Copenhagen)	Wissenberg [8]	2010	1,906	44.9	10.8	32.0	2.4
France (Paris)	Bougouin [9]	2012	3,816	45.0	7.5	25.0	2.4
Netherlands (Amsterdam)	Blom [10]	2012	874	81.2	20.8	41.4	2.7
England	Hawkes [11]	2014	28,729	55.2	7.9	N/A	N/A
Japan	Okubo [12]	2014	97,024	50.6	2.3	N/A	N/A
Denmark	Rajan [13]	2012	N/A	42.8	9.3	35.7	2.3*

*Estimated from the data available; *CPR*: cardiopulmonary resuscitation; *PEA*: pulseless electrical activity; *VF*: ventricular fibrillation; *pVT*: pulseless ventricular tachycardia; *N/A*: not available; *CARES*: Cardiac Arrest Registry to Enhance Survival; *ROC*: Resuscitation Outcomes Consortium

Consortium of 10 North American sites (eight in the United States and two in Canada) showed considerable variation in the incidence and outcome of EMS-assessed OHCA [2]. Across the sites, OHCA incidence ranged from 71.8 to 159.0 per 100,000, while survival to discharge rates ranged from 1.1 to 8.1%. A 2016 analysis of the Cardiac Arrest Registry to Enhance Survival (CARES) database that included 132 US counties showed considerable variation (3.4–22.0%) in survival to hospital discharge [3]. Local rates of both bystander CPR and automated external defibrillator (AED) use were associated with higher survival rates (p < 0.001). The European Registry of Cardiac Arrest (EuReCa) ONE study, published in 2016, included 10,672 patients with OHCA across 248 regions in 27 European countries. It reported an incidence of EMS-treated OHCA ranging from 19.0 to 104.0 per 100,000 people per year, with an overall survival of 10.3% [4].

The majority of survivors of cardiac arrest have an initial rhythm of ventricular fibrillation (VF) or pulseless ventricular tachycardia (pVT). However, only around 15% of OHCAs occur in a public location, with the rest occurring in the home (75%) or in other residential facilities (10%) [5]. Data from nearly 13,000 OHCAs in the US show that over half of cardiac arrests occurring in public places are bystander-witnessed (55%), compared to only 35% of those in the home. Subsequently, the initial monitored rhythm was VF/pVT in 51% of OHCA in public places, compared with 22% of those in the home. The reflection of these differences in the rate of survival to hospital discharge is profound: 6% for cardiac arrests occurring at home, compared to 17% for those occurring in public places.

Trends

The incidence of EMS-treated OHCA is decreasing over time, whereas the survival rate is increasing. A Danish study of 19,468 EMS-treated cardiac arrests with a likely cardiac cause, between 2001 and 2010, documented a decrease in the incidence of EMS-treated OHCA from 40 to 34 per 100,000 people, while 30-day survival increased from 3.5 to 10.8% [8]. A substantial increase in bystander CPR rates (21.1 to 44.9%) likely contributed significantly to the increased survival rate. There has been an extensive national initiative in Denmark to try and increase the rates of bystander CPR rates, including mandatory resuscitation training in elementary schools and mandatory resuscitation training before acquiring a driving license.

Combined with several other interventions, these factors may have contributed to the increase in bystander CPR rates.

In the US, a large study of 1,190,860 patients, hospitalized with a diagnosis of cardiac arrest between 2001 and 2009, documented that in-hospital mortality decreased each year from 69.6 in 2001 to 57.8% in 2009 [14]. Also in North America, the Resuscitation Outcomes Consortium reported an increasing rate of survival to discharge (8.2 to 10.4%) for treated OHCA between 2006 and 2010, from 47,148 cases [7], and a CARES review of 70,027 cases between 2005 and 2012 also found an increase in adjusted-survival from 5.7 to 8.3%, with an unadjusted survival increase to 9.8% [6]. Adjusted survival was used to correct for changes over time in patient, EMS and event characteristics, each of which is known to affect survival. For example, adjustments were made for the increased rate of bystander CPR and EMS-witnessed events seen over time, and for the reduced rate of VT/pVT as the initial rhythm.

Investigators report relatively low survival rates following OHCA in Asia, but there is evidence that survival rates are improving in Japan. An analysis of 861,756 cases in the All-Japan registry identified an increase in neurologically favorable survival from 1.1 to 2.3% between 2005 and 2014 for patients with OHCA of medical origin [12]. For patients who had a bystander-witnessed cardiac arrest, the neurologically favorable survival rates increased from 2.4 to 5.1%. In an analysis of the All-Japan registry that included 547,153 bystander-witnessed VF OHCAs between 2005 and 2009, the neurologically favorable survival rate increased from 9.8 to 20.6% (p < 0.001) [15].

The London Ambulance Service documented an increase in survival rates from EMS-treated OHCA from 3.7% in 2007/8 to 9% in 2015/16. In a subset of patients with a likely cardiac cause, in VF or VT, which was bystander-witnessed (the so called 'Utstein' subgroup), the survival rates rose from 5% in 2001/2, to 12% in 2007/8, to 31.5% in 2015/16 [16].

In the UK, retrospective analysis of the Intensive Care National Audit and Research Centre (ICNARC) database between 2004 and 2014 for all critical care admissions following CPR, identified 29,621 patients with OHCA [17]. Among the 116 intensive care units (ICUs) that contributed throughout this period, the absolute number of admissions for OHCA increased from 1,582 in 2004 to 4,147 in 2014. During this time, the hospital mortality decreased from 70.1 to 66.4% (P = 0.024), with a case mix-adjusted odds ratio per year of 0.96 (p < 0.001).

Neurological Outcomes

Survival is a broad term and many studies now focus on patient-centered outcomes, such as neurological outcomes. The two main methods of assessing neurological outcomes are the Cerebral Performance Category (CPC) (Table 2), and the Modified Rankin Scale (mRS) (Table 3).

Most studies define a CPC of 1–2 or a mRS of 0–3 as good neurological outcome. However, both of these scales are relatively crude tools with which to measure neurological outcome. Although many studies conclude that approximately 75% of OHCA survivors have a good neurological outcome based on these scales, many of these patients will have subtle impairment of cognitive function that is not detected by the CPC or mRS [18].

Although cardiac arrest is often considered to be particularly associated with poor neurological outcomes, it is important to recognize that other acute medical conditions may also impact neurological outcome. In a secondary analysis of the Targeted Temperature Management (TTM) trial, long-term neurological outcomes in the two groups of OHCA patients treated with TTM at a target temperature of 33 °C or 36 °C were compared with ST-segment-elevation myocardial infarction (STEMI) patients who had not had a cardiac arrest [19]. Cognitive impairment, specifically memory, assessed using the Rivermead Behavioral Memory Test, and executive functions, assessed using the Frontal Assessment Battery, were similarly affected in cardiac arrest survivors and STEMI control groups, with roughly 80% of patients either normal or mildly impaired (Fig. 1).

Several investigators have looked in more detail at neurological outcomes using the mRS tool. The Resuscitation Outcomes Consortium group assessed 799 survivors from cardiac arrest at the point of hospital discharge [20]. They found that 72.9% of survivors had mRS scores of 0–3, and 46.3% of these had mRS scores of 0–1. The second study, investigating amiodarone, lidocaine or placebo for OHCA, included 709 survivors; 74.1% had mRS scores of 0–3 and 40.4% had scores of 0–1 [21]. Finally, a trial comparing continuous with interrupted chest com-

Table 2 Cerebral Performance Category (CPC) scale

1	Conscious and alert with normal function or only slight disability
2	Conscious and alert with moderate disability
3	Conscious with severe disability
4	Comatose or persistent vegetative state
5	Brain dead or death from other causes

Table 3 The Modified Rankin Scale (mRS)

0	No symptoms
1	Some symptoms but able to do usual activities
2	Slight disability; unable to do all previous activities, but independent
3	Moderate disability; requiring some help, but able to walk without help
4	Moderately severe disability; unable to walk or attend to bodily needs without assistance
5	Severe disability; bedridden, incontinent and needs constant nursing care
6	Dead

pressions, which included more patients at an earlier stage in cardiac arrest, assessed 2,268 survivors; 76% had mRS scores of 0–3 and 50.6% had scores of 0–1 [22].

What is clear throughout these studies is that, when assessed using CPC or mRS, the majority of survivors will have 'good' neurological recovery. Furthermore, the functional state of many of these survivors improves over time. In a trial that retrospectively assessed functional outcome among 681 survivors over a 6-month period, 30% showed a significant change in functional outcome between one and six months after OHCA, with 12% improving, 1% deteriorating and 17% dying [23]. Of the patients who were CPC 2 at one month, 52% had improved to CPC 1 by six months. Of the patients who were CPC 3 at one month, 38% had improved by six months (Fig. 2).

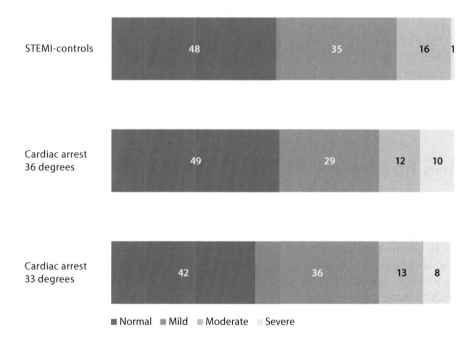

Fig. 1 Rivermead Behavior Memory Test at 180 days, comparing cardiac arrest patients with ST-elevation myocardial infarction (STEMI)-control patients without cardiac arrest. Adapted from [19]

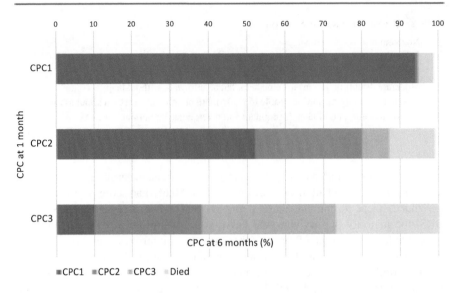

Fig. 2 Cerebral Performance Category (CPC) at six months, grouped by CPC at one month. For example, for those who were CPC 2 at one month (middle row), by six months 52% were CPC 1, 28% CPC 2, 7% CPC 3, and 12% had died. Data from [23]

The trend in neurological outcomes is also improving with time. In Oslo, all OHCAs during three distinct 2-year periods, 1996–1998, 2001–2003 and 2004–2005, were analyzed, with over 400 patients in each period [24]. Overall survival increased from 7% in the first period to 13% in the last (p = 0.002), and survival with favorable neurological outcome, defined as CPC 1–2, also increased (6%, 9%, 12% for the three periods, respectively, p = 0.001). For those admitted to ICU, favorable neurological survival was 26, 30 and 43% in the three periods, respectively (p = 0.005).

Long-Term Survival

With increasing numbers of patients surviving to hospital discharge, and surviving with good neurological function, the long-term outcomes of these patients is important.

In Denmark, among 796 cardiac arrest survivors between 2001 and 2011 who had been employed before suffering a cardiac arrest, 610 (76.6%) returned to work in a median time of 4 months [25]. Of these survivors, 74.6% remained employed without using any sick leave for the first 6 months after returning to work, and the proportion of survivors returning to work increased over time, from 66.1% in 2001–2005, to 78.1% in 2006–2011 (p = 0.002). Those patients more likely to return to work were younger male patients in the later years of the study, with bystander witnessed collapse and bystander CPR.

A recent large Australian study of 3,449 OHCA survivors between 2000 and 2014 identified a mean survival of 11.9 years, with a one-year survival rate of 92.2% [26]. Ten- and 15-year survival rates were 70.1 and 62.3%. After the first 5 years post-arrest, the standardized mortality rate of the survivors had approached that of the standard population.

In-Hospital Cardiac Arrest

Incidence

IHCA rates are difficult to establish, as they are rarely published. A 2007 review of the available literature on IHCA studies estimated the incidence to be 1–5 events per 1,000 hospital admissions [27]. It also identified the survival to hospital discharge rate to be reported most commonly as 15–20%. The American Heart Association Get with the Guidelines-Resuscitation (AHA GWTG-R) registry includes much data on IHCA in the US [28]. From this, the incidence of IHCA has been estimated as 4.0 per 1,000 admissions and the initial cardiac arrest rhythm was asystole or pulseless electrical activity (PEA) in 79.3% of cases, with VF/pVT in the remainder [29, 30]. The risk-adjusted rate of survival to discharge was 22.3%. Hospitals with higher case-survival rates also had lower cardiac arrest incidence (p = 0.003), possibly contributed to by the hospital's nurse-to-bed ratio (p = 0.03) [30]. It is possible that hospitals with the highest survival rates are better at preventing cardiac arrest, or more likely to implement do-not-attempt CPR decisions for patients with the lowest chances of survival.

The majority of hospitals in the UK collect data on IHCA and submit it to the UK National Cardiac Arrest Audit (NCAA), which is the largest registry of IHCA after the GWTG-R. The NCAA includes IHCAs that trigger a resuscitation team alert, and in whom either chest compressions or defibrillation are delivered (in contrast to the GWTG-R, which attempts to capture all IHCAs). Cardiac arrests will not therefore be captured by NCAA if no resuscitation team is called, for example some occurring in ICUs or operating rooms, where they may be managed without the resuscitation team. The cardiac arrest incidence would therefore be expected to be lower than that documented by the GWTG-R registry. The first analysis of the NCAA registry, covering 144 acute hospitals over two years (2011–2013), including 22,628 patients, found an overall cardiac arrest incidence of 1.6 per 1,000 hospital admissions [31]. The overall unadjusted survival to hospital discharge was 18.4%, but was 49.0% in those with VF/pVT as the first monitored rhythm, compared with 10.5% in those with asystole/PEA as the first monitored rhythm. VF/pVT was the presenting rhythm in 16.9% of cases.

In China, a recent study prospectively evaluated the incidence and outcome of IHCA over a 1-year period from 12 hospitals in Beijing. Of 582,242 hospital admissions, the IHCA incidence was 17.5 per 1,000 admissions, with a treated cardiac arrest incidence of 4.6 per 1,000 admissions [32]. The initial rhythm was VF/pVT in 24.0% of cases and, overall, 9.1% of patients survived to hospital discharge.

Trends

An analysis of the US GWTG-R registry from 2000 to 2009 documented an increase in risk-adjusted survival to discharge from 13.7 to 22.3% (p < 0.001) [30]. Roughly 80% of IHCAs were due to asystole or PEA and this proportion has been increasing over time (p < 0.001). Another recent study in the US that assessed solely IHCA in 235,959 patients aged 18–64 documented an increase in survival to hospital discharge from 27.4% in 2007 to 32.8% in 2012 (p < 0.001), with 23.3% of patients having an initial shockable rhythm [33]. Lack of health insurance and weekend admissions were both associated with lower adjusted odds of survival.

In the UK, retrospective analysis of the ICNARC database between 2004 and 2014 for all critical care admissions following CPR identified 33,796 patients with IHCA [17]. During this time, the hospital mortality decreased from 70.4 to 60.3% (p < 0.001). The number of ICUs contributing data increased during the study period, but 116 hospitals contributed data throughout. From these, the contribution of IHCA to the total number of ICU admissions rose from 2.1 to 2.7% between 2004 and 2014, while OHCA and IHCA combined contributed 13.2% of all ventilated admissions in 2014, up from 9.3% in 2004. During this time, length of hospital stay decreased for IHCA survivors, from 27.0 to 22.0 days (p < 0.001), but the ICU stay increased for survivors (3.5 to 5.0 days; p < 0.001) and non-survivors (1.3 to 2.2 days; p < 0.001). This increase in ICU stay for non-survivors is likely at least partly due to implementation of guidelines stating that prognostication is not reliable until at least 72 h after cardiac arrest [34].

Long-term outcomes from IHCA have been assessed and compared with matched controls in a single-institution study. Of the 20% of IHCA patients who survived to discharge, 59% survived one year, versus 82% for the matched controls (p < 0.0001) [35]. The highest mortality rate was within 90 days of discharge (hazard ratio [HR] 2.9; p < 0.0001), but this varied significantly by discharge destination. Patients who were discharged home without care services had the same survival rate as non-IHCA controls. However, patients discharged to long-term hospital care or hospice had a much higher mortality than non-IHCA controls (HR 3.9 and 20.3 respectively; p < 0.0001).

Conclusion

The incidence of EMS-treated OHCA is decreasing and survival is increasing. Survival to hospital discharge for OHCA is roughly 10% for all rhythms, and significantly higher when VF/pVT is the initial rhythm. Neurologically favorable survival is documented in roughly 75% of survivors at hospital discharge, and 10–15% of these patients will show improvement over time. Roughly three quarters of survivors who were working prior to their cardiac arrest will return to work, but mortality rates remain higher than non-cardiac arrest controls for a number of years.

Survival from IHCA is also increasing, with a survival rate currently of approximately 20% for all rhythms, but approximately 50% for those in whom VF/pVT is the initial rhythm. The one-year survival of discharged patients is roughly 60%, but is similar to non-cardiac arrest controls in survivors with good neurological recovery who do not need additional care services.

References

1. Berdowski J, Berg RA, Tijssen JG, Koster RW (2010) Global incidences of out-of-hospital cardiac arrest and survival rates: systematic review of 67 prospective studies. Resuscitation 81:1479–1487
2. Nichol G, Thomas E, Callaway CW et al (2008) Regional variation in out-of-hospital cardiac arrest incidence and outcome. JAMA 300:1423–1431
3. Girotra S, van Diepen S, Nallamothu BK et al (2016) Regional variation in out-of-hospital cardiac arrest survival in the United States. Circulation 133:2159–2168
4. Grasner JT, Lefering R, Koster RW et al (2016) EuReCa ONE-27 Nations, ONE Europe, ONE Registry: a prospective one month analysis of out-of-hospital cardiac arrest outcomes in 27 countries in Europe. Resuscitation 105:188–195
5. Weisfeldt ML, Everson-Stewart S, Sitlani C et al (2011) Ventricular tachyarrhythmias after cardiac arrest in public versus at home. N Engl J Med 364:313–321
6. Chan PS, McNally B, Tang F, Kellermann A, Group CS (2014) Recent trends in survival from out-of-hospital cardiac arrest in the United States. Circulation 130:1876–1882
7. Daya MR, Schmicker RH, Zive DM et al (2015) Out-of-hospital cardiac arrest survival improving over time: results from the Resuscitation Outcomes Consortium (ROC). Resuscitation 91:108–115
8. Wissenberg M, Lippert FK, Folke F et al (2013) Association of national initiatives to improve cardiac arrest management with rates of bystander intervention and patient survival after out-of-hospital cardiac arrest. JAMA 310:1377–1384
9. Bougouin W, Lamhaut L, Marijon E et al (2014) Characteristics and prognosis of sudden cardiac death in greater paris : population-based approach from the paris sudden death expertise center (paris-SDEC). Intensive Care Med 40:846–854
10. Blom MT, Beesems SG, Homma PC et al (2014) Improved survival after out-of-hospital cardiac arrest and use of automated external defibrillators. Circulation 130:1868–1875
11. Hawkes C, Booth S, Ji C et al (2017) Epidemiology and outcomes from out-of-hospital cardiac arrests in England. Resuscitation 110:133–140
12. Okubo M, Kiyohara K, Iwami T, Callaway CW, Kitamura T (2017) Nationwide and regional trends in survival from out-of-hospital cardiac arrest in Japan: A 10-year cohort study from 2005 to 2014. Resuscitation 115:120–128
13. Rajan S, Folke F, Hansen SM et al (2017) Incidence and survival outcome according to heart rhythm during resuscitation attempt in out-of-hospital cardiac arrest patients with presumed cardiac etiology. Resuscitation 114:157–163
14. Fugate JE, Brinjikji W, Mandrekar JN et al (2012) Post-cardiac arrest mortality is declining: a study of the US National Inpatient Sample 2001 to 2009. Circulation 126:546–550
15. Kitamura T, Iwami T, Kawamura T et al (2012) Nationwide improvements in survival from out-of-hospital cardiac arrest in Japan. Circulation 126:2834–2843
16. Virdi G, Picton S, Fothergill R, Whitbread M (2016) Cardiac arrest annual report: 2015/16. London Ambulance Service, London
17. Nolan JP, Ferrando P, Soar J et al (2016) Increasing survival after admission to UK critical care units following cardiopulmonary resuscitation. Crit Care 20:219
18. Cronberg T, Lilja G, Horn J et al (2015) Neurologic function and health-related quality of life in patients following targeted temperature management at 33 degrees C vs 36 degrees C after out-of-hospital cardiac arrest: a randomized clinical trial. JAMA Neurol 72:634–641

19. Lilja G, Nielsen N, Friberg H et al (2015) Cognitive function in survivors of out-of-hospital cardiac arrest after target temperature management at 33 degrees C versus 36 degrees C. Circulation 131:1340–1349

20. Stiell IG, Nichol G, Leroux BG et al (2011) Early versus later rhythm analysis in patients with out-of-hospital cardiac arrest. N Engl J Med 365:787–797

21. Kudenchuk PJ, Brown SP, Daya M et al (2016) Amiodarone, lidocaine, or placebo in out-of-hospital cardiac arrest. N Engl J Med 374:1711–1722

22. Nichol G, Leroux B, Wang H et al (2015) Trial of continuous or interrupted chest compressions during CPR. N Engl J Med 373:2203–2214

23. Arrich J, Zeiner A, Sterz F et al (2009) Factors associated with a change in functional outcome between one month and six months after cardiac arrest: a retrospective cohort study. Resuscitation 80:876–880

24. Lund-Kordahl I, Olasveengen TM, Lorem T, Samdal M, Wik L, Sunde K (2010) Improving outcome after out-of-hospital cardiac arrest by strengthening weak links of the local Chain of Survival; quality of advanced life support and post-resuscitation care. Resuscitation 81:422–426

25. Kragholm K, Wissenberg M, Mortensen RN et al (2015) Return to work in out-of-hospital cardiac arrest survivors: a nationwide register-based follow-up study. Circulation 131:1682–1690

26. Andrew E, Nehme Z, Wolfe R, Bernard S, Smith K (2017) Long-term survival following out-of-hospital cardiac arrest. Heart 103:1104–1110

27. Sandroni C, Nolan J, Cavallaro F, Antonelli M (2007) In-hospital cardiac arrest: incidence, prognosis and possible measures to improve survival. Intensive Care Med 33:237–245

28. Peberdy MA, Kaye W, Ornato JP et al (2003) Cardiopulmonary resuscitation of adults in the hospital: a report of 14720 cardiac arrests from the National Registry of Cardiopulmonary Resuscitation. Resuscitation 58:297–308

29. Chen LM, Nallamothu BK, Spertus JA, Li Y, Chan PS (2013) Association between a hospital's rate of cardiac arrest incidence and cardiac arrest survival. JAMA Intern Med 173:1186–1195

30. Girotra S, Nallamothu BK, Spertus JA et al (2012) Trends in survival after in-hospital cardiac arrest. N Engl J Med 367:1912–1920

31. Nolan JP, Soar J, Smith GB et al (2014) Incidence and outcome of in-hospital cardiac arrest in the United Kingdom National Cardiac Arrest Audit. Resuscitation 85:987–992

32. Shao F, Li CS, Liang LR et al (2016) Incidence and outcome of adult in-hospital cardiac arrest in Beijing, China. Resuscitation 102:51–56

33. Mallikethi-Reddy S, Briasoulis A, Akintoye E et al (2017) Incidence and survival after in-hospital cardiopulmonary resuscitation in nonelderly adults: US experience, 2007 to 2012. Circ Cardiovasc Qual Outcomes 10:e003194

34. Nolan JP, Soar J, Cariou A et al (2015) European resuscitation council and European Society of Intensive Care Medicine guidelines for post-resuscitation care 2015: section 5 of the European Resuscitation Council Guidelines for Resuscitation 2015. Resuscitation 95:202–222

35. Feingold P, Mina MJ, Burke RM et al (2016) Long-term survival following in-hospital cardiac arrest: a matched cohort study. Resuscitation 99:72–78

Medico-economic Evaluation of Out-of-hospital Cardiac Arrest Patient Management

G. Geri

Introduction

Each year, about 360,000 adult people in the United States suffer an out-of-hospital cardiac arrest (OHCA) [1]. The OHCA incidence rate varies from 35 up to 84.0 per 100,000 population in European and North-American countries [2]. While survival has increased in the past years, global outcome remains poor due to both neurological damage and post-cardiac arrest organ failure.

The management of OHCA patients requires the coordination of prehospital, in-hospital and post-discharge teams. In most health systems, Emergency Medical Services (EMS) personnel, including firefighters and paramedics, are involved in the prehospital assessment and treatment of these patients [3, 4], while interventions, such as targeted temperature management (TTM) or percutaneous coronary angiography, are delivered by in-hospital clinicians [5–8]. Although increased coordination of care is widely believed to have led to significant improvements in the survival of cardiac arrest patients, these systems have additional financial cost as well. In addition to survival and qualitative indicators of health-related quality of life, costs related to OHCA management should be part of research as OHCA care requires many, very specific interventions and is associated with poor long-term outcomes. The need to include costs in research about cardiac arrest has been highlighted recently [9] and costs should be considered as a primary outcome or as a secondary outcome in both randomized controlled trials and observational studies.

G. Geri (✉)
Medical Intensive Care Unit, Assistance Publique Hôpitaux de Paris, Ambroise Paré Hospital
Boulogne-Billancourt, France
Renal and Cardiovascular Epidemiology Team, Centre de recherché en Epidémiologie et Santé des Populations, INSERM U1018
Villejuif, France
Versailles Saint Quentin University
Versailles, France
e-mail: guillaume.geri@aphp.fr

© Springer International Publishing AG 2018   165
J.-L. Vincent (ed.), *Annual Update in Intensive Care and Emergency Medicine 2018*,
Annual Update in Intensive Care and Emergency Medicine,
https://doi.org/10.1007/978-3-319-73670-9_14

To date, few studies have quantified costs of cardiac arrest care, usually focusing on individual components of care or specific costs or subgroups of care. In this chapter, I describe reported economic data related to OHCA care.

What Costs to Include in a Medico-economic Evaluation of OHCA Care?

Different approaches may be used in the description of costs related to OHCA care depending on what the purpose of the research is. A global evaluation including every cost – prehospital, in-hospital and post-discharge (i.e., rehabilitation, long-term care facilities and outpatient costs) – seems attractive but some components may be hard to collect (Table 1). A more focused approach, reporting the evaluation of a specific intervention (e.g., TTM, coronary angiography) is also important as it usually provides an accurate overview of the technique.

The biggest difficulty in such a medico-economic evaluation is the definition of the different economic components. The best – but most difficult – approach is the bottom-up strategy. In such a strategy, each component of management is added to

Table 1 Types of costs that should be included in a global medico-economic evaluation of out-of-hospital cardiac arrest care

Prehospital setting	
Costs common to all emergency services	
Basic life support equipment (defibrillators, defibrillator pads, defibrillator batteries, oxygen, bag valve masks) and maintenance	
Vehicles	
Fixed costs not attributable to cardiac arrests (facilities, radio systems, computers and information technology)	
Management	
Fire services	First aid and cardiopulmonary resuscitation training
Emergency medical services	Advanced life support equipment and maintenance Advanced training in resuscitation
Physician on scene – mobile ICU	Advanced life support equipment and maintenance Physician's salary
In-hospital setting	
Emergency department	
Inpatient costs	In-hospital procedures (coronary angiography, targeted temperature management/therapeutic hypothermia, bypass surgery, implantable cardioverter defibrillator) Visits (neurologists, cardiologists) ICU/ward hospitalization
Post-discharge setting	
Rehabilitation	
Long-term care facilities	
Outpatient costs	Laboratory tests Visits Physiotherapy

provide a very detailed and accurate description of the total cost. However, it may be very difficult to retrieve all this information and a more granular approach might be preferred. For example, it may be easier to use prehospital costs based on an hourly rate rather than the sum of direct and indirect costs. Indeed, indirect costs related to prehospital care include many components, which may be difficult to individualize.

Reported Medico-economic Data

Prehospital and Resuscitation Costs

Retrieval of prehospital costs is probably the most difficult and the least comparable part of a medico-economic evaluation of OHCA care as it includes many different components and varies across the different healthcare delivery systems.

Ideally, all the direct and indirect costs related to the intervention of firefighters, paramedics and physicians on scene should be reported. However, it is difficult to retrieve all these costs at an individual level as most of the indirect costs cover not only material for cardiac arrest care but also all the other medical emergencies. Moreover, most of the recent published papers reported average prehospital costs based on annual EMS costs and assumed that the cost per hour for a unit in the EMS service was virtually constant [10–12].

Studies published since 2000 have reported a prehospital cost of OHCA care ranging from 2015-adjusted US $300 up to $915 per patient [10–12]. Interestingly, these costs did not vary according to survival [10, 13].

Valenzuela et al. showed almost 30 years ago that OHCA treatment by paramedics in the USA was more cost-effective than heart, liver, bone marrow transplantation or curative chemotherapy for acute leukemia, with a total cost of US $8,886 per life saved [14]. More interestingly, improvement in prehospital healthcare delivery has been shown to be cost-effective. Bystander cardiopulmonary resuscitation (CPR) was shown to be cost-effective with a cost-effectiveness ratio less than US $50,000 per quality-adjusted life year (QALY) in a US cohort [15]. Nichol et al. reported a cost-effectiveness ratio of $53,000 per QALY for improved response time in a two-tier EMS system by the addition of more basic life support providers/defibrillators to firefighter vehicles and of $40,000 per QALY for a change from a one-tier to a two-tier EMS system by the addition of initial basic life support/defibrillators in the first tier [16]. Sund et al. reported similar results in the Swedish system with a cost-effectiveness ratio of € 13,000 per QALY and € 60,000 per life saved of a dual dispatch defibrillation by ambulance and fire services [17]. In addition to the improvement of the prehospital healthcare delivery system itself, the strategic placement of automatic external defibrillators (AED) to improve AED coverage and widely distribute AED in an urban area has also been demonstrated as cost-effective [18–20]. Such a strategic placement is probably one of the most important aspects of the deployment of AED in a specific area, as it is more cost-effective than a national public access defibrillation program, which would not target locations with the highest incidence of OHCA [21]. Accordingly, providing in-home AEDs to all adults 60-years old of age is not cost-effective, whereas such a strategy may be interesting in patients with multiple risks for OHCA [22]. All these results highlight the necessity to include costs related to bystander and general public training in these evaluations.

To date, no economic comparison has been conducted between the two major types of prehospital healthcare delivery systems – the North American system using the *"scoop and run"* strategy versus the Franco-German *"stay and play"* strategy. A prospective medico-economic comparison of critical care teams and standard advanced life support teams in the United Kingdom is planned and could provide interesting insights in the field [23].

Emergency Department and Inpatient Costs

Emergency department and inpatient costs represent the large majority of costs in OHCA care, even though about 75% of the patients who have an OHCA are pronounced dead at the scene. Indeed, it is during this phase that all the costly pro-

Table 2 Main economic results published since 2010 in OHCA care

Author [ref]	Country	Cost perspective	Inpatient costs		
			Total	Survivors	Non-survivors
Liu, 2011 [39]	Taiwan	Hospital	n.a.	$18,889	$6,404
Berdowski, 2010 [2]	Netherlands	Hospital	n.a.	$32,923	$2,611
Swor, 2010 [27]	USA (NJ)	Hospital	$22,059	$51,365	n.a.
Kazaure, 2014 [26]	USA	3rd party	$20,713	n.a.	n.a.
Kazaure, 2013 [40]	USA	3rd party	n.a.	$34,393	$15,735
Kolte, 2015 [41]	USA	3rd party	$16,086	n.a.	n.a.
Fukuda, 2013 [42]	Japan	Public payer	n.a.	$33,418/$37,062[a]	$2,063/$5,791[b]
Chan, 2014 [43]	USA	Public payer	$41,184	n.a.	n.a.
Petrie, 2015 [29]	UK	Public payer	$18,730	$21,964	$10,426
Moulaert, 2016 [44]	Netherlands	Societal	–	$1,214/$1,727[c]	–

[a]Patient alive discharged home and other than home, respectively
[b]Patient resuscitated, dead on admission day and after at least two days of hospitalization, respectively
[c]Patients randomized in the "early rehabilitation" group and in the control group, respectively
n.a.: not available

cedures attempted after restoration of a spontaneous circulation are performed. The distinction of emergency department and inpatient costs relies on different health-care delivery systems in which OHCA patients may be either directly admitted to the ICU ("bypass procedure") or admitted first to the emergency department (ED) and then transferred to the ICU.

These costs widely vary according to vital status at hospital discharge, as survival and length of stay are strongly associated with increased costs (Table 2). Accordingly, the mean inpatient costs for OHCA patients discharged alive from hospital range from 2015 inflation-adjusted US $15,000 up to $40,000 per patient. On the other hand, the mean inpatient costs for OHCA patients who die within the hospital stay range from $2,500 up to $15,000 per patient [10, 24–29]. These costs are quite informative even if the variation may simultaneously reflect differences in diagnostic and therapeutic algorithms, cost per procedure *per se* or more importantly the different perspective from which costs have been calculated. Moreover, most of the published studies have been performed in the USA, where the economic healthcare system is very complicated because what the hospital charges and what the hospital receives (i.e., the real cost from the societal/3rd party perspective) are different.

Regarding in-hospital procedures, Merchant et al. modeled the cost effectiveness ratio of therapeutic hypothermia after cardiac arrest (external cooling with blankets) and found an incremental cost-effectiveness ratio of US $47,168 per QALY, which is lower that the well-accepted threshold of US $50,000 per QALY [30].

Hospitalization charges and costs increased significantly over time between 2001 and 2013 in the USA [31].

Post-discharge Costs

Post-discharge costs include outpatient costs, rehabilitation and long-term care facility-related costs. Very few data about outpatient costs have been reported so far. Hsu et al. [25] looked at outpatient costs in a cohort of patients discharged alive after one episode of life-threatening ventricular arrhythmia, according to the antiarrhythmic treatment (i.e., amiodarone or implantable cardioverter-defibrillator [ICD]). The total outpatient cost within the first 24 months after the index hospitalization was US $5,164 for patients who received an ICD and US $5,534 for patients treated with amiodarone. These costs were mostly related to the follow-up visits.

Wide variations may be observed in rehabilitation costs. Chan et al. evaluated rehabilitation costs at about US $40,000 per patient discharged alive from hospital [28, 32], whereas two European studies reported much lower costs of about US $2,000 [10, 33]. Moulaert et al. recently reported a randomized controlled trial-based economic evaluation of an early neurologically-focused follow-up after cardiac arrest. The intervention added to usual care screening for cognitive and emotional problems, provision of support and information on cardiac arrest and potential neurological consequences, promotion of self-management and referral to specialized care if indicated. The mean additional cost of such an intervention compared to usual care was €127 while healthcare costs and costs related to productivity loss were comparable in the two groups. The intervention was evaluated as cost-effective in all the sensitivity analyses performed in this study [33]. These results are very encouraging and strongly support active management of OHCA survivors in terms of neurological rehabilitation. This may be explained by the lack of discrimination of minor neurological sequelae of neurological scales used at hospital discharge (like the Cerebral Performance Category [CPC] scale [34]) as these minor consequences may have significant impact in daily personal and professional life [35].

Few data have been reported about long-term care facility-related costs and the generalizability strongly depends on the healthcare delivery system. The two most recent papers reporting costs related to long-term care facilities estimated the total cost at between US $30,000 and $50,000 [28, 32].

Readmission Costs

To date, only one study has evaluated inpatient costs related to readmissions of OHCA patients discharged alive after the index hospitalization [28]. In this American study, the mean cumulative incidence of readmission was 185/100 patients at one-year of follow-up (mainly related to cardiovascular and pulmonary diseases). The mean cost for readmission was US $7,741 at 30 days and US $18,629 at one-year.

Futility Costs

Regarding the large proportion of patients who suffer an OHCA and who are pronounced dead at the scene, some authors have evaluated the costs related to the management of these patients and especially those who meet the termination of resuscitation criteria used by the paramedics to stop resuscitation at the scene without transport to the hospital. In 1993, Bonnin et al. evaluated that less than 1% of patients who had suffered an OHCA related to an unshockable rhythm without any return of spontaneous circulation (ROSC) after at least 25 min of advanced life support were discharged alive. The total estimated costs related to the management of these patients meeting the termination of resuscitation criteria were about US $2,000 per patient. At that time, this could be extrapolated to US $500 million at a national level [36]. In the same manner, Suchard et al. evaluated the total cost related to the management of patients who suffered an OHCA with no prehospital ROSC and were pronounced dead on arrival at the emergency department. The extrapolation reached US $58 million per year [37].

Perspectives

Further research is needed to better evaluate global costs related to OHCA from the scene until discharge and post-discharge at an individual level. Indeed, results from model studies and partial evaluation of real costs preclude generalization and do not allow decision makers to have a good overview of such management. A bottom-up strategy, i.e., including all the components of the management at each step would also be of great value even though such a design may be difficult in view of the complexity of medico-economic healthcare delivery systems. The loss of productivity for OHCA patients discharged alive from hospital and supposed to return to work should be included as well. Moreover, we need non-US studies to better describe costs in different healthcare delivery systems.

These medico-economic evaluations should be considered in the perspective of the willingness to regionalize OHCA care [38]. Indeed, societal resources are limited and health care must be allocated efficiently. As resuscitation interventions are associated with better outcomes, costs related to complex multifaceted interventions are likely to be associated with increased costs. This increase would be related to EMS providing emergent interfacility transfers as well as receiving hospitals that provide the bulk of post-cardiac arrest care. If the system of care delivers better quality of care, these additional costs should be acceptable to society.

Conclusion

Medico-economic evaluation of OHCA care is mandatory as many complex interventions and human resources and skills are required. Further research is needed to consider total costs more globally to help decision makers to improve the healthcare delivery system.

References

1. Benjamin EJ, Blaha MJ, Chiuve SE et al (2017) Heart disease and stroke statistics-2017 update: a report from the American Heart Association. Circulation 135:1851–1867
2. Berdowski J, Berg RA, Tijssen JGP, Koster RW (2010) Global incidences of out-of-hospital cardiac arrest and survival rates: systematic review of 67 prospective studies. Resuscitation 81:1479–1487
3. Pozner CN, Zane R, Nelson SJ, Levine M (2004) International EMS systems: the United States: past, present, and future. Resuscitation 60:239–244
4. Symons P, Shuster M (2004) International EMS systems: Canada. Resuscitation 63:119–122
5. Geri G, Dumas F, Bougouin W et al (2015) Immediate percutaneous coronary intervention is associated with improved short- and long-term survival after out-of-hospital cardiac arrest. Circ Cardiovasc Interv 8:e2303
6. Dumas F, Cariou A, Manzo-Silberman S et al (2010) Immediate percutaneous coronary intervention is associated with better survival after out-of-hospital cardiac arrest: insights from the PROCAT (Parisian Region Out of hospital Cardiac ArresT) registry. Circ Cardiovasc Interv 3:200–207

7. Dumas F, White L, Stubbs BA, Cariou A, Rea TD (2012) Long-term prognosis following resuscitation from out of hospital cardiac arrest: role of percutaneous coronary intervention and therapeutic hypothermia. J Am Coll Cardiol 60:21–27

8. Sunde K, Pytte M, Jacobsen D et al (2007) Implementation of a standardised treatment protocol for post resuscitation care after out-of-hospital cardiac arrest. Resuscitation 73:29–39

9. Becker LB, Aufderheide TP, Geocadin RG et al (2011) Primary outcomes for resuscitation science studies: a consensus statement from the American Heart Association. Circulation 124:2158–2177

10. Næss AC, Steen PA (2004) Long term survival and costs per life year gained after out-of-hospital cardiac arrest. Resuscitation 60:57–64

11. van Alem AP, Dijkgraaf MGW, Tijssen JGP, Koster RW (2004) Health system costs of out-of-hospital cardiac arrest in relation to time to shock. Circulation 110:1967–1973

12. Yen ZS, Chen YT, Ko PCI et al (2006) Cost-effectiveness of Different advanced life support providers for victims of out-of-hospital cardiac arrests. J Formos Med 105:1001–1007

13. Cheung M, Morrison L, Verbeek PR (2001) Prehospital vs. emergency department pronouncement of death: a cost analysis. CJEM 3:19–25

14. Valenzuela TD, Criss EA, Spaite D, Meislin HW, Wright AL, Clark L (1990) Cost-effectiveness analysis of paramedic emergency medical services in the treatment of prehospital cardiopulmonary arrest. Ann Emerg Med 19:1407–1411

15. Geri G, Fahrenbruch C, Meischke H et al (2017) Effects of bystander CPR following out-of-hospital cardiac arrest on hospital costs and long-term survival. Resuscitation 115:129–134

16. Nichol G, Laupacis A, Stiell IG et al (1996) Cost-effectiveness analysis of potential improvements to emergency medical services for victims of out-of-hospital cardiac arrest. Ann Emerg Med 27:711–720

17. Sund B, Svensson L, Rosenqvist M, Hollenberg J (2012) Favourable cost-benefit in an early defibrillation programme using dual dispatch of ambulance and fire services in out-of-hospital cardiac arrest. Eur J Health Econ 13:811–818

18. Folke F, Lippert FK, Nielsen SL et al (2009) Location of cardiac arrest in a city center: strategic placement of automated external defibrillators in public locations. Circulation 120:510–517

19. Cram P, Vijan S, Fendrick AM (2003) Cost-effectiveness of automated external defibrillator deployment in selected public locations. J Gen Intern Med 18:745–754

20. Cappato R, Curnis A, Marzollo P et al (2006) Prospective assessment of integrating the existing emergency medical system with automated external defibrillators fully operated by volunteers and laypersons for out-of-hospital cardiac arrest: the Brescia Early Defibrillation Study (BEDS). Eur Heart J 27:553–561

21. Moran PS, Teljeur C, Masterson S et al (2015) Cost-effectiveness of a national public access defibrillation programme. Resuscitation 91:48–55

22. Cram P, Vijan S, Katz D, Fendrick AM (2005) Cost-effectiveness of in-home automated external defibrillators for individuals at increased risk of sudden cardiac death. J Gen Intern Med 20:251–258

23. von Vopelius-Feldt J, Powell J, Morris R, Benger J (2016) Prehospital critical care for out-of-hospital cardiac arrest: An observational study examining survival and a stakeholder- focused cost analysis. BMC Emerg Med 16:1–7

24. Graf J, Mühlhoff C, Doig GS et al (2008) Health care costs, long-term survival, and quality of life following intensive care unit admission after cardiac arrest. Crit Care 12:R92

25. Hsu J, Uratsu C, Truman A et al (2002) Life after a ventricular arrhythmia. Am Heart J 144:404–412

26. Kazaure HS, Roman SA, Sosa JA (2014) A population-level analysis of 5620 recipients of multiple in-hospital cardiopulmonary resuscitation attempts. J Hosp Med 9:29–34

27. Swor R, Lucia V, McQueen K, Compton S (2010) Hospital costs and revenue are similar for resuscitated out-of-hospital cardiac arrest and ST-segment acute myocardial infarction patients. Acad Emerg Med 17:612–616

28. Chan PS, McNally B, Tang F, Kellermann A (2014) Recent trends in survival from out-of-hospital cardiac arrest in the United States. Circulation 130:1876–1882
29. Petrie J, Easton S, Naik V, Lockie C, Brett SJ, Stumpfle R (2015) Hospital costs of out-of-hospital cardiac arrest patients treated in intensive care; a single centre evaluation using the national tariff-based system. BMJ Open 5:e5797
30. Merchant RM, Becker LB, Abella BS, Asch DA, Groeneveld PW (2009) Cost-effectiveness of therapeutic hypothermia after cardiac arrest. Circ Cardiovasc Qual Outcomes 2:421–428
31. Eid SM, Abougergi MS, Albaeni A, Chandra-Strobos N (2017) Survival, expenditure and disposition in patients following out-of-hospital cardiac arrest: 1995–2013. Resuscitation 113:13–20
32. Chan PS, McNally B, Nallamothu BK et al (2016) Long-term outcomes among elderly survivors of out-of-hospital cardiac arrest. J Am Heart Assoc 5:e2924
33. Moulaert VRM, van Heugten CM, Winkens B et al (2015) Early neurologically-focused follow-up after cardiac arrest improves quality of life at one year: a randomised controlled trial. Int J Cardiol 193:8–16
34. Jennett B, Bond M (1975) Assessment of outcome after severe brain damage. Lancet 1:480–484
35. Peskine A, Rosso C, Picq C, Caron E, Pradat-Diehl P (2010) Neurological sequelae after cerebral anoxia. Brain Inj 24:755–761
36. Bonnin MJ, Pepe PE, Kimball KT, Clark PS (1993) Distinct criteria for termination of resuscitation in the out-of-hospital setting. JAMA 270:1457–1462
37. Suchard JR, Fenton FR, Powers RD (1999) Medicare expenditures on unsuccessful out-of-hospital resuscitations. J Emerg Med 17:801–805
38. Nichol G, Aufderheide TP, Eigel B et al (2010) Regional systems of care for out-of-hospital cardiac arrest: a policy statement from the American Heart Association. Circulation 121:709–729
39. Liu WL, Lai CC, Hii CH et al (2011) Outcomes and cost analysis of patients with successful in-hospital cardiopulmonary resuscitation. Int J Gerontol 5:196–199
40. Kazaure HS, Roman SA, Sosa JA (2013) Epidemiology and outcomes of in-hospital cardiopulmonary resuscitation in the United States, 2000–2009. Resuscitation 84:1255–1260
41. Kolte D, Khera S, Aronow WS et al (2015) Regional variation in the incidence and outcomes of in-hospital cardiac arrest in the United States. Circulation 131:1415–1425
42. Fukuda T, Yasunaga H, Horiguchi H et al (2013) Health care costs related to out-of-hospital cardiopulmonary arrest in Japan. Resuscitation 84:964–969
43. Chan PS, Nallamothu BK, Krumholz HM et al (2014) Readmission rates and long-term hospital costs among survivors of an in-hospital cardiac arrest. Circ Cardiovasc Qual Outcomes 7:889–895
44. Moulaert VRM, Goossens M, Heijnders ILC, Verbunt JA, Heugten CMV (2016) Early neurologically focused follow-up after cardiac arrest is cost-effective: A trial-based economic evaluation. Resuscitation 106:30–36

Part V
Respiratory Support

A Systematic Review of the High-flow Nasal Cannula for Adult Patients

Y. Helviz and S. Einav

Introduction

Awareness of the potential damage associated with the use of invasive ventilation (e.g., ventilator-associated pneumonia [VAP], excessive pulmonary stress and strain) and increasing sophistication in patient-ventilator interfaces have led to development of several interesting new modes of delivering non-invasive ventilation (NIV), not least of which is the high-flow nasal cannula (HFNC).

The HFNC was first developed for use in neonates. Although many adult patients found the use of a close-fitting mask not particularly tolerable, the most common issue in the adult population usually remained clearance of airway secretions [1]. In the neonatal population however, severe pressure sores became a major concern with the use of a tight face mask [2]. The HFNC was thus originally developed with the intention of maintaining the benefit of high oxygen flows (and thus the increased end-expiratory pulmonary pressures) without compromising blood flow to skin areas susceptible to pressure sores [3]. The first cannulas developed to this end were, therefore, designed to match the internal diameter of the neonatal nasal orifice, and for this reason were also constructed from materials that are softer than their predecessors [3].

HFNC devices allow modification of only two variables – the percentage of oxygen being delivered and the rate of gas flow. There are at this time only two such devices on the market. Both are capable of delivering a mix of air and oxygen with an inspired oxygen fraction (FiO_2) ranging between 0.21–1.0. The two differ some-

Y. Helviz
The Intensive Care Unit of the Shaare Zedek Medical Centre
Jerusalem, Israel

S. Einav (✉)
The Intensive Care Unit of the Shaare Zedek Medical Centre
Jerusalem, Israel
The Faculty of Medicine of the Hebrew University
Jerusalem, Israel
e-mail: einav_s@szmc.org.il

© Springer International Publishing AG 2018
J.-L. Vincent (ed.), *Annual Update in Intensive Care and Emergency Medicine 2018*,
Annual Update in Intensive Care and Emergency Medicine,
https://doi.org/10.1007/978-3-319-73670-9_15

what in the range of possible gas flows; one can deliver 5–40 l/min while the other has a slightly greater range of 1–60 l/min. Regardless of the device being used, the gas undergoes 100% humidification and is heated to approximately normal body temperature.

Over the last 10 years, HFNCs have had widespread uptake in the adult population. The idea that one may provide NIV with little discomfort to the patient is conceptually attractive. However, there is still much debate regarding the role of the HFNC in the management of critically ill patients and only recently has some better quality research emerged on the topic. This review covers the potential beneficial and deleterious effects of the HFNC and the latest evidence regarding its use in some of the more common clinical settings.

Literature Search

Using the services of a professional librarian, we conducted an online search for relevant publications in PubMed, Embase and Web of Science. The search was restricted to articles written in English or Spanish. We searched all articles from January 2007 to June 2017 that referred to adults treated with the HFNC using the key words "*humans*" together with "*adult*", "*mature*" or "*grown*". Publications with the key words "*high flow nasal cannula*", "*high flow nasal therapy*", "*high flow nasal oxygen*", "*high flow oxygen therapy*", "*high flow therapy*", "*optiflow (respiration)*" and "*nasal highflow*" were then tabulated in Excel along with a link to their abstracts and the list was manually searched for repeat publications. The main journals most likely to contain publications in this area (i.e., intensive care and emergency medicine journals) were also identified using content experts in the area and hand searched if they were locally available.

For information relevant to elucidation of mechanisms of action with their associated potential benefits/harms, both human (pediatric or adult) and animal studies qualified for inclusion. For evidence regarding clinical use, only adult human studies qualified for inclusion. Reviews, randomized controlled trials (RCTs), case-control studies and case series and reports were all extracted (title and abstract) in order to screen for relevant content. The references appearing in each of the relevant papers were also hand searched.

Abstracts from the selected articles were read, and if considered eligible for further review by the authors, the complete article was obtained. Articles with information relevant to either one of the two aims of the review (elucidation of mechanisms of action with their associated potential benefits/harms and or clinical uses) qualified for inclusion. As noted above, the references of the selected articles that had been retrieved were also screened for additional possible references. Fig. 1 shows the flowchart for study selection. After determining the relevance of each paper, the articles were divided into two main files according to their relevance to each aim (mechanism of action or clinical uses) and then again subdivided in accordance to subtopic within that aim (potentially beneficial/detrimental and clinical scenario – see below). Finally, the data from each topic file were summarized.

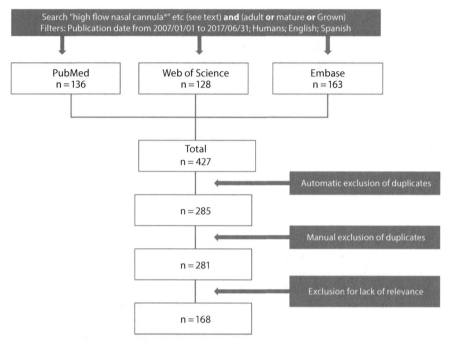

Fig. 1 Flowchart for systematic review study selection

Potential Beneficial and Deleterious Effects

Potential Benefits

It has been proposed that the HFNC can provide several benefits. Among these are maintenance of a constant FiO_2, generation of a positive end-expiratory pressure (PEEP), reduction of the anatomical dead space, improvement of mucociliary clearance and reduction in the work of breathing.

Maintenance of Constant FiO_2
Standard hospital gas delivery systems provide oxygen at 50–55 pounds per square inch (PSI). Such pressures, when released, form dangerously high flows. All NIV devices therefore include a mechanism (usually a series of valves) to modify the flow eventually delivered to the patient. Regular nasal cannulas are connected to the hospital gas delivery system via flowmeters, most of which allow delivery of gas flows up to 15 l/min. However, provision of unregulated and constant flows through standard nasal cannulas has traditionally been limited not only due to the internal diameter of the cannula but also by the discomfort generated by the lack of heating and humidification of the inspired gas. Provision of flows exceeding standard oxygen delivery (15 l/min) may be important in a dyspneic patient; tachypnea is ac-

companied by rapid inspiratory flows which may reach 50 l/min. When inspiratory flow rates exceed the flow of delivered oxygen, the additional flow is recruited from the surrounding air (with its FiO_2 of 0.21). In this situation, the inspired FiO_2 is significantly lower than the delivered gas [3, 4]. In other words, as the respiratory rate of the patient increases, the actual FiO_2 being delivered decreases. Ventilators providing NIV overcome this issue via adaptation of the provided flow to the phases of the respiratory cycle. The HFNC, a simpler device, provides a constant flow. However, it overcomes the issue of air-mixing by enabling delivery of oxygen at particularly high flows, which facilitates maintenance of a constant delivered FiO_2.

Generation of a Positive End-expiratory Pressure

A study performed in human volunteers demonstrated that high flows delivered through a HFNC generated positive airway pressures in the nasopharynx [5]. Animal models have also shown that these pressures are translated to increased intra-alveolar volumes. While these pressures were relatively low compared to those generated easily in closed systems ($< 3 \, cmH_2O$), they could potentially suffice to prevent alveolar closure. The question often asked in this context is whether such pressures are also generated when the mouth is open. A study conducted in adult men and women demonstrated that although increased HFNC flows generated a greater increase in pressure with a closed mouth, a proportionate increase was observed with the mouth open as well [6]. Furthermore, the presence of a constant leak (such as that created by maximal mouth opening) seems to affect the initial pressure but not the pressure increment generated by an increase in flow [5, 7].

Decrease in Anatomical Dead Space

The high flow rates provided by the HFNC wash the expired volume of carbon dioxide (CO_2) from the airway, replacing it with oxygen-enriched gas. In a swine model simulating the human airway, the partial pressure of CO_2 was studied in high leak and low leak conditions. When the leak was low, the partial pressure of CO_2 was significantly lower, suggesting that the inspiratory dead-space had been washed out by the constant flow of high oxygen gas [7]. As patients using the HFNC may open or close their mouth at will, the clinical significance of this finding is unclear. However, it does suggest that washout may contribute to the observed increase in PaO_2.

Improved Mucociliary Clearance

Studies of the percent of tracheobronchial deposition as a function of radioaerosol inhalation (without medication) show a gradual decrease in deposition as the time from the last inhalation increases [8]. This suggests that as the airway dries, patients find it more difficult to clear the airway of secretions. Although there are no studies demonstrating such an effect with the HFNC, it is commonly assumed that contact with an inspired gas that has been warmed to body temperature and contains humidification will cause less mucociliary dessication and thus maintain mucociliary clearance to a greater degree than other methods of delivering oxygen that do not have these characteristics.

Decreased Work of Breathing

Whether the HFNC decreases the work of breathing is still unclear, but there are studies suggesting this may indeed be the case. One study of thoraco-abdominal coordination during breathing showed an improvement in subjective measures of asynchrony over time. In this study, patients diagnosed clinically as having poor thoraco-abdominal coordination during breathing were also more likely to undergo intubation [9]. Another study of 40 adult intensive care unit (ICU) patients with mild to moderate respiratory failure treated with the HFNC after thoracotomy demonstrated similar findings [10]. A strong correlation between airway pressure and end-expiratory lung impedance (a marker of end-respiratory lung volume) was demonstrated in a study using electrical impedance tomography (EIT) to study the respiratory mechanics of adult patients treated with HFNC after cardiothoracic surgery (n = 20). The patients included had at least one sign of respiratory distress (PaO_2/FiO_2 < 300, subjective dyspnea, increased use of accessory muscles or increase in respiratory rate). Compared with conventional oxygen therapy, delivery of oxygen via the HFNC increased the end-expiratory lung impedance by 25.6%, reduced the respiratory rate and increased the tidal volume, allowing the authors to conclude that the HFNC does seem to decrease the work of breathing [11].

Potential Deleterious Effects

The main concern that has arisen regarding the HFNC has been that overuse of this modality may lead to unnecessary and potentially precarious delays in intubation. In 2004, Esteban et al. published a seminal paper describing a multicenter trial that was terminated ahead of time due to an increased risk of death in ICU patients treated post-extubation with non-invasive positive pressure ventilation (NIPPV) compared with those receiving conventional oxygen therapy. The authors attributed the increased mortality in the NIPPV group to the length of time elapsing between respiratory failure and reintubation, which was significantly longer in patients receiving NIPPV [12]. About 10 years later, Kang et al. suggested a similar association in patients treated with the HFNC; in a single ICU, after matching, patients who were intubated early had lower ICU mortality rates [13].

Clinical Uses of the HFNC

The HFNC is very versatile and user friendly. It can be used in a low-monitoring environment, with almost no knowledge of mechanical ventilation. However, most patients treated with the HFNC are extremely hypoxemic, which raises important questions regarding whether it should be used in such conditions. Regardless of this controversy, several potential clinical uses for the HFNC have emerged in recent years. Among these are included the respiratory support of patients with acute hypoxemic respiratory failure or respiratory distress syndrome (ARDS), with respiratory compromise induced by heart failure and with respiratory compromise post-extubation. In this review, we also address the HFNC as an adjunct during airway instrumentation, for immune compromised patients, and as a means of reducing suffering at the end of life.

ARDS and Acute Hypoxemic Respiratory Failure

In 2012, Rello et al. described a series of patients with severe hypoxemia as a result of H1N1 pneumonitis (O_2Sat $< 92\%$ on more than 9 l/min of oxygen via face mask). Among the patients receiving oxygen therapy via a HFNC, almost half (9/20) never required intubation and non-responders were obvious within 6 h of initiating HFNC therapy. Importantly, despite the high flows being used, none of the treating medical and nursing staff were infected with the viral disease [14].

Frat et al. randomized 310 patients with acute respiratory failure (PaO_2/FiO_2 < 300) in 23 medical centers to treatment with either a face mask, NIPPV or HFNC. There was no difference in the intubation rate between the groups but patients treated with the HFNC had more ventilator-free days (if intubated) and better survival rates even after adjustment for simplified acute physiology score II (SAPS II) and a history of cardiac insufficiency [15]. This paper was subject to several criticisms: that the trial was not powered to detect a difference in mortality [16], that an excessive number of patients were excluded (only 313 of the 2,506 screened patients were randomized) [17], that treatment with NIV was suboptimal [18], that there was significant treatment overlap between the groups [18] and finally that the fragility index was low (i.e., it would take only 5 events to change the significance of the results) [16]. Frat et al. emphasized the advantage of the homogeneity of their study groups in their response to comments regarding patient exclusion, noted that five more deaths would represent almost 40% of the patients who died and stated that the treatment provided with NIV (median 8 h daily for the first two days) was hardly suboptimal and that the fact that the NIV group received HFNC support between NIV sessions only strengthens the argument for the benefit of HFNC [19].

Three meta-analyses have studied the literature comparing HFNC to conventional oxygen therapy and NIV in patients with acute hypoxemic respiratory failure. These are presented in Table 1. To summarize, mortality remains unaffected but the HFNC seems to be better tolerated than conventional oxygen therapy by the patients. Although there seems to be a signal suggesting that the HFNC may reduce intubation rate this issue remains controversial; one of the papers suggested this finding may be specific to high-risk patients (as defined by APACHE II or SAPS II scores) [20], whereas another included a trial sequential analysis which demonstrated that more studies on the topic are required [21].

Hypoxemia Induced by Severe Heart Failure

Roca et al. studied 10 patients with New York Heart Association (NYHA) class III heart failure during treatment with HFNC (baseline, 20 l/min, 40 l/min and post-

Table 1 Meta-analyses of the use of high-flow nasal cannulas (HFNCs) in hypoxemic respiratory failure

Reference	Inclusion criteria	Number of studies	Number of patients	Comparators to the HFNC	Intubation rate	Mortality	Other outcomes
Ni et al. [51]	Adults with PaO_2/FiO_2 ≤ 300 mmHg OR $SpO_2 <92\%$ on 10–12 l/min O_2	18	3,881	NIV or conventional oxygen therapy	Lower compared to conventional oxygen therapy but similar to NIV	Similar	Lower RR with HFNC compared to both conventional oxygen therapy and NIV. PaO_2/FiO_2 better than with conventional oxygen therapy. No difference in ICU LOS. No effect on $PaCO_2$ or pH
Ou et al. [20]	Adults with acute hypoxemic respiratory failure ($PaO_2/FiO_2 \leq 300$)	6	1,892	NIV or conventional oxygen therapy	Lower compared to conventional oxygen therapy in high-risk patients, but similar to NIV	Similar	
Monro-Somerville [21]	Adults with respiratory failure	9	2,507	Conventional oxygen therapy	Similar	Similar	Better tolerance of HFNC

NIV: non-invasive ventilation; *LOS*: length of stay; *ICU*: intensive care unit; *RR*: respiratory rate

treatment). The degree of inferior vena cava (IVC) collapse decreased in proportion to the gas flow provided, returning to baseline after treatment discontinuation (median 37, 28, 21 and 39% respectively). At the same time, respiratory rates nearly halved. The researchers concluded that the HFNC reduces preload reduction and thus may benefit patients with heart failure [22]. This study was criticized later by Esquinas and Papakados who noted that IVC collapsibility may be affected by multiple factors that had not been controlled for by the investigators (e.g., airway leaks, peak inspiratory and expiratory pressures, respiratory breathing patterns, airway resistance and flow characteristics) and that preload reduction should have also affected the pulmonary artery pressure and right and/or left ventricular ejection fraction, all of which remained unaffected, making the assumption regarding mechanism void [23].

In another study of the same issue (i.e., whether the HFNC generates a continuous positive airway pressure [CPAP] effect), five female and five male healthy volunteers were connected to a HFNC at flows ranging between 0–60 l/min. The pressure generated inside the pharynx (measured using a catheter) showed that an increase in flow of 10 l/min produced a 0.8 cmH$_2$O increase in expiratory pressures. Additional factors increasing this pressure were mouth closure (2 cmH$_2$O), female sex (0.6 cmH$_2$O), and greater height (0.5 cmH$_2$O per every 10 cm) [6].

Post-extubation Respiratory Compromise

The rate of failed extubation is very variable but may range up 20% or more [24, 25] and the ideal treatment for prevention of reintubation has yet to be determined. Whether HFNC is beneficial post-extubation has been studied in patients after cardiothoracic surgery, abdominal surgery and in general ICU patients at both high- and low-risk for reintubation.

Stéphan et al. randomized high-risk patients from six medical centers who developed hypoxemia after cardiothoracic surgery to either HFNC (n = 414) or NIV (n = 416). Patients were included only if they had failed a spontaneous breathing trial or extubation previously, or had other risk factors for failed extubation (body mass index [BMI] > 30 or left ventricular ejection fraction [LVEF] < 40%). The authors concluded that the HFNC is a valid treatment option in this selective population after finding that the HFNC was non-inferior to NIV in terms of treatment failure, reintubation rate, time to treatment failure and mortality and that this treatment caused less pressure sores and skin breakdown and decreased respiratory rates [26]. A meta-analysis comparing HFNC with conventional oxygen therapy via face mask in the same patient population, adults extubated after cardiac surgery, found only two studies [27, 28] appropriate for inclusion (overall 495 patients). The HFNC was associated with less "escalation of therapy" (e.g., the need to increase HFNC flow, crossover to NIV) but the eventual reintubation rate was similar [29].

In the OPERA (Optiflow® to prevent Post-Extubation hypoxemia after Abdominal surgery) trial, Futier et al. randomized patients after abdominal surgery in three medical centers to preemptive application of either HFNC (n = 108) or conventional oxygen therapy via face mask (n = 112). No significant differences were found in patient outcomes [30]. Maggiore et al. randomized general ICU patients at risk of hypoxemia ($PaO_2/FiO_2 < 300$ immediately before extubation) to preemptive use of either the HFNC (n = 53) or a Venturi mask (n = 52). Patients treated with the HFNC had higher PaO_2/FiO_2 ratios and less interface displacement. They also desaturated less, underwent fewer reintubations and required less ventilator support. Contrary to Futier et al. these authors concluded that the HFNC should have a role in pre-emptive post-extubation management [31].

These inconclusive results drove others to try to determine which patients would benefit from a HFNC after extubation. Patients from seven sites were classified as either high- or low-risk for reintubation. Elderly patients (> 65 years old) and those with a high burden of disease (APACHE II score > 12 points on extubation day, or > 1 comorbidity), risk factors for failed extubation (BMI > 30, heart failure as the primary indication for mechanical ventilation, moderate to severe chronic obstructive pulmonary disease [COPD]) or respiratory issues potentially affecting weaning (airway patency problems, inadequate management of secretions, difficult/prolonged weaning, mechanical ventilation > 7 days) were defined as high risk. The high-risk patients were randomized to either NIV (n = 314) or HFNC (n = 290). The low-risk patients were randomized to either conventional oxygen therapy (n = 263) or HFNC (n = 264). The high-risk group demonstrated non-inferiority of the HFNC compared to NIV regarding reintubation rate and mortality. Only patient comfort was improved with the HFNC [32]. The low-risk group demonstrated a lower rate of reintubation within 72 h with the HFNC, mainly attributable to a decrease in respiratory problems. The number needed to treat in this group was calculated as 1 per 14 (95% confidence interval 8.14) [33].

In conclusion, in post-extubation respiratory failure, the HFNC is consistently better tolerated than NIV. However, although the HFNC seems non-inferior to NIV with regards to intubation and mortality after cardiothoracic surgery and in high-risk ICU patients, its status remains controversial after abdominal surgery. It remains to be elucidated whether these dissimilarities stem from a variable effect on thoraco-abdominal coordination or other causes. In low-risk hypoxemic patients, support with the HFNC seems to prevent intubation to a certain degree compared to conventional oxygen therapy. The specific subgroups of patients that will benefit from this treatment after extubation require further research.

Airway Instrumentation

The HFNC has been studied as an adjunct to airway instrumentation during manipulation of the airway (e.g., bronchoscopy, intubation) in patients with both low and high risk (i.e., hypoxemia, morbid obesity).

Simon et al. randomized hypoxemic patients ($PaO_2/FiO_2 < 300$) undergoing bronchoscopy in the critical care setting to HFNC or NIV (20 patients per group). The FiO_2 was set initially to 1.0 and then adjusted to achieve SaO_2 of above 90%. The HFNC was set to deliver 50 l/min and NIV was set to a PEEP of 3–10 cmH$_2$O and a pressure support of 15–20 cmH$_2$O. The authors found that the HFNC was inferior to NIV for maintenance of oxygenation during bronchoscopy of critical care patients with moderate to severe hypoxemia [34].

Lucangelo et al. compared delivery of 50% oxygen before and during bronchoscopy using either a HFNC (40 or 60 l/min) or a Venturi mask in stable patients (SaO$_2$ > 90% while breathing room air) undergoing bronchoscopy. Fifteen patients in each group contributed data at baseline (while breathing room air), at the end of bronchoscopy (during which they had received 50% oxygen using the assigned treatment modality) and 10 min after bronchoscopy (at which time they were receiving 35% oxygen through a Venturi mask). Patients receiving 60 l/min via HFNC maintained higher PaO$_2$ values, higher arterial-alveolar oxygen tensions and higher PaO$_2$/FiO$_2$ ratios both during and after the procedure. In an attempt to explain their findings, the authors measured airway pressures in healthy volunteers; at a flow rate of 60 l/min the median pressure measured was 3.6 cmH$_2$O whereas at a flow rate of 40 l/min, the median pressure measured was 0 cmH$_2$O. Although interesting, this finding does not necessarily mean that HFNC at 60 l/min must be used to maintain oxygenation during bronchoscopy in patients with mild respiratory dysfunction as suggested by the authors [35].

Induction of sedation/anesthesia for intubation requires (ideally) pre-oxygenation followed by administration of medications (sedatives and/or neuromuscular blockers). The resultant apnea provides better conditions for vocal cord visualization [36] but at the same time may be accompanied by downward spiraling hypoxemia [37]. Although oxygenating face masks must be removed for intubation, the HFNC may be left in place, theoretically maintaining CPAP and thereby prolonging the non-hypoxemic apnea time. Vourc'h et al. assigned adult patients with respiratory failure (PaO$_2$/FiO$_2$ < 300, respiratory rate > 30) in six ICUs to one of two groups during intubation: either 100% FiO$_2$/60 l/min delivered by HFNC (n = 63) or 15 l/min O$_2$ delivered by a face mask (n = 61). The HFNC was kept in place during intubation whereas the face mask was removed after induction of general anesthesia. Pre-oxygenation parameters, the duration of the intubation procedure and the quality of airway visualization were similar in the two groups. Despite randomization, the two groups had similar "lowest SaO$_2$s" and mortality rates. The authors therefore concluded that "using HFNC without discontinuation during an apneic period was not more effective than face mask in preventing desaturation regardless of the severity of respiratory distress" [37].

Jaber et al. randomized hypoxemic patients undergoing intubation in a single ICU (hypoxemia defined as SaO$_2$ < 90% on 0.5 FiO$_2$, respiratory rate > 30, PaO$_2$/FiO$_2$ < 300 within the four hours before inclusion) to pre-oxygenation with either a combination of NIV and HFNC (n = 25) or NIV alone (n = 24). The time from induction to secure airway was 120 and 60 s for the intervention and control groups, respectively (calculated as non significant). The outcome was assessor-blinded. No differences were observed between the groups in intubation-related complications. However, during intubation, peripheral capillary oxygen saturation (SpO$_2$) remained constant at 100% with combination treatment but decreased to

96% with NIV alone [38]. Although this difference was statistically significant, its clinical importance is doubtful.

Simon et al. also randomized patients with hypoxemic respiratory failure who required intubation to pre-oxygenation with either a HFNC with 50 l/min of 100% oxygen (n = 20) or a bag-valve-mask with 10 l/min of 100% oxygen (n = 20). In the 1 min of apnea after induction of anesthesia, saturation dropped significantly more in the bag-valve-mask group than with the HFNC [39]. The authors observed that only patients that had not been pre-treated with HFNC or NIV prior to pre-oxygenation demonstrated an increase in SpO_2. This led them to conclude that pre-oxygenation with a HFNC prior to intubation should be considered only in patients with mild-moderate hypoxemia. In contrast to other authors who have published on this topic, these authors also calculated the power required to detect a 3% difference in SpO_2 between the groups and concluded that their study had been underpowered to detect the difference they had sought.

Obese patients have a particularly low functional residual capacity (FRC), which increases the likelihood and severity of hypoxemia during apnea when compared to other patients [40]. Heinrich et al. randomized obese patients (BMI > 35) undergoing intubation for bariatric surgery to receive FiO_2 1.0 in one of three modes (11 per group): HFNC (flow 50 l/min), face mask connected to an anesthesia ventilator (flow 12 l/min) and CPAP (7 cmH$_2$O). PaO_2 increased significantly in all the groups within one minute of initiating pre-oxygenation. However, after five minutes, patients treated with a HFNC had a significantly higher PaO_2 than those treated with a face mask and, after intubation (at 8.5 min), SpO_2 decreased significantly with the face mask and CPAP but not with the HFNC [40].

To summarize, HFNCs may have a role in decreasing apneic hypoxemia during airway instrumentation but multicenter trials that include a greater number of patients are required to establish this claim.

Immune Compromise

Immune compromised patients have higher mortality rates than those with no immune compromise when intubated for respiratory failure [41, 42]. Studies have provided conflicting results regarding mortality and intubation rates when NIV (as a modality to prevent intubation) is used in this population [43]. Coudroy et al. reviewed the files of immune compromised patients with respiratory failure (i.e., tachypnea or respiratory distress and $PaO_2/FiO_2 \leq 300$). The patients were treated with either HFNC (n = 60), NIV alternating with HFNC (n = 30), or conventional oxygen therapy (25 patients). The rates of both intubation and mortality were higher with NIV than with the HFNC [43]. Lee et al. retrospectively studied all patients with hematological malignancy treated with HFNC in a single medical center (n = 45); one third recovered and the rest eventually received invasive mechanical ventilation due to treatment failure. The mortality rate was 62.2%. Patients who needed endotracheal intubation had higher rates of bacterial pneumonia and death than those who required HFNC treatment alone [44]. Another post-hoc analysis of adult ICU patients admitted with respiratory failure yielded quite the opposite result; the intubation rate among patients treated with HFNC was 80% and the mortality rate was 73% vs. 26.7% in intubated patients. The major reason for HFNC failure was pneumonia [45]. None of these studies adjusted for variables that may have driven the choice of treatment (e.g., selection of NIV in patients who were a-priori worse or avoidance of intubation due to futility). Thus, the data regarding use of the HFNC in immune compromised patients are not only conflicting but also of poor quality.

End-of-Life Care

In 2004, the expert working group of the scientific committee of the association of palliative medicine proposed that oxygen therapy be prescribed for patients with advanced cancer if it can alleviate the symptom of breathlessness [46]. Epstein et al. searched the database of a single hospital and identified 183 cancer patients, 55% with a do-not-attempt-resuscitation (DNAR) order, who had been treated with HFNC (median treatment time 3 days): 41% improved, 44% remained stable and 15% deteriorated during therapy. The overall mortality rate was 55% [47]. In another retrospective cohort of hypoxemic ICU patients with a 'do-not-intubate' order (n = 50), the authors noted a significant increase in oxygenation and a decrease in respiratory rate despite the eventual 60% mortality rate (median treatment time 30 h) [48]. The justification for palliative therapy with the HFNC includes both ethical considerations (beneficence) and economic considerations (justice). The benefit to be considered is alleviation of suffering. The justice to be considered is the cost of care. Fealy et al. studied ICU patients treated with a HFNC (n = 35) versus historical controls treated with a high-flow face mask (n = 48). The device cost per patient was reduced from $32.56 to $17.62 [49].

Conclusion

Rabbat et al. [50] summarized the evidence regarding HFNC post-extubation nicely, and this summary holds true for the use of the HFNC in almost every clinical scenario. Difficulties in blinding of the treatment arm constitute a major source of bias in all of the comparative studies on the HFNC; only one study attempted blinding [38]. The HFNC is consistently better tolerated by patients than NIV. The advantage of this, apart from patient comfort, is that the patient can probably remain connected to the device for longer periods. However, this can also be a disadvantage if it leads to dangerous delays in intubation.

The HFNC seems more effective than conventional oxygen therapy and noninferior to NIV in most studies. The quality of data on the HFNC is slightly better regarding patients post-extubation, but there is need for more studies even in this clinical setting to generate a clearer signal. The HFNC seems to hold promise for apneic oxygenation during airway instrumentation but the studies performed on this topic have largely been underpowered. With regards to provision of HFNC therapy to immune compromised patients and those requiring palliative care, the retrospective nature of the studies performed thus far precludes determination of any causative association between patient management and outcome. However, there may be ethical considerations for providing this treatment in some cases.

Acknowledgement

We are indebted to Dr. Iris Arad for the hours she spend performing the online search. Without her professional help this article could have never been written.

References

1. Ozyilmaz E, Ugurlu AO, Nava S (2014) Timing of noninvasive ventilation failure: causes, risk factors, and potential remedies. BMC Pulm Med 14:19
2. Shoemaker M, Pierce M, Yoder B, DiGeronimo R (2007) High flow nasal cannula versus nasal CPAP for neonatal respiratory disease: a retrospective study. J Perinatol 27:85–91
3. Ward JJ (2013) High-flow oxygen administration by nasal cannula for adult and perinatal patients. Respir Care 58:98–122
4. Nishimura M (2016) High-flow nasal cannula oxygen therapy in adults. J Intensive Care 3:15
5. Parke RL, Eccleston ML, McGuinness SP (2011) The effects of flow on airway pressure during nasal high-flow oxygen therapy. Respir Care 56:1151–1155
6. Groves N, Tobin A (2007) High flow nasal oxygen generates positive airway pressure in adult volunteers. Aust Crit Care 20:126–131
7. Frizzola M, Miller TL, Rodriguez ME et al (2011) High-flow nasal cannula: Impact on oxygenation and ventilation in an acute lung injury model. Pediatr Pulmonol 46:67–74
8. Hasani A, Chapman T, McCool D et al (2008) Domiciliary humidification improves lung mucociliary clearance in patients with bronchiectasis. Chron Respir Dis 5:81–86
9. Sztrymf B, Messika J, Bertrand F et al (2011) Beneficial effects of humidified high flow nasal oxygen in critical care patients: a prospective pilot study. Intensive Care Med 37:1780–1786
10. Itagaki T, Okuda N, Tsunano Y et al (2014) Effect of high-flow nasal cannula on thoraco-abdominal synchrony in adult critically ill patients. Respir Care 59:70–74
11. Corley A, Caruana LR, Barnett AG et al (2011) Oxygen delivery through high-flow nasal cannulae increase end-expiratory lung volume and reduce respiratory rate in post-cardiac surgical patients. Br J Anaesth 107:998–1004
12. Esteban A, Frutos-Vivar F, Ferguson ND et al (2004) Noninvasive positive-pressure ventilation for respiratory failure after extubation. N Engl J Med 350:2452–2460
13. Kang BJ, Koh Y, Lim C-M et al (2015) Failure of high-flow nasal cannula therapy may delay intubation and increase mortality. Intensive Care Med 41:623–632
14. Rello J, Pérez M, Roca O et al (2012) High-flow nasal therapy in adults with severe acute respiratory infection. J Crit Care 27:434–439
15. Frat JP, Thille AW, Mercat A et al (2015) High-flow oxygen through nasal cannula in acute hypoxemic respiratory failure. N Engl J Med 372:2185–2196
16. Belley-Côté EP, Duceppe E, Whitlock RP (2015) High-flow nasal cannula oxygen in respiratory failure. N Engl J Med 373:1373
17. Wawrzeniak IC, Moraes RB, Fendt LCC (2015) High-flow nasal cannula oxygen in respiratory failure. N Engl J Med 373:1373
18. Sehgal IS, Dhooria S, Agarwal R (2015) High-flow nasal cannula oxygen in respiratory failure. N Engl J Med 373:1374

19. Frat JP, Ragot S, Thille AW (2015) High-flow nasal cannula oxygen in respiratory failure. N Engl J Med 373:1373–1375
20. Ou X, Hua Y, Liu J et al (2017) Effect of high-flow nasal cannula oxygen therapy in adults with acute hypoxemic respiratory failure: a meta-analysis of randomized controlled trials. CMAJ 189:E260–E267
21. Monro-Somerville T, Sim M, Ruddy J et al (2017) The effect of high-flow nasal cannula oxygen therapy on mortality and intubation rate in acute respiratory failure. Crit Care Med 45:e449–e456
22. Roca O, Pérez-Terán P, Masclans JR et al (2013) Patients with New York Heart Association class III heart failure may benefit with high flow nasal cannula supportive therapy: high flow nasal cannula in heart failure. J Crit Care 28:741–746
23. Esquinas AM, Papadakos PJ (2014) High-flow nasal cannula supportive therapy in chronic heart failure: a partial or completed "CPAP-like effect"? J Crit Care 29:465
24. Krinsley JS, Reddy PK, Iqbal A (2012) What is the optimal rate of failed extubation? Crit Care 16:111
25. Kulkarni AP, Agarwal V (2008) Extubation failure in intensive care unit: predictors and management. Indian J Crit Care Med 12:1–9
26. Stéphan F, Barrucand B, Petit P et al (2015) High-flow nasal oxygen vs noninvasive positive airway pressure in hypoxemic patients after cardiothoracic surgery. JAMA 313:2331
27. Parke R, McGuinness S, Dixon R, Jull A (2013) Open-label, phase II study of routine high-flow nasal oxygen therapy in cardiac surgical patients. Br J Anaesth 111:925–931
28. Corley A, Bull T, Spooner AJ et al (2015) Direct extubation onto high-flow nasal cannulae post-cardiac surgery versus standard treatment in patients with a BMI≥30: a randomised controlled trial. Intensive Care Med 41:887–894
29. Zhu Y, Yin H, Zhang R, Wei J (2017) High-flow nasal cannula oxygen therapy vs conventional oxygen therapy in cardiac surgical patients: a meta-analysis. J Crit Care 38:123–128
30. Futier E, Paugam-Burtz C, Godet T et al (2016) Effect of early postextubation high-flow nasal cannula vs conventional oxygen therapy on hypoxaemia in patients after major abdominal surgery: a French multicentre randomised controlled trial (OPERA). Intensive Care Med 42:1888–1898
31. Maggiore SM, Idone FA, Vaschetto R et al (2014) Nasal high-flow versus venturi mask oxygen therapy after extubation. Effects on oxygenation, comfort, and clinical outcome. Am J Respir Crit Care Med 190:282–288
32. Hernández G, Vaquero C, Colinas L et al (2016) Effect of postextubation high-flow nasal cannula vs noninvasive ventilation on reintubation and postextubation respiratory failure in high-risk patients. JAMA 316:1565
33. Hernández G, Vaquero C, González P et al (2016) Effect of postextubation high-flow nasal cannula vs conventional oxygen therapy on reintubation in low-risk patients. JAMA 315:1354
34. Simon M, Braune S, Frings D et al (2014) High-flow nasal cannula oxygen versus non-invasive ventilation in patients with acute hypoxaemic respiratory failure undergoing flexible bronchoscopy - a prospective randomised trial. Crit Care 18:712
35. Lucangelo U, Vassallo FG, Marras E et al (2012) High-flow nasal interface improves oxygenation in patients undergoing bronchoscopy. Crit Care Res Pract 2012:506382
36. Neilipovitz DT, Crosby ET (2007) No evidence for decreased incidence of aspiration after rapid sequence induction. Can J Anesth 54:748–764
37. Vourc'h M, Asfar P, Volteau C et al (2015) High-flow nasal cannula oxygen during endotracheal intubation in hypoxemic patients: a randomized controlled clinical trial. Intensive Care Med 41:1538–1548
38. Jaber S, Monnin M, Girard M et al (2016) Apnoeic oxygenation via high-flow nasal cannula oxygen combined with non-invasive ventilation preoxygenation for intubation in hypoxaemic patients in the intensive care unit: the single-centre, blinded, randomised controlled OPTINIV trial. Intensive Care Med 42:1877–1887

39. Simon M, Wachs C, Braune S et al (2016) High-flow nasal cannula versus bag-valve-mask for preoxygenation before intubation in subjects with hypoxemic respiratory failure. Respir Care 61:1160–1167
40. Heinrich S, Horbach T, Stubner B et al (2014) Benefits of heated and humidified high flow nasal oxygen for preoxygenation in morbidly obese patients undergoing bariatric surgery: a randomized controlled study. J Obes Bariatrics 1:1–7
41. Azoulay E, Lemiale V, Mokart D et al (2014) Acute respiratory distress syndrome in patients with malignancies. Intensive Care Med 40:1106–1114
42. Ewig S, Torres A, Riquelme R et al (1998) Pulmonary complications in patients with haematological malignancies treated at a respiratory ICU. Eur Respir J 12:116–122
43. Coudroy R, Jamet A, Petua P et al (2016) High-flow nasal cannula oxygen therapy versus noninvasive ventilation in immunocompromised patients with acute respiratory failure: an observational cohort study. Ann Intensive Care 6:45
44. Lee HY, Rhee CK, Lee JW (2015) Feasibility of high-flow nasal cannula oxygen therapy for acute respiratory failure in patients with hematologic malignancies: a retrospective single-center study. J Crit Care 30:773–777
45. Harada K, Kurosawa S, Hino Y et al (2016) Clinical utility of high-flow nasal cannula oxygen therapy for acute respiratory failure in patients with hematological disease. Springerplus 5:512
46. Booth S, Anderson H, Swannick M et al (2004) The use of oxygen in the palliation of breathlessness. A report of the expert working group of the scientific committee of the association of palliative medicine. Respir Med 98:66–77
47. Epstein AS, Hartridge-Lambert SK, Ramaker JS et al (2011) Humidified high-flow nasal oxygen utilization in patients with cancer at Memorial Sloan-Kettering Cancer Center. J Palliat Med 14:835–839
48. Peters SG, Holets SR, Gay PC (2013) High-flow nasal cannula therapy in do-not-intubate patients with hypoxemic respiratory distress. Respir Care 58:597–600
49. Fealy N, Osborne C, Eastwood GM et al (2016) Nasal high-flow oxygen therapy in ICU: a before-and-after study. Aust Crit Care 29:17–22
50. Rabbat A, Blanc K, Lefebvre A, Lorut C (2016) Nasal high flow oxygen therapy after extubation: the road is open but don't drive too fast! J Thorac Dis 8:E1620–E1624
51. Ni YN, Luo J, Yu H et al (2017) Can high-flow nasal cannula reduce the rate of endotracheal intubation in adult patients with acute respiratory failure compared with conventional oxygen therapy and noninvasive positive pressure ventilation?: a systematic review and meta-analysis. Chest 151:764–775

Role of Tissue Viscoelasticity in the Pathogenesis of Ventilator-induced Lung Injury

A. Protti and E. Votta

Introduction

Biomechanics is mechanics applied to biology. One of its goals is to quantify the effect of mechanical stimuli on living organs and tissues, based on the relationship between the *microscopic* structure and the *macroscopic* function of these biological systems [1].

Ventilator-induced lung injury (VILI) can be defined as damage to the lungs (the biological system) triggered by physical forces (the mechanical stimuli) generated by an external ventilator. Biomechanical concepts could then be used to understand and predict the harm of mechanical ventilation. Based on this rationale, we and other authors have started to refer to the amplitude of lung inflation as "volumetric strain", the velocity of lung inflation as "strain rate", the reactive pulmonary tissue tension as "stress" and lung inhomogeneities as "stress risers" [2–6]. Ventilator-induced air leaks, such as pneumothorax, pneumomediastinum, subcutaneous emphysema or gaseous embolism, could then be interpreted as the rupture of one lung region that has been stretched above its upper physiological limit, or "ultimate tensile stress" [7]. Other lung injuries induced by less extreme inflation, including pulmonary edema, apparently develop as cumulative damage or "fatigue". They start from microscopic structural discontinuities, slowly propagate and then suddenly grow into macroscopic defects [7]. The probability of developing these other lung injuries increases with the number of cycles of deformation, that is with the respiratory rate and the overall duration of mechanical ventilation [8]. As a general rule, the larger the mechanical stimulus, the lower the number of cycles to failure [7].

A. Protti (✉)
Dipartimento di Anestesia, Rianimazione ed Emergenza-Urgenza, Fondazione IRCCS Ca' Granda-Ospedale Maggiore Policlinico
Milan, Italy
e-mail: alessandro.protti@policlinico.mi.it

E. Votta
Dipartimento di Elettronica, Informazione e Bioingegneria, Politecnico di Milano
Piazza Leonardo da Vinci, Milan, Italy

© Springer International Publishing AG 2018   193
J.-L. Vincent (ed.), *Annual Update in Intensive Care and Emergency Medicine 2018*,
Annual Update in Intensive Care and Emergency Medicine,
https://doi.org/10.1007/978-3-319-73670-9_16

The aim of this chapter is to use biomechanical concepts to understand the effects of mechanical ventilation on the lungs. Our final objective is to identify easy-to-measure variables that will hopefully improve our ability to recognize injurious ventilator settings and allow better allocation to alternative, putatively more protective, modes of support (including extracorporeal ones). First, we will review the microscopic structural features that are relevant for the macroscopic mechanical behavior of the lungs (or other connective tissues), with special emphasis on viscoelasticity. Second, we will discuss the reasons why ventilator settings that amplify the viscoelastic behavior of the lungs can produce tissue damage. Finally, we will introduce the hypothesis that the slow post-occlusion airway pressure decay (P1–P2), that somehow reflects lung viscoelasticity, predicts risks of mechanical ventilation. We will report preliminary observations from our swine model of VILI [4, 5].

The Microscopic Structure of the Lungs

The lung fibrous skeleton is the structure that directly bears the forces applied by mechanical ventilation. It mainly consists of two fiber systems: an axial system anchored to the hilum and running along the branching airways down to the alveolar ducts, and a peripheral system anchored to the visceral pleura and going centrally to the lung parenchyma. The two systems join together in the alveolar septa and form a continuum, from the hilum to the visceral pleura [9].

The microscopic structure of the lung fibrous skeleton can be described as an intricate network of elastin and collagen fibers, embedded in a hydrophilic gel known as ground substance. Both elastin and collagen fibers are formed by monomeric units that aggregate into polymeric structures of increasing complexity (the fibrils, the fibers, the three-dimensional matrix). For elastin, the basic unit is tropoelastin deposited onto a scaffold of fibrillin-rich microfibrils; for collagen, it is the triple poly amino-acidic helix [10]. In human lungs, the tissue densities of elastin and collagen fibers are 7 and 10%, respectively [11]. Elastin fibers impart the properties of extensibility and reversible recoil. They behave as thin strands of rubbery material or extensible springs and can be easily deformed and stretched (their strain at rupture is > 100%). Collagen fibers provide tissue with tensile strength. They work as stiff strings with non-linear mechanical properties: they cannot sustain large elongation (strain at rupture is only 10–15%) and become stiffer when they are progressively stretched. As a result, they strongly resist further deformation when lung volume approaches total capacity (tension at rupture is around 100 MPa). The ground substance is mainly formed by proteoglycans, macromolecules consisting of a protein core and glycosaminoglycan side chains [10].

These individual constituents of the lung fibrous skeleton form a complex three-dimensional matrix. Alveolar elastin and collagen fibers, which are largely entangled and interconnected, form a continuum with elastin and collagen fibers in pulmonary blood vessels and in the pleura [11, 12]. Collagen molecules form hydrogen bonds with the surrounding water molecules. Proteoglycans interact, chemically and physically, with all other constituents and thus influence the way the lung fibrous skeleton reacts to tensile stress [13].

When there is no load, elastin and collagen fibers appear wavy and crimped; they form a 'spaghetti'-like network. In response to progressive loading, elastic fibers elongate smoothly while collagen fibers are gradually oriented along the direction of tension, uncrimp and get stretched. Thereafter, elastin and collagen fibrils and fibers start to slide against each other, while hydrogen bonds start to fail. Tension slowly relaxes and falls to a lower value. Beyond this stage, if the ultimate tensile stress is exceeded, fibers will break [14].

It is this ultrastructural arrangement of the fibrous skeleton, and not the mechanical characteristic of its individual microscopic components, that primarily determines the macroscopic mechanical behavior of the lungs. Depending on how tissue fibers, cells and the extracellular matrix are organized, the properties of the tissue vary [15]. In line with this conclusion, factors that affect the interaction between elastin, collagen and interstitial fluids, such as body temperature or inflammation, all influence lung mechanics [16].

The Macroscopic Mechanical Behavior of the Lungs

Viscoelasticity is the property of materials that exhibit both *elastic* and *viscous* characteristics when undergoing deformation (Fig. 1).

Elastic materials attain equilibrium instantaneously after the application of an external load: they immediately strain when stressed and quickly return to their original state once the load has been removed. Elastic materials accumulate energy and entirely return it, so that their stress-strain relationship is exactly the same during loading and unloading. Most elastic soft tissues display non-linear, biphasic, stress-strain relationships. If strain is below a critical threshold, the stress-strain response will be reasonably linear but quite flat; if it is beyond that threshold, the stress-strain response will be reasonably linear but much steeper. This behavior depends neither on the strain rate nor on the specific sequence of events experienced by the material, unless the ultimate tensile stress is exceeded [17].

Viscoelastic materials are different. Their response to loads is not instantaneous: elongation is delayed and impeded by *internal viscous resistances*. When a viscoelastic body is suddenly stressed and then the stress is kept constant, the body continues to deform until it reaches a plateau value. This phenomenon is called 'creep'. When a viscoelastic body is suddenly strained and the strain is kept constant afterwards, the corresponding stress induced in the body decreases over time, again progressively approaching a plateau value. This phenomenon is called 'stress relaxation'. Viscoelastic materials only partly return energy during unloading, because internal friction leads to energy dissipation in the form of heat. As a result, the stress-strain plots describing loading and unloading differ from each other, with stress being lower during unloading at any given strain. The extent of the area limited by the two limbs of the plot corresponds to the energy that has been dissipated.

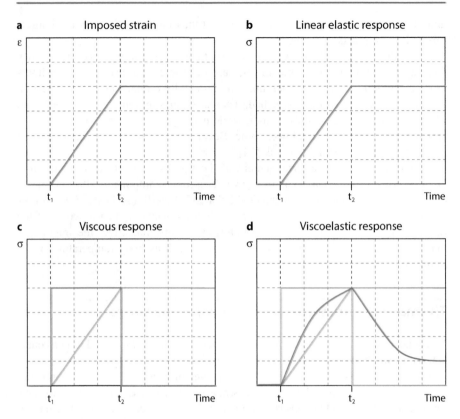

Fig. 1 Stress-strain relationship for linear elastic, viscous and viscoelastic materials. Deformation (strain, ε) is progressively increased at a constant rate (dynamic phase) and then kept constant over time (static phase) (panel **a**). In a linear elastic body, internal tension (stress, σ) is proportional to strain: it increases during the dynamic phase and remains constantly high during the static phase (panel **b**). In a viscous body, stress is proportional to the velocity of deformation: it is high during the dynamic phase, but returns to zero when elongation ceases, irrespective of the residual static deformation (panel **c**). In a viscoelastic body, which combines the properties of linear elastic and viscous materials, stress is high during the dynamic phase, but slowly declines during the static state, down to a plateau value (stress relaxation) (panel **d**). Reproduced from [23] with permission

This property of dissipating energy during cyclic loading and unloading is called 'hysteresis' [17].

The simplest models to describe the mechanical response of viscoelastic materials consist of networks of linear elastic springs and linear viscous dashpots. The stress-strain relationship of the springs is:

$$\text{stress} = k \times \text{strain}$$

where k is a proportionality constant and strain is the amplitude of deformation.

The stress-strain relationship of the dashpots is:

$$\text{stress} = \eta \times \text{strain rate}$$

where η is a proportionality constant and strain is the velocity of deformation [17]. K and η are usually derived from experimental data.

Mechanically ventilated lungs behave as polymeric viscoelastic bodies undergoing cyclic loading and unloading. During inflation and deflation, the individual constituents of the lung fibrous skeleton unfold and refold, lengthen and shorten, change orientation, slip against each other, while their physical and chemical interactions break and form again. These phenomena occur primarily in sites of contact between fibers and, to some extent, even within the elastin and collagen fibers and into the ground substance [18]. Scanning electron micrographs clearly demonstrate that collagen fiber networks differ considerably between collapsed and inflated (rat) lungs. In the collapsed lung, collagen fibers show a wavy, disordered morphology whereas in the inflated lung, they are straight and oriented along the direction of stretching [12]. During inflation and deflation, lungs exhibit creep, stress relaxation and hysteresis [19, 20]. Viscous forces resist against the structural rearrangement described above and retard elongation. Energy that is spent to overcome these internal frictions during inflation cannot be recovered during deflation.

Like elastic bodies, lungs change their shape according to the force applied and recover their original shape when the force is released; stress depends on the amplitude of strain. Unlike elastic bodies, lungs irreversibly loose some energy in their internal structure during inflation, as a consequence of their viscoelastic components.

According to Bachofen and Hildebrand [21], quasi-static lung hysteresis, which is recorded after stress relaxation, can be defined as:

$$\text{lung hysteresis} = \text{k} \times \text{volume} \times \text{pressure}$$

where k is the hysteresis constant of lung tissue. Energy dissipation is proportional to strain (volume inflated) and strain rate. In fact, for any given strain, pressure is proportional to the velocity of deformation. Of note, dynamic lung hysteresis, which is recorded before stress relaxation, is greater than quasi-static lung hysteresis, because viscoelastic phenomena dissipate energy [22].

Role of Tissue Viscoelasticity in the Pathogenesis of Ventilator-induced Lung Injury

Tissue viscoelasticity can explain the harmful effects of large (and fast, if respiratory rate is kept constant) lung deformations [23]. First, large and rapid strain increases viscous resistance: time for ultrastructural rearrangement is short, so that individual fibers carry more stress, and more energy is lost as heat. According to the kinetic molecular theory, heating a material increases the amount of kinetic energy of its constituents. Molecular vibrations become large and fast and the distance between molecules increases. In addition, heat can change the protein conformation, so that weak intermolecular bonds may fail. The fibrous skeleton becomes more fragile, also because of ensuing inflammation. In fact, fragmentation of extracellular matrix constituents, such as hyaluronan, stimulates the expression of chemokines in macrophages that recruit neutrophils into the lungs [24]. Second, large and fast strain promotes the formation of entanglements or 'nodes' where lines of force will concentrate. It is in the immediate proximity of these discontinuities, where stress gets amplified, that microstructural defects will initially form. From there, damage will propagate to the surrounding regions to finally become macroscopically evident [25]. Third, if the interval between two inflations is very short, the lung tissue will not have enough time to return to its initial conformation, with the microstructure arranged at its best to tolerate the next elongation, and to disperse the heat that has been previously generated. Immediate reloading and incomplete unloading reduce the number of cycles a polymer can withstand.

Lung tissue viscoelasticity also explains why limiting tidal volume (and inspiratory flow) can be of benefit. In fact, small and slow strain allows smooth and complete adaptation of the lung fibrous skeleton. It generates low stress so that the risk of rupture is reduced. In addition, it diminishes the amount of energy converted into heat and allows the tissue to fully rearrange in time for the next deformation.

Monitoring Lung Viscoelastic Behavior: The Slow Post-occlusion Airway Pressure Decay (P1–P2)

Since creep, stress relaxation and hysteresis all reflect the intimate structure of the tissue, monitoring these three features provides insight into the mechanical behavior of the lungs. The interrupter technique enables measurement of stress relaxation quite easily, even at the bedside. This is the reason why we will focus on this specific technique.

The 'interrupter technique', or 'end-inflation occlusion method', was originally developed to measure airway resistance. It involves making a sudden interruption of gas flow at the mouth, during constant flow inflation, while measuring the pressure just distal to the point of occlusion [26, 27]. If the interruption is instantaneous, the airway is completely rigid and the gas in the system is incompressible, then the airway pressure and the alveolar pressure will equilibrate immediately on interruption. If the alveolar pressure immediately prior to and after the interruption remains the same, then the instantaneous pressure drop recorded just distal to the point of occlusion will reflect the resistive pressure drop existing across the airways at the instant before interruption (that is, the airway resistance).

In the real word, however, the pressure signal observed following an end-inspiratory occlusion invariably exhibits two distinct phases (Fig. 2; [26, 27]). The first phase is a very rapid drop, which occurs immediately on interruption of flow: airway pressure jumps from its peak value, recorded at the time of occlusion, down to P1, the airway pressure recorded when flow becomes zero. This is the pressure

Fig. 2 The slow post-occlusion airway pressure decay (P1–P2). Decay in airway pressure (*upper panel*) and gas flow (*lower panel*) following rapid occlusion during constant inspiratory flow inflation. P1 is the airway pressure when flow becomes zero; P2 is the plateau airway pressure. In subjects with healthy lungs, P1–P2 mainly reflects viscoelastic stress relaxation. Reproduced from [39] with permission

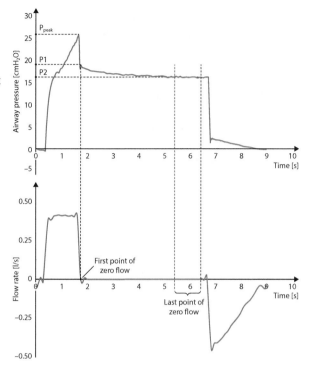

change that can be used to compute airway resistance:

$$\text{airway resistance} = (\text{peak airway pressure} - \text{P1})/\text{gas flow}$$

where gas flow refers to the time immediately preceding the occlusion. The second phase is a further pressure change in the same direction as the first one but it evolves over a few seconds. Airway pressure keeps on declining, from P1 to P2, the (plateau) airway pressure that corresponds to the static equilibrium elastic recoil of the respiratory system. This second, nearly exponential, pressure change reflects 'additional resistance'. It is due to viscoelastic pressure dissipation (stress relaxation) and gas redistribution between regions of the lung at different pressures at the time of occlusion (a phenomenon often referred to as "pendelluft") [28]:

$$\text{additional respiratory system resistance} = (\text{P1} - \text{P2})/\text{gas flow}$$

Bates and colleagues measured alveolar pressure directly from capsules glued to the lung surface in open-chest ventilated dogs. They demonstrated that, in normal lungs, this second pressure change was almost entirely due to the stress relaxation of the alveolar tissue [26]. The role of pendelluft becomes relevant in highly inhomogeneous lungs [29]. There, fast alveolar units receive most of the tidal volume during inflation. Following interruption of flow, gas will redistribute from these over-distended – with higher pressure – units towards the others, which are under-inflated – with lower pressure [28]. This phenomenon will decrease airway pressure and widen P1–P2.

In humans with healthy lungs, undergoing elective surgery, additional resistance of the respiratory system is around 1.7 ± 0.7 cmH$_2$O/s/l [30] or 2.1 ± 0.8 cmH$_2$O/s/l [31]. In patients with acute respiratory distress syndrome (ARDS), resistance increases with severity of disease, up to 4.7 ± 1.1 cmH$_2$O/s/l [31]. On average, additional respiratory system resistance is around 50% of the total respiratory system resistance; additional lung resistance is around 50–70% of additional respiratory system resistance [30, 31].

Several aspects related to the measurement of P1–P2 deserve a comment. First, it is not possible to separate the contributions of stress relaxation and gas redistribution to the overall signal. Second, determination of P1 can be difficult. The transition between the first and the second phase of pressure decline is very rapid; high frequency recording systems are required. In addition, airway pressure can largely oscillate immediately after the interruption of gas flow, due to the inertia and compressibility of the air column in the airways. This is one reason why linear [32] or curvilinear [33] extrapolation of airway pressure back to the time of interruption has been suggested. Third, airway pressure decline due to lung volume loss by continuing oxygen uptake is ignored. This seems reasonable as the whole registration requires only a few seconds. Fourth, some stress relaxation occurs out of the lung tissue: (1) at the air-liquid interface of the alveolar spaces, as a result of the reversible movement of surfactant between the surface and the sublayer [34]; (2) in contractile tissue associated with the airways [35]; (3) as a result of alveolar recruitment and de-recruitment [36]; (4) in the blood contained in the pulmonary vasculature [37]. Of note, excised and bloodless parenchymal strips, in which the air-liquid interface has been removed and/or the basal tone has been ablated, still exhibit substantial viscoelasticity [38].

P1–P2 provides at least some insight on how lung tissue behaves during *ongoing* ventilation, in response to one specific ventilator setting. Other variables commonly recorded describe the respiratory system during *static* pauses, which never occur during ventilation.

High P1–P2 as a Risk Factor for Ventilator-induced Lung Injury: Preliminary Observations in Healthy Pigs

We have recently reported on 30 healthy pigs ventilated for 54 h with different combinations of tidal volume (strain) and inspiratory flow (strain rate), resulting in P1–P2 ranging between 1.8 and 10.2 cmH$_2$O. P1 was simply defined as the airway pressure recorded when gas flow stopped following an end-inspiratory occlusion maneuver (back-extrapolation was not used). Inspiratory flow was adjusted based on the inspiratory-to-expiratory time ratio; respiratory rate was always 15 breaths per minute. None of the animals assigned to combinations resulting in P1–P2 less than 3.4 cmH$_2$O (n = 13), including those receiving large (expectedly injurious) tidal volume but low inspiratory flow, developed pulmonary edema by the end of the study. By contrast, all of the animals assigned to combinations resulting in P1–P2 greater than $3.8 \, cmH_2O$ (n = 13), including those receiving small (expectedly protective) tidal volume but very high inspiratory flow, always did. Intermediate settings were not consistently associated with outcome ('gray zone') [5]. These findings suggest that P1–P2 predicts VILI independently from tidal volume and respiratory rate. That high inspiratory flow contributes to the risks of mechanical ventilation is consistent with the model described above. Viscoelastic bodies poorly tolerate very fast elongation: they require some time to rearrange their internal structure and they dissipate more energy when the strain rate is high.

Reasons why high P1–P2 should predict lung damage include the following. First, as long as we are concerned with the airway pressure reached by the end of inspiration, P1 should be certainly preferred over plateau airway pressure. In fact, plateau airway pressure totally ignores the (additional) pressure gradient due to the viscoelastic properties of the respiratory system and to inhomogeneous gas distribution. Both these phenomena occur during ongoing ventilation but they rapidly disappear during an (artefactual) end-inspiratory pause. Second, as long as we are concerned with driving airway pressure, this should be computed as P1 – positive end-expiratory pressure (PEEP), as P1 is the airway pressure that really distends the respiratory system at the end of inspiration [39]. Third, P1–P2 tends to change in line with the energy delivered per cycle to the lungs [8], the respiratory system hys-

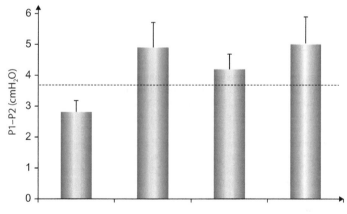

Tidal volume (ml)	500	750	500	500
Inspiratory flow (ml/s)	500	500	900	500
PEEP (cmH₂O)	0	0	0	12

Fig. 3 Ventilator settings associated with high P1–P2. In healthy, mechanically ventilated pigs, large tidal volume, high inspiratory flow or high positive end-expiratory pressure (PEEP), which usually induce pulmonary edema within 54 h, are associated with P1–P2 values above the probable threshold for harm, herein indicated with the *dashed line* (n = 3)

teresis [5] and the amount of energy dissipated at the tissue level during mechanical ventilation [8]. Moreover, it increases with the extent of lung inhomogeneities that can act as stress risers [8]. Unpublished data from our laboratory also suggest that P1–P2 rises when PEEP is increased up to potentially injurious levels while tidal volume is kept constant (Fig. 3).

Conclusion

The lung fibrous skeleton is composed of elastin fibers, collagen fibers and the extracellular matrix. Even so, the mechanical properties of the lungs are not equivalent to those of the individual fibers. The complex interactions between the microstructural components of the fibrous skeleton are responsible for frictional, or viscous, energy loss during cyclic deformation (as for ongoing mechanical ventilation). Energy that is not recovered by the end of expiration can have been spent to disrupt physical and chemical bonds that ensure the structural and functional integrity of the tissue and/or to trigger inflammation.

Stress relaxation can be monitored as P1–P2 even at the bedside. Biomechanical concepts and preliminary experimental findings in healthy pigs undergoing prolonged mechanical ventilation suggest that high P1–P2 predicts pulmonary edema.

As P1–P2 changes in line with tidal volume, inspiratory flow and PEEP, it may easily describe the safety profile of one specific ventilator setting, considering the interplay between all these major variables.

References

1. Fung YC (1993) Introduction: a sketch of the history and scope of the field. In: Fung YC (ed) Biomechanics: mechanical properties of living tissues, 2nd edn. Springer, New York, pp 1–22
2. Gattinoni L, Carlesso E, Cadringher P, Valenza F, Vagginelli F, Chiumello D (2003) Physical and biological triggers of ventilator-induced lung injury and its prevention. Eur Respir J Suppl 47:15s–25s
3. Chiumello D, Carlesso E, Cadringher P et al (2008) Lung stress and strain during mechanical ventilation for acute respiratory distress syndrome. Am J Respir Crit Care Med 178:346–355
4. Protti A, Cressoni M, Santini A et al (2011) Lung stress and strain during mechanical ventilation: any safe threshold? Am J Respir Crit Care Med 183:1354–1362
5. Protti A, Maraffi T, Milesi M et al (2016) Role of strain rate in the pathogenesis of ventilator-induced lung edema. Crit Care Med 44:e838–e845
6. Cressoni M, Cadringher P, Chiurazzi C et al (2014) Lung inhomogeneity in patients with acute respiratory distress syndrome. Am J Respir Crit Care Med 189:149–158
7. Hoeppner DW (1998) Industrial significance of fatigue problems. In: Lampman SR (ed) Fatigue and fracture, 2nd edn. ASM Handbook, vol 19. ASM International, Ohio, pp 10–36
8. Cressoni M, Gotti M, Chiurazzi C et al (2016) Mechanical power and development of ventilator-induced lung injury. Anesthesiology 124:1100–1108
9. Weibel ER (1984) The lung's mechanical support. In: Weibel ER (ed) The pathway for oxygen: structure and function in the mammalian respiratory system, 1st edn. Harvard University Press, Cambridge, pp 302–338

10. Muiznieks LD, Keeley FW (2013) Molecular assembly and mechanical properties of the extracellular matrix: a fibrous protein perspective. Biochim Biophys Acta 1832:866–875
11. Mercer RR, Crapo JD (1990) Spatial distribution of collagen and elastin fibers in the lungs. J Appl Physiol 69:756–765
12. Toshima M, Ohtani Y, Ohtani O (2004) Three-dimensional architecture of elastin and collagen fiber networks in the human and rat lung. Arch Histol Cytol 67:31–40
13. Al Jamal R, Roughley PJ, Ludwig MS (2001) Effect of glycosaminoglycan degradation on lung tissue viscoelasticity. Am J Physiol Lung Cell Mol Physiol 280:L306–L315
14. Yang W, Sherman VR, Gludovatz B et al (2015) On the tear resistance of skin. Nat Commun 6:6649
15. Suki B, Barabási AL, Lutchen KR (1994) Lung tissue viscoelasticity: a mathematical framework and its molecular basis. J Appl Physiol 76:2749–2759
16. Rubini A, Carniel EL (2014) A review of recent findings about stress-relaxation in the respiratory system tissues. Lung 192:833–839
17. Fung YC (1993) Bioviscoelastic solids. In: Fung YC (ed) Biomechanics: mechanical properties of living tissues, 2nd edn. Springer, New York, pp 242–320
18. Mijailovich SM, Stamenović D, Brown R, Leith DE, Fredberg JJ (1994) Dynamic moduli of rabbit lung tissue and pigeon ligamentum propatagiale undergoing uniaxial cyclic loading. J Appl Physiol 76:773–782
19. Bayliss LE, Robertson GW (1939) The viscoelastic properties of the lungs. Q J Exp Physiol 29:27–47
20. Sugihara T, Hildebrandt J, Martin CJ (1972) Viscoelastic properties of alveolar wall. J Appl Physiol 33:93–98
21. Bachofen H, Hildebrandt J (1971) Area analysis of pressure-volume hysteresis in mammalian lungs. J Appl Physiol 30:493–497
22. Bachofen H (1968) Lung tissue resistance and pulmonary hysteresis. J Appl Physiol 24:296–301
23. Protti A, Votta E, Gattinoni L (2014) Which is the most important strain in the pathogenesis of ventilator-induced lung injury: dynamic or static? Curr Opin Crit Care 20:33–38
24. Jiang D, Liang J, Fan J et al (2005) Regulation of lung injury and repair by Toll-like receptors and hyaluronan. Nat Med 11:1173–1179
25. Cressoni M, Chiurazzi C, Gotti M et al (2015) Lung inhomogeneities and time course of ventilator-induced mechanical injuries. Anesthesiology 123:618–627
26. Bates JH, Ludwig MS, Sly PD et al (1988) Interrupter resistance elucidated by alveolar pressure measurement in open-chest normal dogs. J Appl Physiol 65:408–414
27. D'Angelo E, Calderini E, Torri G et al (1989) Respiratory mechanics in anesthetized paralyzed humans: effects of flow, volume, and time. J Appl Physiol 67:2556–2564
28. Otis AB, McKerrow CB, Bartlett RA et al (1956) Mechanical factors in distribution of pulmonary ventilation. J Appl Physiol 8:427–443
29. Similowski T, Bates JH (1991) Two-compartment modelling of respiratory system mechanics at low frequencies: gas redistribution or tissue rheology? Eur Respir J 4:353–358
30. Pesenti A, Pelosi P, Rossi N, Virtuani A, Brazzi L, Rossi A (1991) The effects of positive end-expiratory pressure on respiratory resistance in patients with the adult respiratory distress syndrome and in normal anesthetized subjects. Am Rev Respir Dis 144:101–107
31. Pelosi P, Cereda M, Foti G, Giacomini M, Pesenti A (1995) Alterations of lung and chest wall mechanics in patients with acute lung injury: effects of positive end-expiratory pressure. Am J Respir Crit Care Med 152:531–537
32. Carter ER (1997) It is time to consider standardizing the interrupter technique. Eur Respir J 10:1428–1429
33. Jackson AC, Milhorn HT Jr, Norman JR (1974) A reevaluation of the interrupter technique for airway resistance measurement. J Appl Physiol 36:264–268
34. Lorino AM, Harf A, Atlan G, Lorino H, Laurent D (1982) Role of surface tension and tissue in rat lung stress relaxation. Respir Physiol 48:143–155

35. Martin HB, Proctor DF (1958) Pressure-volume measurements on dog bronchi. J Appl Physiol 13:337–343
36. Smaldone GC, Mitzner W, Itoh H (1983) Role of alveolar recruitment in lung inflation: influence on pressure-volume hysteresis. J Appl Physiol Respir Environ Exerc Physiol 55:1321–1332
37. Peták F, Fodor GH, Babik B, Habre W (2016) Airway mechanics and lung tissue viscoelasticity: effects of altered blood hematocrit in the pulmonary circulation. J Appl Physiol 121:261–267
38. Salerno FG, Kurosawa H, Eidelman DH, Ludwig MS (1996) Characterization of the anatomical structures involved in the contractile response of the rat lung periphery. Br J Pharmacol 118:734–740
39. Santini A, Votta E, Protti A, Mezidi M, Guérin C (2017) Driving airway pressure: should we use a static measure to describe a dynamic phenomenon? Intensive Care Med 43:1544–1545

Alveolar Recruitment in Patients with Assisted Ventilation: Open Up the Lung in Spontaneous Breathing

A. Lovas and Z. Molnár

Introduction

Hypoxemic respiratory failure, especially its most severe form, acute respiratory distress syndrome (ARDS), is one of the leading reasons for implementing mechanical ventilation in the critically ill [1]. ARDS is a life-threatening condition precipitated by disorders that frequently result in intensive care unit (ICU) admission. All of these disorders causing either direct pulmonary or indirect extrapulmonary tissue damage feature a systemic inflammatory response. Released cytokines, such as interleukin (IL)-1, IL-6, IL-8 and tumor necrosis factor (TNF), activate neutrophils in the lung throughout the inflammatory cascade [2]. Thereafter, injurious substances, such as free oxygen radicals and proteolytic enzymes, are secreted by the activated immune cells leading to alveolar endothelium and epithelium destruction. The latter pathophysiological mechanism induces impaired permeability in the lung resulting in alveolar flooding by protein-rich edema fluid [3]. Surfactant, which has a major role in the modulation of the surface tension of the alveoli, is also washed out. Most importantly, surfactant excretion is also diminished due to the dysfunction of type II epithelial cells. As a net result of the pathophysiological cascade, pulmonary atelectasis develops as the alveoli collapse.

Pulmonary atelectasis is accompanied by arterial hypoxemia from the increased right-to-left shunt in the lungs ([4]; Fig. 1)). As severe acute hypoxemia is a potential danger for all vital organs, its resolution is of paramount importance. However, in the most severe cases this may require high oxygen concentrations, high pressures and/or volumes, which are far above physiological values. This is a therapeutic conflict, as on the one hand systemic hypoxemia can be dangerous to all vital organs and tissues, but non-physiological ventilator settings may be harmful for the lung. Therefore, finding the balance between maintaining adequate oxygenation

A. Lovas · Z. Molnár (✉)
Department of Anesthesiology and Intensive Care, University of Szeged
Szeged, Hungary
e-mail: zsoltmolna@gmail.com

© Springer International Publishing AG 2018   205
J.-L. Vincent (ed.), *Annual Update in Intensive Care and Emergency Medicine 2018*,
Annual Update in Intensive Care and Emergency Medicine,
https://doi.org/10.1007/978-3-319-73670-9_17

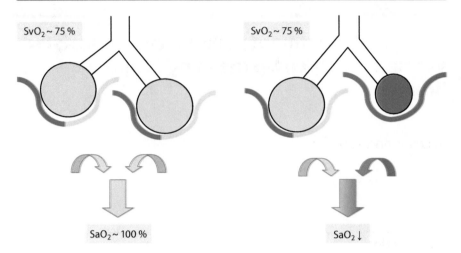

Fig. 1 Intrapulmonary shunt as a result of atelectasis of alveoli. The figure demonstrates, that under normal circumstances (*left panel*) alveoli are open and gas exchange takes place continuously, hence resulting in almost 100% saturation of the hemoglobin. On the *right panel*, there is a shunt phenomenon in the dark alveolus, hence venous admixture takes place, resulting in lower arterial oxygen content, which is indicated by decreasing arterial oxygen saturation (SaO_2). SvO_2: mixed venous oxygen saturation

with the least injurious ventilator settings is of utmost importance. Several therapeutic interventions have been tested and described to serve this purpose, such as extracorporeal membrane oxygenation (ECMO) [5], high frequency oscillatory ventilation (HFOV) [6], and prone positioning [7]. However, these interventions require special equipment, extra manpower and can be costly and time consuming to set up. Another alternative is the lung recruitment maneuver, which does not require any special equipment and can be performed simply by adjusting certain settings on the ventilator.

The Rationale and Basic Principles of Lung Recruitment

In normal conditions, we breathe 21% oxygen from the air, which is satisfactory to maintain adequate oxygenation to our cells. This statement applies only when almost all of our alveoli are open, where gas exchange takes place continuously. Regarding lung mechanics, under physiological conditions our lungs operate with very small pressure changes. With these minimal pressure alterations, tidal volumes (V_T) of around 4 to 6 ml/kg are generated. The question arises as to why has this evolved according to these substructures? The answer must lie in the fact that 'it's good for us'! Therefore, parameters that are different from those of physiology must be assumed to be harmful.

In hypoxemic respiratory failure, because of the right-to-left shunt (induced by atelectasis, secretions, edema fluid, etc.), we have to apply inspired oxygen fraction

(FiO_2) levels greater than physiological values and high pressures to restore adequate arterial oxygenation. In the case of atelectasis, when we recruit non-aerated lung regions (hence reducing intrapulmonary shunt and improving oxygen uptake) this enables us to reduce FiO_2, which means that the whole scenario moves closer to the physiological normal ranges. This forms the pathophysiological rationale of lung recruitment.

Theoretically, atelectatic lung areas can be opened up with the help of a transient increase in transpulmonary pressure over a short period of time, which can decrease the right-to-left shunt ratio and hence improve arterial oxygenation [8]. The intervention is called the lung recruitment maneuver (Fig. 2). It can be accompanied by titration of the 'optimal' positive end-expiratory pressure (PEEP), a process which Lachmann called by the broader term "open lung concept" in 1992 [8].

Several methods have described the execution of this procedure and discussing them is beyond the scope of the current article. Nevertheless, most of the studies were performed under controlled mechanical ventilation (CMV). However, intermittent positive pressure ventilation (IPPV) contradicts physiological breathing in several ways, whereas maintaining and/or assisting spontaneous breathing during mechanical ventilation may have some theoretical benefits. According to a recent large international survey, around 30% of patients with ARDS in general, and more than 20% with severe ARDS, are managed with spontaneous ventilation modes [9]. This important observation raises two questions. First, which is the safest and most advantageous mode of ventilation in these patients? Second, should lung recruit-

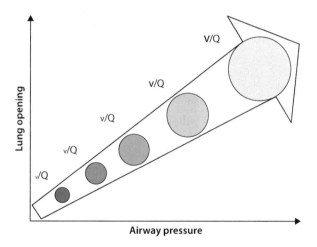

Fig. 2 Recruitment of alveoli with increasing airway pressures and consecutive improvement in ventilation/perfusion (V/Q) ratio. If the lung is recruitable, by increasing inspiratory pressure, more and more atelectatic alveoli can be opened up (indicated by the increasing size of the "V"), without necessarily impairing perfusion, hence improving V/Q ratios. Theoretically, with this approach, the whole lung could become aerated. However, it is important to note (not shown on the figure), that at certain high inspiratory pressures overdistension and impaired perfusion of the overstretched alveoli can also take place causing V/Q mismatch

ment be performed during assisted spontaneous ventilation (ASV) or is this the privilege of CMV modes only?

Controlled Versus Assisted Spontaneous Mechanical Ventilation

First of all, it is useful to give a brief summary of the pros and cons between CMV and ASV.

Diaphragmatic Dysfunction

One of the potential side effects of CMV is related to the loss of respiratory muscle strength. In an animal investigation, CMV induced diaphragmatic dysfunction compared to ASV [10]. This is most likely the result of diaphragm inactivity, which – as with skeletal muscles – leads to atrophy, which is certainly an important issue during ASV modes. Furthermore, spontaneous diaphragm movement plays an important role in ventilation-perfusion mismatch. In CMV, especially when the muscles are relaxed, in supine patients the majority of the V_T is delivered into the less perfused, smaller pressure, ventral, non-dependent regions of the lungs, which are also smaller in volume. By contrast, in spontaneous breathing the dorsal part of the diaphragm moves more actively, shifting the air more effectively into the dependent, larger in volume lung areas, consequently resulting in better ventilation-perfusion match, hence better oxygenation [11]. Spontaneous breathing also promotes alveolar recruitment with the redistribution of ventilation and also reduces cyclic alveolar shearing [11].

Atelectotrauma

Cycling alveolar shearing along with the repetitive collapse and re-opening of the unstable alveoli in ARDS facilitates further stress injury of the inflamed lung. This mechanically induced dysfunction of the alveoli is called atelectotrauma [12]. The resultant tissue damage is proportional to the amplitude of the cyclic shearing caused by the mechanical ventilation [13].

It has been known for decades, that IPPV can itself cause further lung injury even in normal lungs. Therefore, applying the open lung concept with lung protective ventilation while the patient is breathing spontaneously may prevent further deleterious effects resulting in alveolar collapse.

Additional Effects

In addition to the effects of the different ventilation modes on lung mechanics and gas exchange, there are other important issues to be considered. The reduced requirement of sedation hence better patient-ventilator interaction is an important potential benefit [14]. Another concern could be the use of neuromuscular blocking agents, which is obviously impossible during ASV. In a randomized controlled trial, early administration of neuromuscular blocking agents in severe ARDS improved the 90-day adjusted survival [15]. However, patients undergoing pharmacological paralysis during mechanical ventilation are at higher risk of developing myopathy, and may require prolonged weaning [16–18].

Limitations of ASV

Despite the above mentioned theoretical benefits, ASV and especially pressure support ventilation (PSV) may also have undesired effects. Spontaneous breathing efforts in patients with markedly distressed ventilation can generate large negative pleural pressure, hence the transpulmonary pressure (see below) can be extremely high, causing severe lung stretching [19]. Furthermore, significant patient-ventilator asynchrony may also be present during seemingly synchronous PSV [20, 21].

Regarding lung recruitment, there are very limited data in spontaneously breathing patients, therefore comparison of the efficacy of recruitment during CMV and ASV is not possible at present. Nevertheless, performing lung recruitment during spontaneous modes of ventilation certainly has some rationale.

Lung Recruitment in the Spontaneously Breathing Patient

Theoretically, any lung recruitment maneuver can be applied during ASV, and there are certain ventilator settings and modes of ventilation that inevitably recruit lung areas without any further intervention.

Airway Pressure Release Ventilation

Airway pressure release ventilation (APRV) is *per se* a controlled ventilation mode, but at the same time it allows unrestricted spontaneous breathing as well. APRV performs on two levels of continuous positive airway pressure (CPAP), P_{high} and P_{low}; when there is a mandatory step in pressure change that is time-cycled and time-triggered, the inspiratory time is called T_{high} and the expiratory one T_{low}. APRV is an inverse ratio pressure control with which the patient is allowed to breath spontaneously at any time during the ventilator cycle on two different levels of pressure [22]. Considering the features of APRV, it is an optimal modality for the open lung concept with its prolonged CPAP duration recruiting the lung and the short release duration preventing lung collapse.

Another potential benefit of APRV is that spontaneous breathing improves the functional residual capacity (FRC) and respiratory system compliance hence reducing the elastic work of breathing (WOB) [23]. However, WOB is markedly dependent on the pre-settings made by the operator, as this ventilator mode cannot adapt to the patient's WOB. Any increase or decrease in the patient's WOB will be left to the operator to detect, and to adjust the settings. Accordingly, use of APRV at the bedside requires a high level of vigilance by the operator to optimize and correct each setting according to the current condition of the patient.

Pressure Support Ventilation

PSV can provide all the previously specified advantages of preserved spontaneous breathing in ARDS, such as increased ventilation of dependent lung regions, redistribution of intrapulmonary blood flow, hence improved ventilation/perfusion ratio, reduced damage of the alveolar cells [24], maintained activation of diaphragm muscles [10, 11] and lowered sedation requirements [14]. However, we should note that most of the benefits of assisted ventilation were observed in mild-to-moderate level of ARDS and the impact of spontaneous breathing in severe ARDS may be significantly different.

To avoid further damage of the alveoli during PSV, the level of the generated transpulmonary pressure should be considered. During CMV the transpulmonary pressure (airway pressure – pleural pressure) is kept constant. Conversely, when the patient has spontaneous breathing efforts in ARDS, the actual transpulmonary pressure represents the sum of the pressure generated by the ventilator and by the patient's respiratory muscles. Thus, the real driving pressure is higher than the airway pressure indicated by the ventilator [25]. When the patient is switched from CMV to PSV often a lower level of peak pressure is required to maintain the same level of V_T as in the controlled mode. However, at the same time the diaphragm generates a higher transpulmonary pressure with the presence of active muscle effort. Accordingly, the transpulmonary pressure may encompass very high rates if the level of support is not adequately reduced and/or the V_T is not properly monitored and reduced [26].

Lung Recruitment in PSV

Theoretically, with the transient increase in inflation pressure (i.e., pressure support), atelectatic lung regions may be opened up in PSV. However, the question arises as to whether we should switch back to CMV to perform the recruitment maneuver, or if it is safe and effective to execute the procedure when the patient is ventilated in PSV?

In one of our recent studies, we demonstrated that lung recruitment (see later) improved the PaO_2/FiO_2 ratio by more than 20% in half of the patients with moderate-to-severe hypoxemic respiratory failure ventilated in PSV [27]. Serious adverse effects of recruitment maneuvers, such as pneumothorax and worsening hemodynamic instability, were not detected during the study so the intervention could be performed safely.

In the study protocol, PEEP was first increased by $5\,cmH_2O$ from baseline to investigate any effect of PEEP-induced recruitment. Thereafter, for the alveolar re-

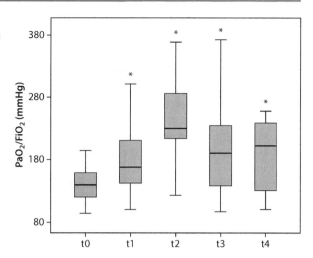

Fig. 3 Recruitment maneuver performed under pressure support ventilation improves oxygenation significantly and persistently among responders. *t0*, baseline; *t1*, increasing positive end-expiratory pressure (PEEP) by 5 H_2Ocm; *t2*, after recruitment; *t3* and *t4*, 15 and 30 min after recruitment; * $p < 0.05$ compared to baseline measurements. Boxplots are presented as 5th–95th percentile, interquartile range and median. For explanation, see text. Modified from [27]

cruitment procedure, pressure support was increased to 40 cmH_2O for 40 s to limit the undesirable side effects of volutrauma. Peak inspiratory pressure was then reduced to the initial baseline value while maintaining the increased level of PEEP (by 5 cmH_2O) according to the open lung concept [8]. The primary outcome parameter was the change in oxygenation (PaO_2/FiO_2) following recruitment. Patients were considered as non-responders if the difference in PaO_2/FiO_2 was < 20% and as responders if the difference in PaO_2/FiO_2 was ≥ 20% between baseline and following recruitment measurements. These are arbitrary thresholds to differentiate between responders and non-responders, but reflect the literature where there is no consensus that agrees on clearly defined limits.

In the responder group, PaO_2/FiO_2 significantly improved after the recruitment manoeuver as compared to baseline results and remained elevated throughout the observation period (Fig. 3). Although it is not the most accurate way to assess lung recruitment, measuring changes in arterial oxygenation is one of the commonly used methods to detect the efficacy of recruitment [28]. It is important to note that the improvement in arterial oxygenation among the responders lasted longer than in studies where controlled ventilation was applied. In a study by Oczenski et al., after the initial improvement, PaO_2/FiO_2 returned to baseline values after 30 min [29], whereas in recruitment performed under PSV, the significant improvement in oxygenation persisted throughout, suggesting that the effects of recruitment may last longer in spontaneous assisted modes compared to controlled modes of ventilation in hypoxemic respiratory failure.

Assessing Recruitability in PSV

It is also well known that not every lung responds to recruitment maneuvers [30]. Even the transient increment in transpulmonary pressure may have deleterious side effects, such as pneumothorax and significantly reduced venous return resulting in diminished cardiac index [31]. Therefore, it is of paramount importance to assess whether the injured lung is responding to the instantly increased airway pressure or not.

Recruitability means a positive reaction to recruitment in which the atelectatic lung regions open up, hence improving the ventilation-perfusion ratio. In most cases, the severity of the alveolar damage in ARDS is not homogenous among the lung sections. Moreover, healthy lung regions can persist alongside damaged ones. In these pulmonary areas, the increased airway pressures and/or the elevated PEEP levels, according to the open lung concept, can cause undesired overdistension of the alveoli resulting in strain of the alveolar wall, hence causing attenuated capillary flow leading to further hypoxemia.

Absolute improvement in oxygenation can be detected in almost 75% of patients with moderate-to-severe lung injury when recruitment is performed under PSV [27]. To differentiate responders from non-responders it was found that improve-

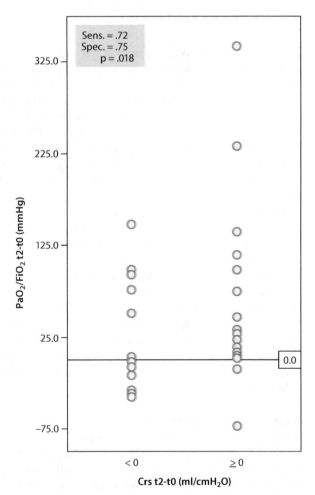

Fig. 4 Absolute change in dynamic compliance is a good predictor of responding patients following recruitment maneuver in pressure support ventilation. *Crs*: dynamic compliance; *t0*: baseline; *t2*: after recruitment in PSV; *Sens*: sensitivity; *Spec*: specificity. For explanation, see text. Reproduced from [27]

ment or deterioration of dynamic compliance had high sensitivity and specificity with a positive predictive value of 0.89 when differentiating patients with worsening compared to improving PaO_2/FiO_2 (Fig. 4).

Theoretically, in patients with recruitable lungs, increasing pressures will increase volume hence compliance should improve or remain unchanged. In nonrecruitable lungs, increased pressures during recruitment can lead to overdistension without gaining lung volumes, and hence result in a consecutive fall in respiratory compliance [32]. This could be a simple, bedside alternative to the 'gold standard', namely visualization of the recruitable lung tissue by CT scan [30].

Recruitment Without Pressure

Conducting spontaneous breathing trials (SBT) with a T-piece to identify patients ready for extubation has been broadly applied [33], but it may also be used as a weaning tool by alternating periods of ventilator support and SBT on the T-piece. Ayre's T-piece is a simple, non-rebreathing circuit first used in pediatric anesthesia [34]. Its potential advantages in the critical care setting are the minimal dead space, the low airway resistance and activation of the breathing muscles. The FiO_2 can be adjusted with high flow oxygen/air mixers or by the application of a Venturi injector on the inspiratory limb. PEEP can also be applied with the help of a PEEP-valve at the end of the expiratory limb thereby establishing a high flow CPAP circuit [35]. Compared with mechanical ventilation, the disadvantages are lack of pressure support, monitoring airway pressure and V_T.

In a recent investigation it was found that with the same FiO_2 and PEEP setting, breathing via a T-piece improved oxygenation compared to PSV in tracheostomized patients [36]. Furthermore, this significant impact on arterial oxygenation was explained by activation of the breathing muscles without interference of the ventilator. In patients who fulfill 'ready to be weaned' criteria, breathing via a T-piece may be beneficial compared to several ventilation modes in which the patient has to trigger the ventilator by either flow or pressure. During T-piece trials, respiratory muscle movements may promote immediate alveolar recruitment [37] with a prompt benefit on gas exchange. Therefore, we can conclude that further decrement of pressure support to zero along with switching to a T-piece CPAP circuit may have additional advantages for improving the ventilation-perfusion ratio.

Conclusion

CMV often appears the obvious choice of ventilation mode in patients with ARDS. It provides a precisely controlled ventilation cycle, adequately managed airway pressures and V_T, but these advantages might be counterbalanced by the features of the spontaneous modes. Furthermore, spontaneous modes are frequently applied as clinical routine, even in severe ARDS all around the world. In spontaneous assisted modes, diaphragmatic function and ventilation-perfusion match are adequately maintained and sedation requirements are also decreased. Performing recruitment maneuvers in these patients seems easily achievable by simply manipulating the level of PEEP and pressure support and by observing the changes in the V_T, compliance and the resultant effects on the blood gases. We believe that this safe and simple approach can help to optimize FiO_2, PEEP and pressure support settings within minutes in patients on ASV and helps to minimize the risk of inducing further damage by ventilating our patients outside the physiological parameter ranges.

References

1. Eastwood G, Bellomo R, Bailey M et al (2012) Arterial oxygen tension and mortality in mechanically ventilated patients. Intensive Care Med 38:91–98
2. Lee WL, Downey GP (2001) Neutrophil activation and acute lung injury. Curr Opin Crit Care 7:1–7
3. Han S, Mallampalli RK (2015) The acute respiratory distress syndrome: from mechanism to translation. J Immunol 194:855–860
4. Pelosi P, de Abreu MG (2015) Acute respiratory distress syndrome: we can't miss regional lung perfusion! BMC Anesth 15:35
5. Leligdowicz A, Fan E (2015) Extracorporeal life support for severe acute respiratory distress syndrome. Curr Opin Crit Care 21:13–19
6. Ferguson ND, Cook DJ, Guyatt GH et al (2013) High-frequency oscillation in early acute respiratory distress syndrome. N Engl J Med 368:795–805
7. Guérin C, Reignier J, Richard JC et al (2013) Prone positioning in severe acute respiratory distress syndrome. N Engl J Med 368:2159–2168
8. Lachmann B (1992) Open up the lung and keep the lung open. Intensive Care Med 18:319–321
9. Bellani G, Laffey JG, Pham T et al (2016) Epidemiology, patterns of care, and mortality for patients with acute respiratory distress syndrome in intensive care units in 50 countries. JAMA 315:788–800
10. Sassoon CS, Zhu E, Caiozzo VJ (2004) Assist-control mechanical ventilation attenuates ventilator-induced diaphragmatic dysfunction. Am J Respir Crit Care Med 170:626–632
11. Putensen C, Muders T, Varelmann D, Wrigge H (2006) The impact of spontaneous breathing during mechanical ventilation. Curr Opin Crit Care 12:13–18
12. Fisher AB, Chien S, Barakat AI, Nerem RM (2001) Endothelial cellular response to altered shear stress. Am J Physiol Lung Cell Mol Physiol 281:L529–L533
13. Tschumperlin DJ, Oswari J, Margulies AS (2000) Deformation-induced injury of alveolar epithelial cells. Effect of frequency, duration, and amplitude. Am J Respir Crit Care Med 162:357–362
14. Putensen C, Zech S, Wrigge H et al (2001) Long-term effects of spontaneous breathing during ventilatory support in patients with acute lung injury. Am J Respir Crit Care Med 164:43–49
15. Papazian L, Forel JM, Gacouin A et al (2010) Neuromuscular blockers in early acute respiratory distress syndrome. N Engl J Med 363:1107–1116
16. Leatherman JW, Fluegel WL, David WS, Davies SF, Iber C (1996) Muscle weakness in mechanically ventilated patients with severe asthma. Am J Respir Crit Care Med 153:1686–1690
17. Garnacho-Montero J, Madrazo-Osuna J, Garcia-Garmendia JL et al (2001) Critical illness polyneuropathy: risk factors and clinical consequences: a cohort study in septic patients. Intensive Care Med 27:1288–1296
18. Peñuelas Ó, Thille AW, Esteban A (2015) Discontinuation of ventilatory support: new solutions to old dilemmas. Curr Opin Crit Care 21:74–81

19. Slutsky AS, Ranieri VM (2013) Ventilator-induced lung injury. N Engl J Med 369:2126–2136
20. Piquilloud L, Tassaux D, Bialais E et al (2012) Neurally adjusted ventilatory assist (NAVA) improves patient-ventilator interaction during non-invasive ventilation delivered by face mask. Intensive Care Med 38:1624–1631
21. Sehgal IS, Dhooria S, Aggarwal AN, Behera D, Agarwal R (2016) Asynchrony index in pressure support ventilation (PSV) versus neurally adjusted ventilator assist (NAVA) during non-invasive ventilation (NIV) for respiratory failure: systematic review and meta-analysis. Intensive Care Med 42:1813–1815
22. Mireles-Cabodevila E, Kacmarek RM (2016) Should airway pressure release ventilation be the primary mode in ARDS? Respir Care 61:761–773
23. Calzia E, Lindner KH, Witt S et al (1994) Pressure-time product and work of breathing during biphasic continuous positive airway pressure and assisted spontaneous breathing. Am J Respir Crit Care Med 150:904–910
24. Neumann P, Wrigge H, Zinserling J et al (2005) Spontaneous breathing affects the spatial ventilation and perfusion distribution during mechanical ventilatory support. Crit Care Med 33:1090–1095
25. Rittayamai N, Brochard L (2015) Recent advances in mechanical ventilation in patients with acute respiratory distress syndrome. Eur Respir Rev 24:132–140
26. Petitjeans F, Pichot C, Ghignone M, Quintin L (2016) Early severe acute respiratory distress syndrome: what's going on? Part II: controlled vs. spontaneous ventilation? Anaesthesiol Intensive Ther 48:339–351
27. Lovas A, Németh MF, Trásy D, Molnár Z (2015) Lung recruitment can improve oxygenation in patients ventilated in continuous positive airway pressure/pressure support mode. Front Med (Lausanne) 2:25
28. Esan A, Hess DR, Raoof S et al (2010) Severe hypoxemic respiratory failure: part 1–ventilator strategies. Chest 137:1203–1216
29. Oczenski W, Hörmann C, Keller C et al (2004) Recruitment maneuvers after a positive end-expiratory pressure trial do not induce sustained effects in early adult respiratory distress syndrome. Anesthesiology 101:620–625
30. Gattinoni L, Caironi P, Cressoni M et al (2006) Lung recruitment in patients with the acute respiratory distress syndrome. N Engl J Med 354:1775–1786
31. Lovas A, Szakmány T (2015) Haemodynamic effects of lung recruitment manoeuvres. Biomed Res Int 2015:478970
32. Schumann S, Vimlati L, Kawati R et al (2011) Analysis of dynamic intratidal compliance in a lung collapse model. Anesthesiology 114:1111–1117
33. Boles J-M, Bion J, Connors A et al (2007) Weaning from mechanical ventilation. Eur Respir J 29:1033–1056
34. Ayre P (1937) Anaesthesia for intracranial operations: a new technique. Lancet 229:561–563
35. Lawrence JC (1978) PEEP and the Ayre's T-Piece system. Anaesth Intensive Care 6:359
36. Lovas A, Molnár Z (2013) T-piece improves arterial and central venous oxygenation in trachestomized patients as compared to continuous positive airway pressure/pressure support ventilation. Minerva Anestesiol 79:492–497
37. Westerdahl E, Lindmark B, Eriksson T et al (2003) The immediate effects of deep breathing exercises on atelectasis and oxygenation after cardiac surgery. Scand Cardiovasc J 37:363–367

Close Down the Lungs and Keep them Resting to Minimize Ventilator-induced Lung Injury

P. Pelosi, P. R. M. Rocco, and M. Gama de Abreu

Introduction

Mechanical ventilation is needed to support respiratory function in different clinical conditions, from healthy to diseased lungs. However, in recent years, research has shown that mechanical ventilation may promote acute and chronic damage to pulmonary structures, the so-called ventilator-induced lung injury (VILI), especially in patients with acute respiratory distress syndrome (ARDS) [1]. ARDS is characterized by a loss of aerated lung tissue as a result of edema and atelectasis, which reduces respiratory system compliance and impairs gas exchange. Several mechanisms have been identified that may underlie VILI. Those considered most important are alveolar overdistension and the continuous opening and closing of atelectatic lung units during breath cycles [2]. As a consequence, clinical use of lower tidal volume (V_T) to achieve reduced inspiratory stress and strain ('gentle' ventilation of the aerated lung), combined with higher levels of positive end-expiratory pressure (PEEP) to avoid repetitive collapse and reopening of alveolar units, have been suggested as a protective ventilatory strategy [3–5]. Furthermore, use of inspiratory pressures to open up atelectatic lung regions (so-called recruitment maneuvers) before setting PEEP has been proposed [6].

P. Pelosi (✉)
Department of Surgical Sciences and Integrated Diagnostics, San Martino Policlinico Hospital, IRCCS for Oncology, University of Genoa
Genoa, Italy
e-mail: ppelosi@hotmail.com

P. R. M. Rocco
Laboratory of Pulmonary Investigation, Carlos Chagas Filho Institute of Biophysics, Federal University of Rio de Janeiro
Rio de Janeiro, Brazil

M. Gama de Abreu
Department of Anesthesiology and Intensive Care Medicine, Pulmonary Engineering Group, University Hospital Carl Gustav Carus, Technische Universität Dresden
Dresden, Germany

© Springer International Publishing AG 2018   217
J.-L. Vincent (ed.), *Annual Update in Intensive Care and Emergency Medicine 2018*,
Annual Update in Intensive Care and Emergency Medicine,
https://doi.org/10.1007/978-3-319-73670-9_18

From a pathophysiological perspective, the "open lung approach" as originally recommended by Lachmann [7], now combined with protective V_T, is considered the optimal ventilation strategy to minimize VILI in moderate to severe ARDS. However, clinical data regarding application of the open lung approach in patients with ARDS are conflicting. One meta-analysis showed that application of higher PEEP levels, as compared to low PEEP, was not associated with improved outcome (mortality rate before hospital discharge), did not affect barotrauma and only improved oxygenation within the first week of treatment in ARDS patients [8]. On the other hand, a more recent meta-analysis [9] showed that the open-lung strategy might reduce hospital mortality, 28-day mortality, and intensive care unit (ICU) mortality among patients with ARDS. However, the control group included studies with a combination of high V_T and low PEEP, hindering any direct comparison of the potential beneficial effects of low V_T and/or higher PEEP.

In the present chapter, we will discuss and address: 1) the ARDS lung and its characteristics; 2) controversial issues related to the open lung approach; and 3) the alternative concept of 'permissive atelectasis'.

The ARDS Lung

The ARDS lung is characterized by different degrees of damage to the alveolar-capillary membrane, depending on the pathogenetic pathway, which leads to increased lung edema [10]. The model that most comprehensively explains the pathophysiologic consequences of ARDS on the lungs is the so-called "sponge model". The amount of edema depends on the severity of the injury, i.e., the worse the injury, the greater the alveolar edema, and *vice versa* [11]. Interstitial and alveolar edema promote collapse of the most dependent alveoli, as a result of increased superimposed pressure according to the density of fluids (plasma and blood) and the height of the lung. In general, the ARDS lung may be described as a 'sponge' filled with water, with best aeration of the non-dependent lung regions (the so-called "baby lung"), the dependent lung regions characterized by atelectatic areas, and consolidated lung regions widely distributed along the pulmonary structure or mainly localized in dependent areas [12]. Interestingly, even the aerated, non-dependent lung regions exhibit increased density, which suggests generalized, equally distributed injury of the alveolar-capillary barrier [13]. Additionally, small airway closure occurs mainly in the middle lung regions [14]. The reduction in aeration yields decreased lung compliance, while the presence of atelectatic and consolidated alveoli as well as peripheral airway closure might promote more or less severe alterations in gas exchange. These alterations are the result of a lower ventilation–perfusion ratio and the presence of true pulmonary shunt, according to the redistribution of regional perfusion. In fact, data suggest that regional perfusion is altered in ARDS as a result of intravascular clotting, collapse of capillaries and peripheral vessels, as well as edema of the endothelium and extracellular matrix [15].

Hubmayr [16] proposed an alternative mechanism for reduction in lung volume in ARDS, namely the presence of liquid and foam in conducting airways. In this model, increased edema occurs in the alveoli because of alterations in the alveolar-capillary barrier, rather than a predominance of alveolar collapse. This model completely changes and challenges the hypothesis that higher pressures in the lungs may be able to effectively re-open collapsed alveoli. In fact, if the model holds true, higher pressures may promote overstretching of partially aerated pulmonary zones.

The Open Lung Approach: Controversial Issues

The putative beneficial effects of higher PEEP and the open lung approach in ARDS are the following: 1) maintenance of full opening of the lungs; 2) reduction of interfaces between open and closed lung regions; 3) minimization of injurious effects caused by continuous opening and closing of collapsed alveolar units during tidal breath, which promotes lung injury and inflammation leading to systemic release of inflammatory biomarkers, distal organ failure and death.

Lung Edema: Controversial Effects of PEEP

Most experimental studies have shown an increase in lung edema after application of increasing levels of PEEP [17, 18]. However, other studies reported possible protective effects of PEEP against edema formation, which seem to be mediated by decreased cardiac output and/or reduced pulmonary blood volume, and not by an action of PEEP *per se* [19, 20].

Reduced Injury in Atelectatic-Collapsed Areas

In contrast to widespread belief, several experimental studies have shown less lung injury in atelectatic areas. Tsuchida et al. [21] investigated histological damage in lavaged rats subjected to non-injurious (with V_T 8 ml/kg and PEEP 14 cmH$_2$O) and injurious (V_T 25 ml/kg and PEEP 4–7 cmH$_2$O) mechanical ventilation. During injurious mechanical ventilation, lung injury was higher in non-dependent than in dependent lung regions. This finding was explained by the fact that injurious ventilation, and more particularly higher V_T, was distributed mainly in non-dependent lung regions with potential risk of overdistension, while dependent lung regions were relatively protected because of possible intra-alveolar edema. Interestingly, the greatest damage was observed in peripheral airways, which were likely subjected to higher stress during injurious mechanical ventilation. In line with these findings, Wakabayashi et al. [22] investigated three different settings of mechanical ventilation in isolated, perfused lungs: 1) low V_T (7 ml/kg) with PEEP (5 cmH$_2$O) and regular sustained inflation; 2) high-stretch strategy consisting of high V_T (30–32 ml/kg) with PEEP (3 cmH$_2$O) and sustained inflation; and 3) atelectasis strategy with low tidal volume but no PEEP or sustained inflation. They found that the high-stretch strategy, but not atelectrauma (atelectasis), activated monocytes within the pulmonary vasculature, leading to cytokine release into the systemic circulation. Finally, Chu et al. [23] ventilated *ex vivo* rat lungs with an opening and closing strategy without PEEP (V_T 7 ml/kg), opening and closing strategy with PEEP (V_T 7 ml/kg and PEEP 5 cmH$_2$O), and resting atelectasis. While the inflammatory process was more pronounced in animals ventilated with no PEEP, no differences were found between the PEEP-treated vs. resting atelectasis groups. Furthermore, the authors found that, at high volumes, cyclic stretch increased inflammatory mediators in the lungs compared to continuous stretch at a pressure equivalent to the mean airway pressure, but had no additional effect compared with continuous stretch at a pressure equal to the peak inspiratory pressure. These experimental data indicate that the degree of alveolar overdistension is a more important contributor to the release of pro-inflammatory cytokines than the cyclic nature of the ventilatory pattern. The authors suggested that "closing the lungs and keeping them closed" might be protective against VILI. These results differed from previous studies that observed increases in chemokines in the presence of overstretch of the lung, most likely because they used two-hit models, in which the lungs were injured before overstretch [24, 25].

In conclusion, experimental evidence suggests that atelectatic-collapsed lung regions, when not subjected to repetitive opening and closing, are not characterized by more tissue inflammation.

Reduced Inflammation in Atelectatic-Collapsed Areas

A recent study investigated the severity of inflammation in atelectatic and non-atelectatic lung regions by using the 18F-fluorodesoxyglucose (FDG) positron emission tomography (PET) technique [26]. FDG-PET has been proposed as a means of evaluating the activation of lung neutrophils, which are a key feature of pathophysiologic mechanisms and inflammatory cell activity in ARDS [27]. In fact, pulmonary FDG kinetics are altered during both experimental and clinical ARDS. Therefore, FDG-PET has been proposed as a potential non-invasive method to provide comprehensive understanding of the mechanisms of ARDS, and help for early diagnosis and for evaluation of different therapeutic interventions [28]. Other techniques used PET with a sialic acid-binding immunoglobulin-like lectin 9 (siglec-9)-based imaging agent targeting vascular adhesion protein-1 (VAP-1) for quantification of regional pulmonary inflammation [29]. In anesthetized sheep receiving intravenous endotoxin, FDG-PET was performed during protective ventilation with low V_T (8 ml/kg) and PEEP 17 cmH$_2$O and compared with injurious ventilation with high V_T (18 ml/kg) and no PEEP. During protective ventilation, there was a reduction in the amount and heterogeneity of pulmonary-cell metabolic activity, namely, inflammation formed mainly in the dependent lung regions [30]. In ARDS patients, independent of the type of mechanical ventilation, Bellani et al. [31] reported that lung metabolic activity was not directly related to the amount of atelectasis, being higher in the boundary areas between aerated and non-aerated lung regions (perhaps those with presence of airway closure) in most patients.

In conclusion, there is compelling experimental evidence suggesting that:

1) excessive inspiratory pressure and volume translate into overdistension and lung damage, stimulating inflammatory and fibrogenic responses;
2) studies in favor of a protective ventilatory strategy including low V_T and higher PEEP, thus minimizing lung collapse and repetitive closing and opening of alveolar units with less inflammatory response, were always compared with strategies consisting of high or extremely high V_T and no or low levels of PEEP. Thus, the possible beneficial effects of lower V_T could not be separated from those of higher PEEP (or both). In other words, our hypothesis is that the beneficial effects of the so-called "open lung" strategy in different experimental models were mainly due to a reduction in V_T and not to PEEP;
3) most of the studies were performed in models with apparently high recruitability. However, even in this case, conflicting results were observed regarding the beneficial effects for minimizing VILI;
4) hemodynamic impairment and its possible role in reducing lung injury was not considered in the majority of these experimental studies.

Recent Experimental Evidence of 'Permissive Atelectasis' to Minimize VILI

Low PEEP Combined with Low V_T, Plateau Pressure and Transpulmonary Pressure Minimizes Lung Injury

Recently, experimental studies challenged the common belief that atelectasis might be detrimental to protective ventilation, provided lungs are kept at rest. This protective strategy includes the following elements: 1) a minimal PEEP level to assure adequate gas exchange (a certain level of 'permissive hypoxemia' to allow for an oxygen saturation not below 88%) associated with low V_T or a V_T able to ventilate only the aerated lungs, while minimizing any detrimental effect on the collapsed alveoli and peripheral airways; and 2) the respiratory rate should be set to keep pHa within physiologic ranges, or even to allow a certain degree of permissive hypercapnia. This strategy of so-called "permissive atelectasis" should combine protective effects on the lungs as well as mitigate possible hemodynamic impairment. In endotoxin-induced lung ARDS, Samary et al. [32] investigated the impact of different mechanical ventilation strategies combining different V_T and PEEP, aiming to reach different driving transpulmonary pressures (ΔP): 1) low ΔP ($V_T = 6$ ml/kg, PEEP $= 3$ cmH$_2$O); high ΔP ($V_T = 22$ ml/kg, PEEP $= 3$ cmH$_2$O) and mean ΔP with a V_T to reach a mean between low and high ΔP ($V_T = 13$ ml/kg, PEEP $= 3$ cmH$_2$O). Other groups, with low V_T and moderate (9.5 cmH$_2$O) and high (11 cmH$_2$O) PEEP, were also investigated. In these experimental settings, PEEP was adjusted to obtain an inspiratory plateau pressure of the respiratory system similar to that achieved with mean and high ΔP while using high V_T. This was the first experimental study to evaluate the individual effects of V_T, PEEP, plateau pressure (Pplat) and ΔP on

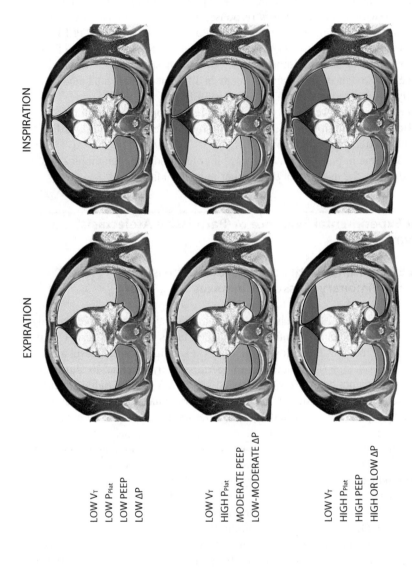

Fig. 1 Lung aeration at expiration (*left*) and inspiration (*right*) using different ventilation strategies. *Very light blue*: normally aerated regions; *light blue*: poorly aerated regions; *middle blue*: collapsed regions; *dark blue*: hyper-aerated regions. V_T: tidal volume; *PEEP*: positive end-expiratory pressure; *Pplat*: plateau pressure; ΔP: driving transpulmonary pressure

lung inflammation, fibrogenic response, endothelial and epithelial cell injury, and activation of cell stress. Ventilation with low V_T and low PEEP was associated with greater atelectasis, while increased V_T and low PEEP reduced the amount of atelectasis and low V_T and higher PEEP promoted a progressive increase in hyperinflation, to similar degrees as with high V_T with low PEEP.

The first question is, therefore, whether it is more injurious to the lungs to adopt a ventilation strategy with more atelectasis but lower inspiratory pressures with low V_T, designed to ventilate only the aerated lungs without promoting excessive opening and closing of alveolar units or stressing the peripheral airways? In agreement with our primary hypothesis, ventilation with low V_T, low PEEP and low ΔP resulted in reduced expression of interleukin (IL)-6, receptor for advanced glycation end products (RAGE), and amphiregulin. Interestingly, mechanical ventilation with low V_T and higher PEEP combined with higher ΔP and plateau pressure, a situation in which lungs were fully open, resulted in reduced expressions of IL-6 and RAGE, but was associated with increased amphiregulin expression and lung hyperinflation. Therefore, our data suggest that a ventilation strategy aimed to keep the lung fully open and then gently ventilated with low V_T might effectively reduce lung inflammation, However, mechanical ventilation with low V_T but a PEEP level not high enough to keep the lung fully open induced alveolar instability, thus resulting in increased expression of IL-6, RAGE and amphiregulin. Overall, IL-6 and amphiregulin expressions correlated better with plateau pressure and ΔP, highlighting the major influence of inspiratory stress as compared to other pressures in determining VILI. In a secondary analysis of these data, we investigated the impact of energy and power on VILI. IL-6 and amphiregulin expressions correlated better with power compared to energy of mechanical ventilation [33]. In conclusion, in experimental pulmonary ARDS, both mechanical ventilation strategies – 1) low V_T and PEEP, yielding low transpulmonary ΔP, plateau pressure, energy, and power, and 2) low V_T combined with a PEEP level sufficient to keep the lungs fully open – mitigated VILI. It is noteworthy that non-optimal PEEP might have negative effects on lung injury (Fig. 1).

Low Static Strain Is Less Injurious

Another important and underevaluated effect of PEEP is its possible injurious effects related to excessive static strain. In fact, as discussed above, only dynamic strain (such as ΔP) has been considered as a potential factor determining lung injury. In a study by Güldner et al. [34], pigs that had undergone saline lung lavage were separately ventilated with a double-lumen tube: the left lung with a very low V_T (3 ml/kg predicted body weight [PBW]) according to an atelectrauma or volutrauma strategy, while the right lung was ventilated with a continuous positive airway pressure (CPAP) of $20 \, \text{cmH}_2\text{O}$. The volutrauma strategy included high PEEP set above the level where dynamic compliance increased more than 5% during a PEEP trial, and the atelectrauma strategy included low PEEP to achieve driving pressures comparable with those of volutrauma. The potential increase in CO_2

and decrease in pHa due to the extremely low V_T was controlled by extracorporeal removal. This experiment separated the potential beneficial or detrimental effects of higher or lower static strain on VILI, i.e., higher or lower PEEP. In both conditions, atelectrauma and volutrauma, the tidal breath was extremely low. Regional lung aeration was assessed by computed tomography (CT), and inflammation by FDG-PET. Contrary to general belief regarding ultraprotective ventilation, volutrauma (i.e., higher static strain) yielded higher inflammation as compared to atelectrauma (i.e., lower static strain). Volutrauma decreased the blood fraction at similar perfusion and increased normally and hyperaerated lung compartments and tidal hyperaeration. Atelectrauma yielded more poorly and non-aerated lung compartments, and tidal recruitment, as well as increased ΔP. These data suggested that volutrauma and static strain may promote even greater lung inflammation than atelectrauma at comparable low V_T values and lower driving pressures, suggesting again that static stress and strain are major determinants of VILI. Mechanical power was higher in volutrauma compared to atelectrauma groups. However, the intensity, i.e., mechanical power normalized to lung tissue, was comparable between volutrauma and atelectrauma, with negligible differences. Thus, we exclude any influence of differences in intensity to explain our results regarding the potential injurious effects of excessive static strain. In conclusion, higher PEEP increases static strain, thus promoting lung inflammation.

Low PEEP Minimally Impairs Lymphatic Drainage

Higher PEEP may also have negative effects on fluid drainage from pulmonary structures. The dynamic of fluids in the pulmonary interstitium is carefully regulated by the pressures inside and outside the capillaries, the extracellular matrix, and pulmonary lymphatics, and differs between spontaneous breathing and mechanical ventilation. The lymphatics collect fluids through three routes: hilar, transpleural, and transabdominal [35]. In normal conditions, a continuous leak of fluids occurs from the capillaries to the interstitium, because of the overall balance between hydrostatic and oncotic pressures in the capillaries and interstitium. The lymphatics maintain a negative pressure in the interstitium, which is important to prevent changes in the mechanical and functional properties of the respiratory system. Furthermore, fluids are also drained from the pleural space to the interstitium in the parietal side through specific foramina or, again, a combination of hydrostatic and oncotic pressures. Finally, drainage occurs through lymphatics positioned in the diaphragm, which play a relevant role during spontaneous breathing and mechanical ventilation.

Unlike the situation for more central diaphragmatic lymphatic vessels, optimization of lymphatic drainage through the diaphragm depends on anatomical location and functional physiological properties. In fact, central diaphragmatic lymphatic vessels are passively activated by muscular contraction, and thus become partially ineffective during controlled mechanical ventilation. On the other hand, lymphatic loops located at the extreme diaphragmatic periphery additionally require an intrinsic pumping mechanism to propel lymph centripetally [36]. Such active lymph propulsion is attained by means of a complex interplay among sites and is able to organize lymph flow in an ordered way. More recently, it has been shown that spontaneous contraction of lymphatics located in the extreme diaphragmatic periphery might involve hyperpolarization-activated cyclic nucleotide-gated channels in lymphatics equipped with muscle cells [37]. Hence, the three-dimensional arrangement of the diaphragmatic lymphatic network seems to be finalized to efficiently exploit the stresses exerted by muscle fibers during the contracting inspiratory phase to promote lymph formation in superficial submesothelial lymphatics and its further propulsion in deeper intramuscular vessels [38]. In the presence of diffuse damage of the alveolar capillary membrane, the role of lymphatics is even more important, to avoid progression and provide at least partial cleaning of lung edema. The increase in pressure in the alveoli, with increased inspiratory, mean or end-expiratory pressure, may markedly impair the function of lymphatics, determining a reduction in fluid drainage capability. During spontaneous breathing, the pressure in the interstitium is higher than the pressure in the lymphatics, resulting in a negative gradient (around 3–4 mmHg) which facilitates continuous drainage of fluids [39]. By contrast, during positive pressure, an increase in interstitial and lymphatic pressures occurs, to a similar degree (10 mmHg). In this case, the gradient between the interstitium and lymphatics becomes around zero or even positive, impairing possible fluid drainage. In addition, the increase in pressure in the respiratory system increases pressures in the pulmonary vessels and, as a consequence, on the venous side. This increase in hydrostatic pressures promotes fluid leak from capillaries on the abdominal and diaphragmatic side, thus potentially increasing pressure in the abdomen and further worsening respiratory and circulatory function as well as lymphatic drainage from the lungs (Fig. 2). In conclusion, mechanical ventilation with higher PEEP negatively affects lymphatic drainage from the lung, possibly impairing fluid exchange from the interstitial lung tissue.

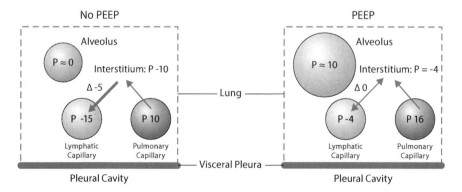

Fig. 2 Relation between alveolar, capillary, lymphatic and interstitial pressures in a lung ventilated without (*left*) or with (*right*) positive end-expiratory pressure (PEEP)

Low PEEP Improves Right Ventricular Function

Patients with ARDS are characterized by a moderate-to-severe impairment of right ventricular (RV) function, which impacts on systemic hemodynamics [40]. Several devices and modalities, such as echocardiography, are now available to monitor respiratory settings according to RV tolerance. Acute *cor pulmonale* is defined as a persistent increase in pulmonary vascular resistance and, from an echocardiographic point of view, is characterized by paradoxical septal motion [40]. In patients with ARDS, the severity of the pulmonary disease involving the microvasculature influences development of acute *cor pulmonale*, which may also be caused or exacerbated by an aggressive ventilatory strategy. In fact, even minor overload in pulmonary vascular resistance may impair RV function. In this context, the use of lower V_T has been associated with a decreased rate of RV impairment and acute *cor pulmonale*, with possible beneficial effects on outcome [41]. However, PEEP may negatively affect RV function [42]. In fact, the decrease in cardiac output is more often associated with a preload decrease and no change in RV contractility, whereas the increased RV volumes with PEEP may be associated with a reduction in RV myocardial performance. Acidosis and hypercapnia induced by V_T reduction and increase in PEEP with constant plateau pressure have been found to be associated with impaired RV function despite positive effects on oxygenation and alveolar recruitment [43]. It has been suggested that respiratory system $\Delta P \geq 18\,cmH_2O$, $PaCO_2 \geq 48\,mmHg$, and $PaO_2/FiO_2 < 150\,mmHg$ are three factors independently associated with acute *cor pulmonale*. Thus, extended sessions of prone positioning instead of increasing PEEP have been proposed in patients with moderate to severe ARDS [44]. In conclusion: 1) increased RV afterload during ARDS may induce acute *cor pulmonale*; 2) higher PEEP and plateau pressure, as well as increased ΔP, worsens RV function and systemic hemodynamics.

PEEP and CT Scan

As discussed above, it is likely that it is necessary to keep the lungs fully open to achieve the potential positive effects of the 'open-lung' strategy. CT scan studies in ARDS patients have shown that the potential of recruitment in this population varies widely [45]. Moreover, the level of PEEP required to keep the lungs fully open is extremely high, especially in moderate to severe ARDS [46]. Additionally, even 15 cmH_2O PEEP has been shown not to be enough to keep the lung open [47] and to be associated with overdistension [48]. In conclusion, therefore, CT scan studies have shown that high PEEP levels ($> 15\,cmH_2O$) are needed to keep the lungs fully open and are always associated with increased overdistension and hemodynamic impairment.

Conclusion

Several studies have reported that the open lung approach, as achieved with high PEEP and recruitment maneuvers, is important to reduce VILI and improve outcomes. However, experimental and clinical evidence does not fully support the hypothesis that PEEP *per se* might reduce lung injury. Indeed, PEEP may have negative effects resulting in overdistension, edema formation, poor lymphatic drainage and impairment of RV function, as well as an impact on systemic hemodynamics. Furthermore, atelectatic lung regions exhibit reduced lung inflammation if kept at rest. Most studies have compared ventilatory strategies with high PEEP combined with low V_T to high V_T and no PEEP. Thus, it was impossible to separate the possible protective effects of low V_T from those of PEEP or the combination thereof. Moreover, moderate PEEP levels might induce even greater injury as compared to high PEEP. Thus, we propose the following ventilation strategies:

1) keep the lungs partially collapsed;
2) avoid opening and closing of collapsed alveoli;
3) mitigate injury in the peripheral airways, thus resulting in gentle ventilation of the aerated lungs while keeping collapsed and consolidated lung tissues at rest.

We believe that permissive atelectasis might be at least as effective as a strategy aimed at opening the lungs and keeping them open, but with the advantage of minimizing overstretch of the lung parenchyma and mitigating hemodynamic consequences. In short, we believe that, in order to minimize VILI, we should consider moving away from the classical concept of 'open up the lungs and keep them open' towards 'close down the lungs and keep them closed'. A ventilatory strategy that leaves as much lung derecruited as possible, so that gas exchange is still adequate and opening and closing of collapsed alveoli is avoided could potentially minimize lung injury.

References

1. Thompson BT, Chambers RC, Liu KD (2017) Acute respiratory distress syndrome. N Engl J Med 377:562–572
2. Rocco PRM, Dos Santos C, Pelosi P (2012) Pathophysiology of ventilator-associated lung injury. Curr Opin Anaesthesiol 25:123–130
3. Putensen C, Theuerkauf N, Zinserling J, Wrigge H, Pelosi P (2009) Meta-analysis: ventilation strategies and outcomes of the acute respiratory distress syndrome and acute lung injury. Ann Intern Med 151:566–576
4. Bellani G, Laffey JG, Pham T et al (2016) Epidemiology, patterns of care, and mortality for patients with acute respiratory distress syndrome in intensive care units in 50 countries. JAMA 315:788–800
5. Esteban A, Frutos-Vivar F, Muriel A et al (2013) Evolution of mortality over time in patients receiving mechanical ventilation. Am J Respir Crit Care Med 188:220–230
6. Constantin JM, Godet T, Jabaudon M, Bazin JE, Futier E (2017) Recruitment maneuvers in acute respiratory distress syndrome. Ann Transl Med 5:290

7. Lachmann B (1992) Open up the lung and keep the lung open. Intensive Care Med 18:319–321
8. Cruz SR, Rojas JI, Nervi R, Heredia R, Ciapponi A (2013) High versus low positive end-expiratory pressure (PEEP) levels for mechanically ventilated adult patients with acute lung injury and acute respiratory distress syndrome. Cochrane Database Syst Rev CD009098
9. Lu J, Wang X, Chen M et al (2017) An open lung strategy in the management of acute respiratory distress syndrome: a systematic review and meta-analysis. Shock 48:43–53
10. Rezoagli E, Fumagalli R, Bellani G (2017) Definition and epidemiology of acute respiratory distress syndrome. Ann Transl Med 5:282
11. Gattinoni L, Marini JJ, Pesenti A, Quintel M, Mancebo J, Brochard L (2016) The "baby lung" became an adult. Intensive Care Med 42:663–673
12. Gattinoni L, Pesenti A, Carlesso E (2013) Body position changes redistribute lung computed-tomographic density in patients with acute respiratory failure: impact and clinical fallout through the following 20 years. Intensive Care Med 39:1909–1915
13. Pelosi P, D'Andrea L, Vitale G, Pesenti A, Gattinoni L (1994) Vertical gradient of regional lung inflation in adult respiratory distress syndrome. Am J Respir Crit Care Med 149:8–13
14. Pelosi P, Rocco PRM (2007) Airway closure: the silent killer of peripheral airways. Crit Care 11:114
15. Pesenti A, Musch G, Lichtenstein D et al (2016) Imaging in acute respiratory distress syndrome. Intensive Care Med 42:686–698
16. Hubmayr RD (2002) Perspective on lung injury and recruitment: a skeptical look at the opening and collapse story. Am J Respir Crit Care Med 165:1647–1653
17. Caldini P, Leith JD, Brennan MJ (1975) Effect of continuous postive-pressure ventilation (CPPV) on edema formation in dog lung. J Appl Physiol 39:672–679
18. Demling RH, Staub NC, Edmunds LH (1975) Effect of end-expiratory airway pressure on accumulation of extravascular lung water. J Appl Physiol 38:907–912
19. Colmenero-Ruiz M, Fernández-Mondéjar E, Fernández-Sacristán MA, Rivera-Fernández R, Vazquez-Mata G (1997) PEEP and low tidal volume ventilation reduce lung water in porcine pulmonary edema. Am J Respir Crit Care Med 155:964–970
20. Russell JA, Hoeffel J, Murray JF (1982) Effect of different levels of positive end-expiratory pressure on lung water content. J Appl Physiol 53:9–15
21. Tsuchida S, Engelberts D, Peltekova V et al (2006) Atelectasis causes alveolar injury in nonatelectatic lung regions. Am J Respir Crit Care Med 174:279–289
22. Wakabayashi K, Wilson MR, Tatham KC, O'Dea KP, Takata M (2014) Volutrauma, but not atelectrauma, induces systemic cytokine production by lung-marginated monocytes. Crit Care Med 42:e49–e57
23. Chu EK, Whitehead T, Slutsky AS (2004) Effects of cyclic opening and closing at low- and high-volume ventilation on bronchoalveolar lavage cytokines. Crit Care Med 32:168–174
24. Narimanbekov IO, Rozycki HJ (1995) Effect of IL-1 blockade on inflammatory manifestations of acute ventilator-induced lung injury in a rabbit model. Exp Lung Res 21:239–254
25. Takata M, Abe J, Tanaka H et al (1997) Intraalveolar expression of tumor necrosis factor-alpha gene during conventional and high-frequency ventilation. Am J Respir Crit Care Med 156:272–279
26. Bellani G, Rouby JJ, Constantin JM, Pesenti A (2017) Looking closer at acute respiratory distress syndrome: the role of advanced imaging techniques. Curr Opin Crit Care 23:30–37
27. Ball L, Vercesi V, Costantino F, Chandrapatham K, Pelosi P (2017) Lung imaging: how to get better look inside the lung. Ann Transl Med 5:294
28. Rodrigues RS, Bozza FA, Hanrahan CJ et al (2017) (18)F-fluoro-2-deoxyglucose PET informs neutrophil accumulation and activation in lipopolysaccharide-induced acute lung injury. Nucl Med Biol 48:52–62
29. Retamal J, Sörensen J, Lubberink M et al (2016) Feasibility of (68)Ga-labeled Siglec-9 peptide for the imaging of acute lung inflammation: a pilot study in a porcine model of acute respiratory distress syndrome. Am J Nucl Med Mol Imaging 6:18–31
30.

de Prost N, Costa EL, Wellman T et al (2013) Effects of ventilation strategy on distribution of lung inflammatory cell activity. Crit Care 17:R175

31. Bellani G, Messa C, Guerra L et al (2009) Lungs of patients with acute respiratory distress syndrome show diffuse inflammation in normally aerated regions: a [18F]-fluoro-2-deoxy-D-glucose PET/CT study. Crit Care Med 37:2216–2222

32. Samary CS, Santos RS, Santos CL et al (2015) Biological impact of transpulmonary driving pressure in experimental acute respiratory distress syndrome. Anesthesiology 123:423–433

33. Samary CS, Silva PL, Gama de Abreu M, Pelosi P, Rocco PRM (2016) Ventilator-induced lung injury: power to the mechanical power. Anesthesiology 125:1070–1071

34. Güldner A, Braune A, Ball L et al (2016) Comparative effects of volutrauma and atelectrauma on lung inflammation in experimental acute respiratory distress syndrome. Crit Care Med 44:e854–e865

35. Malbrain M, Pelosi P (2006) Open up and keep the lymphatics open: they are the hydraulics of the body! Crit Care Med 34:2860–2862

36. Moriondo A, Solari E, Marcozzi C, Negrini D (2013) Spontaneous activity in peripheral diaphragmatic lymphatic loops. Am J Physiol Heart Circ Physiol 305:H987–H995

37. Negrini D, Marcozzi C, Solari E et al (2016) Hyperpolarization-activated cyclic nucleotide-gated channels in peripheral diaphragmatic lymphatics. Am J Physiol Heart Circ Physiol 311:H892–H903

38. Moriondo A, Solari E, Marcozzi C, Negrini D (2015) Diaphragmatic lymphatic vessel behavior during local skeletal muscle contraction. Am J Physiol Heart Circ Physiol 308:H193–H205

39. Moriondo A, Mukenge S, Negrini D (2005) Transmural pressure in rat initial subpleural lymphatics during spontaneous or mechanical ventilation. Am J Physiol Heart Circ Physiol 289:H263–H269

40. Repessé X, Charron C, Vieillard-Baron A (2015) Acute cor pulmonale in ARDS: rationale for protecting the right ventricle. Chest 147:259–265

41. Mekontso Dessap A, Boissier F et al (2016) Acute cor pulmonale during protective ventilation for acute respiratory distress syndrome: prevalence, predictors, and clinical impact. Intensive Care Med 42:862–870

42. Dambrosio M, Fiore G, Brienza N et al (1996) Right ventricular myocardial function in ARF patients. PEEP as a challenge for the right heart. Intensive Care Med 22:772–780

43. Mekontso Dessap A, Charron C, Devaquet J et al (2009) Impact of acute hypercapnia and augmented positive end-expiratory pressure on right ventricle function in severe acute respiratory distress syndrome. Intensive Care Med 35:1850–1858

44. Repessé X, Vieillard-Baron A (2017) Right heart function during acute respiratory distress syndrome. Ann Transl Med 5:295

45. Gattinoni L, Caironi P, Cressoni M et al (2006) Lung recruitment in patients with the acute respiratory distress syndrome. N Engl J Med 354:1775–1786

46. Gattinoni L, Pelosi P, Crotti S, Valenza F (1995) Effects of positive end-expiratory pressure on regional distribution of tidal volume and recruitment in adult respiratory distress syndrome. Am J Respir Crit Care Med 151:1807–1814

47. Cressoni M, Chiumello D, Algieri I et al (2017) Opening pressures and atelectrauma in acute respiratory distress syndrome. Intensive Care Med 43:603–611

48. Puybasset L, Cluzel P, Gusman P, Grenier P, Preteux F, Rouby JJ (2000) Regional distribution of gas and tissue in acute respiratory distress syndrome. I. Consequences for lung morphology. CT Scan ARDS Study Group. Intensive Care Med 26:857–869

Diaphragm Dysfunction during Weaning from Mechanical Ventilation: An Underestimated Phenomenon with Clinical Implications

M. Dres and A. Demoule

Introduction

Weaning failure is defined as the inability to liberate a patient from the ventilator. Therefore, the term 'weaning failure' encompasses the failure of a spontaneous breathing trial (SBT) or the need to resume mechanical ventilation after extubation within 48 h to seven days [1]. The majority of patients are safely weaned from the ventilator after a first attempt, some are even extubated without any SBT [2]. Thereby, weaning failure occurs in a minority of patients but represents an important burden in term of days of mechanical ventilation, intensive care unit (ICU) lengths of stay and morbi-mortality [2]. Investigating the causes of weaning failure is therefore crucial because the duration of mechanical ventilation for those who fail the SBT [2] and the reintubation for those in whom reintubation is needed [3, 4] have both been associated with poor outcomes. Ultimately, identifying the reason why a patient fails the weaning process might help to reduce the duration of mechanical ventilation and hence to improve patient outcomes.

Recent findings suggest that diaphragm dysfunction is frequently involved during weaning failure [5, 6] and that it is associated with poor prognosis at time of liberation from mechanical ventilation [7, 8]. Until recently, exploration of the diaphragm has not been convenient to achieve at the bedside. This factor may explain the growing interest in ultrasound. Diaphragm ultrasound provides non-invasive indices that describe the structure and the function of the muscle. Herein, we summarize the mechanisms of diaphragm dysfunction in the critically ill and describe current approaches aimed at assessing diaphragm function at the bedside.

M. Dres (✉) · A. Demoule
UPMC Univ Paris 06, INSERM, UMRS1158 Neurophysiologie respiratoire expérimentale et clinique, Sorbonne Universités
Paris, France
Groupe Hospitalier Pitié-Salpêtrière Charles Foix, Service de Pneumologie et Réanimation Médicale (Département "R3S"), AP-HP
Paris, France
e-mail: martin.dres@aphp.fr

© Springer International Publishing AG 2018
J.-L. Vincent (ed.), *Annual Update in Intensive Care and Emergency Medicine 2018*,
Annual Update in Intensive Care and Emergency Medicine,
https://doi.org/10.1007/978-3-319-73670-9_19

We discuss some recent aspects of the epidemiology and risk factors for diaphragm dysfunction at the time of weaning from mechanical ventilation. Finally, latest advances regarding preventive and curative strategies for diaphragm dysfunction are presented.

Mechanisms of Diaphragm Function

A comprehensive review describing the mechanisms of diaphragm dysfunction in the ICU has been published recently [9]. In the following lines, we briefly summarize the existing literature on this topic. The main experimental model of diaphragm dysfunction comes from experimental studies where ventilator-induced diaphragm inactivity was used as the promoter. From these studies, ventilator-induced diaphragm dysfunction was defined in 2004 as loss of diaphragmatic force-generating capacity specifically related to the use of mechanical ventilation [10]. Elucidating the mechanisms leading to diaphragm dysfunction requires biopsies, an option rarely used in the ICU. Nevertheless, in recent years, better understanding has been achieved by obtaining diaphragm specimens from very specific populations, such as brain dead organ donors [11] and thoracic surgery patients [12]. It is now established that diaphragm dysfunction is accompanied by two landmark pathophysiological features: disuse atrophy and microstructural changes [9]. The first study reporting evidence of diaphragm atrophy in adults was published by Levine and coworkers [11]. This group established, in 14 brain dead organ donors, that disuse atrophy occurred shortly after the start of controlled mechanical ventilation [11]. In addition, muscle fiber atrophy was associated with signs of increased oxidative stress and with an increase in muscle proteolysis biomarkers. Oxidative stress, downregulation of protein synthesis and activation of proteolytic pathways represent the biochemical changes of diaphragm dysfunction. Interestingly, no such atrophy or sign of oxidative stress has been noted in the pectoralis [11] or latissimus dorsi [12] muscles.

Detection of Diaphragm Dysfunction in ICU Patients

Several methods are now available to detect the presence of diaphragm dysfunction in critically ill patients (Fig. 1). Although bilateral anterior magnetic phrenic stimulation (BAMPS) is considered as the reference method [13], it must be pointed out that it is a relatively recent technique, used in the ICU only in the last 20 years [14, 15]. Physiologically speaking, diaphragm dysfunction can be defined as a reduced ability of the diaphragm to generate a negative intrathoracic pressure, regardless of the origin of the observation. BAMPS elicits an isolated contraction of the diaphragm and enables the change (twitch) in endotracheal pressure (Pet,tw) or in transdiaphragmatic pressure (Pdi,tw) to be measured [15]. Based on this method, diaphragm dysfunction is defined as a decrease in its capacity to generate a negative intrathoracic pressure, usually less than $11\,cmH_2O$ [13]. Although this method

Diaphragm Pressure Generating Capacity

An isolated contraction of the diaphragm is elicited by a magnetic supramaximal stimulation (twitch). The negative airway pressure is measured at the tip of the endotracheal tube.
A twitch endotracheal pressure less than 11 cmH$_2$O defines diaphragm dysfunction.

Advantage:
- Reference method

Disadvantages:
- Only available in expert centers

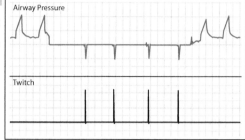

Diaphragm Electrical Activity (EAdi)

EAdi is obtained continuously through a dedicated nasogastric feeding tube and displayed on the ventilator screen. Airway pressure waveform and EAdi are therefore provided synchronously.

Advantages:
- Continuous assessment of EAdi
- EAdi-derived indices estimate neuromechanical coupling

Disadvantages:
- Not available on all ventilators
- Requires a dedicated catheter

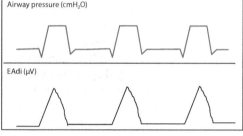
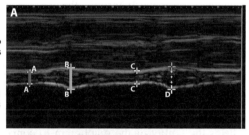

Diaphragm Ultrasound

Structure, movement and function of the diaphragm are provided by ultrasound through two distinct approaches. Intercostal approach provides end-expiratory thickness (dark blue bar) and peak inspiratory thickness (light blue bar) enabling the calculation of the thickening fraction of the diaphragm (Panel A). Subcostal approach provides excursion of the diaphragm, the diaphragm moves caudally toward the probe during inspiration (light blue arrows) (Panel B).

Advantages:
- Widely available at the bedside
- Non-invasive

Disadvantages:
- Operator dependent
- Not continuous monitoring

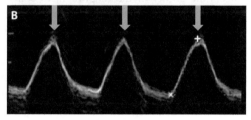

Fig. 1 Techniques to investigate diaphragm function in the ICU

provides a rigorous assessment of diaphragm function, it is only available in expert centers and requires costly equipment, precluding its generalization.

By contrast, ultrasound is widely available in every ICU and, furthermore, it is totally non-invasive. The use of ultrasound is growing in the ICU and may become a key player in the evaluation of diaphragm function during weaning. From two distinct approaches, diaphragm ultrasound provides structural and functional assessment of the muscle, the right side being the most frequently evaluated. Using the intercostal approach, the diaphragm is examined on its zone of apposition to the rib cage. At this location, ultrasound enables measurement of the end-expiratory (Tee) and peak inspiratory (Tei) diaphragm thickness. The diaphragm thickening fraction (TFdi) is computed as the difference between Tei and Tee, divided by Tee. TFdi is tightly correlated with transdiaphragmatic pressure [16], an estimator of diaphragm function [13]. Only one study has compared diaphragm ultrasound and BAMPS and reported a good correlation between TFdi and the change in tracheal pressure generated by the phrenic nerves stimulation ($r = 0.87$), provided that patients trigger the ventilator [7]. According to this study, a TFdi cut-off of 29% is an optimal value to identify diaphragm dysfunction [7]. With the subcostal approach, the diaphragm is assessed by the excursion of the dome. Using transdiaphragmatic pressure as a reference, Lerolle et al. identified a diaphragm excursion cut-off less than 2.5 cm to define diaphragm dysfunction [17].

Electromyography (EMG) of the diaphragm was first described more than 50 years ago. It provides diaphragm electrical activity (EAdi), which is the spatial and temporal summation of neural impulses. Diaphragm EMG can be obtained easily and continuously through the use of a dedicated nasogastric feeding catheter equipped with multiarray electrodes. EAdi is tightly correlated to a patient's inspiratory effort and is a good estimate of diaphragm function. Combining EAdi with the breathing pattern provide indices that evaluate the diaphragm's contribution to the generation of tidal volume (V_T). For example, the ratio of V_T to EAdi (V_T/EAdi) represents the neuroventilatory efficiency of the diaphragm. When V_T/EAdi is high, it indicates that a patient generates a large V_T with a relatively low EAdi, whereas when V_T/EAdi is low, this indicates that despite a high EAdi, V_T is low. This index reflects the ability of the diaphragm to convert respiratory drive into ventilation. A low V_T/EAdi suggests severe impairment of neuromechanical coupling. EAdi-derived indices have been used to discriminate patients with weaning failure [18, 19]. Interestingly, monitoring neuroventilatory efficiency during an SBT enables very early (after 3 min) detection of patients likely to fail the test [18]. However, the performance of EAdi-derived indices to predict weaning failure is not better than the performance of the rapid shallow breathing index [18], a popular weaning predictor that is not specific to the diaphragm.

Risk Factors and Population Concerned by Diaphragm Dysfunction at Time of Weaning

Several risk factors are associated with the occurrence of diaphragm dysfunction in the ICU. In the sickest patients, it is likely that multiple factors hit simultaneously. Some are present before the ICU admission (sepsis, shock) while others develop during the stay (mechanical ventilation) (Fig. 2). Confirming a previous report showing that sepsis induced preferential diaphragm atrophy [20], Demoule et al. established that, on admission, sepsis is an independent risk factor for diaphragm dysfunction [21]. An important but not elucidated question is whether the delay between sepsis onset and ICU admission is correlated with the severity of the dysfunction. In the same study [21], disease severity, as assessed with Simplified Acute Physiology Score (SAPS) II, was also independently associated with diaphragm dysfunction, suggesting that diaphragm dysfunction behaves as any other organ failure. Shock states, in particular of cardiogenic origin, are associated with diaphragm dysfunction [22]. The imbalance between oxygen supply and demand during cardiogenic shock can ultimately result in diaphragm fatigue [22]. Although these findings performed in animals have not been replicated in humans, they are based on a strong methodology and have a strong 'face validity' for clinicians.

After ICU admission, patients may be exposed to prolonged mechanical ventilation, a risk factor for diaphragm dysfunction [10]. Two studies used BAMPS to serially investigate diaphragm function in a limited number of patients [23, 24]. Both reported a time-dependent deterioration in diaphragm function with increased duration of mechanical ventilation [23, 24]. Speculating that atrophy would constitute a meaningful marker of diaphragm function, these findings were confirmed by Grosu et al. who observed a time-dependent decline in diaphragm thickness by ultrasound in seven patients receiving mechanically ventilation [25]. Larger cohorts [26, 27] have now confirmed this very preliminary observation [25]. As expected, in a series of medical ICU patients undergoing mechanical ventilation in whom di-

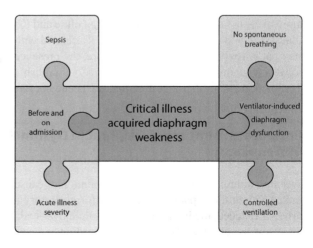

Fig. 2 Main factors contributing to diaphragm weakness before and on ICU admission and after exposure to mechanical ventilation

aphragm function was investigated by the phrenic nerve stimulation technique at the time of weaning, the duration of mechanical ventilation from intubation to weaning was associated with the occurrence of diaphragm dysfunction [6]. Nevertheless, this effect was not retained in a multivariable analysis incorporating other risk factors [6]. These findings support the hypothesis that rather than mechanical ventilation *per se*, it is the inactivity of the diaphragm that is the critical determinant of dysfunction. This assumption was incidentally confirmed by Goligher et al. who reported that changes in diaphragm thickness were modulated by a patient's inspiratory efforts: the lower the inspiratory effort, the greater the atrophy [26]. In a subsequent study, the same team also demonstrated that diaphragm atrophy developing during the ICU stay was associated with prolonged duration of mechanical ventilation, increased risk of reintubation and tracheostomy [28]. In addition to mechanical ventilation, some drugs, such as corticosteroids and neuromuscular blocking agents, may generate diaphragm dysfunction but their effects are not univocal.

Critical illness polyneuropathy and myopathy are frequently observed in patients with weaning failure [29] and coexist with respiratory muscle weakness [5, 30]. Since the detection of diaphragm dysfunction is a challenge in daily practice, it would be tempting to use critical illness polyneuropathy and myopathy as a surrogate. However, accumulating evidence indicates that it would be a cursory glance. First, as demonstrated by experimental and clinical studies [11, 31], the consequences of prolonged unloading of the diaphragm are distinct from the consequences of unloading limb muscles. Second, the diaphragm seems preferentially affected compared to limb muscles in septic patients [20] and to the latissimus dorsi muscle in mechanically ventilated patients [12]. Whether diaphragm dysfunction is a respiratory component of critical illness polyneuropathy and myopathy is therefore not established. Hence, diaphragm dysfunction is not always present in patients with critical illness polyneuropathy and myopathy [5] and the correlation between the two diseases is weak [6] or lacking [5]. In addition, there is a distinct difference between diaphragm dysfunction and critical illness polyneuropathy and myopathy, as the latter condition is often associated with conduction abnormalities in electrophysiological studies [9]. The prognosis of both diseases is also clearly different as diaphragm dysfunction is more likely to be associated with weaning failure and ICU mortality, whereas critical illness polyneuropathy and myopathy is associated with prolonged duration of ICU stay but not with mortality [6]. Therefore, the presence of critical illness polyneuropathy and myopathy is not sufficient to establish the presence of diaphragm dysfunction and further investigations are needed before confirming the diagnosis.

Presence and Impact of Diaphragm Dysfunction at the Time of Weaning

Weaning failure is provoked by a constellation of causes, some of them potentially linked. When the capacity of the system (respiratory muscle strength, respiratory drive) is reduced, the load (lung disease, fluid overload, cardiac dysfunction, abnormality of the chest wall) is increased, leading to respiratory load/capacity imbalance. The weight of the diaphragm in the load/capacity balance is heavy but it is important to remember that decreased capacity of the respiratory system can also be the consequence of impaired respiratory drive or neuromuscular dysfunction. Impaired respiratory drive is an obvious cause of weaning failure. It can be easily identified by a simple physical examination showing signs of encephalitis or stroke. Since weaning from the ventilator in this category of patients is a specific issue, it is not addressed in the present review.

As noted earlier, exploring diaphragm function is not straightforward in the critically ill, which may explain why some investigators opted rather to investigate global respiratory function [30]. Thus, respiratory muscle weakness has been reported to be associated with delayed weaning in some studies [30], but not in all [5]. This discrepancy may be explained by differences in duration of mechanical ventilation and by population characteristics in the two studies [5, 30]. Looking at diaphragm function, there is now compelling evidence to establish a relationship between diaphragm dysfunction and weaning failure [6, 8, 17]. However, the incidence of diaphragm dysfunction is not yet completely established and may depend on the population that is investigated and on the diagnostic method that is employed. Accordingly, the incidence of diaphragm dysfunction ranges from 23 to 80% (Table 1). Using diaphragm ultrasound, Kim et al. identified diaphragm dysfunction in 24/82 medical ICU patients (29%) undergoing a first SBT [8]. Diaphragm dysfunction was associated with a longer total duration of mechanical ventilation (576 vs. 203 h, $p < 0.01$) and a longer weaning duration (401 vs. 90 h, $p < 0.01$) [8]. Using BAMPs at the time of weaning, diaphragm dysfunction was present in 48/76 (63%) non-selected ICU patients [6] and in 32/40 (80%) patients with critical illness polyneuropathy and myopathy [5]. In the first study, diaphragm dysfunction was associated with difficult weaning, prolonged duration of mechanical ventilation, prolonged ICU stay and greater ICU and hospital mortality [6]. In the

Table 1 Prevalence of diaphragm dysfunction at weaning from mechanical ventilation

Author [ref]	Populations	Prevalence
Studies using ultrasound		
Kim et al. [8]	Medical ICU	24/82 (29%)
Jiang et al. [47]	Medical ICU	20/55 (36%)
DiNino et al. [34]	Medical ICU	15/66 (23%)
Lu et al. [48]	Prolonged MV	14/41 (34%)
Studies using pressure generating capacity		
Watson et al. [15]	Medical ICU	26/33 (79%)
Supinski et al. [49]	Medical ICU	48/57 (84%)
Jung et al. [5]	Medical-surgical ICU-AW	32/40 (80%)
Laghi et al. [50]	Prolonged MV – COPD	12/16 (75%)
Dres et al. [6]	Medical ICU	48/76 (63%)
Lerolle et al. [17]	Post-cardiac surgery	19/28 (68%)

ICU: intensive care unit; *MV*: mechanical ventilation; *ICU-AW*: ICU-acquired weakness; *COPD*: chronic obstructive pulmonary disease

Table 2 Diaphragm ultrasound findings in patients with successful and failed weaning

	Weaning test	Successful weaning	Failed weaning	Cut-off to predict successful weaning
Diaphragm thickening fraction				
DiNino et al. [34]	PSV 8-0	–	–	>36%
	T-tube	–	–	>27%
Ferrari et al. [33]	T-tube	–	–	>36%
Blumhof et al. [32]	PSV 5-5	38%	18%	>20%
Farghaly et al. [35]	PSV 8-0	60%	31%	>34%
Dres et al. [6]	PSV 7-0	35%	19%	>29%
Jung et al. [5]	PSV 7-0	20%	9%	–
	T-tube	20%	12%	–
Diaphragm excursion				
Dres et al. [6]	PSV 7-0	1.10 cm	0.80 cm	0.95 cm
Kim et al. [8]	–	–	–	1.00 cm
Carrie et al. [51]	PSV 7-0	4.10	3.0	2.70 cm
Jiang et al. [47]	T-tube	1.45	0.84	1.10 cm

PSV: pressure support ventilation

second study [5], among the 13 patients who died during the ICU stay, 10 (77%) had diaphragm dysfunction on the day of the SBT.

Because of its negative impact on weaning, it may be worthwhile to use diaphragm function as a predictor of weaning failure. Patients with weaning failure consistently have a lower TFdi compared to patients with successful weaning ([5, 6, 32–35]; Table 2). From these studies, the optimal Tfdi cut-off to predict successful weaning ranges from 20 to 36% depending on the ventilator support provided during the measurement; the higher the support, the lower the Tfdi.

Management of Weaning Failure as a Result of Diaphragm Dysfunction

As soon as diaphragm dysfunction is diagnosed in a patient failing the weaning process, there is a need for caregivers to develop strategies aimed at reducing the duration of mechanical ventilation. However, efforts have to be taken before this step by applying preventive strategies.

Preventive Strategies

Maintaining spontaneous breathing under mechanical ventilation alleviates diaphragm dysfunction in animals [36, 37]. Accordingly, a first preventive task may be to favor spontaneous inspiratory effort in patients exposed to mechanical ventilation. This could be achieved by optimizing the level of ventilator assistance and by enhancing sedation strategy. The balance between diaphragm unloading and diaphragm loading is, however, difficult to determine. Although no data are available at this time, the use of ultrasound may be useful to monitor diaphragm activity and to tailor ventilator support in this context. Another interesting option, although not yet investigated in humans, is to cause intermittent contraction of the diaphragm in order to prevent atrophy [38]. Diaphragm pacing can be applied through a transvenous phrenic nerve pacing system designed to be percutaneously placed in the left subclavian vein. This technique has been employed in pigs exposed to mechanical ventilation. Mechanically ventilated (but not paced) pigs suffered significant diaphragm atrophy and loss of endurance. In contrast, pigs that received transvenous phrenic nerve pacing in synchrony with ventilation exhibited less diaphragm atrophy [38]. Whether preventive diaphragm pacing would be possible and effective in patients receiving mechanically ventilation has yet to be proved. Targeting the population who could benefit from this strategy will be the next challenge.

Curative Strategies

There is no specific treatment for diaphragm dysfunction. Management of patients failing the weaning process in whom diaphragm dysfunction has been identified require global evaluation and a multi-approach strategy. We will first review the possible tasks that could be applied in daily practice and then briefly discuss some promising research developments.

All potential causes of weaning failure need to be looked for and removed before resuming the weaning process. Notably, attention has to be paid to the occurrence of weaning-induced cardiac dysfunction, a frequent and treatable cause of weaning failure [39]. Several methods exist to detect weaning-induced cardiac dysfunction [39, 40] and the use of nitrates or diuretics is a good option in this context. Whether diaphragm dysfunction may worsen or alleviate underlying cardiac dysfunction is unclear and the coexistence of these two frequent causes of weaning failure has to be investigated further. Although pleural effusion is not particularly associated with weaning failure [41], some data suggest that removing large pleural effusions may improve diaphragm function [42]. However, the impact of such an intervention on weaning has not yet been established.

If diaphragm dysfunction is identified as a reason for weaning failure, improving respiratory muscle function is a meaningful option. In the ICU, muscle-directed therapies have used various forms of volitional or electrically-induced exercises. The most promising therapy seems to be inspiratory muscle training but only a few studies have been conducted. When looking at studies on inspiratory muscle training, two factors must be considered. First, the modalities of the 'control' arm to which inspiratory muscle training is compared should be carefully examined because there is considerable heterogeneity in practice. Second, the impact of the intervention should have clinical relevance. There is no real benefit of improving inspiratory muscle force itself, attention has to be paid to clinical outcomes, such as shortened duration of mechanical ventilation, successful extubation or greater survival. The largest study enrolled 69 long-term ventilated patients and randomized them to receive either inspiratory muscle training or control training [43]. Inspiratory muscle training consisted of a 5-day-a-week program with four sets of 6 to 10 breaths per day. During each set, patients breathed through a threshold inspiratory muscle trainer and patients in the control group used a resistive inspiratory muscle training device set at the largest opening. In this study, inspiratory muscle training significantly improved maximal inspiratory pressure and successful weaning was more likely [43]. In another study, it was recently reported that inspiratory muscle training performed after successful extubation improved respiratory muscle function but without any clinical benefit [44]. Furthermore, the intervention group had a trend toward greater mortality (12 vs. 0%, p = 0.051). In summary, inspiratory muscle training appears to be effective by improving markers of respiratory muscle function but fails to produce any clinical benefits, in particular on the duration of mechanical ventilation. In the future, the optimal timing to start inspiratory muscle training will need to be determined as well as the target population likely to benefit from this therapy.

Since anabolic steroids increase muscle force in healthy individuals, there is a rationale for their use in patients with diaphragm dysfunction. Although several trials have been conducted in patients with chronic disease, no clear clinical benefits have been identified and they are not indicated in ICU patients. Conversely, the use of inotropes may be of interest to restore diaphragm function. Levosimendan is a cardiac inotrope that exerts positive effects on the contractility of muscle fibers. In healthy subjects, levosimendan reverses diaphragm fatigue and improves neuromechanical efficiency of the diaphragm [45]. However, in a recent trial in which levosimendan was tested to prevent acute organ dysfunction in sepsis, patients who received the drug were more likely to fail weaning from mechanical ventilation (95%CI 0.60 to 0.97, p = 0.03) [46]. Further studies are therefore needed to elucidate the potential indication of levosimendan in patients with diaphragm dysfunction.

As described above, diaphragm pacing is a novel method that can stimulate the diaphragm. This method could be viewed as an effort to support, maintain and strengthen the diaphragm in patients with weaning failure. A phrenic nerve stimulator has been developed as a temporary, minimally invasive, percutaneously-placed, transvenous pacing system intended for use in conjunction with mechanical ventilation. A randomized controlled trial is currently investigating the effect of diaphragm pacing on weaning outcome (NCT03107949).

As re-intubation is associated with increased mortality, any strategy aimed at reducing the rate of post-extubation respiratory failure and avoiding re-intubation deserves consideration. The benefits of early application of non-invasive ventilation soon after extubation have been assessed in unselected patients and in at-risk patients (i.e., > 65 years old or patients with underlying cardiac or respiratory disease). Whether diaphragm dysfunction constitutes an additional risk factor for extubation failure has yet to be determined. If this is shown to be the case, further studies may investigate the use of prophylactic non-invasive ventilation in patients with diaphragm dysfunction who are undergoing extubation.

Conclusion

There is compelling evidence that diaphragm dysfunction is a frequent and serious clinical concern in critically ill patients. In recent years, important progress has been made in the assessment of diaphragm function at the bedside. Whether use of ultrasound is achievable and beneficial beyond the scope of research is an important question that needs to be addressed. Ultrasound may help to better recognize and manage diaphragm dysfunction during weaning from mechanical ventilation. Some preventive strategies may be implemented to tailor ventilatory assistance and maintain diaphragm function while patients are ventilated. Finally, some innovative approaches could also enhance the prognosis of patients; in this context, the use of diaphragm pacing is a promising development.

References

1. Thille AW, Cortés-Puch I, Esteban A (2013) Weaning from the ventilator and extubation in ICU. Curr Opin Crit Care 19:57–64
2. Béduneau G, Pham T, Schortgen F et al (2017) Epidemiology of weaning outcome according to a new definition. The WIND study. Am J Respir Crit Care Med 195:772–783
3. Epstein SK, Ciubotaru RL, Wong JB (1997) Effect of failed extubation on the outcome of mechanical ventilation. Chest 112:186–192
4. Thille AW, Harrois A, Schortgen F et al (2011) Outcomes of extubation failure in medical intensive care unit patients. Crit Care Med 39:2612–2618
5. Jung B, Moury PH, Mahul M et al (2016) Diaphragmatic dysfunction in patients with ICU-acquired weakness and its impact on extubation failure. Intensive Care Med 42:853–861
6. Dres M, Dubé BP, Mayaux J et al (2017) Coexistence and impact of limb muscle and diaphragm weakness at time of liberation from mechanical ventilation in medical intensive care unit patients. Am J Respir Crit Care Med 195:57–66
7. Dubé BP, Dres M, Mayaux J, Demiri S, Similowski T, Demoule A (2017) Ultrasound evaluation of diaphragm function in mechanically ventilated patients: comparison to phrenic stimulation and prognostic implications. Thorax 72:811–818
8. Kim WY, Suh HJ, Hong SB et al (2011) Diaphragm dysfunction assessed by ultrasonography: influence on weaning from mechanical ventilation. Crit Care Med 39:2627–2630
9. Berger D, Bloechlinger S, von Haehling S et al (2016) Dysfunction of respiratory muscles in critically ill patients on the intensive care unit. J Cachexia Sarcopenia Muscle 7:403–412
10. Vassilakopoulos T, Petrof BJ (2004) Ventilator-induced diaphragmatic dysfunction. Am J Respir Crit Care Med 169:336–341
11. Levine S, Nguyen T, Taylor N et al (2008) Rapid disuse atrophy of diaphragm fibers in mechanically ventilated humans. N Engl J Med 358:1327–1335
12. Welvaart WN, Paul MA, Stienen GJM et al (2011) Selective diaphragm muscle weakness after contractile inactivity during thoracic surgery. Ann Surg 254:1044–1049
13. American Thoracic Society, European Respiratory Society (2002) ATS/ERS Statement on respiratory muscle testing. Am J Respir Crit Care Med 166:518–624
14. Moxham J, Goldstone J (1994) Assessment of respiratory muscle strength in the intensive care unit. Eur Respir J 7:2057–2061
15. Watson AC, Hughes PD, Harris LM et al (2001) Measurement of twitch transdiaphragmatic, esophageal, and endotracheal tube pressure with bilateral anterolateral magnetic phrenic nerve stimulation in patients in the intensive care unit. Crit Care Med 29:1325–1331
16. Vivier E, Mekontso Dessap A, Dimassi S et al (2012) Diaphragm ultrasonography to estimate the work of breathing during non-invasive ventilation. Intensive Care Med 38:796–803

17. Lerolle N, Guérot E, Dimassi S et al (2009) Ultrasonographic diagnostic criterion for severe diaphragmatic dysfunction after cardiac surgery. Chest 135:401–407

18. Dres M, Schmidt M, Ferre A et al (2012) Diaphragm electromyographic activity as a predictor of weaning failure. Intensive Care Med 38:2017–2025

19. Rozé H, Repusseau B, Perrier V et al (2013) Neuro-ventilatory efficiency during weaning from mechanical ventilation using neurally adjusted ventilatory assist. Br J Anaesth 111:955–960

20. Jung B, Nougaret S, Conseil M et al (2014) Sepsis is associated with a preferential diaphragmatic atrophy: a critically ill patient study using tridimensional computed tomography. Anesthesiology 120:1182–1191

21. Demoule A, Jung B, Prodanovic H et al (2013) Diaphragm dysfunction on admission to icu: prevalence, risk factors and prognostic impact – a prospective study. Am J Respir Crit Care Med 188:213–219

22. Aubier M, Trippenbach T, Roussos C (1981) Respiratory muscle fatigue during cardiogenic shock. J Appl Physiol 51:499–508

23. Jaber S, Petrof BJ, Jung B et al (2011) Rapidly progressive diaphragmatic weakness and injury during mechanical ventilation in humans. Am J Respir Crit Care Med 183:364–371

24. Hermans G, Agten A, Testelmans D et al (2010) Increased duration of mechanical ventilation is associated with decreased diaphragmatic force: a prospective observational study. Crit Care 14:R127

25. Grosu HB, Lee YI, Lee J et al (2012) Diaphragm muscle thinning in patients who are mechanically ventilated. Chest 142:1455–1460

26. Goligher EC, Fan E, Herridge MS et al (2015) Evolution of diaphragm thickness during mechanical ventilation: impact of inspiratory effort. Am J Respir Crit Care Med 192:1080–1088

27. Zambon M, Beccaria P, Matsuno J et al (2016) Mechanical ventilation and diaphragmatic atrophy in critically ill patients: an ultrasound study. Crit Care Med 44:1347–1352

28. Goligher EC, Dres M, Fan E et al (2017) Mechanical ventilation-induced diaphragm atrophy strongly impacts clinical outcomes. Am J Respir Crit Care Med. https://doi.org/10.1164/rccm.201703-0536OC (Sep 20 Epub ahead of print)

29. Garnacho-Montero J, Amaya-Villar R, García-Garmendía JL et al (2005) Effect of critical illness polyneuropathy on the withdrawal from mechanical ventilation and the length of stay in septic patients. Crit Care Med 33:349–354

30. De Jonghe B, Bastuji-Garin S, Durand MC et al (2007) Respiratory weakness is associated with limb weakness and delayed weaning in critical illness. Crit Care Med 35:2007–2015

31. Mrozek S, Jung B, Petrof BJ et al (2012) Rapid onset of specific diaphragm weakness in a healthy murine model of ventilator-induced diaphragmatic dysfunction. Anesthesiology 117:560–567

32. Blumhof S, Wheeler D, Thomas K et al (2016) Change in diaphragmatic thickness during the respiratory cycle predicts extubation success at various levels of pressure support ventilation. Lung 194:519–525

33. Ferrari G, De Filippi G, Elia F, Panero F, Volpicelli G, Aprà F (2014) Diaphragm ultrasound as a new index of discontinuation from mechanical ventilation. Crit Ultrasound J 6:8

34. DiNino E, Gartman EJ, Sethi JM, McCool FD (2014) Diaphragm ultrasound as a predictor of successful extubation from mechanical ventilation. Thorax 69:423–427

35. Farghaly S, Hasan AA (2017) Diaphragm ultrasound as a new method to predict extubation outcome in mechanically ventilated patients. Aust Crit Care 30:37–43

36. Sassoon CSH, Zhu E, Caiozzo VJ (2004) Assist-control mechanical ventilation attenuates ventilator-induced diaphragmatic dysfunction. Am J Respir Crit Care Med 170:626–632

37. Gayan-Ramirez G, Testelmans D, Maes K et al (2005) Intermittent spontaneous breathing protects the rat diaphragm from mechanical ventilation effects. Crit Care Med 33:2804–2809

38. Reynolds SC, Meyyappan R, Thakkar V et al (2017) Mitigation of ventilator-induced diaphragm atrophy by transvenous phrenic nerve stimulation. Am J Respir Crit Care Med 195:339–348

39. Dres M, Teboul JL, Monnet X (2014) Weaning the cardiac patient from mechanical ventilation. Curr Opin Crit Care 20:493–498
40. Dres M, Teboul JL, Anguel N et al (2014) Extravascular lung water, B-type natriuretic peptide, and blood volume contraction enable diagnosis of weaning-induced pulmonary edema. Crit Care Med 42:1882–1889
41. Dres M, Roux D, Pham T et al (2017) Prevalence and impact on weaning of pleural effusion at the time of liberation from mechanical ventilation: a multicenter prospective observational study. Anesthesiology 126:1107–1115
42. Umbrello M, Mistraletti G, Galimberti A et al (2017) Drainage of pleural effusion improves diaphragmatic function in mechanically ventilated patients. Crit Care Resusc J 19:64–70
43. Martin AD, Smith BK, Davenport PD et al (2011) Inspiratory muscle strength training improves weaning outcome in failure to wean patients: a randomized trial. Crit Care 15:R84
44. Bissett BM, Leditschke IA, Neeman T et al (2016) Inspiratory muscle training to enhance recovery from mechanical ventilation: a randomised trial. Thorax 71:812–819
45. Doorduin J, Sinderby CA, Beck J et al (2012) The calcium sensitizer levosimendan improves human diaphragm function. Am J Respir Crit Care Med 185:90–95
46. Gordon AC, Perkins GD, Singer M et al (2016) Levosimendan for the prevention of acute organ dysfunction in sepsis. N Engl J Med 375:1638–1648
47. Jiang JR, Tsai TH, Jerng JS et al (2004) Ultrasonographic evaluation of liver/spleen movements and extubation outcome. Chest 126:179–185
48. Lu Z, Xu Q, Yuan Y, Zhang G, Guo F, Ge H (2016) Diaphragmatic dysfunction is characterized by increased duration of mechanical ventilation in subjects with prolonged weaning. Respir Care 61:1316–1322
49. Supinski GS, Callahan LA (2013) Diaphragm weakness in mechanically ventilated critically ill patients. Crit Care 17:R120
50. Laghi F, Cattapan SE, Jubran A et al (2003) Is weaning failure caused by low-frequency fatigue of the diaphragm? Am J Respir Crit Care Med 167:120–127
51. Carrie C, Gisbert-Mora C, Bonnardel E et al (2017) Ultrasonographic diaphragmatic excursion is inaccurate and not better than the MRC score for predicting weaning-failure in mechanically ventilated patients. Anaesth Crit Care Pain Med 36:9–14

Part VI
Monitoring: New Aspects

Emerging Technology Platforms for Optical Molecular Imaging and Sensing at the Alveolar Level in the Critically ill

T. H. Craven, T. S. Walsh, and K. Dhaliwal

Introduction

Advances in the understanding of various disease processes have outstripped the clinical care of critically ill patients. Diagnosis, quantification, monitoring and management are often determined through pattern recognition of clinical features rather than reliance on 'true' pathological sampling. There is a great deal of uncertainty surrounding the true presence of disease in many organ systems and especially in pulmonary critical care in diseases such as pneumonia and acute respiratory distress syndrome (ARDS). Formal pulmonary biopsy may provide certainty regarding the diagnosis but is not often performed due to perceived peril, patchy nature of a single sample and the absence of serial biopsy to facilitate monitoring. New developments in biophotonics, fiberoptics, chemistry and image analysis may provide the opportunity to perform real time *in vivo* optical molecular biopsy at the bedside. Healthcare biophotonics is a relatively novel, interdisciplinary science that uses light-based technology to image, detect and characterize the interplay between light and biological materials, including cells and tissues in living organisms (Table 1; [1]).

Optical Molecular Imaging

Molecular imaging has been defined as "the direct and indirect monitoring and recording of the spatiotemporal distribution of molecular or cellular processes for biochemical, biological, diagnostic or therapeutic application" [2]. Molecular imaging includes a wide spectrum of imaging modalities ranging from nuclear medicine and ultrasound to magnetic resonance and optical imaging, all utilized to capture

T. H. Craven (✉) · T. S. Walsh · K. Dhaliwal
Edinburgh Critical Care Research Group, University of Edinburgh
Edinburgh, UK
EPSRC IRC Proteus Hub, MRC Centre for Inflammation Research, University of Edinburgh
Edinburgh, UK
e-mail: Thomas.craven@ed.ac.uk

© Springer International Publishing AG 2018   247
J.-L. Vincent (ed.), *Annual Update in Intensive Care and Emergency Medicine 2018*,
Annual Update in Intensive Care and Emergency Medicine,
https://doi.org/10.1007/978-3-319-73670-9_20

Table 1 Glossary of key terms

Biophotonics	Novel interdisciplinary science using light-based technology to image, detect, and characterize the interplay between light (photons) and biological materials, including cells and tissues in living organisms [1]
Fluorescence	Absorption and subsequent emission of photons, usually at different wavelengths
Fluorophore	A molecule that exhibits fluorescence
Fluorescence lifetime	The time taken for photons to be emitted by a fluorophore after they have been absorbed
Confocal microscopy	A microscope that uses a pinhole to eliminate out of focus light. Sectioning is 'optical', rather than requiring the physical preparation of thin specimens
Optical endomicroscope	Any endoscopically delivered system that is capable of returning images at micron resolution using visual and near visual wavelengths of the electromagnetic spectrum
Optical molecular imaging agent	Exogenously applied compound capable of identifying a specific biological target when combined with an optical imaging device

molecular processes by some means and present them to the eye of the user. Imaging modalities can be used in isolation, relying on the structural properties of the target tissue to produce an image. They can also be used in conjunction with an exogenously administered agent, designed to identify a specific biological process or target in order for it to become detectable and quantifiable.

Optical imaging employs photons from the visible range of the electromagnetic spectrum, and by convention also includes photons from the near visible spectrum, i.e., ultraviolet and near-infrared light. When light illuminates biological tissue it can undergo a variety of physical processes. A substantial fraction of the light may, for example, be immediately reflected from the surface of the tissue. In this situation, a lens can be used to focus this light to some position in space to create an image of the tissue, which can then be permanently recorded using a device such as a multi-pixel detector array (as in a digital camera), or photographic film.

From this simple description, it is immediately clear that the technique of imaging an object, such as a biological tissue, provides information about the spatially distributed physical properties of the object. But light can also undergo a variety of other processes when interacting with tissue. In general, there are four basic processes that can occur when a photon (a particle of light) is incident on tissue; these are reflection, absorption, transmission and scattering. In the same way that the reflective properties of the tissue can be used to create an image of the tissue, so can the other properties, and these images each provide different information about the tissue. The absorption properties of tissue are, for example, directly determined by its spatially dependent molecular composition. Since a molecule only absorbs a photon if it has just the right energy (or wavelength) to excite it from one state to another, an image dominated by absorption, such as a transmission-mode microscope image of a tissue slide, can reveal information about the detailed composition of the tissue – particularly if viewed using light at different wavelengths to provide differential contrast. Scattering can be used to reveal different information, such as the refractive index boundaries at structures such as cell nuclei and cell organelles during dark-field microscopy. In addition to these four basic mechanisms, images can be produced by fluorescence or phosphorescence. In this case, an incident photon with just the right energy (or wavelength) is absorbed by a molecule, and a second photon of a different wavelength is emitted a short time later. As with the other imaging modalities that exploit absorption, scattering and reflection, fluorescence imaging can provide a range of different types of information – particularly if the tissue is stained with a fluorophore to reveal structures that are not visible in other types of imaging.

A huge amount of information is therefore available from the photons returning from the tissue target and the measurements of these data and the implications for clinical practice are only just beginning to be explored. Of the many techniques used to derive information from tissue, fluorescence intensity is the most commonly exploited in optical molecular imaging but other techniques are coming to the fore, such as fluorescence lifetime imaging, which reveal information about the environment surrounding the fluorophore (e.g., pH) and more advanced vibrational imaging modes, such as coherent anti-stokes Raman spectroscopy and stimulated Raman spectroscopy, which, in effect, enable imaging of the chemical bonds present across the tissue [3].

Fluorescence Intensity and Confocal Microscopy

Fluorescence occurs when susceptible molecules within a biological sample absorb photons at one wavelength, and emit photons at another wavelength a few nanoseconds later. Typically, the energy of the emitted photon is lower (i.e., the wavelength is longer) than that of the absorbed photon (Stokes shift), but if two or more photons are absorbed simultaneously the emitted photon may have higher energy and shorter wavelength (anti-Stokes shift). Fluorescence can originate from endogenous fluorophores within the tissue sample or can originate from exogenously applied fluorophores. The selection of different fluorophores with separate excitation and emission spectra permits detection of multiple biological targets within one image.

The modern incarnation of fluorescence and laboratory microscopy is the confocal laser-scanning microscope. Unlike standard widefield microscopy, confocal microscopy adds a pinhole to the light path taken as it is emitted from the sample towards the detector. Out of focus light is blocked and the sectioning is optical rather than relying on thin sample preparation. In a confocal laser scanning microscope, numerous lasers at numerous wavelengths can be scanned across a sample sequentially to build up a multi-color image of an image. Lateral resolution is specified by the user through a selection of pixel number but physically limited by a function of the wavelength of light used to illuminate the sample, known as Abbe's diffraction limit (at which the separation between two adjacent points on a sample can no longer be resolved; for example, approximately 250 nm for blue light), and the axial resolution specified by the pinhole diameter and the focusing lens, but physically limited by the penetration of light through and back from the sample.

This technology is widely used in scientific laboratories and permits a huge amount of *in vitro* investigation, but the bulk of the equipment, the high power of the lasers in question, and the lack of tissue penetration at these wavelengths (approximately 90% of light is lost for every 1 cm travelled [4]) more or less prevents *in vivo* work with this format of the technology, especially in humans. The lack of tissue penetration has been overcome for many decades using fiberoptic light transmission during endoscopic examination, permitting simple visualization of surface features from internal tissue surfaces. As fiberoptic technology develops, optical molecular imaging with all its advanced modalities is becoming a reality in any endoscopically accessible organ system.

Optical Endomicroscopy

Optical endomicroscopy describes the use of any endoscopically delivered system that is capable of returning images at micron resolution utilizing visual and near visual wavelengths of the electromagnetic spectrum. The term covers a range of optical technologies such as confocal laser endomicroscopy, fiber-based optical coherence tomography [5] and fiber-based widefield fluorescence microscopy [6]. Conventional optical fibers consist of a single high refractive index guiding core, around which there is a low refractive index cladding region. Light propagates down the core by the phenomenon of total internal reflection at the core-cladding boundary due to the refractive index difference. These conventional single-core fibers would be of little use for endomicroscopy because they would not transmit an image of the tissue to the proximal end. To transmit an image, endomicroscopy relies on the use of a coherent fiber bundle, a single-optical fiber designed and fabricated in such a way that light can be transmitted down the fiber in a spatially selective manner using thousands of individual cores in the same fiber. Unfortunately, these cores are always 'coupled', and light can tunnel from one core to another, smearing out the image of interest. To reduce this effect, the coherent fiber bundles are carefully optimized to control the refractive indices of the cores and also their spacing. One approach in commercial coherent fiber bundles has been to use high refractive index glass for the cores, but this results in very expensive fibers, that are necessarily re-used for cost-efficiency with subsequent impact of disinfection and wear and tear of fibers. A recent important advance has been to arrange the cores into a square pattern and to use a variety of glasses with different refractive indices for the cores. This approach allows the fabrication of coherent fiber bundles with comparable imaging performance to commercial coherent fiber bundles, but without the expense of high refractive index glass [7]. This is a crucial step for future medical applications of endomicroscopy, as the advent of low-cost coherent fiber bundles will enable new endomicroscopy modalities that would benefit from single-use low cost disposable fibers.

Confocal Laser Endomicroscopy

Confocal laser endomicroscopy is achieving widespread clinical application and there is now a great deal of *in vivo* experience with commercially available systems that are contributing to clinical decision-making, but experience in critical care is lacking. The images generated by confocal laser endomicroscopy are confocal because the narrow aperture of each core in the fiber acts as the pinhole to reject returning out of focus light. To reduce motion artefact during *in vivo* imaging, the acquisition speed of the image needs to be rapid, and acquisition is limited by the speed at which the laser scans across each individual core in turn and therefore also by the number of cores in the fiber bundle. Even though the laser-scanning unit is housed proximally, it is sometimes still necessary to design the fiber tip to adequately focus light onto the sample and facilitate the collection of reflected or fluorescent light. In order to make this distal tip as small as possible, tiny gradient index lenses can be used but this adds bulk and reduces flexibility at the fiber tip [8].

At the time of writing there is only one commercially available range meeting the design and construction requirements for clinical use. The Cellvizio (Mauna Kea Technologies, Paris) [9] system consists of a laser-scanning unit, a selection of fiber imaging bundles and proprietary software for processing the raw data presenting the processed image and manipulating or interacting with the processed image using a variety of tools. The device produces blue argon 488 nm laser light, and collects returning light from the fiber bundle in the 505–700 nm range by passing it through a dichroic mirror and onto a photodetector. Each scanning unit can be paired with any one of a number of different fiberoptic bundles, each with a unique set of characteristics making it more or less suitable for any particular clinical application [10, 11].

Confocal laser endomicroscopy is particularly well established in the field of gastrointestinal investigation, where it has been used to image inflammatory lesions or lesions with suspicion of malignancy in the esophagus and stomach [12, 13], pancreas [14, 15], biliary tree [16, 17] and large bowel [18, 19], and enjoys widespread clinical use internationally.

The use of confocal laser endomicroscopy in respiratory medicine is becoming more extensive [20]. The alveoflex™ fiber bundle is widely used for respiratory imaging, housing 30,000 optical fibers in a stiff casing with a tip diameter of 1.4 mm. It returns an image with a field of view of 600 μm, a lateral resolution of 3.5 μm, and an axial resolution of 0–50 μm, at a frame rate of 12 per second [20]. As with other applications, respiratory imaging relies on the autofluorescent characteristics of lung tissue [21], predominantly due to elastin [22, 23], with lower contributions from other connective tissues, such as collagen [20]. In smokers, brightly autofluorescent cells can often be seen, with features suggesting they are alveolar macrophages [21]. The system has been used clinically for the assessment of pulmonary nodules [24, 25], following lung transplantation [26], and in asthma [27], emphysema [28], *Pneumocystis* pneumonia [29], alveolar proteinosis [30, 31] and amiodarone-associated pneumonia [32]. The technique appears to have a good

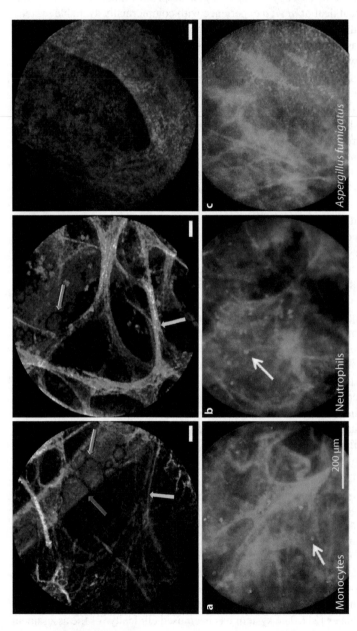

Fig. 1 Examples of optical endomicroscopy images of the lung. *Top row*: confocal laser endomicroscopy images. *Left image* – healthy alveolar tissue; *yellow arrow*: alveolar wall; *blue arrow*: pulmonary capillary; *red arrow*: fluid bubbles. *Center image* – diseased lung from a mechanically ventilated patient with a pulmonary infiltrate. *Right image* – endobronchial imaging, the opening of a respiratory bronchiole can be seen surrounded by smooth muscle. Scale bar 50 μm. *Bottom row* (reproduced from [6] with permission): multicolor widefield optical endomicroscopy. Images show *ex vivo* lung tissue with similar endogenous tissue autofluorescent architecture as confocal laser endomicroscopy images. Monocytes, neutrophils, and *Aspergillus* have been labelled and added to tissue. The potential strength of multicolor imaging is demonstrated

safety profile although there has been no directed research searching for adverse events. There is a learning curve associated with conducting the technique and interpreting the images. To date, there have been very few published reports of the use of the technique in patients undergoing positive pressure ventilation via endotracheal tube and there are no systematic interrogations of confocal laser endomicroscopy images correlating images with histological findings or clinical features. The main limitations of the produced images are the reliance on tissue autofluorescence, the single excitation wavelength, cost, and the inability to discriminate the wavelength of emitted photons. All images are single color and all excited fluorophores whose emissions pass within the wide filter will be presented in that one color, indistinguishable from one another – the 'green-on-green' discrimination problem (Fig. 1).

The reliance on intensity-based tissue autofluorescence can be addressed through the development of targeted optical molecular imaging agents permitting a diverse range of biological targets to be examined, and the future use of additional photonic properties, such as fluorescence lifetime or multiple illumination sources with multiple filters will address the 'green-on-green' imaging problem.

The manufacturers of Cellvizio have developed a two-wavelength device but it is yet to be authorized for human application [33]. Another potential strategy is to use light emitting diodes rather than laser sources. Filters and timers are used to permit multiple illumination sources simultaneously, for a fraction of the cost of a laser-based device [6]. Blue illumination can be used to identify tissue autofluorescence and, therefore, tissue architecture, whilst other channels can be reserved for exogenously applied agents, where there is little or no tissue autofluorescence (Fig. 1, bottom row).

Optical Molecular Imaging Agents

A molecular imaging agent is a chemical entity applied to a biological sample to facilitate the visualization, characterization and quantification of biological processes in living systems [34]. To identify a specific target, the agent will usually comprise a contrast generating moiety and a targeting moiety. Other moieties may be present to add specificity and improve pharmacodynamic/pharmacokinetic properties. In the case of optical imaging, the contrast moiety is typically a fluorescent molecule. Molecular agents for optical molecular imaging are widely used in *in vitro* and *ex vivo* assays, have been so for many decades, and are responsible for some of the most breathtaking and insightful scientific images. The vast majority of these laboratory stains use a simple ligand as their targeting moiety, and are flooded across a suitably prepared sample before unbound stain is washed away and imaging proceeds. This technique is not immediately suitable for *in vivo* work and more consideration needs to be given to the development of the agent.

For *in vivo* work, there are two main strategies for identifying a specific biological target: affinity-based agents and activity-based agents. Affinity-based agents rely on the simple ligand target moieties followed by accumulation as described above, but the agent must be resilient to the pharmacodynamic/pharmacokinetic rigors of the human body, provide sufficient signal to noise, and be compatible with a clinical imaging platform. Activity-based agents still contain a contrast and target moiety but must employ some strategy to 'turn on' in the presence of the target of interest, making use of a change in fluorescent signal upon processing or binding to the target [35]. They are often referred to as "SmartProbes" for this reason [36], although we prefer to avoid the use of this term as fiberoptic bundles are also often referred to as probes and confusion abounds. This ability to report signal only when acted on by a target allows rapid imaging, as there is no need to remove, or wait for the removal of, the unbound agent. The commonest strategy to keep the agent 'off' in the absence of the target is to quench the signal moiety, and quenching can be achieved through a variety of dynamic mechanisms that can be released to reveal fluorescence in the presence of the target. Most activity-based agents use a peptide sequence as the target moiety; they are easy and cheap to work with, confer chemical properties to the agent that can be manipulated, and are very specific because of their complementary shape, charge, and hydrophilic/phobic characteristics [37].

Bacterial Imaging Using Optical Endomicroscopy

The diagnosis of infectious pneumonia seems simple to describe: inflammation of the lung parenchyma as a result of infection by an invading microorganism. But the diagnosis is much more difficult to make in reality. A combination of clinical markers and radiological findings are often relied upon to guide the prescription of antibiotics long before microbiological sampling and confirmation is available. *In vivo* optical imaging of bacterial infection is a developing field with many potential bacterial targets and imaging modalities [38]. For pneumonia, sufficiently bright and specific imaging agents have the potential to be combined with OEM to achieve direct bacterial imaging in the alveolar space. In one example, conjugates of the environmental fluorophore nitrobenzoxadiazole (NBD) have been used to detect bacteria in models of suspected pneumonia [39]. Here, NBD is conjugated to a variant of the innate antimicrobial peptide ubiquicidin or variants of antibiotics. The antibiotic targets the bacteria and once inserted into the hydrophobic bacterial membrane, the NBD fluorophore becomes fluorescent. The agents therefore can be used to identify bacterial infection in general or Gram-negative bacterial infection, respectively (Fig. 2).

Activated Neutrophils Using Optical Endomicroscopy

To confirm the presence of acute inflammation one potential target is the activated neutrophil. These cells flood into the lungs of critically ill patients in certain conditions such as ARDS [41], a condition surrounded by a huge amount of diagnostic doubt and error [42, 43]. An optical imaging agent designed to identify activated neutrophils in mechanically ventilated patients has shown promise in a completed phase 1 study (NCT01532024) and is now undergoing phase 2

Fig. 2 Bacterial imaging with optical endomicroscopy. *Staphylococcus aureus* with *ex vivo* human lung tissue without (*top*) and with (*bottom*) ubiquicidin nitrobenzoxadiazole (NBD) imaging agent. The bacteria appear as punctate dots, which twinkle in and out of focus during live imaging. *Yellow arrows*: alveolar walls; *magenta arrow*; optical signal from labeled bacteria. Reproduced and modified from [40] under creative commons attribution 3.0 unported license

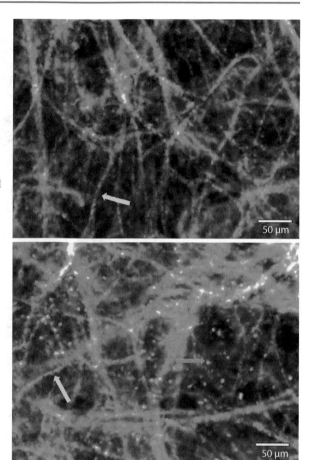

assessment (NCT02804854). Example images from *ex vivo* lung ventilation and perfusion, a routine pre-clinical assessment of pulmonary optical molecular imaging techniques, are shown in Fig. 3.

Fiber Tip Location

One of the main criticisms facing the use of optical endomicroscopy in human lungs is the extremely small field of view generated by the device, compared to the whole surface area of the alveoli in general. How can one be certain that the field of view is representative of the lungs, lobes or segments? This question can be resolved in part with a rigorous sampling procedure and good technical bronchoscopy skills in directing the optical fiber. But the direction of the tips of the current generation of fibers is not controllable once the fiber exits the working channel of the bronchoscope, and the tip will follow the path of least resistance to the alveolus so the final

Fig. 3 Optical endomicroscopy with activated neutrophil imaging agent during ovine *ex vivo* lung ventilation and perfusion. **a** No inflammation. **b** Inflammation with *Pseudomonas aeruginosa*. **c** Sterile inflammation with endotoxin. *Yellow arrows*: alveolar walls; *magenta arrow*: optical signal from activated neutrophils

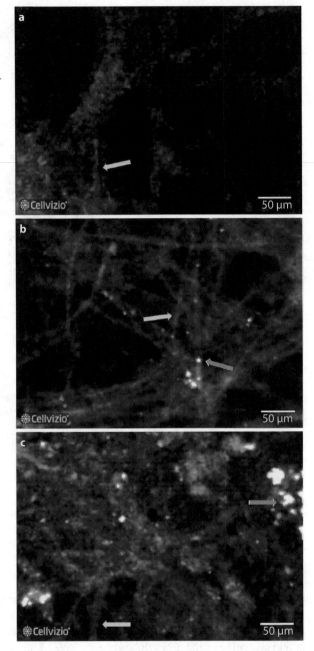

resting place of the tip of optical fiber is not directly visualized. Additional optical properties can be exploited to perform imaging and localization of the fiber tip, in a manner similar to screening for interventional radiology, but without the need for ionizing radiation. If the fiber tip in the alveolus contains an infrared light source, photons from this source will travel sufficiently far without being absorbed by body tissues that some will be detectable outside the body. Most of these photons will be heavily scattered by body tissues but some will travel relatively unperturbed in a straight line – so-called ballistic photons. A sufficiently time-resolved photon detector placed outside the body will be able to differentiate the unperturbed ballistic photons from those heavily scattered photons arriving later, whose location origin cannot be accurately determined. Multiple detectors would be able to triangulate the fiber tip position with sufficient accuracy and the technique has been demonstrated during *ex vivo* lung perfusion and in other tissue models [44]. The technique also has potential applications for static and dynamic confirmation of intravascular device placement.

Fluorescence Lifetime

Fluorescent lifetime is a physical phenomenon related to generation of fluorescence. The detection of fluorescence is determined by the number of photons at a particular wavelength arriving at a detector, and their associated energy. Fluorescent lifetime refers to the time taken for a susceptible molecule to eject a fluorescent photon after absorbing an incident photon from a light source. To quantify fluorescent lifetime a pulsed lased and time gated detector are required. The laser pulses on for only a fraction of every time period. Incident light strikes the sample, photons are absorbed by the fluorophore and after a short period of time, fluorescent photons are emitted. The detector is synchronized to the pulse of the laser and begins counting. Each photon that hits the detector is time stamped and so a decay curve of arrival times is produced. The fluorescent lifetime of a sample (τ) is taken at $1/e$, a standard mathematical action for exponential functions. If the detector is pixelated, an image can be produced. Although fluorescence varies considerably with fluorophore concentration, fluorescent lifetime varies only with changes in environmental conditions [45]. Fluorescent lifetime could prove extremely important *in vivo* where the delivery of exact quantities of fluorophore to a particular field of view cannot necessarily be guaranteed, and so quantification using fluorescent intensity may be flawed. Fluorescence lifetime imaging may also address one of the main current limitations of confocal laser endomicroscopy, where all imaging is 'green-on-green', by providing an additional level of contrast: two different fluorophores may emit photons at the same wavelength but with different fluorescent lifetimes.

Raman Spectroscopy

In contrast to fluorescence microscopy with which molecules absorb photons to become electronically excited, Raman scattering occurs when a molecule absorbs a photon and undergoes vibrational excitement. Typically when this occurs, the molecule will emit a photon at the same wavelength of the absorbed photon (elastic or Rayleigh scattering) without delay. Much less frequently, when the molecule absorbs a photon it will emit a photon with a different wavelength (fewer than 1 in 1^{10} of all incident photons), either longer (Stokes shifted) or shorter (anti-Stokes shifted). The precise emission of Stokes or anti-Stokes shifted photons is unique to each molecule under investigation and can be used to build a unique 'fingerprint' spectrum. The information derived from the Raman spectrum from a particular point in the sample can be overlaid on traditional light microscopy images to give additional label free information about the nature of the biological sample [46]. Raman spectroscopy could provide label free live imaging of inflammatory cells, but is currently being developed for sensing physiological parameters, using devices small enough to work in the alveolar space. Coherent techniques such as coherent anti-Stokes Raman spectroscopy and stimulated Raman spectroscopy can also enable Raman imaging, but at a greatly enhanced efficiency and speed.

Pulmonary Optical Sensing

Many of the optical technologies described here can be used not only for imaging but also for physiological sensing at the alveolar level. The technology is conceptually simpler, as bundles of fibers are not required and no image reconstruction is necessary. Innovative chemistry is applied at the fiber tip in the form of tiny molecular agents, such as surface-enhanced Raman spectroscopy reporters or fluorescent modifiable reporters, detecting physiological parameters and transmitting via a single optic fiber to a proximal detector. The technology has been used to monitor alveolar changes in pH ([47, 48]; Fig. 4) and oxygen tension with time, and may be useful in measuring the physiological effects of acute lung disease. Such miniaturized solutions to sensing could be easily multiplexed with imaging technology to record multiple parameters simultaneously at the bedside.

Conclusion

A non-destructive optical molecular biopsy of lung tissue is tangible, can be feasibly carried out at the bedside, and has the potential to be repeated as often as clinically indicated. The technology and research are well established *in vitro* but there is currently limited experience in the clinical environment. The use of multiple colors and additional technologies, exploiting additional properties of reflected photons for the purposes of imaging and sensing, are in development and will, in the future, be multiplexed together to provide a dynamic bedside assessment of the lungs of critically ill patients.

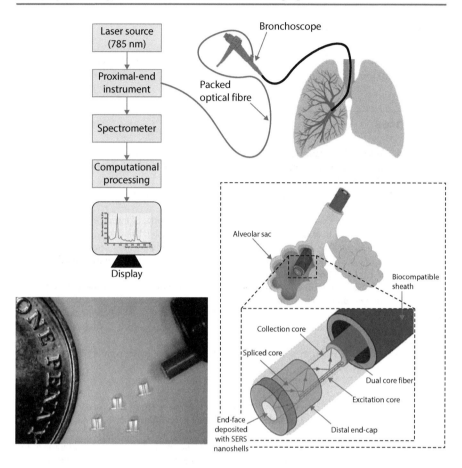

Fig. 4 Sensing alveolar pH. Schematic illustration of the fiberoptic sensing system for measuring alveolar pH. Inset photograph: 4 distal end-caps containing the pH sensors are also shown alongside a one-penny coin. *SERS*: surface enhanced Raman spectroscopy. Reproduced from [47] with permission

The ultimate aim is to provide cheap, safe, and minimally invasive dynamic *in vivo* molecular pathology that can be repeated frequently in mechanically ventilated patients or, in the future, potentially 'left in place' to provide telemetry. Clinical studies examining the utility and promise of combining optical endomicroscopy and specific optical molecular agents are underway including the visualization of alveolar bacteria, class of bacteria, and whether pulmonary inflammation (alveolar neutrophils) is present either in combination with bacteria (true alveolar infection) or in isolation (pure inflammation/lung injury). This will enable a precision approach to guide antimicrobial use and/or anti-inflammatory therapies and could open a new chapter in precision trials in pulmonary critical care that could address the acknowledged limitations of the existing literature and trial designs.

Acknowledgements

The authors are grateful to Professor Robert Thomson of Heriot-Watt University for his comments on the manuscript.

References

1. Coda S, Siersema PD, Stamp GWH, Thillainayagam AV (2015) Biophotonic endoscopy: a review of clinical research techniques for optical imaging and sensing of early gastrointestinal cancer. Endosc Int Open 3:E380–E392
2. Thakur M, Lentle BC (2005) Report of a summit on molecular imaging. Radiology 236:753–755
3. Pezacki JP, Blake JA, Danielson DC et al (2011) Chemical contrast for imaging living systems: molecular vibrations drive CARS microscopy. Nat Chem Biol 7:137–145
4. Dorward DA, Lucas CD, Rossi AG et al (2012) Imaging inflammation: molecular strategies to visualize key components of the inflammatory cascade, from initiation to resolution. Pharmacol Ther 135:182–199
5. Carignan CS, Yagi Y (2012) Optical endomicroscopy and the road to real-time, in vivo pathology: present and future. Diagn Pathol 7:98
6. Krstajic N, Akram AR, Choudhary TR et al (2016) Two-color widefield fluorescence microendoscopy enables multiplexed molecular imaging in the alveolar space of human lung tissue. J Biomed Opt 21:46009
7. Stone JM, Wood HAC, Harrington K, Birks TA (2017) Low index contrast imaging fibers. Opt Lett 42:1484
8. Lane PM, Lam S, McWilliams A et al (2009) Confocal fluorescence microendoscopy of bronchial epithelium. J Biomed Opt 14:24008
9. Laemmel E, Genet M, Le Goualher G et al (2004) Fibered confocal fluorescence microscopy (Cell-viZio^{TM}) facilitates extended imaging in the field of microcirculation. J Vasc Res 41:400–411
10. Osdoit A, Lacombe F, Cavé C et al (2007) To see the unseeable: confocal miniprobes for routine microscopic imaging during endoscopy. In: Tearney GJ, Wang TD (eds) Endoscocpic Microscopy II. Proceedings of the SPIE, vol 6432. (Article id. 64320F)
11. Paull PE, Hyatt BJ, Wassef W, Fischer AH (2011) Confocal laser endomicroscopy: a primer for pathologists. Arch Pathol Lab Med 135:1343–1348
12. Dunbar KB, Okolo P, Montgomery E, Canto MI (2009) Confocal laser endomicroscopy in Barrett's esophagus and endoscopically inapparent Barrett's neoplasia: a prospective, randomized, double-blind, controlled, crossover trial. Gastrointest Endosc 70:645–654
13. Kiesslich R, Gossner L, Goetz M et al (2006) In vivo histology of barrett's esophagus and associated neoplasia by confocal laser endomicroscopy. Clin Gastroenterol Hepatol 4:979–987
14. Napoléon B, Lemaistre AI, Pujol B et al (2014) A novel approach to the diagnosis of pancreatic serous cystadenoma: needle-based confocal laser endomicroscopy. Endoscopy 47:26–32
15. Napoleon B, Lemaistre AI, Pujol B et al (2016) In vivo characterization of pancreatic cystic lesions by needle-based confocal laser endomicroscopy (nCLE): proposition of a comprehensive nCLE classification confirmed by an external retrospective evaluation. Surg Endosc 30:2603–2612
16. Loeser CS, Robert ME, Mennone A et al (2011) Confocal endomicroscopic examination of malignant biliary strictures and histologic correlation with lymphatics. J Clin Gastroenterol 45:246–252

17. Kahaleh M, Giovannini M, Jamidar P et al (2015) Probe-based confocal laser endomicroscopy for indeterminate biliary strictures: refinement of the image interpretation classification. Gastroenterol Res Pract 2015:675210

18. Hlavaty T, Huorka M, Koller T et al (2011) Colorectal cancer screening in patients with ulcerative and crohn's colitis with use of colonoscopy, chromoendoscopy and confocal endomicroscopy. Eur J Gastroenterol Hepatol 23:680–689

19. Kiesslich R, Duckworth CA, Moussata D et al (2012) Local barrier dysfunction identified by confocal laser endomicroscopy predicts relapse in inflammatory bowel disease. Gut 61:1146–1153

20. Thiberville L, Salaün M, Lachkar S et al (2009) Confocal fluorescence endomicroscopy of the human airways. Proc Am Thorac Soc 6:444–449

21. Thiberville L, Salaün M, Lachkar S et al (2009) Human in vivo fluorescence microimaging of the alveolar ducts and sacs during bronchoscopy. Eur Respir J 33:974–985

22. Gabrecht T, Andrejevic-Blant S, Wagnières G (2007) Blue-violet excited autofluorescence spectroscopy and imaging of normal and cancerous human bronchial tissue after formalin fixation. Photochem Photobiol 83:450–459

23. Thiberville L, Moreno-Swirc S, Vercauteren T et al (2007) In vivo imaging of the bronchial wall microstructure using fibered confocal fluorescence microscopy. Am J Respir Crit Care Med 175:22–31

24. Hassan T, Piton N, Lachkar S, Salaün M, Thiberville L (2015) A novel method for in vivo imaging of solitary lung nodules using navigational bronchoscopy and confocal laser microendoscopy. Lung 193:773–778

25. Seth S, Akram AR, McCool P et al (2016) Assessing the utility of autofluorescence-based pulmonary optical endomicroscopy to predict the malignant potential of solitary pulmonary nodules in humans. Sci Rep 6:31372

26. Yserbyt J, Dooms C, Decramer M, Verleden GM (2014) Acute lung allograft rejection: diagnostic role of probe-based confocal laser endomicroscopy of the respiratory tract. J Heart Lung Transpl 33:492–498

27. Yick CY, von der Thüsen JH, Bel EH, Sterk PJ, Kunst PW (2011) In vivo imaging of the airway wall in asthma: fibered confocal fluorescence microscopy in relation to histology and lung function. Respir Res 12:85

28. Newton RC, Kemp SV, Yang GZ et al (2012) Imaging parenchymal lung diseases with confocal endomicroscopy. Respir Med 106:127–137

29. Shafiek H, Fiorentino F, Cosio BG et al (2016) Usefulness of bronchoscopic probe-based confocal laser endomicroscopy in the diagnosis of Pneumocystis jirovecii pneumonia. Respiration 92:40–47

30. Salaün M, Roussel F, Hauss PA, Lachkar S, Thiberville L (2010) In vivo imaging of pulmonary alveolar proteinosis using confocal endomicroscopy. Eur Respir J 36:451–453

31. Danilevskaya O, Averyanov A, Lesnyak V et al (2015) Confocal laser endomicroscopy for diagnosis and monitoring of pulmonary alveolar proteinosis. J Bronchology Interv Pulmonol 22:33–40

32. Salaün M, Roussel F, Bourg-Heckly G et al (2013) In vivo probe-based confocal laser endomicroscopy in amiodarone-related pneumonia. Eur Respir J 42:1646–1658

33. Marien A, Rock A, El Maadarani K et al (2017) Urothelial tumors and dual-band imaging: a new concept in confocal laser endomicroscopy. J Endourol 31:538–544

34. Chen K, Chen X (2010) Design and development of molecular imaging probes. Curr Top Med Chem 10:1227–1236

35. Garland M, Yim JJ, Bogyo M (2016) A Bright future for precision medicine: advances in fluorescent chemical probe design and their clinical application. Cell Chem Biol 23:122–136

36. Blum G, Weimer RM, Edgington LE et al (2009) Comparative assessment of substrates and activity based probes as tools for non-invasive optical imaging of cysteine protease activity. PLoS One 4:e6374

37. Ha Y (2009) Structure and mechanism of intramembrane protease. Semin Cell Dev Biol 20:240–250
38. Mills B, Bradley M, Dhaliwal K (2016) Optical imaging of bacterial infections. Clin Transl Imaging 4:163–174
39. Akram AR, Avlonitis N, Craven T et al (2016) Structural modifications of the antimicrobial peptide ubiquicidin for pulmonary imaging of bacteria in the alveolar space. Lancet 387(suppl 1):S17 (abst)
40. Akram AR, Avlonitis N, Lilienkampf A et al (2015) A labelled-ubiquicidin antimicrobial peptide for immediate in situ optical detection of live bacteria in human alveolar lung tissue. Chem Sci 6:6971–6979
41. Williams AE, Chambers RC (2014) The mercurial nature of neutrophils: still an enigma in ARDS? Am J Physiol Lung Cell Mol Physiol 306:L217–L230
42. Thille AW, Esteban A, Fernández-Segoviano P et al (2013) Comparison of the Berlin definition for acute respiratory distress syndrome with autopsy. Am J Respir Crit Care Med 187:761–767
43. Bellani G, Laffey JG, Pham T et al (2016) Epidemiology, patterns of care, and mortality for patients with acute respiratory distress syndrome in intensive care units in 50 countries. JAMA 315:788–800
44. Tanner MG, Choudhary TR, Craven TH et al (2017) Ballistic and snake photon imaging for locating optical endomicroscopy fibres. Biomed Opt Express 8:4077
45. Berezin MY, Achilefu S (2010) Fluorescence lifetime measurements and biological imaging. Chem Rev 110:2641–2684
46. Movasaghi Z, Rehman S, Rehman IU (2007) Raman spectroscopy of biological tissues. Appl Spectrosc Rev 42:493–541
47. Choudhury D, Tanner MG, McAughtrie S et al (2017) Endoscopic sensing of alveolar pH. Biomed Opt Express 8:243
48. Mohamad F, Tanner MG, Choudhury D et al (2017) Controlled core-to-core photo-polymerisation – fabrication of an optical fibre-based pH sensor. Analyst 41:918–926

Contributors to Differences between Mixed and Central Venous Oxygen Saturation

T. D. Corrêa, J. Takala, and S. M. Jakob

Introduction

Mixed venous oxygen saturation (SvO_2) represents the relationship between systemic oxygen delivery (DO_2) and consumption (VO_2) and, therefore, the adequacy of oxygen supply to the tissues [1]. SvO_2 reflects the total amount of oxygen contained in the blood that returns to the right heart through the superior vena cava, inferior vena cava (IVC) and coronary sinus [1]. Whereas SvO_2 can only be obtained by right heart catheterization, central venous oxygen saturation ($ScvO_2$) can be measured using a central venous catheter (CVC), which is easier to place, cheaper, and is assumed to have fewer complications than a pulmonary artery catheter (PAC) [2]. Since the use of PAC in critically ill patients has declined [3], $ScvO_2$ has been used as a surrogate of SvO_2 [4]. $ScvO_2$ represents the blood oxygen saturation at the drainage from the superior or the inferior vena cava into the right atrium, depending on catheter position [5, 6].

The underlying assumption for using $ScvO_2$ as a surrogate for SvO_2 is that differences between the two saturations [$\Delta(ScvO_2\text{-}SvO_2)$] are rather small or relatively constant [7] and that changes in $ScvO_2$ reflect changes in SvO_2 [8]. This assumption, although true sometimes, cannot be generalized for the hemodynamic management of unstable patients [9]. Very large differences between central and mixed venous oxygen saturations exist in individual subjects [10, 11]. The reasons for these differences can be understood when the regional distribution of blood flow and metabolic demands in individual organs and tissues are considered [12].

T. D. Corrêa
Department of Intensive Care Medicine, Inselspital, Bern University Hospital, University of Bern
Bern, Switzerland
Intensive Care Unit, Hospital Israelita Albert Einstein
São Paulo, Brazil

J. Takala · S. M. Jakob (✉)
Department of Intensive Care Medicine, Inselspital, Bern University Hospital, University of Bern
Bern, Switzerland
e-mail: stephan.jakob@insel.ch

© Springer International Publishing AG 2018   263
J.-L. Vincent (ed.), *Annual Update in Intensive Care and Emergency Medicine 2018*,
Annual Update in Intensive Care and Emergency Medicine,
https://doi.org/10.1007/978-3-319-73670-9_21

For example, compared to systemic oxygen extraction, the oxygen extraction of the kidney is typically lower and of the splanchnic region higher [13]. In critically ill patients, both femoral venous and hepatic venous saturations can be substantially lower than the mixed venous saturation [14]. Obviously, this contributes to central-mixed venous oxygen gradients.

In this chapter, we try to improve the understanding of differences between central venous and mixed venous oxygen saturation in different, frequent diseases in critically ill patients. This may help intensivists to judge the relevance of $ScvO_2$ at the bedside. In order to complement the relatively few data in the literature with simultaneous, repeated SvO_2 and $ScvO_2$ measurements, we review some of our own, unpublished data from previous, clinically relevant animal experiments.

$ScvO_2$ and SvO_2: General Considerations

$ScvO_2$ is highly dependent on the site of measurement. The ideal positioning for the CVC tip is in the lower superior vena cava, near its junction with the right atrium [15]. Nevertheless, it has been shown that nearly one in four CVC tips inserted through the subclavian or right internal jugular vein is not properly located [15]. If positioned in the right atrium, central venous blood, which should contain only blood draining from the brain, neck and upper limbs, will be mixed with variable amounts of blood from the IVC.

In healthy persons, $ScvO_2$ is less than SvO_2 due to higher oxygen extraction in the brain compared to abdominal organs, especially the kidneys [16]. Conversely, in shock, $ScvO_2$ usually exceeds SvO_2 as a result of increasing oxygen extraction by intraabdominal organs, such as gut and liver, and lower limbs [4, 10, 11, 17]. Treatments may also interfere with $\Delta(ScvO_2\text{-}SvO_2)$ [18]. For example, most hypnotic anesthetic agents commonly used in critically ill patients, such as benzodiazepines, propofol and barbiturates, reduce the cerebral metabolic rate [19]. If cerebral blood flow does not decrease to the same extent, oxygen saturation of blood returning from the brain to the right atrium is increased. This may enlarge the $\Delta(ScvO_2\text{-}SvO_2)$. Furthermore, at least during anesthesia for cardiac surgery, $\Delta(ScvO_2\text{-}SvO_2)$ seems to be dependent on systemic oxygen extraction, exhibiting negative values at low and positive values at high oxygen extraction [20].

Hypothermia during cardiopulmonary bypass (CPB) can serve as a model of how $\Delta(ScvO_2\text{-}SvO_2)$ is influenced at extreme physiological conditions: in a study with an uneventful clinical course in all patients, oxygen saturation in the IVC was lower than $ScvO_2$ and SvO_2 with a maximal difference of 17% during hypothermia (28 °C) and 24% during rewarming [21]. While SvO_2 and saturation in the IVC correlated significantly, $ScvO_2$ and SvO_2 did not [21]. Hypothermia reduced backflow from the superior in favor of the inferior vena cava. Interestingly, all the changes occurred while SvO_2 remained within the normal range [21]. Similar discrepancies between $ScvO_2$ and SvO_2 were also observed during cardiac surgery using mild hypothermia (34–35 °C) [22]. Based on the frequently observed large inter-individual variability in the difference between $ScvO_2$ and SvO_2, many authors agree that neither absolute values nor trends in $ScvO_2$ should replace SvO_2 in situations with expected large variability in physiological parameters [10, 22–24].

Comparison Between SvO_2 and $ScvO_2$ in Critically Ill Patients

Several studies have evaluated the agreement and correlation between $ScvO_2$ and SvO_2 in medical-surgical critically ill patients [4, 8, 17]. Taken together, these studies have shown poor agreement albeit a good correlation between the two saturations [4, 8, 17]. For example, Chawla et al. reported a mean bias between SvO_2 and $ScvO_2$ of −5.2%, with 95% limits of agreement ranging from −15.5 to 5.2% ($r = 0.88$, $p < 0.001$) in a mixed sample of 53 medical-surgical critically ill patients [17].

Since absolute values of $ScvO_2$ and SvO_2 can vary considerably in different clinical situations, some authors hypothesized that trends in $ScvO_2$ could more closely reflect changes in SvO_2 [4, 8]. Reinhart et al. demonstrated in a cohort of ICU patients that $\Delta(ScvO_2\text{-}SvO_2)$ was highest in patients with elevated increased intracranial pressure (mean = 11%), lowest in postoperative (7%) and intermediate in sepsis patients (8%), but that changes in $ScvO_2$ tracked changes in SvO_2 values in approximately 90% of the occasions where SvO_2 changed more than 5% [4]. Considering the substantial bias (7.7%) and wide 95% limits of agreement between the changes (−2.9 to 18.4%), this conclusion seems questionable.

Severe Sepsis and Septic Shock

When $ScvO_2$ and SvO_2 are compared in these patients, the most usual finding is a mostly moderate (< 10%) bias with very wide 95% limits of agreement ranging from −20 to +15% and more [10, 11, 25]. This makes changes in individual patients very difficult to interpret, and potentially misleading.

In a study in septic shock, the authors reported a significant correlation between $\Delta(ScvO_2\text{-}SvO_2)$ with both norepinephrine dose ($r = 0.41$, $p = 0.012$) and oxygen extraction ratio ($r = 0.43$, $p < 0.01$) suggesting that blood flow redistribution secondary to catecholamine infusion and varying oxygen extraction, especially in splanchnic organs, may affect the gradient between the two saturations [25].

Low Cardiac Output

Wide gradients and poor correlation between $ScvO_2$ and SvO_2 have been shown in patients with heart failure or established shock [7]. The agreement between the two saturations appears better in patients with stable hemodynamics, whereas $ScvO_2$ reflects SvO_2 poorly in critically ill patients with heart failure or frank shock [7].

The consistently higher $ScvO_2$ as compared to SvO_2 values in heart failure have been attributed to regional blood flow redistribution [7]. It has been argued that shock and heart failure produce a reduction in renal blood flow and therefore reduce the contribution of the (highly saturated) renal vein flow to IVC flow. At the same time, preferential maintenance of cerebral blood flow in shock would keep the saturation in the internal jugular vein relatively unaltered. As a result, $ScvO_2$ would be higher than IVC saturation and SvO_2 [7].

Low cardiac output also reduces blood flow to the extremities and the splanchnic region. Indeed, patients with low cardiac output after cardiac surgery had high femoral and splanchnic oxygen extractions, which substantially exceeded the systemic oxygen extraction. This would inevitably lead to dissociation between $ScvO_2$ in the superior vena cava and the SvO_2 [26]. Finally, Ho et al. demonstrated in 20 critically ill patients under mechanically ventilation with cardiogenic ($n = 7$) or septic shock ($n = 13$) a mean bias between $ScvO_2$ (CVC tip placed in the lower part of the superior vena cava) and SvO_2 of 6.9% (95% limits of agreement -5.0 to 18.8%) [27]. Although the authors did not analyze the gradient between $ScvO_2$ and SvO_2 according to the type of shock, it seems that especially in low output states, the ranges of $ScvO_2$ and $\Delta(ScvO_2\text{-}SvO_2)$ were large [27].

Hypoxia

Few clinical studies have evaluated the impact of hypoxemia on $\Delta(ScvO_2\text{-}SvO_2)$ [25]. In patients with septic shock (46% with pneumonia) receiving mechanical ventilation with fraction of inspired oxygen (FiO_2) of 64% on average, agreement between SvO_2 [mean (SD); 70.2% (± 11.4)] and $ScvO_2$ [78.6% (± 10.2)] was -8.45% (95% limits of agreement -20.23 to 3.33%) [25]. The authors did not separate patients fulfilling criteria of acute respiratory distress syndrome (ARDS) from other patients.

In a study in patients with moderate to severe ARDS (mean PaO_2/FiO_2 approximately 120) a low mean $ScvO_2$ was reported (52–58%, depending on ventilatory mode) [28]. These values are similar to those reported in cardiogenic shock [27]. Because patients with ARDS usually have normal or high cardiac output, regional blood flow redistribution according to changing oxygen demand is less likely and therefore $\Delta(ScvO_2\text{-}SvO_2)$ can be expected to be smaller/less variable than in low cardiac output states.

Experimental Data

Most of the available literature from critically ill patients with the above discussed diseases does not provide explanations for the observed differences between $ScvO_2$ and SvO_2 and respective changes of the two in individual patients. We previously conducted a series of experiments in clinical relevant animal models to address these questions.

Here, we present original, unpublished data from these experiments in which systemic and regional blood flows and regional, central and mixed venous oxygen saturations were measured [12, 29]. These data enable calculation of the contribution of carotid blood flow, femoral vein oxygen saturation and oxygen efflux from kidney and liver on $\Delta(ScvO_2\text{-}SvO_2)$. The studies were performed in accordance with the National Institutes of Health guidelines for the care and use of experimental animals and with the approval of the Animal Care Committee of the Canton of Bern, Switzerland.

Severe Sepsis

Sepsis was induced in anesthetized pigs either with endotoxin or by fecal peritonitis and the animals were resuscitated using two different fluid administration protocols [24]. Cardiac output was measured with thermodilution, regional blood flows by Doppler ultrasound and oxygen saturation using co-oximetry. The animals were monitored for 24 h or until death occurred. Blood samples for co-oximetry

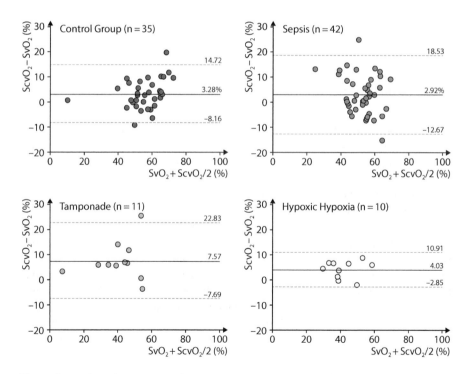

Fig. 1 Comparisons between central venous oxygen saturation (ScvO$_2$) and mixed venous oxygen saturation (SvO$_2$) measurements using the Bland-Altman method in the different experimental models. The *solid line* indicates the mean difference (bias) and the *broken lines* the bias ±2 standard deviations (SD)

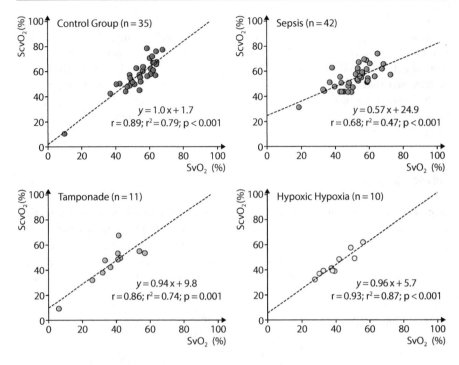

Fig. 2 Paired samples of central venous oxygen saturation ($ScvO_2$) and mixed venous oxygen saturation (SvO_2) and their correlation the different experimental models

were taken every 6 h. Hepatic venous oxygen efflux was determined as hepatic arterial + portal venous blood flow times hepatic venous oxygen content, and renal venous oxygen efflux as twice renal artery blood flow times renal venous oxygen content [12, 29].

Forty-two paired blood samples were obtained from septic animals in our study. We observed a mean bias of 2.92 (95% limits of agreement −12.67 to 18.53%; Fig. 1) and a positive correlation ($r = 0.68$, $p < 0.001$; Fig. 2) between $ScvO_2$ and SvO_2. A multiple linear regression analysis with backward elimination procedure was undertaken to define contributions of the variables to $\Delta(ScvO_2\text{-}SvO_2)$. From the initial model containing four predictors (hepatic and renal venous oxygen efflux, femoral oxygen saturation and carotid artery blood flow), the backward elimination procedure yielded a 'best' model containing hepatic venous oxygen efflux ($r = -0.46$, $p < 0.01$) and carotid artery blood flow ($r = 0.58$, $p < 0.01$) (Table 1). This final model accounted for 66% ($R^2 = 0.66$) of variation in $\Delta(ScvO_2\text{-}SvO_2)$ (Table 1).

Table 1 Predictors of the difference between central venous and mixed venous oxygen saturation [$\Delta(ScvO_2\text{-}SvO_2)$] in septic animals (n = 42)

Model	Predictors[#]	β value*	P value	R^2
1	Carotid artery blood flow index	0.60	< 0.01	0.66
	Hepatic venous oxygen efflux	−0.44	< 0.01	
	Femoral vein oxygen saturation	−0.22	0.83	
	Renal venous oxygen efflux	−0.07	0.50	
2	Carotid artery blood flow index	0.59	< 0.01	0.66
	Hepatic venous oxygen efflux	−0.44	< 0.01	
	Renal venous oxygen efflux	−0.08	0.42	
3	Carotid artery blood flow index	0.58	< 0.01	0.66
	Hepatic venous oxygen efflux	−0.46	< 0.01	

[#]Dependent variable: $\Delta[ScvO_2\text{-}SvO_2]$; *standardized beta values

Cardiogenic Shock

Cardiac tamponade was induced by filling the pericardial sac with hydroxyethyl starch through a catheter, aiming for a cardiac output of 60 ml/min/kg (at 6 h), 50 ml/min/kg (at 12 h), 40 ml/min/kg (at 18 h), and 30 ml/min/kg (at 24 h) [12]. Eleven paired blood samples were obtained from animals submitted to cardiac tamponade. We observed a mean bias of 7.57 (95% limits of agreement −7.69 to 22.83%; Fig. 1) and positive correlation (r = 0.86, p = 0.001; Fig. 2) between $ScvO_2$ and SvO_2. In contrast to the findings in the sepsis model, $\Delta(ScvO_2\text{-}SvO_2)$ was not explained by hepatic and renal venous oxygen efflux, femoral oxygen saturation or carotid artery blood flow (data not shown), also explained by the small number of observations.

Severe Hypoxia

Hypoxic hypoxia was established by decreasing the FiO_2 from 21 to 16% during a 24-h period [12]. Ten paired blood samples were obtained from animals submitted to hypoxic hypoxia. We observed a mean bias of 4.03 (95% limits of agreement −2.85 to 10.91%; Fig. 1) and positive correlation (r = 0.93, p < 0.001; Fig. 2) between $ScvO_2$ and SvO_2. Similarly to the findings in cardiogenic shock, $\Delta(ScvO_2\text{-}SvO_2)$ in this small sample was not explained by any of the other parameters reflecting regional oxygen transport (data now shown).

In agreement with our findings, Reinhart et al. reported a mean bias of 5.9% with a maximal difference of 20%, and a correlation coefficient of 0.78 between SvO_2 and $ScvO_2$ in hypoxemic anesthetized dogs [30].

Determinants of $\Delta(ScvO_2\text{-}SvO_2)$

As outlined above, a multiple linear regression analysis with backward elimination procedure was undertaken to define contributions of the variables to $\Delta(ScvO_2\text{-}SvO_2)$. In the pooled sample (n = 98), the backward elimination procedure yielded a 'best' model containing hepatic venous oxygen efflux (r = −0.46, p < 0.01) and carotid artery blood flow (r = 0.52, p < 0.01). This final model accounted for 45% of the variation in $\Delta(ScvO_2\text{-}SvO_2)$ (Table 2 and Fig. 3).

There were no relevant differences between the 'best' models for septic (Table 1) and control (Table 3) animals, the two groups with a sufficiently large number of observations, suggesting that also in anesthetized, otherwise healthy subjects, there are significant, potentially varying contributors to $\Delta(ScvO_2\text{-}SvO_2)$.

Table 2 Predictors of the difference between central venous and mixed venous oxygen saturation [$\Delta(ScvO_2\text{-}SvO_2)$] in the pooled sample (n = 98)

Model	Predictors[#]	β value*	p value	R^2
1	Carotid artery blood flow index	0.55	< 0.01	0.45
	Hepatic venous oxygen efflux	−0.42	< 0.01	
	Femoral vein oxygen saturation	−0.04	0.64	
	Renal venous oxygen efflux	−0.08	0.40	
2	Carotid artery blood flow index	0.53	< 0.01	0.45
	Hepatic venous oxygen efflux	−0.42	< 0.01	
	Renal venous oxygen efflux	−0.09	0.30	
3	Carotid artery blood flow index	0.52	< 0.01	0.45
	Hepatic venous oxygen efflux	−0.46	< 0.01	

[#]Dependent variable: $\Delta[ScvO_2\text{-}SvO_2]$; *standardized beta values

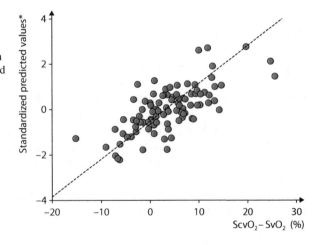

Fig. 3 Scatterplot of standardized predicted values against the difference between central venous oxygen saturation ($ScvO_2$) and mixed venous oxygen saturation (SvO_2). *standardized predicted values [(predicted value − mean of predicted values) divided by the standard deviation of the predicted values]

Table 3 Predictors of the difference between central venous and mixed venous oxygen saturation [$\Delta(ScvO_2\text{-}SvO_2)$] in control animals (n = 35)

Model	Predictors[#]	β value*	P value	R^2
1	Carotid artery blood flow index	0.62	<0.01	0.58
	Hepatic venous oxygen efflux	−0.32	0.03	
	Femoral vein oxygen saturation	0.17	0.27	
	Renal venous oxygen efflux	−0.05	0.73	
2	Carotid artery blood flow index	0.61	<0.01	0.58
	Hepatic venous oxygen efflux	−0.34	0.01	
	Renal venous oxygen efflux	0.16	0.28	
3	Carotid artery blood flow index	0.70	<0.01	0.56
	Hepatic venous oxygen efflux	−0.29	0.02	

[#]Dependent variable: $\Delta[ScvO_2\text{-}SvO_2]$; *standardized beta values

Applications in the Critically Ill

The results from this analysis indicate that carotid artery blood flow and hepatic but not renal venous oxygen efflux can predict more than half of the differences between mixed and central venous oxygen saturation, depending on the model. The experimental models included cardiogenic shock, hypodynamic sepsis with increasing lactate concentrations, and severe hypoxic hypoxemia which, when combined with the data from control animals, resulted in a wide range of central and mixed venous oxygen saturations between < 10 and > 70%.

In principle, our results support the impact of blood flow redistribution on the saturation gradient and that the hepatosplanchnic rather than the renal venous efflux of oxygen is important for $\Delta(ScvO_2\text{-}SvO_2)$. A study in animals with abdominal sepsis and shock demonstrated that renal perfusion and oxygen consumption were maintained despite a decrease in renal perfusion pressure [31]. This should result in largely unaltered renal vein oxygen saturation, and could therefore explain the limited influence on renal vein oxygen efflux on the $ScvO_2\text{-}SvO_2$ gradient in sepsis. Since significant changes in $ScvO_2$ occur without parallel changes in systemic DO_2 [32], varying oxygen demands should also be considered when assessing $ScvO_2$ and SvO_2. Indeed, splanchnic blood flow and VO_2 increase in hyperdynamic sepsis, both during hypotension and when a vasopressor is infused [33].

Femoral vein oxygen saturation was not associated with $\Delta(ScvO_2\text{-}SvO_2)$ in our study. Since the femoral blood flow was not measured, we cannot quantify the influence of femoral oxygen efflux on the saturation gradient. However, in ICU patients, differences of > 5% between femoral and central vein oxygen saturation can be found in > 50% of the cases [6].

Our model could explain roughly half of the differences between central and mixed venous oxygen saturation. We did not measure the contribution of femoral and lower abdominal organ oxygen efflux or of blood drained by sinus coronarius. Furthermore, inherent variability in the methods used to measure flow and oxygen saturation could also have contributed to unexplained differences, although we used established methods, calibration (flow probes) and correct animal species module for the assessment of oxygen saturations.

Conclusions

Agreement between central venous and mixed venous oxygen saturation has been shown to be poor in different, but frequent diseases of critically ill patients. Therefore, using $ScvO_2$ as a surrogate for SvO_2 in this population of patients may be misleading. Carotid artery blood flow and hepatic but not renal venous oxygen efflux predict some of the differences between mixed and central venous oxygen saturation. This suggests that it is difficult or impossible to predict SvO_2 from $ScvO_2$ alone.

References

1. Bloos F, Reinhart K (2005) Venous oximetry. Intensive Care Med 31:911–913
2. Wheeler AP, Bernard GR, Thompson BT et al (2006) Pulmonary-artery versus central venous catheter to guide treatment of acute lung injury. N Engl J Med 354:2213–2224
3. Pandey A, Khera R, Kumar N, Golwala H, Girotra S, Fonarow GC (2016) Use of pulmonary artery catheterization in US patients with heart failure, 2001–2012. JAMA Intern Med 176:129–132
4. Reinhart K, Kuhn HJ, Hartog C, Bredle DL (2004) Continuous central venous and pulmonary artery oxygen saturation monitoring in the critically ill. Intensive Care Med 30:1572–1578
5. Reinhart K, Bloos F (2005) The value of venous oximetry. Curr Opin Crit Care 11:259–263
6. Davison DL, Chawla LS, Selassie L et al (2010) Femoral-based central venous oxygen saturation is not a reliable substitute for subclavian/internal jugular-based central venous oxygen saturation in patients who are critically ill. Chest 138:76–83
7. Scheinman MM, Brown MA, Rapaport E (1969) Critical assessment of use of central venous oxygen saturation as a mirror of mixed venous oxygen in severely ill cardiac patients. Circulation 40:165–172
8. Dueck MH, Klimek M, Appenrodt S, Weigand C, Boerner U (2005) Trends but not individual values of central venous oxygen saturation agree with mixed venous oxygen saturation during varying hemodynamic conditions. Anesthesiology 103:249–257
9. Mozina H, Podbregar M (2010) Near-infrared spectroscopy during stagnant ischemia estimates central venous oxygen saturation and mixed venous oxygen saturation discrepancy in patients with severe left heart failure and additional sepsis/septic shock. Crit Care 14:R42
10. Varpula M, Karlsson S, Ruokonen E, Pettila V (2006) Mixed venous oxygen saturation cannot be estimated by central venous oxygen saturation in septic shock. Intensive Care Med 32:1336–1343
11. van Beest PA, van Ingen J, Boerma EC et al (2010) No agreement of mixed venous and central venous saturation in sepsis, independent of sepsis origin. Crit Care 14:R219
12. Regueira T, Djafarzadeh S, Brandt S et al (2012) Oxygen transport and mitochondrial function in porcine septic shock, cardiogenic shock, and hypoxaemia. Acta Anaesth Scand 56:846–859
13. Gorrasi J, Eleftheriadis A, Takala J et al (2013) Different contribution of splanchnic organs to hyperlactatemia in fecal peritonitis and cardiac tamponade. Biomed Res Int 2013:251084
14. Ruokonen E, Takala J, Uusaro A (1991) Effect of vasoactive treatment on the relationship between mixed venous and regional oxygen saturation. Crit Care Med 19:1365–1369

15. Ahn JH, Kim IS, Yang JH, Lee IG, Seo DH, Kim SP (2017) Transoesophageal echocardiographic evaluation of central venous catheter positioning using Peres' formula or a radiological landmark-based approach: a prospective randomized single-centre study. Br J Anaesth 118:215–222
16. Barratt-Boyes BG, Wood EH (1957) The oxygen saturation of blood in the venae cavae, right-heart chambers, and pulmonary vessels of healthy subjects. J Lab Clin Med 50:93–106
17. Chawla LS, Zia H, Gutierrez G, Katz NM, Seneff MG, Shah M (2004) Lack of equivalence between central and mixed venous oxygen saturation. Chest 126:1891–1896
18. Shepherd SJ, Pearse RM (2009) Role of central and mixed venous oxygen saturation measurement in perioperative care. Anesthesiology 111:649–656
19. Kaisti KK, Langsjo JW, Aalto S et al (2003) Effects of sevoflurane, propofol, and adjunct nitrous oxide on regional cerebral blood flow, oxygen consumption, and blood volume in humans. Anesthesiology 99:603–613
20. Sander M, Spies CD, Foer A et al (2007) Agreement of central venous saturation and mixed venous saturation in cardiac surgery patients. Intensive Care Med 33:1719–1725
21. Schmid FX, Philipp A, Foltan M, Jueckstock H, Wiesenack C, Birnbaum D (2003) Adequacy of perfusion during hypothermia: regional distribution of cardiopulmonary bypass flow, mixed venous and regional venous oxygen saturation – hypothermia and distribution of flow and oxygen. Thorac Cardiovasc Surg 51:306–311
22. Soussi MS, Jebali MA, Le MY et al (2012) Central venous saturation is not an alternative to mixed venous saturation during cardiopulmonary bypass in coronary artery surgery patients. Perfusion 27:300–306
23. Lorentzen AG, Lindskov C, Sloth E, Jakobsen CJ (2008) Central venous oxygen saturation cannot replace mixed venous saturation in patients undergoing cardiac surgery. J Cardiothorac Vasc Anesth 22:853–857
24. Lequeux PY, Bouckaert Y, Sekkat H et al (2010) Continuous mixed venous and central venous oxygen saturation in cardiac surgery with cardiopulmonary bypass. Eur J Anaesthesiol 27:295–299
25. Kopterides P, Bonovas S, Mavrou I, Kostadima E, Zakynthinos E, Armaganidis A (2009) Venous oxygen saturation and lactate gradient from superior vena cava to pulmonary artery in patients with septic shock. Shock 31:561–567
26. Ruokonen E, Takala J, Kari A (1993) Regional blood flow and oxygen transport in patients with the low cardiac output syndrome after cardiac surgery. Crit Care Med 21:1304–1311
27. Ho KM, Harding R, Chamberlain J, Bulsara M (2010) A comparison of central and mixed venous oxygen saturation in circulatory failure. J Cardiothorac Vasc Anesth 24:434–439
28. Li JQ, Li N, Han GJ et al (2016) Clinical research about airway pressure release ventilation for moderate to severe acute respiratory distress syndrome. Eur Rev Med Pharmacol Sci 20:2634–2641
29. Brandt S, Regueira T, Bracht H et al (2009) Effect of fluid resuscitation on mortality and organ function in experimental sepsis models. Crit Care 13:R186
30. Reinhart K, Rudolph T, Bredle DL, Hannemann L, Cain SM (1989) Comparison of central-venous to mixed-venous oxygen saturation during changes in oxygen supply/demand. Chest 95:1216–1221
31. Chvojka J, Sykora R, Krouzecky A et al (2008) Renal haemodynamic, microcirculatory, metabolic and histopathological responses to peritonitis-induced septic shock in pigs. Crit Care 12:R164
32. Pearse R, Dawson D, Fawcett J, Rhodes A, Grounds RM, Bennett ED (2005) Changes in central venous saturation after major surgery, and association with outcome. Crit Care 9:R694–R699
33. Ruokonen E, Takala J, Kari A, Saxen H, Mertsola J, Hansen EJ (1993) Regional blood flow and oxygen transport in septic shock. Crit Care Med 21:1296–1303

Bioelectrical Impedance Analysis in Critical Care

P. Formenti, L. Bolgiaghi, and D. Chiumello

Introduction

Bioelectrical impedance analysis (BIA) is the collective term that describes the non-invasive methods to measure the electrical body responses to the introduction of a low-level, alternating current. BIA was conceptually developed more than 100 years ago, but was only applied in humans using a validated method in the early 1980s [1]. BIA has been used for estimation of body cell mass and total body water (TBW) over the last three decades [2, 3]. More recently, advances in BIA technology have enabled detailed and sophisticated data analyses and targeted applications in clinical practice, including in the critical care environment. Among the different methodologies available, single-frequency BIA (SF-BIA) [4] and multi-frequency bioelectrical impedance spectroscopy (MF-BIS) [5] offer similar readings for bioelectrical parameters with a wide variation in the quantification of volume and body mass depending on the equation used for calculation [6, 7]. The bioelectric impedance vector analysis (BIVA) is today a widely used approach for body composition measurements and assessment of clinical condition and has recently been developed to assess both nutritional status and tissue hydration [8–10]. In this chap-

P. Formenti
Unità Operativa Complessa di Anestesia e Rianimazione, Ospedale San Paolo-Azienda Socio Sanitaria Territoriale Santi Paolo e Carlo
Milan, Italy

L. Bolgiaghi
Dipartimento di Scienze della Salute, Università degli Studi di Milano
Milan, Italy

D. Chiumello (✉)
Unità Operativa Complessa di Anestesia e Rianimazione, Ospedale San Paolo-Azienda Socio Sanitaria Territoriale Santi Paolo e Carlo
Milan, Italy
Dipartimento di Scienze della Salute, Università degli Studi di Milano
Milan, Italy
e-mail: davide.chiumello@unimi.it

© Springer International Publishing AG 2018   275
J.-L. Vincent (ed.), *Annual Update in Intensive Care and Emergency Medicine 2018*,
Annual Update in Intensive Care and Emergency Medicine,
https://doi.org/10.1007/978-3-319-73670-9_22

ter, we will discuss briefly the methodologies and the clinical critical settings in which BIA can be applied.

How Bioelectrical Impedance Works

BIA measures the opposition of body tissues to the flow of a small alternating current (i.e., the impedance). The classical BIA method consists of four electrodes attached to the hands, wrist, feet and ankles in which a painless electrical current at a fixed or multiple frequency is introduced in the organism [11]. Thus, BIA only measures the end to-end voltage across the entire path between the voltage-sensing electrodes. This voltage is the energy expended per unit of charge for the total current path and does not provide any direct information with respect to the amount of current traveling through intracellular versus extracellular volumes, in blood versus muscle, or in fat versus fat-free media. The impedance is a function of two components (or vectors): the 'resistance' (R) of the tissues themselves and the additional opposition or 'reactance' (Xc).

BIA Measurement Parameters

- Impedance (Z): the total resistance of a biological conductor to alternating current is called impedance. There are two components that form impedance:
  1. The resistance (R), which is a pure resistance of the electrolyte-containing total body water
  2. The reactance (Xc), which is present due to the condenser-like properties of the body cells.
- Resistance (R): the pure resistance of a conductor to alternating current. Whereas fat mass has high resistance, lean body mass is a good conductor of electrical current, as proportionally it contains higher amounts of water and electrolytes. In healthy, normal weight individuals, the resistance is an excellent measure to calculate body water. The R of a homogeneous material of uniform cross-sectional area is proportional to its length (L) and inversely related to its cross sectional area (A) ([12]; Fig. 1). The sum of the arm, trunk and leg volumes can be modeled as a cylinder with uniform conductivity [2, 13]. However, this assumption is reductive as many independent factors – environmental (such as temperature, infusion, and humidity) and anthropometric (such as sex, height, weight, age and impedance value) – act together or separately to modify the dynamic state of the human body. As the human body is a 'dynamic system' with hourly changes in body water, a BIA current can be considered as a snapshot of the condition at that point in time, requiring several repeat measurements to provide a more accurate assessment of body composition.
- Reactance (Xc): represents the resistance that a condenser exerts to an alternating current. Due to their protein-lipid layers, all cell membranes of the body act like mini-condensers and reactance is therefore an assessment of the body cell mass.

Total body water (TBW)		It represents approximately 60% of body weight. To be measured the muscle mass, described by BCM, is necessary
Lean body mass (LBM)		It refers to the tissue mass of the body that contains no fat (inner organs, muscles, the skeletal system and the central nervous system). LBM contains BCM and ECM. Since it contains 73% of water, LBM = TBW/0.73
Body cell mass (BCM)		It represents the sum of cells that are actively involved in the metabolic processes (the smooth muscles, the cells of the skeletal muscle system, the inner organs, the cardiac muscles, the blood, the gastrointestinal tract, the nervous systems). It describes better the nutritional status.
Extracellular mass (ECM)		It includes the LBM that exists outside the cells of the BCM (such as skin, elastin, collagen, tendons, bone and fasciae). Trans-cellular water is the description of fluids that are present in the body cavities (i.e. the contents of the gastro-intestinal lumen and the spinal fluid) while non-physiological transcellular fluids appear as ascites, or as pericardial or pleural effusions.
Body fat (BF)		It is calculated as the difference between body weight and LBM. Body fat performs as an insulator to alternating current, having hardly any capacitive resistance.

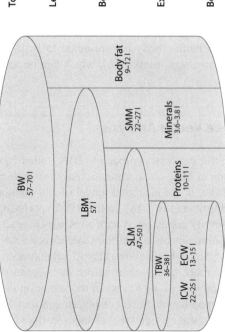

Fig. 1 Body composition in a healthy subject. The figure shows the body composition (five compartments) in a healthy subject as analyzed by bioimpedance. In this model, the human body is composed of fat mass; lean body mass, which consists of extracellular (ECW, divided into interstitial and intravascular fluid) and intracellular (ICW) water. The *left panel* describes the main parameters related to the body composition derived from bioelectrical impedance analysis (BIA). *SLM:* soft lean mass = TBW + protein of muscles (skeletal and smooth muscle); *SMM:* skeletal muscle mass; *LBM:* SLM + minerals; *BW:* body weight = LBM + body fat; units are expressed in liters

- Phase angle: used as a general measure of cellular membrane integrity. The phase angle represents the relationship between resistance and reactance and provides information about the state of a cell and the overall condition of a patient's body. Each metabolically active cell has an electrical membrane potential of about 50–100 mV at the cell membrane and this potential permits the cell to act like a spherical condenser in an alternating electrical field. Alternating current has a sinus wave, therefore the shift is measured in ° (degrees). Pure electrolyte water has a phase angle of 0° (i.e., no cell membrane), while a cell membrane mass would have a phase angle of 90°. In contrast, fat cells have hardly any metabolic activity and cannot be detected by phase sensitive measurements because of their minimal membrane potential. A high phase angle is observed in healthy individuals, representing a large amount of cell membrane and body cell mass with high reactance; whereas a low phase angle is generally observed in critically ill patients [14, 15].
- Multi-frequency measurements: frequency plays an important role in the resistance of a biological conductor. As the frequency increases, the phase angle increases with increasing reactance. Use of multi-frequency analysis provides improved differentiation with regard to cell loss or water displacement, by assessing variations in mass of the extracellular mass and the body cellular mass.

Body Composition Parameters

The elements of a human body include protein, water, fat, minerals and other important constituents in a certain ratio to each other. While in healthy subjects the body composition is quite homogeneous, in sick patients the body composition is significantly modified. The human body is considered to be divided into five inhomogeneous segments (arms, legs, trunk) [16], which can be analyzed by the bioimpedance (Fig. 2).

Bioelectrical Impedance Vector Analysis

By contrast to classic BIA, the vectorial approach to BIA, called BIVA, does not provide any absolute estimate of body compartments, makes no assumptions about body geometry, hydration state, or the electrical model of cell membranes, and is unaffected by regression adjustments [17, 18]. In the BIVA approach, soft tissues, hydration status and cell integrity are assessed with a resistance–reactance (R–Xc) graph, using the two direct components of the impedance vector standardized by height (Fig. 3). Impedance vector analysis allows classification (under-, normal and overhydration) and ranking (more or less than before intervention) of hydration for an individual by examining the two directions of the vector on the R–Xc plane relative to a healthy reference population. Vector displacements parallel to the major axis of the tolerance ellipse indicate progressive changes in tissue hydration; low hydration is associated with long vectors outside of the upper region of the 50%

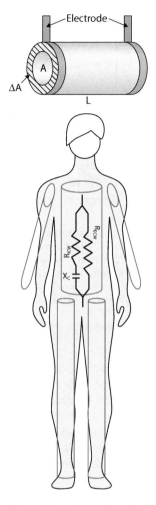

Fig. 2 Bioelectrical model of bioimpedance. Analysis of body composition by bioelectrical impedance analysis (BIA) assumes that resistance to a determined electrical current is inversely proportional to the distribution of total body water (TBW) and electrolytes. And this resistance (R) of the length of a conductor of homogeneous material and uniform cross-sectional area is proportional to its length (L) and inversely proportional to its cross-sectional area (A). Although the body is not a uniform cylinder and its conductivity is not constant, an empirical relation can be established between the coefficient of impedance (L2/R) and the volume of water that contains electrolytes, which conduct the electrical current through the body. In practice, it is easier to measure the height rather than the length of the conductor, which usually is from the wrist to the ankle. Thus, the empirical relation is between the lean mass (typically 73% of water) and height^2/R. Because of the lack of inherent homogeneity of the body, the term height^2/R describes a cylindrical equivalent that must be adapted to the real geometry using an appropriate coefficient

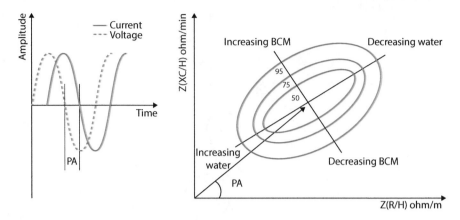

Fig. 3 Diagram of the phase angle (PA) and bioelectrical impedance vector analysis (BIVA). The phase angle correlation between resistance (R), reactance (Xc), impedance (Z), and the frequency of the electrical current: $Z = (x2 + R2)1/2$; normal phase angle is $4–15°$; $= -\tan\text{-}1$ (X/R). The right panel shows an ideal BIVA graph with R on the x-axis and X on the y-axis. The center point refers to the healthy population. The increasing water profile includes sepsis, fluid overload, capillary leak syndrome; decrease in body cell mass (BCM) includes muscle wasting, weight reduction, malnutrition, cell damage; increase in BCM includes increase in muscle mass, in weight, a good supply of nutrients, a reduction in water retention, a sufficient recovery

tolerance ellipse, and fluid overload with apparent edema is characterized with short vectors outside the lower pole of the 50% ellipse. Peripheral vectors to the left or right side of the major axis of the tolerance ellipse indicate more or less cell mass, respectively. The length of the impedance vector is inversely related to TBW, and the combination of the vector length and its direction, the phase angle, is an indicator of tissue hydration status. On this basis, a statement can be made with regards to water balance and nutritional status [19].

Bioimpedance in the Critical Care Setting

Patients with severe critical illness initially require large amounts of fluid as part of resuscitation, which may later lead to complications, such as increased time on the ventilator and kidney damage. Moreover, associated factors, such as systemic inflammation, corticosteroids and neuromuscular blocking agents, electrolyte disturbances and immobility, result in loss of muscle mass strength, all implicated in prognosis [20]. Thus, fluid and nutritional assessment represent a crucial aspect of evaluation and treatment of critically ill patients. Although in healthy subjects (who have no fluid imbalance, no body shape abnormalities and who are within a certain body mass index [BMI] range) BIA offers reliable information on body composition, in patients with disturbed hydration or altered distribution of extracellular and intracellular water and their ratio (normally < 1), it may provide poorly reliable measures of fluid and nutritional status. In several clinical conditions, free fat mass or phase angle (lower than normal) has been associated with clinical outcome as it reflects the intracellular status (i.e., intracellular to extracellular water distribution). Table 1 summarizes the main clinical studies that have evaluated BIA for nutritional, volemic, perioperative and prognostic assessments in the critical care setting.

Nutritional Assessment

The metabolic response to critical illness is characterized by increased energy expenditure, proteolysis, gluconeogenesis and miolysis with an increment that exceeds 100% of predicted energy expenditure [21]. This prediction can be influenced by volume overload, since body weight is often used in equations to predict energy needs. Increased proteolysis leads to accelerated protein loss, which occurs despite provision of exogenous protein and non-protein intake. Thus, muscle wasting often occurs due to increased metabolic demands on the body, determining major losses of lean tissue due to severity of illness and organ dysfunction, prolonged immobility and malnutrition [22]. The variability of BIA measurements has often been cited as a major limitation for their clinical use in evaluating nutritional status [13]. Moreover, the oldest studies were performed using classical BIA to determine body composition, whereas more recent studies have focused on the use of BIVA and phase angle analysis.

In one of the first studies, Robert et al. [23] investigated the utility of BIA in determining nutritional status in 33 mechanically ventilated medical and surgical intensive care unit (ICU) patients requiring nutrition as part of their care. BIA, with subsequent calculation of body-composition indexes, was performed every day for the duration of the ICU stay as well as measurements of height, actual body weight, fluid intake and output, daily protein and energy intake, albumin, total protein and nitrogen balance. The authors showed how the body composition changes correlated with energy and protein intakes. Other investigations explored the role of phase angle in the assessment of nutritional status. In a recent multicenter prospective study, Kuchnia et al. [24] tested whether phase angle derived from MF-BIA could be used to assess low muscularity and predict clinical outcomes compared with computed tomography (CT) scans analyzed for skeletal muscle cross-sectional area that defined low muscularity in 71 critically ill patients. The phase angle's area under the receiver operating characteristic (ROC) curve to predict CT-defined low muscularity was 0.67 and patients with lower phase angles had longer lengths of ICU stay. Similar results have been shown comparing the phase angle values delivered by MF-BIA with traditional nutrition assessment tools (BMI, serum albumin levels, total lymphocyte counts) in 89 adult patients admitted to a medical ICU [25]. Patients with phase angles less than the median value (3.5°) had significantly lower nutritional status, increased duration of mechanical ventilation and increased length of ICU stay. There is only one study that investigated the use of BIA to estimate the nutritional status of 51 patients with chronic obstructive pulmonary disease (COPD) and acute respiratory failure compared with measurements of anthropometric par-

Table 1 Principal studies regarding bioelectrical impedance analysis (BIA) in the critical care setting

Fields	First author, year of publication [ref]	Type of study, number of patients	Parameters	Main remarks
Nutrition assessment	Robert et al. 1993 [23]	Prospective n = 33 MV	BIA; BCM	Changes in BCM correlated with protein and energy intakes ($r^2 = 0.82$). Represented a valid method to evaluate the nutritional status in critically ill
	Faisy et al. 2000 [26]	Retrospective n = 51 COPD	Two frequency BIA; ACM, ECW, ECW/ICW	BIA-derived ACM reduction was a good indicator of malnutrition in patients with COPD exacerbation
	Lee et al. 2015 [27]	Prospective n = 66	BIVA; PA, ECW, ECW/TBW	Phase angle was higher in well-nourished patients, whereas the edema index (ECW/TBW) was higher in malnourished patients. Furthermore BIA-derived indexes represented prognostic factors in critically ill patients
	Kim et al. 2015 [25]	Prospective n = 89	SMF BIA; PA vs. BMI, albumin, NSI	PA correlated with BMI, albumin and NSI. PA <3.6° = increment in mortality, LOS, MV days
	Kuchnia et al. 2016 [24]	Multicenter prospective n = 71	MF BIA vs. CT MCSA; PA, IR	PA and IR were potential markers able to identify patients with low muscularity who may benefit from early and rigorous intervention
Perioperative assessment	Gonzalez et al. 1995 [47]	Prospective n = 18 CPB	BIA; R vs. weight, fluid balance	The measurement of whole body resistance detected acute changes in total body water and fluid distribution in the body. Evaluation of day-to-day change in whole body resistance was better than absolute fluid changes over time
	Tatara et al. 1998 [35]	Prospective n = 30 abdominal surgery	MF BIA; SMF vs. whole Body BIA; ECW	SMF BIA ΔECW was similar to net fluid balance whereas whole body MF BIA resulted in considerable underestimation of ΔECW. SMF BIA was better in prediction of ECW changes
	Bracco et al. 1998 [34]	Observational n = 26 cardiac surgery	MF BIA in whole body vs. segmental BIA in the arm and in the trunk	Fluid accumulation resulted in a reduction in whole-body and segmental bioelectrical impedance
	Ernstbrunner et al. 2014 [38]	Prospective n = 71	Whole-body BIA spectroscopy, total body fluid volume, ECW, ICW, fluid overload	Increase in ECW was paralleled by an increase in total body fluid volume; ICW increased without statistical significance. Net perioperative fluid balance associated with change in ECW
	Chong 2016 [39]	Retrospective review n = 36 hepato-pancreato-biliary surgery	BIA; TBW, ECW, ECW/TBW, ICW	TBW, ECW, ECW/TBW, ICW did not change significantly in fluid-balanced patients. ECW, ECW/TBW, and ICW showed significant postoperative increases, causing development of ascites

Table 1 (Continued)

Fields	First author, year of publication [ref]	Type of study, number of patients	Parameters	Main remarks
Fluids & volemia	Foley, 1999 [31]	Prospective controlled n = 50 (healthy vs. sick)	S-BIA vs. whole body BIA; TBW	In the patients, S-BIA contributed more to total body impedance as indication of TBW, but was not accurate enough
	Piccoli, 2000 [10]	Cross-sectional n = 121	BIVA; R and Xc vs. CVP	CVP significantly and inversely correlated with individual R and Xc, with both vector components together. Patients with higher CVP agreed with BIVA variables. Combined BIVA and CVP useful in therapy planning
	House, 2011 [48]	Retrospective n = 34 MV	BIVA vs. CVP vs. BNP vs. O_2I	CVP and BIVA were weakly correlated; only BNP was significantly associated with O_2I; no correlation BIVA and volume status
	Basso, 2013 [49]	Retrospective n = 64	BIVA; measurements for 5 days	Overhydration was detected by BIVA on admission, persisted during the ICU stay. Patients who required CRRT were more likely to be overhydrated
	Chen, 2015 [45]	Prospective n = 89 CRRT	BIVA vs. NT-pro-BNP	Significant difference in fluid status detected by BIVA before and after CRRT
	Rochwerg, 2016 [32]	Prospective n = 64	BIVA; VL vs. pro BNP vs. CVP and probability of intubation	Increment in VL correlated with decreased probability of intubation; baseline VL correlated with pro-BNP and CVP
	Dewitte, 2016 [29]	Observational n = 25 MV	BIA spectroscopy; TBW and fluid balance	BIA without real weight was unreliable; daily change in TBW correlated with fluid balance

Table 1 (Continued)

Fields	First author, year of publication [ref]	Type of study, number of patients	Parameters	Main remarks
Prognostic value	Visser, 2012 [41]	Prospective n = 325 cardiac surgery	BIA spectroscopy; PA vs. BMI, weight loss, FFM, C-reactive protein and albumin	Low phase angle (<5.38°) associated with low BMI and low FFM but not with weight loss or immune function. Low PA was associated with prolonged LOS
	Basso, 2013 [49]	Retrospective n = 64	BIVA; measurements for 5 days	Strong and significant correlation between mean/maximum hydration reached and mortality, independently and after correcting for severity
	Rhee, 2015 [44]	Retrospective review n = 208 AKI in CRRT	MF-BIA;	TBW/H^2 and low serum albumin were independently associated with higher in-hospital mortality
	Chen, 2015 [45]	Prospective n = 89 CRRT	BIVA vs. NT-pro-BNP	The stratification of patient fluid status, made by measurements of BIVA and NT-pro-BNP, was associated with outcome in patients receiving CRRT
	Da Silva, 2015 [42]	Cohort n = 95	BIVA; PA vs. SOFA vs. APACHE II	Weak correlation between PA and APACHE II score
	Thibault, 2016 [43]	Multicenter prospective n = 931	BIVA; PA and FFM vs. outcome	Low FFM at ICU admission (PA 4.1° ± 2°) was associated with 28-day mortality

MV: mechanical ventilation; *MF-BIA*: multifrequency bioimpedance analysis; *SMF*: segmental multifrequency; *BMI*: body mass index; *NSI*: nutritional score index; *BCM*: body cell mass; *LOS*: length of stay; *ACM*: active cell mass; *ECW*: extracellular water; *TBW*: total body water; *ICW*: intracellular water; *FFM*: fat free mass; *PA*: phase angle; *IR*: impedance ratio; *CT MSCA*: computed tomography cross-sectional area; *RMA*: resting metabolic activity; *R*: resistance; *Xc*: reactance; *TEB*: thoracic electrical bioimpedance; *NT-pro-BNP*: serum N-terminal pro-B-type natriuretic peptides; *VL*: vector length; *CVP*: central venous pressure; *TD*: pulmonary artery thermodilution; *BNP*: brain natriuretic peptide; *O₂I*: oxygenation index; *CRRT*: continuous renal replacement therapy; *CPB*: cardiopulmonary bypass; *COPD*: chronic obstructive pulmonary disease

ameters and plasma levels of visceral proteins [26]. The BIA results showed lower active cell mass and a higher extracellular-intracellular body ratio suggesting more severe alteration in the nutritional status among patients on mechanical ventilation. More recently, Lee et al. [27] put together clinical, biochemical and BIA data from 66 critically ill patients. The authors compared the BIA results and conventional indicators of nutrition. Phase angle was greater than $4.1°$ in the well-nourished patients, whereas the edema index (expressed as the ratio between extracellular and total body water) was greater than 0.4 in the severely malnourished. Moreover, the phase angle was positively associated with albumin while edema index was not, and negatively associated with hemoglobin and duration of mechanical ventilation. There is currently insufficient validation of the BIA equations in obese individuals because of a relatively increased amount of TBW in these patients and an underestimation of the relative increase in extracellular water [28]. In conclusion, BIA variables, in particular the phase angle, integrated with standard nutritional parameters, seem to be a potentially useful tool for nutritional assessment in ICU patients.

Fluids and Volemia

A reliable assessment of volume status in ICU patients is valuable in guiding fluid management. Conventional BIA can be used to estimate TBW, extracellular and intracellular water by the regression equation and at the same time lean body mass through relationship with soft tissue; however, in patients with abnormal hydration, this estimation is prone to bias. By contrast, using the patterns of the RXc graph, BIVA seems to be able to grade both fluid status and mass. There are a couple of studies that have investigated the feasibility of using BIA in assessment of fluid status. One compared BIA results with fluid balance and TBW in 25 mechanically ventilated patients. Daily changes in TBW were correlated with fluid balance and this correlation was improved after exclusion of patients with a higher sequential organ failure assessment (SOFA) score [29]. The other, more recent study, performed BIVA measurements twice-daily and fluid balance calculations at ICU admission and for 5 days, showing how BIVA-defined hydration between first and last measurements correlated with the corresponding change in fluid balance [30]. Foley et al. [31] used SF-BIA to estimate TBW in patients with multiple organ failure and fluid overload. The authors observed that a change in TBW, calculated from changes in body weight, was overestimated by between 0 and 46%, suggesting that SF-BIA was inaccurate at predicting TBW. Other studies focused the attention on assessing the relationship between central venous pressure (CVP) and BIVA. Piccoli et al. [10] first investigated this relationship in 120 ICU patients and showed that CVP was significantly and inversely correlated with resistance and reactance. Moreover, dividing patients into subgroups according to a low or high CVP (<4 and $>12\,cmH_2O$, respectively), BIVA showed good agreement with higher CVP. Another study investigated the combination of CVP, BIVA and brain natriuretic peptide (BNP) to predict change in oxygenation index and showed a weak correlation between CVP and BIVA. There is only one study in septic patients in which the authors determined the possibility of using vector length in the assessment of postresuscitation volume status. The vector length was chosen as it reflects an individual's overall volume status. The baseline vector length correlated with other measures of volume expansion including CVP and for each 50-unit increase in vector length, there was a 22% increase in the probability of not requiring mechanical ventilation [32]. In conclusion, since fluid therapy is not necessarily dependent on the hydration status – which is based on free fat mass (reduced) and fluid shifts (frequently present) – BIVA alone cannot be considered a sufficient guide to fluid management. Combined use of BIVA with clinical evaluation, serum biomarkers and ultrasound may represent the best multidimensional approach to facilitate the optimal administration of fluids in critical care.

Perioperative Assessment

General anesthesia and surgery are responsible for a systemic stress response characterized by secretion of antidiuretic hormone and cortisol, activation of the renin-angiotensin-aldosterone-system and stimulation of the adrenal axis to maintain hemodynamic stability and to increase fluid retention [33]. Additionally, a local inflammatory reaction controlling the secretion of pro-inflammatory cytokines augments the fluid shifts and increases vascular permeability. BIA has been evaluated in a few studies with the aim to assess and improve pre- and postsurgical clinical condition. Bracco et al. [34] showed good correlation between fluid accumulation measured by MF-BIA and fluid balance after cardiac surgery. Tatara and Tsuzaki [35] compared segmental MF-BIA to whole body BIA with the aim of predicting intraoperative changes in extracellular water before and after abdominal surgery. This parameter from segmental MF-BIA analysis was similar to the net fluid balance, whereas whole body BIA resulted in considerable underestimations. Ackland et al. [36] compared BIA and real body weight in the preoperative period of abdominal surgery, in particular during bowel preparation, when fluid depletion is difficult to assess. TBW was derived from an analyzer algorithm, using the absolute value of foot BIA, weight and sex. The results showed a lack of correlation between BIA and weight. Barbosa-Silva et al. prospectively evaluated 279 patients during the first 72 h after admission for elective gastrointestinal surgery. Body cell mass, extracellular mass/body cell mass and phase angle were compared with a standard subjective global assessment (SGA) score [37]. The results showed only fair overall agreement between SGA and BIA estimates. To determine pre- and postoperative fluid status, Ernstbrunner et al. [38] tested TBW, extracellular and intracellular water and fluid overload as surplus or deficit of 'normal' extracellular volume using whole-body BIA spectroscopy before and after standardized general anesthesia for gynecological procedures. The increase in extracellular water observed was paralleled by the increase in TBW, whereas intracellular water increased only slightly without reaching statistical significance. Finally, Chong et al. [39] explored fluid dynamics with segmental BIA (shift between extracellular to intracellular water) in 36 perioperative patients undergoing operation for hepato-pancreatic-biliary diseases. Extracellular water, the ratio between extracellular water and TBW, and intracellular water showed significant postoperative increases.

In conclusion, the available data suggest that BIA measurement can detect acute changes in TBW and in fluid redistribution through the body. However, determining the relative day-to-day change in whole body resistance seems more appropriate than calculating absolute fluid changes over time. Moreover, the segmental MF-BIA provides a better approach to predicting extracellular water changes in critically ill patients with non-uniform fluid distribution. Further work is likely warranted to determine whether BIA changes may serve as useful indicator of perioperative fluid depletion.

Prognostic Value

The prediction of short-term mortality and ICU outcomes still remains an arduous objective for the intensivist. The prevalence of undernutrition in chronic disease and critically ill patients has increased during the last decade with a negative impact on clinical outcome [40]. This concept represents the rationale for the use of BIA in evaluation of outcome in critically ill patients. Faisy et al. [26] evaluated the use of BIA to estimate the outcome of patients with COPD and reported that a lower active cell mass was associated with a higher death rate (38 vs 0%). Another study [41] analyzed the associations between preoperative phase angle and well-established indicators of undernutrition (i.e., BMI, fatty free mass index and muscle strength) and adverse clinical outcomes. Phase angle was measured in 325 patients before surgery. A phase angle $< 5.38°$ was associated with lower BMI and prolonged ICU length of stay. In a more recent study that investigated the phase angle, there was an association between phase angle $< 5.1°$ and the APACHE II score [42]. To determine the association between fatty free mass and 28-day mortality, Thibault et al. [43] measured fatty free mass assessed by measurement of the phase angle at admission to the ICU. The phase angle was lower in patients who died than in survivors ($4.1 \pm 2.0°$ vs. $4.6 \pm 1.8°$) with an area under the curve (AUC) for 28-day mortality of 0.63 [0.58–0.67]. Rhee et al. [44] studied the application of MF-BIA in a subgroup of 208 female patients with acute kidney injury (AKI), with the aim of defining a correlation between BIA parameters of fluid status and mortality. The results showed that the hospital mortality rate increased with increasing TBW adjusted to the height squared. Each liter excess in the intracellular body water compartment was independently associated with a 56% increase in mortality. Another interesting prospective study [45] investigated whether BIVA could determine fluid status, combined with serum BNP and reported that this was associated with outcome in patients treated with continuous renal replacement therapy (CRRT). Patients were divided into four groups, based on BIVA vector length hydration status and BNP measurements (no overhydration and BNP normal; no overhydration and elevated BNP; overhydration and normal BNP; overhydration and elevated BNP). There were significant differences among patients with different fluid status before CRRT and with a higher mortality rate (64.4%) when the parameters were both indicative of overhydration. Finally, a recent study tried to define the impact of hyperhydration on mortality risk in 150 ICU patients, comparing BIVA with fluid balance [46]. Severe hyperhydration measured by BIVA was the only variable significantly associated with ICU mortality.

In conclusion, measurement of the relative changes in bioelectrical impedance, which reflects alterations in body composition, provides a quantitative estimation of critical illness. In particular, a low preoperative phase angle seems to be associated with undernutrition and an increased risk of adverse clinical outcome.

Conclusion

BIA is a non-invasive and practical tool that can be easily used in ICU patients, but measurements should be interpreted in conjunction with other clinical data. In particular, the BIVA approach with the phase angle calculated from the ratio between various R and Xc measurements is considered to be an indicator of membrane integrity and body cell mass. In fact, low phase angle values in critically ill patients correlate with poorer disease progress and higher mortality. Moreover, this tool is considered to be valid when the hydration status varies in contrast to other parameters used to assess body composition measured by BIA. While its use seems to be well established for nutritional assessment, studies need to explore its use compared to other biochemical parameters commonly used in critical patients and novel approaches, such as muscles ultrasonographic assessment. Considering the wide variability of BIVA parameters found across the different studies, these measurements seem best suited for qualitative comparisons among patients and for quantitative comparison within patients.

References

1. Lukaski HC, Johnson PE, Bolonchuk WW et al (1985) Assessment of fat-free mass using bioelectrical impedance measurements of the human body. Am J Clin Nutr 41:810–817
2. NIH (1996) NIH Consensus statement. Bioelectrical impedance analysis in body composition measurement. National Institutes of Health Technology Assessment Conference Statement. December 12–14, 1994. Nutrition 12:749–762
3. Anonymous (1996) Bioelectrical impedance analysis in body composition measurement. Proceedings of a National Institutes of Health Technology Assessment Conference. Bethesda, Maryland, December 12–14, 1994. Am J Clin Nutr 64(3 Suppl):387S–532S
4. Shafer KJ, Siders WA, Johnson LK et al (2009) Validity of segmental multiple-frequency bioelectrical impedance analysis to estimate body composition of adults across a range of body mass indexes. Nutrition 25:25–32
5. Sun SS, Chumlea WC, Heymsfield SB et al (2003) Development of bioelectrical impedance analysis prediction equations for body composition with the use of a multicomponent model for use in epidemiologic surveys. Am J Clin Nutr 77:331–340
6. Teruel-Briones JL, Fernandez-Lucas M, Ruiz-Roso G et al (2012) Analysis of concordance between the bioelectrical impedance vector analysis and the bioelectrical impedance spectroscopy in haemodialysis patients. Nefrologia 32:389–395

7. Jaffrin MY, Morel H (2008) Body fluid volumes measurements by impedance: a review of bioimpedance spectroscopy (BIS) and bioimpedance analysis (BIA) methods. Med Eng Phys 30:1257–1269

8. Dumler F, Kilates C (2003) Body composition analysis by bioelectrical impedance in chronic maintenance dialysis patients: comparisons to the National Health and Nutrition Examination Survey III. J Renal Nutr 13:166–172

9. Peacock WF 4th (2010) Use of bioimpedance vector analysis in critically ill and cardiorenal patients. Contrib Nephrol 165:226–235

10. Piccoli A, Pittoni G, Facco E et al (2000) Relationship between central venous pressure and bioimpedance vector analysis in critically ill patients. Crit Care Med 28:132–137

11. Ellis KJ, Bell SJ, Chertow GM et al (1999) Bioelectrical impedance methods in clinical research: a follow-up to the NIH Technology Assessment Conference. Nutrition 15:874–880

12. Kyle UG, Bosaeus I, De Lorenzo AD et al (2004) Bioelectrical impedance analysis – part I: review of principles and methods. Clin Nutr 23:1226–1243

13. Khalil SF, Mohktar MS, Ibrahim F (2014) The theory and fundamentals of bioimpedance analysis in clinical status monitoring and diagnosis of diseases. Sensors (Basel) 14:10895–10928

14. Kyle UG, Bosaeus I, De Lorenzo AD et al (2004) Bioelectrical impedance analysis-part II: utilization in clinical practice. Clin Nutr 23:1430–1453

15. Savalle M, Gillaizeau F, Maruani G et al (2012) Assessment of body cell mass at bedside in critically ill patients. Am J Physiol Endocrinol Metab 303:E389–E396

16. Foster KR, Lukaski HC (1996) Whole-body impedance – what does it measure? Am J Clin Nutr 64(3 Suppl):388S–396S

17. Nescolarde L, Garcia-Gonzalez MA, Rosell-Ferrer J et al (2006) Thoracic versus whole body bioimpedance measurements: the relation to hydration status and hypertension in peritoneal dialysis patients. Physiol Meas 27:961–971

18. De Palo T, Messina G, Edefonti A et al (2000) Normal values of the bioelectrical impedance vector in childhood and puberty. Nutrition 16:417–424

19. Lee SY, Gallagher D (2008) Assessment methods in human body composition. Curr Opin Clin Nutr Metab Care 11:566–572

20. Schweickert WD, Hall J (2007) ICU-acquired weakness. Chest 131:1541–1549

21. Rehal MS, Fiskaare E, Tjader I et al (2016) Measuring energy expenditure in the intensive care unit: a comparison of indirect calorimetry by E-sCOVX and Quark RMR with Deltatrac II in mechanically ventilated critically ill patients. Crit Care 20:54

22. Griffiths RD (1996) Muscle mass, survival, and the elderly ICU patient. Nutrition 12:456–458

23. Robert S, Zarowitz BJ, Hyzy R et al (1993) Bioelectrical impedance assessment of nutritional status in critically ill patients. Am J Clin Nutr 57:840–844

24. Kuchnia A, Earthman C, Teigen L et al (2017) Evaluation of bioelectrical impedance analysis in critically ill patients: results of a multicenter prospective study. JPEN J Parenter Enteral Nutr 41:1131–1138

25. Kim HSLE, Lee YJ, Lee JH, Lee CT, Cho YJ (2015) Clinical application of bioelectrical impedance analysis and its phase angle for nutritional assessment of critically ill patients. J Clin Nutr 7:54–61

26. Faisy C, Rabbat A, Kouchakji B et al (2000) Bioelectrical impedance analysis in estimating nutritional status and outcome of patients with chronic obstructive pulmonary disease and acute respiratory failure. Intensive Care Med 26:518–525

27. Lee Y, Kwon O, Shin CS, Lee SM (2015) Use of bioelectrical impedance analysis for the assessment of nutritional status in critically ill patients. Clin Nutr Res 4:32–40

28. Coppini LZ, Waitzberg DL, Campos AC (2005) Limitations and validation of bioelectrical impedance analysis in morbidly obese patients. Curr Opin Clin Nutr Metab Care 8:329–332

29. Dewitte A, Carles P, Joannes-Boyau O et al (2016) Bioelectrical impedance spectroscopy to estimate fluid balance in critically ill patients. J Clin Monit Comput 30:227–233

30. Jones SL, Tanaka A, Eastwood GM et al (2015) Bioelectrical impedance vector analysis in critically ill patients: a prospective, clinician-blinded investigation. Crit Care 19:290
31. Foley K, Keegan M, Campbell I et al (1999) Use of single-frequency bioimpedance at 50 kHz to estimate total body water in patients with multiple organ failure and fluid overload. Crit Care Med 27:1472–1477
32. Rochwerg B, Cheung JH, Ribic CM et al (2016) Assessment of postresuscitation volume status by bioimpedance analysis in patients with sepsis in the intensive care unit: a pilot observational study. Can Rrespir J 2016:8671742
33. Sheeran P, Hall GM (1997) Cytokines in anaesthesia. Br J Anaesth 78:201–219
34. Bracco D, Revelly JP, Berger MM et al (1998) Bedside determination of fluid accumulation after cardiac surgery using segmental bioelectrical impedance. Crit Care Med 26:1065–1070
35. Tatara T, Tsuzaki K (1998) Segmental bioelectrical impedance analysis improves the prediction for extracellular water volume changes during abdominal surgery. Crit Care Med 26:470–476
36. Ackland GL, Singh-Ranger D, Fox S et al (2004) Assessment of preoperative fluid depletion using bioimpedance analysis. Br J Anaesth 92:134–136
37. Barbosa-Silva MC, Barros AJ, Post CL et al (2003) Can bioelectrical impedance analysis identify malnutrition in preoperative nutrition assessment? Nutrition 19:422–426
38. Ernstbrunner M, Kostner L, Kimberger O et al (2014) Bioimpedance spectroscopy for assessment of volume status in patients before and after general anaesthesia. PLoS One 9:e111139
39. Chong JU, Nam S, Kim HJ et al (2016) Exploration of fluid dynamics in perioperative patients using bioimpedance analysis. J Gastrointest Surg 20:1020–1027
40. Pirlich M, Norman K, Lochs H et al (2006) Role of intestinal function in cachexia. Curr Opin Clin Nutr Metab Care 9:603–606
41. Visser M, van Venrooij LM, Wanders DC et al (2012) The bioelectrical impedance phase angle as an indicator of undernutrition and adverse clinical outcome in cardiac surgical patients. Clin Nutr 31:981–986
42. da Silva TK, Berbigier MC, Rubin Bde A, Moraes RB, Corrêa Souza G, Schweigert P (2015) Phase angle as a prognostic marker in patients with critical illness. Nutr Clin Pract 30:261–265
43. Thibault R, Makhlouf AM, Mulliez A et al (2016) Fat-free mass at admission predicts 28-day mortality in intensive care unit patients: the international prospective observational study Phase Angle Project. Intensive Care Med 42:1445–1453
44. Rhee H, Jang KS, Shin MJ et al (2015) Use of multifrequency bioimpedance analysis in male patients with acute kidney injury who are undergoing continuous veno-venous hemodiafiltration. PLoS One 10:e133199
45. Chen H, Wu B, Gong D et al (2015) Fluid overload at start of continuous renal replacement therapy is associated with poorer clinical condition and outcome: a prospective observational study on the combined use of bioimpedance vector analysis and serum N-terminal pro-B-type natriuretic peptide measurement. Crit Care 19:135
46. Samoni S, Vigo V, Resendiz LI et al (2016) Impact of hyperhydration on the mortality risk in critically ill patients admitted in intensive care units: comparison between bioelectrical impedance vector analysis and cumulative fluid balance recording. Crit Care 20:95
47. Gonzalez J, Morrissey T, Byrne T et al (1995) Bioelectric impedance detects fluid retention in patients undergoing cardiopulmonary bypass. J Thorac Cardiovasc Surg 111:111–118
48. House AA, Haapio M, Lentini P et al (2010) Volume assessment in mechanically ventilated critical care patients using bioimpedance vectorial analysis, brain natriuretic Peptide, and central venous pressure. Int J Nephrol 2011:413760
49. Basso F, Berdin G, Virzi GM et al (2013) Fluid management in the intensive care unit: bioelectrical impedance vector analysis as a tool to assess hydration status and optimal fluid balance in critically ill patients. Blood Purif 36:192–199

Part VII
Acute Renal Failure

Acute Kidney Injury and Microcirculatory Shock

P. Guerci, B. Ergin, and C. Ince

Introduction

Acute kidney injury (AKI) is characterized by a rapid deterioration in renal function possibly combining decreased urine excretion with positive fluid balance, electrolyte disturbances and accumulation of metabolic end- or waste products. AKI is among the most frequent shock-related organ failure in critically ill patients [1]. AKI remains one of the leading causes of morbidity and mortality in intensive care medicine and generates high costs [1]. Up to one-third of patients who survive an occurrence of AKI will subsequently develop chronic kidney disease.

Endothelial dysfunction and microcirculation impairment are considered hallmarks of shock and generally precede the occurrence of organ failure [2]. The central role of the microcirculation in the pathogenesis of shock has increasingly come to the forefront over the past decades [3]. However, how microcirculatory dysfunction is related to inflammatory activation, tissue hypoxia and endothelial dysfunction leading to AKI still remains an area of intensive experimental and clinical research. Better understanding of the pathophysiology of AKI in relation to the microcirculatory alterations associated with shock is expected to provide new insights resulting in innovative new therapeutics targeting specific aspects of the

P. Guerci
Department of Anesthesiology and Critical Care Medicine, University Hospital of Nancy
Nancy, France
INSERM U1116, University of Lorraine
Vandoeuvre-Les-Nancy, France
Department of Translational Physiology, Academic Medical Centre
Amsterdam, Netherlands

B. Ergin · C. Ince (✉)
Department of Translational Physiology, Academic Medical Centre
Amsterdam, Netherlands
Department of Intensive Care Medicine, Erasmus MC, University Medical Center
Rotterdam, Netherlands
e-mail: c.ince@amc.uva.nl

© Springer International Publishing AG 2018   293
J.-L. Vincent (ed.), *Annual Update in Intensive Care and Emergency Medicine 2018*,
Annual Update in Intensive Care and Emergency Medicine,
https://doi.org/10.1007/978-3-319-73670-9_23

microcirculation, inflammation or tissue hypoxia. These targeted therapeutics will pave the way to a new era of personalized medicine.

In this chapter, we present an overview of shock-related microcirculatory disturbances and endothelial dysfunction relating to the development of AKI.

The Anatomy of the Kidney: A Unique Microcirculation

The kidneys receive about 20 to 25% of the cardiac output, which in adults is equivalent to 1,000 to 1,200 ml of blood per minute. Twenty percent of the plasma flow – approximately 120 to 140 ml/minute – is filtered by the glomerulus in the cortex and passes into the Bowman capsule. The remaining 80% (about 480 ml/minute) of plasma flows through the efferent arterioles to the peritubular capillaries in the medulla to ensure solute exchange and water resorption. It is estimated that only 5–15% of total renal blood flow (RBF) is directed to the medulla, with the outer medulla having higher blood flow (130–340 ml/100 g tissue/min) than the inner medulla (22–69 ml/100 g tissue/min) [4].

The kidney microcirculation is one of the richest of the human body, having a unique architecture [5]. The renal microcirculation includes the interlobar, arcuate and interlobular arteries and microvessels of smaller branch order, such as arterioles, capillaries and venules. Two types of capillary bed – connected in series – coexist in the kidney; namely the glomerular and the peritubular microcirculations. Both have different functions, which can be affected and/or harmed differently in states of shock. The renal microcirculation is complex and responsible for supplying the kidney with oxygen and ensuring plasma filtration, electrolyte exchange and water reabsorption. The glomerular microcirculation, originating from the afferent arteriole, is located within the Bowman's capsule in the renal cortex. This primary capillary system is responsible for the filtration of the plasma to form ultrafiltrate also known as primary urine. Instead of classically being followed by a venule, this capillary system exits into an efferent arteriole. The peritubular microcirculation emerges from the efferent arteriole and is mainly constituted with the vasa recta in the medulla. Their parallel and counter-flow arrangement to the adjacent tubules creates a countercurrent exchange system with the corticomedullary osmotic gradient resulting in the increase in urine concentration.

The endothelium in the kidney is remarkably heterogeneous in structure and function. For example, various endothelial cell arrangements in the kidney cause varying permeability properties. The endothelial cell lining contains pores and fenestrations defining renal permeability and transport of molecules to the underlying cells and basal membrane. Of all the organs, the kidney and intestines exhibit the highest microvascular permeability. Glomerular endothelial cells are unusually thin. Around capillary loops, they have a cell thickness of approximately 50–150 nm, whereas in other locations, this thickness is approximately 500 nm [6]. Endothelial cells in the glomerulus present large fenestrated areas constituting 20–50% of the entire endothelial surface [7]. These fenestrations are typically 60–70 nm in diameter but, unlike renal peritubular endothelial cell, do not possess a thin (3–5 nm) diaphragm. In general, these fenestrations act as a sieving barrier to control the production of urine in the glomerulus, filtering plasma based on hydrostatic pressure [6].

Systemic hemodynamic (macrocirculation) changes in arterial pressure or RBF do not always cause an equivalent change in the renal microcirculation. The glomerular filtration rate is tightly regulated by autoregulatory mechanism, renal sympathetic nerve activation, the renin-angiotensin-aldosterone system (RAAS) and tubulo-glomerular feedback. The glomerular filtration rate (GFR) is maintained fairly constant over a wide range of arterial pressures between 80 to 180 mmHg. RBF and GFR (and thereby the total tubular sodium reabsorption) do not always change in parallel under physiological conditions, as evidenced by changes in filtration fraction in response to both vasoconstrictor and vasodilator factors. Although changes in RBF can alter the circulatory transit time in the microcirculation of the kidney and, therefore, the time available for diffusive transport of oxygen from arteries to veins, renal tissue oxygenation is maintained constant due to an adaptation of arterio-to-venous shunts [8].

Regulators of Microcirculatory Flow

The glomerular microcirculation in the kidney is regulated upstream by the afferent arteriole and downstream by the efferent arteriole under the influence of autoregulatory mechanisms (myogenic activation), tubulo-glomerular feedback, renal sympathetic nerve activation and the RAAS [9]. All these mechanisms regulate the vascular tone of the glomerular arterioles. During shock and depending on the type of insult inducing AKI, these regulatory systems can become affected and responses to changes of vascular tone may vary in an inappropriate way.

In addition, myogenic activation is mediated by the shear stress caused by blood flow which translates into biochemical signals through mechanotransductors located on endothelial cells, inducing vasorelaxation by vasoactive compounds such as nitric oxide (NO) [10]. Endothelial cells synthesize and release various molecules that upregulate the production of relaxing factors (NO, prostaglandin [PG]I$_2$) that lead to endothelium-mediated vascular smooth muscle relaxation or constriction.

In physiology, the microcirculation is tightly regulated by the RAAS to maintain the GFR constant. The RAAS is activated by tubuloglomerular feedback, which acts as a negative feedback control mechanism driven by distal tubular fluid flow and sodium and chloride reabsorption [9].

Oxygenation Regulation in the Kidney

In addition to being exposed to a corticomedullary osmotic gradient throughout, the renal microcirculation is faced with unique challenges for oxygen regulation [8]. Intrinsically, the filtration function requires that perfusion greatly exceeds the metabolic demand. In addition, the vascular control in the kidney is dominated by mechanisms that regulate glomerular filtration and tubular reabsorption. Thus, the perfusion but also the oxygenation within the microcirculation is continuously altered by these regulatory mechanisms. The tissue oxygen tension ranges from approximately 50–80 mmHg in the cortex to less than 20–40 mmHg in the medulla but is otherwise maintained stable within this physiological range. Arterio-to-venous shunting mechanisms have been suggested to protect the medullar region from excessive oxygen delivery (DO_2) and induced oxidative stress [8]. Diffusive shunting of oxygen from arteries to veins in the cortex and from descending to ascending vasa recta in the medulla limits DO_2 to renal tissue. Oxygen shunting depends on the microcirculatory network, the RBF and the kidney oxygen consumption (VO_2). It has been suggested that preglomerular arterial-venous oxygen shunting might act as anti-oxidant system to protect the kidney from deleterious hyperoxia [11].

To achieve all its complex functions, the kidney needs an adequate amount of oxygen to maintain oxygen-dependent adenosine triphosphate (ATP) production. Tubular sodium reabsorption driven by the Na-K-ATPase pump accounts for most VO_2 (~ 80%) in the kidney [12]. Thus, this renal VO_2 varies with GFR, the need for tubular Na^+ reabsorption, and/or the volume status of the patient. The regulation of appropriate tissue oxygenation is key to sustain kidney functions. There are two mechanisms to maintain normal renal function in case of renal hypoxia; (i) an increment in DO_2 to increase tissue oxygenation, and (ii) a reduction in VO_2 that can protect tissues from hypoxia during moderate to severe arterial hypoxemia. Evans et al., demonstrated that even a 55% reduction in arterial oxygen content did not lead to significant impairment of VO_2 because of the adaptive reduction in oxygen demand following the decrease in tubular sodium reabsorption [13].

Key sensors of tissue hypoxia are the well-known hypoxia inducible factor-1α (HIF-1α) and heme-oxygenase 1 (HO-1). Briefly, HIF-1α is an O_2-sensitive transcription factor that accumulates and binds to the key sequence of the erythropoietin (EPO) gene, the hypoxia-responsive element (HRE), and activates transcription of EPO when oxygen tensions decrease. HIFα possesses two isoforms, HIF-1α and HIF-2α, which are expressed in a cell-type fashion: HIF-1α is expressed in tubular cells and HIF-2α is expressed in interstitial and endothelial cells [14]. HO-1 converts heme to biliverdin via a reaction that produces carbon monoxide and liberates iron. Although these products are considered toxic at high concentrations, they may become cytoprotective molecules at a low level and are involved in several signaling pathways [15]. These processes lead to vasorelaxant, antioxidant, anti-inflammatory and anti-apoptotic effects that are salutary in AKI.

How to Explore Renal Microcirculatory Perfusion and Oxygenation

In experimental studies, several techniques have been developed to explore the microcirculation and oxygenation of the kidney. There are several ways to measure the microcirculation. Both morphological and functional studies are possible. Non-invasive methods are preferred because they do not cause disruption or injury to the microcirculatory architecture and function.

Visualization of the Microcirculation

Intravital Microscopy and Fluorescence Microscopy
Intravital microscopy is considered the gold standard for the evaluation of the microcirculation. Many organs have been explored with this technique but it requires either exposure of the organ surface or the organ to be thin or without a thick capsule. Intravital fluorescence microscopy requires an injection of a fluorescent dye (fluorophore) to image the intravascular lumen or specific cells (e.g., leukocytes), which is subsequently excited at a specific wavelength to allow imaging of the microvasculature. In addition to the visualization of the microcirculation, dyes of different size or that can stain different molecules of the vascular endothelium or glycocalyx can be used. In rodents, measurements of glomerular and cortical peritubular capillary perfusion have been performed.

Handheld Vital Microscopy Techniques
Handheld vital microscopy techniques can be used for direct visualization of the microcirculation on organ surfaces without the need for use of fluorescence microscopy or transillumination. Embedded in handheld microscopes, this epiillumination is accomplished by orthogonal polarization spectral (OPS) imaging, sidestream dark-field (SDF) imaging or more recently incident dark-field (IDF) imaging [16]. These techniques can be used to observe the microcirculation in both experimental animal and human studies. The devices allow a large field of examination and are based on the absorption of green light (530–540 nm) by the hemoglobin within red blood cells (RBCs). Briefly, the tip of the device is placed on the organ surface of interest and the illumination light emerges either down a light guide (OPS imaging) or from a ring of light-emitting diodes placed in close proximity to the tip of the light guide. The illumination light consists of a green light that hits the tissue and is either scattered or reflected to the light guide. The reflected light forms an image of the illuminated area and can be recorded with a video camera or an image sensor. The measurement depth is approximately 500 µm. These methods are, however, sensitive to motion and pressure artifacts as they require the tip of the device to touch the organ surface.

In addition to the recording of images on exposed organ surfaces, the obtained clips require offline analysis for quantification of the microcirculation. This requires specialized software that is not yet fully automatic, thus creating a learning curve; it is also time-consuming [17]. Several scores have been proposed to quantify microvascular flow, characterize the functional capillary density or describe leukocyte behavior and leukocyte-endothelium interactions within the microcirculation. Handheld vital microscopy has been used for the study of renal cortex microcirculation where the tubular capillaries can be visualized.

Laser Doppler Perfusion Imaging

Laser Doppler perfusion imaging uses coherent laser light that undergoes a small shift in frequency because of the Doppler effect when striking moving particles such as RBCs. The average amount of change in frequency, called the Doppler shift, in the reflected light is proportional to the product of average velocity and concentration of RBC. The Doppler shift is the output of laser Doppler flowmetry. Laser Doppler perfusion imaging is normally a single-point technique measuring an average of the microcirculation in about $1 \, mm^3$ of tissue. By combining several single measurements, an image of the perfusion of the microcirculation of the tissue under analysis is created. It can offer a wide image of $50 \times 50 \, cm$. The measurement depth ranges from 1 to 1.5 mm but is dependent on laser wavelength and the nature of the tissue.

Laser Speckle Contrast Imaging

Laser speckle is the result of a phenomenon occurring when laser light illuminates a biological tissue. Laser speckle arises from irregularities in the structure of the tissue, which backscatter the laser light irregularly, creating dark and light interference patterns. A charged coupled device camera then detects these patterns. The speckle pattern is altered with the presence of movement within the tissue, such as those created by flowing RBCs. Therefore, laser speckle contrast imaging provides full-field perfusion maps of the organ surface (e.g., renal cortex) and allows quantification of the average laser speckle contrast imaging perfusion within an arbitrarily set region of interest. Laser speckle contrast imaging has been used to assess renal perfusion heterogeneities [18]. A major advantage of the laser speckle contrast imaging techniques is that it does not require direct contact with the organ. Moreover, it provides the possibility of measuring large areas; however it lacks the detail provided by handheld vital microscopy.

Laser Doppler Flowmetry

The laser Doppler flowmetry probe is usually (but not necessarily) a microprobe and can be inserted in the tissue. Its use has been reported in a large variety of organs including the renal cortex. It measures (invasively) the flow and, as with all the previous laser-based techniques, provides a quantitation of perfusion in arbitrary units. The major drawback of this technique is that it can damage the tissue (insertion) and create microhemorrhages and hematomas that influence local microcirculation.

Contrast-enhanced Ultrasound

Contrast-enhanced ultrasound may be of particular interest for non-invasively assessing the renal microcirculation at the bedside. Contrast-enhanced ultrasound involves the administration of intravenous contrast agents containing microbubbles filled usually with a gas such as nitrogen. Contrast-enhanced ultrasound non-invasively shows the microcirculatory perfusion of an organ. Contrast-enhanced ultrasound has been performed in the critically ill setting to assess the renal cortical microcirculation response to incremental dose of norepinephrine in patients with

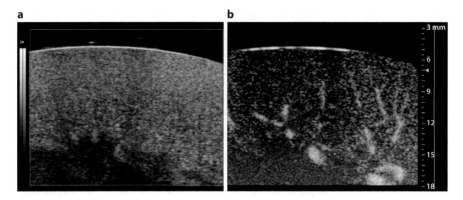

Fig. 1 Longitudinal section of the kidney obtained with contrast enhanced ultrasound. **a** before injection, **b** following bolus injection of ultrasound contrast agent

septic shock [19]. In addition to providing direct visualization of the microcirculation within the cortex kidney, the microcirculatory mean transit time of contrast can be expected to provide information about renal cortex microcirculatory perfusion and its heterogeneity. An example of the images obtained with contrast-enhanced ultrasound are shown in Fig. 1.

Renal Microvascular Oxygenation

Phosphorescence Quenching Methods
Phosphorescence occurs as a result of the delayed emission of photons when a molecule is excited by light, and the absorbed energy is excited into a triplet state before returning to the singlet ground state. A phosphorescent dye (palladium-porphyrin) either emits this energy as photons or transfers this energy to oxygen (the only molecule in a biological system that has this property), which is referred to as oxygen quenching. The phosphorescence decay is time dependent and quantitatively related to the concentration of available oxygen described by the Stern–Volmer relationship. Dual-wavelength phosphorimeters have been developed that allow continuous and simultaneous measurement at two depths. These have been used to measure both cortical and medullary microvascular oxygenation [20]. Recently, light-emitting diode (LED)-based devices have been developed to measure up to 4 wavelengths within one organ giving the possibility of analyzing microvascular oxygenation [21].

Oxygen Electrodes and PO₂ Fluorescence Quenching Probes
The classical Clark electrode (polarographic) has been widely used in experimental studies to measure tissue oxygen tensions. These electrodes can be inserted in every tissue depending on the size of needle. Two major drawbacks of the use of these electrodes are however: (i) that insertion of the electrode causes microtraumatism

disrupting the natural architecture; and (ii) there is uncertainty about the physiological compartment that is being measured, which is most likely the PO_2 of the interstitial fluid. It also should be noted that Clark electrodes consume local oxygen. An alternative electrode is offered by the incorporation of an oxygen-dependent fluorescent dye into the tip. Although offering key advantages over polarographic technology by providing an exact value of tissue oxygen tension ($PtiO_2$), the PO_2 fluorescence quenching probes also suffer the same limitations as the Clark electrode.

Near-Infrared Spectroscopy

The near-infrared spectroscopy (NIRS) technique is a non-invasive optical spectroscopy technique that provides a measure of microcirculatory oxygen availability. The NIRS technique describes blood oxygenation status, by determining hemoglobin saturation according to the difference in absorption of wavelength (presence of oxy- or deoxy-hemoglobin). Classically, the renal oxygen saturation is higher than in other organs ($\sim$ 80–90%) because of its unique arteriolar organization. The assessment of renal oxygenation with NIRS has been performed in infants ($< 10\,kg$) undergoing cardiac surgery with cardiopulmonary bypass, where the light can penetrate the tissues until the kidney [22]. Such measurements are not possible in adult patients due to the limitations of the penetration depth of the optical signal.

Blood Oxygen Level-Dependent Magnetic Resonance Imaging

Blood oxygen level-dependent magnetic resonance imaging (BOLD-MRI) is another non-invasive technique to measure kidney oxygenation *in vivo* in animal models and in humans. BOLD-MRI uses the paramagnetic properties of deoxyhemoglobin to acquire images sensitive to local tissue oxygen concentration. BOLD-MRI has been used to assess kidney oxygenation during sepsis but because of the presence of medullary hypoxia unifying conclusions concerning the role of hypoxia in general could not be drawn [23]. These studies, however, involved a low number of animals or patients. Because of the complexity of the procedure requiring transport of an acutely ill patient to the MRI device, BOLD-MRI cannot reasonably be performed routinely.

To summarize, all these techniques were able to detect changes in microcirculatory perfusion and oxygenation occurring during AKI. With the exception of contrast-enhanced ultrasound, BOLD-MRI and NIRS, most techniques require exposure of the kidney and cannot therefore be used in human studies. The sublingual microcirculation has been studied extensively in shock patients using handheld microscopy. It has been suggested that the sublingual microcirculation could provide a surrogate measure of the visceral microcirculation. To date, however, no study has clearly demonstrated similarity in changes between kidney and sublingual microcirculatory flow and oxygenation during AKI. Only one study reported the use of handheld microscopy using SDF and analysis of the microcirculation on kidney transplants in humans [24]. It should be noted that microcirculatory perfusion or oxygen abnormalities can precede the onset of AKI, implying that all the adaptive mechanisms to limit these dysfunctions have already been jeopardized or overwhelmed.

Microcirculatory Alterations and Renal Tissue Hypoxia During AKI

Microcirculatory alterations and renal tissue hypoxia leading to reduction in GFR are hallmarks of AKI [4]. The interplay between inflammation, hypoxia and microcirculatory dysfunction is not yet completely understood but theories have been proposed highlighting these interactions as being central in the development of AKI [25]. Changes in NO bioavailability and production of reactive oxygen species (ROS) are considered two of the cornerstone mechanisms underlying the pathogenesis of AKI. These events together contribute to endothelial cell dysfunction leading to microcirculatory dysfunction and renal failure. A summary of the actors involved in microvascular alteration and tubular renal damage is given in Fig. 2.

Functional Capillary Density

The functional capillary density (FCD) is defined as the length of red cell-perfused capillaries per observation area, and has been used as a physiological variable describing the capacity of the microcirculation to deliver oxygen carrying RBCs to the tissues. A decrease in FCD has been shown to be the main hemodynamic culprit preceding organ dysfunction. Alterations in the microcirculation are not organ specific in shock; however, the associated clinical pattern is organ specific [2]. Many experimental studies, in various models, focused on microcirculatory dysfunction or renal microcirculatory oxygenation during AKI following either hemorrhagic shock, sepsis or ischemia/reperfusion injury have been performed. Although in prerenal insults with altered systemic hemodynamics (e.g., low cardiac output, profound hypovolemia, low blood pressure) there is a homogenous and intense reduction in single-nephron GFR in virtually all nephrons primarily as a result of reduced RBF [26], it is far more difficult to account for these changes in sepsis-associated AKI [27]. Indeed, the widely held concept of 'renal ischemia' in sepsis-associated AKI due to afferent arteriolar vasoconstriction leading to reduction in GFR has been challenged with accumulating evidence demonstrating that AKI can occur in the presence of normal or even increased RBF [27–29]. In this context pathological microcirculatory heterogeneity in blood flow leading to defects in cortical and medullary perfusion and oxygenation are the primary cause for AKI [18, 30]. Legrand et al. demonstrated that early fluid resuscitation after induction of endotoxemia failed to prevent the development of AKI and microcirculatory defects [18]. Thus, trying to restore the FCD solely by administering fluids in sepsis-associated AKI may not be an adequate option.

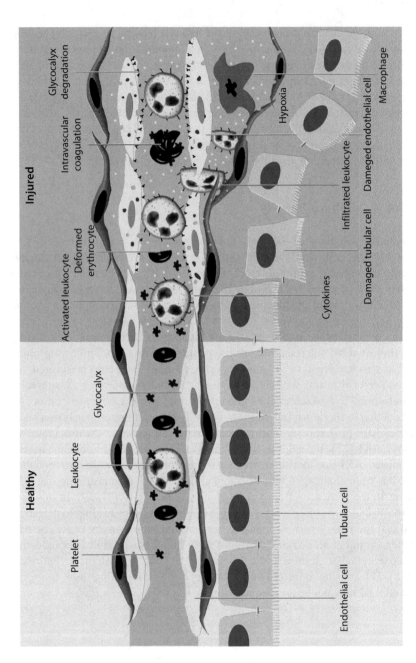

Fig. 2 General overview of key players involved in microvascular dysfunction and occurrence of AKI

The Key Players of Microcirculatory Dysfunction

The Glycocalyx

Endothelial cells play a major role in the progression towards AKI. A thin gel-like layer, the glycocalyx, lining the luminal membrane of endothelial cells protects the endothelium and regulates cellular and macromolecular traffic. The glycocalyx is generally believed to contribute to vascular barrier permeability. During AKI, there is evidence that the glycocalyx is degraded therefore directly exposing the endothelium surface to the blood flow [27, 31, 32]. This sequence of events leads to microcirculation derangement associated with plugged microvessels, functional microcirculatory shunting contributing to reduced O_2 extraction, and renal tissue hypoxemia. Microcirculatory alterations cause heterogeneous flow, which generates microareas of ischemia, leading to functional failure of the kidney.

The compromise of the glycocalyx and the disruption of endothelial cell-to-cell junctions promotes microvascular permeability, increases fluid accumulation in the renal tissue and subsequently contributes to endothelial dysfunction [33, 34]. Thus, compelling evidence has shown that endothelial and glycocalyx damage contribute to albuminuria revealing an alteration in the renal glomerular vascular barrier [35].

Leukocytes, platelets and endothelial cells simultaneously trigger cascades of mediators, causing massive physiological changes. The leukocyte-endothelial cell interaction is mediated by cellular adhesion molecules, which facilitate the adhesion of leukocytes to the endothelium. Cellular adhesion molecules are exposed following glycocalyx shedding due to inflammatory mediators, such as cytokines, ROS and nitrosative species.

Mediators Involved in AKI

Tumor necrosis factor (TNF)-α exerts deleterious effects on renal endothelial cells and plays a key role in AKI [36]. Xu et al. observed in TNF-receptor 1 (TNFR1) knock-out mice submitted to endotoxin challenge that the glomerular endothelial surface layer, endothelial cell fenestrae, GFR, and albuminuria were diminished [36]. These results suggest that sepsis-induced endothelial dysfunction may be mediated by TNF-α activation of TNFR1. In addition, Wu et al. demonstrated that mice lacking expression of intercellular adhesion molecule-1 (ICAM-1) exhibited reduced AKI, leukocyte infiltration and mortality in response to endotoxin [37].

Angiogenic factors, such as vascular endothelial growth factor (VEGF) and angiopoietin-Tie2 systems, are critically involved in vascular barrier permeability, which becomes compromised during sepsis and ischemia/reperfusion injury [31, 38]. Although high levels of VEGF have been shown in septic patients, this was preferentially associated with a more severe form of AKI.

A common pathway in AKI is the generation of oxidative and nitrosative stress. ROS, especially the superoxide (O_2^-), are produced in large amounts in various forms of shock. Both, ROS and nitrosative species alter endothelial cell function and cause lipid peroxidation. In an experimental study in rats, the administration of L-NIL, an inhibitor of inducible NO synthase, ameliorated renal dysfunction and reduced the nitrotyrosine formation, lipid peroxidation and DNA damage [39]. This resulted in the conclusion that the renal damage could be more related to peroxynitrite than to superoxide anion. Similarly, Legrand et al. demonstrated that infusion of L-NIL prevented renal microvascular hypoxia and increased renal VO_2 in a rodent model of renal ischemia/reperfusion injury [40].

Renal Hypoxia During AKI: Cause or Consequence?

Renal hypoxia is considered a central event in the occurrence of AKI, regardless of the initial insult. However, whether hypoxia or microcirculatory alterations and inflammation are the primary cause of AKI, is still a subject of investigation. It is likely that all these events arise more or less at the same time and contribute to a vicious circle. The relationships between inflammation and hypoxia are still unclear [40].

Because of the large oxygen demand needed for tubular sodium reabsorption, inappropriate sodium excretion and subsequent dysregulation of tubulo-glomerular feedback are expected to occur as a result of AKI. A protective role of HIF-1α during ischemia/reperfusion injury of the kidney has been suggested [31]. The mechanisms of activation and regulation of HIF-1α in the kidney are a subject of intense research especially during sepsis [4, 41]. In sepsis-associated AKI models, induced by either endotoxemia or cecal-ligation and puncture, several studies have shown that the expressions of HIF-1α genes and mRNA are upregulated [29, 42]. The cytoprotective properties of HO-1 were first recognized in the kidney, specifically in a rat model of rhabdomyolysis-induced AKI [43]. Protective properties of HO-1 were then demonstrated in AKI induced by ischemia-reperfusion [44], endotoxemia [45] and following renal transplantation [46].

As heterogeneity in microvascular perfusion occurs during AKI and more precisely in sepsis-associated AKI, it is likely to be the same for tissue oxygenation. Indeed, this was demonstrated by Legrand and co-workers who combined phosphorescent measurements for measurement of oxygen and laser speckle contrast imaging for measuring perfusion heterogeneity [18]. In anesthetized dogs subjected to endotoxemia, although renal tissue hypoxia was present, renal venous PO_2 was markedly increased, suggesting an increase in convective a-v shunting of oxygen [47]. Therefore, understanding the underlying mechanisms of hypoxia during AKI is of prime importance. Therapies such as loop diuretics, may increase renal tissue oxygenation by simply lowering the workload of the Na/K-ATPase pump [48]. However, this treatment may not be tailored to the pathogenic mechanisms that are responsible for AKI.

Zafrani et al. recently demonstrated in endotoxemic rats resuscitated with blood transfusion that there was a significant improvement in renal oxygenation but also renal function, mediated in part by the restoration of endothelial NO synthase in the kidney [49].

Considering the concept of increasing the oxygen supply in the microcirculation, hemoglobin-based oxygen carriers (HBOCs) could be a rationale alternative. Indeed, HBOCs have not been contemplated as therapies to increase the bioavailability of oxygen within the microcirculation in the kidney. The development of HBOCs has been hampered because of deleterious effects, mainly of first generations of HBOCs, due to NO scavenging effects [50]. However, new generation HBOCs do not cause such adverse effects and can embed anti-oxidant molecules, which might be interesting to protect the kidney microcirculation.

How to Prevent or Treat Microcirculatory Dysfunction in AKI: A Soup of Drugs?

In the era of personalized medicine and targeted therapies, treating AKI or preventing AKI in a critically ill patient cannot be performed without insight into the pathogenic mechanism underlying microvasculature perfusion and oxygenation alterations in the kidney. A tailored approach based on results of analysis of the microcirculation, the severity and location of hypoxia and the intensity of the leukocyte-endothelium interactions reflecting inflammation, will help the clinician in providing the best treatment. For now, some tools are lacking at the bedside to give a complete picture of the manner in which the kidney has been injured. Handheld vital microscopy may provide some information on the type of microcirculatory dysfunction observed [3] but can only assess the sublingual area at the bedside.

Despite promising experimental research, many human clinical trials have targeted receptors on endothelial cells or blocking/modulating molecules known to promote endothelial cell injury but failed to demonstrate benefit in ischemia/reperfusion injury or sepsis-associated AKI. The need for selection of new endpoints or to perform studies in very homogeneous populations has been advocated. Others have suggested that one drug cannot fit all and proposed that therapies for AKI should target multiple sites. Indeed, a 'soup' of drugs combining an oxygen carrier to sustain oxygenation in the microvasculature, powerful antioxidants to limit damage induced by oxidative stress (ROS and reactive nitrogen species) and modulators of endothelial cell function to restore vasoregulatory functions and restrict leukocyte-endothelium interactions, may provide an alternative strategy to resolve AKI. Nevertheless there is an urgent need for a better understanding of pathophysiology at the bedside, to provide personalized care.

References

1. Hoste EAJ, Bagshaw SM, Bellomo R et al (2015) Epidemiology of acute kidney injury in critically ill patients: the multinational AKI-EPI study. Intensive Care Med 41:1411–1423
2. Ince C (2005) The microcirculation is the motor of sepsis. Crit Care 9(Suppl 4):S13–S19
3. Ince C (2015) Hemodynamic coherence and the rationale for monitoring the microcirculation. Crit Care 19(Suppl 3):S8
4. Evans RG, Ince C, Joles JA et al (2013) Haemodynamic influences on kidney oxygenation: clinical implications of integrative physiology. Clin Exp Pharmacol Physiol 40:106–122

5. Pallone TL, Edwards A, Mattson DL (2012) Renal medullary circulation. Compr Physiol 2:97–140
6. Haraldsson B, Nyström J, Deen WM (2008) Properties of the glomerular barrier and mechanisms of proteinuria. Physiol Rev 88:451–487
7. Satchell SC, Braet F (2009) Glomerular endothelial cell fenestrations: an integral component of the glomerular filtration barrier. Am J Physiol Renal Physiol 296:F947–F956
8. Evans RG, Gardiner BS, Smith DW, O'Connor PM (2008) Intrarenal oxygenation: unique challenges and the biophysical basis of homeostasis. Am J Physiol Renal Physiol 295:F1259–F1270
9. Pallone TL, Silldorff EP, Turner MR (1998) Intrarenal blood flow: microvascular anatomy and the regulation of medullary perfusion. Clin Exp Pharmacol Physiol 25:383–392
10. Aird WC (2003) The role of the endothelium in severe sepsis and multiple organ dysfunction syndrome. Blood 101:3765–3777
11. O'Connor PM, Anderson WP, Kett MM, Evans RG (2006) Renal preglomerular arterial-venous O2 shunting is a structural anti-oxidant defence mechanism of the renal cortex. Clin Exp Pharmacol Physiol 33:637–641
12. Lassen NA, Munck O, Thaysen JH (1961) Oxygen consumption and sodium reabsorption in the kidney. Acta Physiol Scand 51:371–384
13. Evans RG, Goddard D, Eppel GA, O'Connor PM (2011) Factors that render the kidney susceptible to tissue hypoxia in hypoxemia. Am J Physiol Regul Integr Comp Physiol 300:R931–R940
14. Nangaku M, Eckardt K-U (2007) Hypoxia and the HIF system in kidney disease. J Mol Med 85:1325–1330
15. Abraham NG, Cao J, Sacerdoti D, Li X, Drummond G (2009) Heme oxygenase: the key to renal function regulation. Am J Physiol Renal Physiol 297:F1137–F1152
16. Aykut G, Veenstra G, Scorcella C, Ince C, Boerma C (2015) Cytocam-IDF (incident dark field illumination) imaging for bedside monitoring of the microcirculation. Intensive Care Med Exp 3:40
17. Massey MJ, Shapiro NI (2015) A guide to human in vivo microcirculatory flow image analysis. Crit Care 20:35–35
18. Legrand M, Bezemer R, Kandil A, Demirci C, Payen D, Ince C (2011) The role of renal hypoperfusion in development of renal microcirculatory dysfunction in endotoxemic rats. Intensive Care Med 37:1534–1542
19. Schneider AG, Goodwin MD, Schelleman A, Bailey M, Johnson L, Bellomo R (2014) Contrast-enhanced ultrasonography to evaluate changes in renal cortical microcirculation induced by noradrenaline: a pilot study. Crit Care 18:653
20. Johannes T, Mik EG, Ince C (2006) Dual-wavelength phosphorimetry for determination of cortical and subcortical microvascular oxygenation in rat kidney. J Appl Physiol 100:1301–1310
21. Guerci P, Ince Y, Faber D, Ergin B (2017) A LED-based phosphorimeter for measurement of microcirculatory oxygen pressure. J Appl Physiol 122:307–316
22. Ruf B, Bonelli V, Balling G et al (2015) Intraoperative renal near-infrared spectroscopy indicates developing acute kidney injury in infants undergoing cardiac surgery with cardiopulmonary bypass: a case-control study. Crit Care 19:27
23. Zhou HY, Chen TW, Zhang XM (2016) Functional magnetic resonance imaging in acute kidney injury: present status. Biomed Res Int 2016:2027370
24. Snoeijs MG, Vink H, Voesten N et al (2010) Acute ischemic injury to the renal microvasculature in human kidney transplantation. Am J Physiol Renal Physiol 299:F1134–F1140
25. Gomez H, Ince C, De Backer D et al (2014) A unified theory of sepsis-induced acute kidney injury: inflammation, microcirculatory dysfunction, bioenergetics, and the tubular cell adaptation to injury. Shock 41:3–11
26. Matejovic M, Ince C, Chawla LS et al (2016) Renal hemodynamics in AKI: in search of new treatment targets. J Am Soc Nephrol 27:49–58

27. Bellomo R, Kellum JA, Ronco C et al (2017) Acute kidney injury in sepsis. Intensive Care Med 8:R204

28. Maiden MJ, Otto S, Brealey JK et al (2016) Structure and function of the kidney in septic shock: a prospective controlled experimental study. Am J Respir Crit Care Med 194:692–700. https://doi.org/10.1164/rccm.201511-2285OC

29. Langenberg C, Gobe G, Hood S, May CN, Bellomo R (2014) Renal histopathology during experimental septic acute kidney injury and recovery. Crit Care Med 42:e58–e67

30. Johannes T, Mik EG, Nohé B, Raat NJH, Unertl KE, Ince C (2006) Influence of fluid resuscitation on renal microvascular PO2 in a normotensive rat model of endotoxemia. Crit Care 10:R88

31. Bonventre JV, Yang L (2011) Cellular pathophysiology of ischemic acute kidney injury. J Clin Invest 121:4210–4221

32. Ince C, Mayeux PR, Nguyen T et al (2016) The endothelium in sepsis. Shock 45:259–270

33. Molitoris BA (2014) Therapeutic translation in acute kidney injury: the epithelial/endothelial axis. J Clin Invest 124:2355–2363

34. Goldenberg NM, Steinberg BE, Slutsky AS, Lee WL (2011) Broken barriers: a new take on sepsis pathogenesis. Sci Transl Med 3:88ps25–88ps25

35. Salmon AHJ, Satchell SC (2012) Endothelial glycocalyx dysfunction in disease: albuminuria and increased microvascular permeability. J Pathol 226:562–574

36. Xu C, Chang A, Hack BK, Eadon MT, Alper SL, Cunningham PN (2014) TNF-mediated damage to glomerular endothelium is an important determinant of acute kidney injury in sepsis. Kidney Int 85:72–81

37. Wu X, Guo R, Wang Y, Cunningham PN (2007) The role of ICAM-1 in endotoxin-induced acute renal failure. Am J Physiol Renal Physiol 293:F1262–F1271

38. Siner JM, Bhandari V, Engle KM, Elias JA, Siegel MD (2009) Elevated serum angiopoietin 2 levels are associated with increased mortality in sepsis. Shock 31:348–353

39. Noiri E, Nakao A, Uchida K et al (2001) Oxidative and nitrosative stress in acute renal ischemia. Am J Physiol Renal Physiol 281:F948–957

40. Legrand M, Almac E, Mik EG et al (2009) L-NIL prevents renal microvascular hypoxia and increase of renal oxygen consumption after ischemia-reperfusion in rats. Am J Physiol Renal Physiol 296:F1109–F1117

41. Haase VH (2013) Mechanisms of hypoxia responses in renal tissue. J Am Soc Nephrol 24:537–541

42. Castoldi A, Braga TT, Correa-Costa M et al (2012) TLR2, TLR4 and the MYD88 signaling pathway are crucial for neutrophil migration in acute kidney injury induced by sepsis. PLoS One 7:e37584

43. Nath KA, Balla G, Vercellotti GM et al (1992) Induction of heme oxygenase is a rapid, protective response in rhabdomyolysis in the rat. J Clin Invest 90:267–270

44. Shimizu H, Takahashi T, Suzuki T et al (2000) Protective effect of heme oxygenase induction in ischemic acute renal failure. Crit Care Med 28:809–817

45. Tracz MJ, Juncos JP, Grande JP et al (2007) Renal hemodynamic, inflammatory, and apoptotic responses to lipopolysaccharide in HO-1-/- mice. Am J Pathol 170:1820–1830

46. Tullius SG, Nieminen-Kelhä M, Buelow R et al (2002) Inhibition of ischemia/reperfusion injury and chronic graft deterioration by a single-donor treatment with cobalt-protoporphyrin for the induction of heme oxygenase-1. Transplantation 74:591–598

47. Gullichsen E, Nelimarkka O, Halkola L, Niinikoski J (1989) Renal oxygenation in endotoxin shock in dogs. Crit Care Med 17:547–550

48. Brezis M, Agmon Y, Epstein FH (1994) Determinants of intrarenal oxygenation. I. Effects of diuretics. Am J Physiol 267:F1059–F1062

49. Zafrani L, Ergin B, Kapucu A, Ince C (2016) Blood transfusion improves renal oxygenation and renal function in sepsis-induced acute kidney injury in rats. Crit Care 20:406

50. Alayash AI (2014) Blood substitutes: why haven't we been more successful? Trends Biotechnol 32:177–185

Critical Care Ultrasonography and Acute Kidney Injury

R. Wiersema, J. Koeze, and I. C. C. van der Horst

Introduction

Ultrasonography is an essential imaging modality in the intensive care unit (ICU) used for diagnosis and to guide treatment. Critical care ultrasonography is defined as focused echography since it informs specific clinical questions. The examination is performed at point of care and results are combined with clinical and laboratory data. Recently, Narasimhan et al., have suggested that critical care ultrasonography should shift towards a whole-body approach, rather than taking a single-organ approach [1]. Other studies have proposed that a whole-body ultrasonography approach may have benefits in terms of diagnosis, may lead to decreased use of other diagnostic tests and may also decrease costs. Acute kidney injury (AKI) is one of the current challenges in critical care [2] and literature on the role of ultrasound in understanding and diagnosing AKI is scarce. Many overviews on ultrasonography in critical and emergency care have focused on cardiopulmonary evaluations [3]. Here we focus on the evidence concerning use of critical care ultrasonography for the diagnosis and management of AKI in critical care.

Circulatory Failure and AKI

The association between circulatory failure or shock and AKI is well established. Circulatory failure with low blood pressure (mean arterial pressure [MAP] < 65 mmHg) and signs of low perfusion of organs is defined as circulatory shock. Circulatory shock is caused by one or a combination of four categories of mechanisms [4]. While normal hemodynamic physiology is complex and multifactorial, three principles form the basis for an adequate circulation: blood supply to organs

R. Wiersema · J. Koeze · I. C. C. van der Horst (✉)
Department of Critical Care, University Medical Center, University of Groningen
Groningen, Netherlands
e-mail: i.c.c.van.der.horst@umcg.nl

© Springer International Publishing AG 2018   309
J.-L. Vincent (ed.), *Annual Update in Intensive Care and Emergency Medicine 2018*,
Annual Update in Intensive Care and Emergency Medicine,
https://doi.org/10.1007/978-3-319-73670-9_24

and tissues should meet total demands and therefore in a way control/regulate cardiac output. Further, blood flow and cardiac output are in general not strictly related to the blood pressure. These principles are important to consider when evaluating the hemodynamic status of patients with circulatory failure and at risk of AKI. In states of vasodilatation, patients with circulatory failure can suffer from intravascular underload. Observational studies suggest that patients with shock have an increased incidence of AKI [5, 6]. On the other hand, because of circulatory failure patients receive interventions such as fluids, vasopressors and inotropes. Fluid therapy is suggested to be associated with an increased incidence of AKI [7]. Moreover, the use of vasoactive medication is also a predictor for AKI [8, 9]. However, circulatory failure should not be considered the cause of AKI. The underlying causes of shock, such as sepsis, can be associated with AKI by mechanisms such as inflammation. Several tests have been suggested for improved and earlier diagnosis of AKI, including biomarkers [10]. Diagnostics may also elucidate parts of the underlying pathophysiologic mechanisms of AKI in critically ill patients.

Venous Congestion, Fluid Balance and AKI

Venous congestion entails venous fluid overload, manifested by, for example, an increased central venous pressure (CVP) or peripheral edema [11]. Such increased venous volumes may be associated with increased venous pressures, which may in turn, at least theoretically reduce renal venous blood flow. In analogy to the concept of cerebral perfusion pressure, this increased afterload may reduce the driving pressure difference between arterial and venous pressures. Theoretically, venous congestion may also affect renal function. Improved understanding of this concept may contribute to understanding of the pathophysiological changes and potentially guide hemodynamic interventions [12].

As the concept is relatively new, there is no consensus on how to measure venous congestion and/or renal venous pressure. Reliable measurement of the venous return or venous blood flow and the CVP in the vena cavae is complex. Whether CVP as a single measure reflects venous congestion is highly questionable and in the jugular vein probably insufficient. First, the CVP in ICU patients is measured by a central venous catheter (CVC) likely in the vena iliaca or the vena jugularis, and very rarely at both sites at the same time. Second, the CVP can vary in different patients and still be normal in an individual. Clear reference values are lacking, mostly due to the variations associated with positions of patients, positions of the lines, and varying intrathoracic pressures in mechanically ventilated patients. CVP differences may be used for preload assessments but do not reflect the preload directly. Therefore, a reliable variable for assessment of venous congestion is not available [13, 14]. Observational studies have suggested that higher CVP is associated with increased serum creatinine and increased incidence of AKI [11, 15–17]. This observation supports the concept of venous congestion and reduced renal outflow.

Several studies have evaluated associations between fluid balance and AKI in different categories of patients. Mao et al. evaluated the development of AKI in

209 heart valve surgery patients and showed that receiving large volumes of intraoperative fluid was an independent risk factor for AKI (odds ratio [OR] 1.10, CI 1.01–1.21, p = 0.02) [18]. Haase-Fielitz et al. report similar results and noted fluid overload was associated with worse outcomes after cardiac surgery [19]. In a retrospective analysis in 210 patients with early AKI, Raimundo et al. reported that higher fluid intake was an independent risk factor for progression of AKI [20]. More recently, Chen et al. [11] assessed venous congestion in terms of peripheral edema or increased CVP in 2,338 critically ill patients and reported AKI in 27% of patients with peripheral edema at admission compared to 16% of patients without peripheral edema at admission. Their multivariate analyses suggested a 30% higher risk of AKI in patients with peripheral edema. Each centimeter increase in CVP was associated with a 2% adjusted increased risk of AKI [11]. Together these studies suggest that fluid therapy, fluid balance or even venous congestion are associated with renal failure. Importantly, fluid balance refers to the sum of all given fluids (intravascular, extravascular [including third space] and intracellular) and all fluids lost, whereas venous congestion refers only to the intravascular fluid status. When considering measures that might reflect this venous congestion and that influence the kidney, critical care ultrasonography might provide some options. Critical care ultrasonography can be used at three different levels of the circulation, starting from the right heart, down through the inferior vena cava (IVC) and finally the kidneys themselves.

Right Heart Function and AKI

Cardiac preload is defined as the amount of blood that flows into the right heart. Assessment of right ventricular (RV) function might reflect preload. Current gold standard measures to assess RV function with critical care ultrasonography are the tricuspid annular plane systolic excursion (TAPSE) and the right ventricular RV systolic excursion (RV S') [21]. The associations between TAPSE and RV S' and renal failure have not yet been studied. Nohria et al. assessed the association between renal failure (defined by a rise in serum creatinine ≥ 0.3 mg/dl) and right atrial pressure in 433 patients with congestive heart failure. In a subgroup of 194 patients, a pulmonary artery catheter was used to measure right atrial pressure. In these patients, there was a correlation at baseline between right atrial pressure and serum creatinine (r = 0.165, p = 0.03) and estimated glomerular filtration rate (eGFR) (r = −0.195, p = 0.01) [22]. Aronson et al. assessed right atrial pressure as a surrogate for venous congestion in a subgroup of 238 from a total of 475 patients with acute decompensated heart failure. They observed a weak but significant correlation between right atrial pressure and eGFR (r = −0.17, p = 0.009). They also observed that the risk of renal failure (defined by maximal increase in serum creatinine > 0.3 mg/dl from admission until 14 days) increased with a more positive fluid balance. In their study, changes in right atrial pressure were similar in patients with and without renal failure (14 vs. 15 mmHg), which can be interpreted to suggest that fluid loading without an increase in pressure in the right heart is still associated with renal failure [15]. By contrast, Haddad et al. reported that right atrial pressure was independently associated with AKI in 105 patients who had one or more periods of acute right-sided heart failure (OR 1.8 95% CI 1.1–2.4, p = 0.018) [23].

Mukherjee et al. [24] studied the association between right-sided cardiac dysfunction and renal failure in 104 patients with acute decompensated heart failure with preserved ejection fraction. Patients with renal failure (defined as a serum creatinine increase of ≥ 0.3 mg/dl within 72 h of hospitalization) had a significantly lower RV fractional area change, an indicator of overall RV function, compared to patients without renal failure (40.6 ± 0.1 vs 46.9 ± 0.1, p = 0.003) [24]. Guinot et al. [25] investigated RV dysfunction and renal function in 74 patients undergoing cardiac surgery and reported that patients with RV dysfunction (defined as values in the lowest quartile of at least two echocardiographic variables) had an OR of 12.7 (95% CI 2.6–63.4, p = 0.02) for development of renal dysfunction. They found no association between cardiac index and renal failure, suggesting once again the impact of venous congestion [25]. These studies together suggest an association between right heart function and renal failure, but this has not yet been studied in a large unselected population of critically ill patients. Some studies even suggest that right heart failure is more important when compared to cardiac index and left heart function.

Critical Care Ultrasonography of the Inferior Vena Cava

Guinot et al. [25] reported that a dilated vena cava (i.e., increased CVP from 11.5 mm [9.6 to 15.0] to 15.2 mm [11.8 to 19.1], p = 0.004) was associated with renal failure. Thus, critical care ultrasonography of the IVC might provide useful information concerning venous congestion [25]. The diameter can be assessed but Rudski et al. [21] also suggest assessing the IVC collapsibility index (IVCCI). The IVC collapses at different rates depending on the pressure in the surrounding tissues, suggesting that a lower collapsibility would indicate higher surrounding pressures. A normal IVCCI was defined by Rudski as > 50% [21]. Ferrada et al. [26] noted that the IVCCI offered good and rapid assessment of fluid status in 108 acutely admitted critically ill patients. Muniz Pazeli et al. [27] used ultrasonography to evaluate the IVC for assessment of fluid status in 52 patients before hemodialysis and reported that nephrologists obtained reliable measurements after limited ultrasound training. De Vecchis et al. [28] described that the IVCCI may be associated with an increased risk of renal failure in 49 patients with right or biventricular heart failure. These studies suggest that the IVC can provide useful information on fluid status in different fields, as has been described before. Additionally, these measurements may indicate or even precede renal failure. Currently there is little knowledge about the additional value for renal failure of IVC measurements in the critically ill patient.

Critical Care Ultrasonography of the Kidney

Recently, interest in ultrasonography of the kidneys has increased, as illustrated by the number of studies in nephrology stimulating the use of ultrasound in clinical practice [29]. Youngrock and Hongchuen describe how renal ultrasound should gain a place in whole-body ultrasonography to improve the diagnostic certainty of the physician [30]. Wilson and Breyer explain its potential to improve diagnostic accuracy [31]. Renal ultrasonography encompasses focused renal ultrasound for causes of pre- or post-renal pathologies but more specific variables are being used that may provide other information. The Doppler renal resistive index (RRI) has been used for years in a variety of clinical settings [32]. Doppler imaging identifies changes in blood flow at the microvascular level. Evaluation of the vascular impedance at different sites of the renal parenchyma could provide useful diagnostic and prognostic information. An increase in renal vascular resistance may be an early sensitive sign of hemodynamic deterioration, even in seemingly stable patients. An increased Doppler RRI is suggested to not only reflect changes in intrarenal perfusion, but also in systemic hemodynamics. In a meta-analysis, Ninet et al. show that an elevated Doppler RRI may be a predictor of persistent AKI in critically ill patients [32]. In Table 1, studies that have investigated Doppler RRI in the ICU setting are shown. Qin et al. proposed that the RRI might even be used for early detection of AKI, as they demonstrated this in 61 patients who underwent surgery for aortic dissection [33]. Several potential limitations should be mentioned, including whether Doppler RRI can be obtained in such a manner that measures can be reproduced. To establish a more definite role for Doppler RRI, it should be investigated in a large unselected group of critically ill patients.

Challenges

Challenges remain in critical care ultrasonography, including the technical aspects of the measurements but also on its reliability and importance when deliberating diagnosis. There are scarce data evaluating critical care ultrasonography of the right heart, and conventional measurements of RV function have not yet been compared to renal function. Some studies have investigated right atrial pressure, but it is unclear to what extent these measurements reflect the venous function. Critical care ultrasonography variables of the IVC, such as the diameter and IVCCI, are influenced by mechanical ventilation, rendering them less reliable and unsuitable as general variables, in a setting where a large percentage of patients is usually receiving mechanically ventilation. Renal ultrasound represents another technical challenge for which research in the critical care setting has only recently begun and the value of these measurements is unclear but promising. If reliable, these new 'conventional' measurements of renal function should be included in daily practice and most certainly in whole-body ultrasonography. One remaining challenge is that although these measurements may be validated, patients remain variable. Single

Table 1 Critical care ultrasonography: studies investigating Doppler renal resistive index (RRI)

Author, year	Centers	Pts[a]	Population	MV	Vasopressors	Image quality	Validation	Renal dysfunction	Outcome, Doppler RRI
Stevens, 1990 [35]	1	57	Medical ICU	12 AKI 9 transient 15 no AKI	3 AKI 3 transient 0 no AKI	NR	NR	20 AKI 14 transient 23 no AKI	4.39 (3.32–5.46) in AKI 1.96 (1.58–2.34) transient 1.16 (0.99–1.33) no AKI
Lerolle, 2006 [36]	1, 20 beds	35	Septic shock, <24 h on vaso-pressor	91%	63%	2 poor (obesity)	2 intensivists	18 AKI day 5	>0.74 on day 1 LR+ of 3.3 for day 5 AKI
Lauschke, 2006 [37]	1	40	Medical ICU	NR	25% (NE)	NR	NR	30 AKI	0.75 ± 0.05 in AKI with NE 0.81 ± 0.07 in AKI no NE 0.69 ± 0.08 in no AKI
Deruddre, 2007 [38]	1	11	Septic shock <12 h after admission	100%	100% (NE)	NR	NR	NR	0.75 ± 0.07 at MAP 65 mmHg 0.71 ± 0.06 at MAP 75 mmHg 0.71 ± 0.05 at MAP 85 mmHg
Darmon, 2011 [39]	1, 24 beds	51	No severe chronic renal dysfunction or diuretics	100%	6%	1 Doppler not possible	NR	22 persistent 13 transient 16 no AKI	0.82 (0.80–0.89) persistent 0.71 (0.62–0.77) transient 0.71 (0.66–0.77) no AKI
Bossard, 2011 [40]	1	65 of 316	Elective cardiopulmonary bypass surgery	100%	49%	NR	3 investigators	18 AKI 47 no AKI	0.79 ± 0.08 AKI 0.68 ± 0.06 no AKI
Schnell, 2012 [41]	2	58	Severe sepsis or polytrauma	60%	50% (NE)	1 poor (obesity)	NR	40 AKI stage 0–1 18 AKI stage 2–3	0.66 (0.62–0.70) AKI stage 0–1 0.80 (0.72–0.82) AKI stage 2–3
Dewitte, 2012 [42]	1, 22 beds	94	Severe sepsis or septic shock	64%	50% (NE)	2 poor	2 investigators	55% AKI	0.74 (0.66–0.78) AKI 0.72 (0.68–0.77) no AKI
Schnell, 2013 [43]	3	35	Receiving MV and a fluid challenge	100%	85% (NE)	NR	NR	13 AKI 13 transient 9 no AKI	Before fluid challenge: 0.76 (0.67–0.80) AKI 0.71 (0.70–0.73) transient 0.66 (0.65–0.70) no AKI

Table 1 (Continued)

Author, year	Centers	Pts[a]	Population	MV	Vasopressors	Image quality	Validation	Renal dysfunction	Outcome, Doppler RRI
Schnell, 2014 [44]	3	69	Medical ICU	100%	49%	1 poor	Junior and senior operators, ICC 89%	48 AKI 21 AKI	Junior operator: 0.76 (0.66–0.82) AKI 0.67 (0.62–0.72) no AKI Senior operator: 0.75 (0.69–0.81) AKI 0.70 (0.64–0.74) no AKI
Lahmer, 2016 [45]	1	30 of 53	Sepsis, AKI and requiring volume challenge	53% responders 43% non-responders	100% (NE)	NR	NR	100% by inclusion	0.71 (0.66–0.76) responders 0.72 (0.69–0.76) non-responders
Marty, 2016 [46]	1	48 of 72	Hip fracture surgery, 2 or more known risk factors for AKI	NR	NR	24 poor or arrhythmia	1 observer, interobserver variability 2.7%	60% presented with postoperative AKI	Preoperative: 0.72 (0.70–0.73) AKI 0.68 (0.67–0.71) no AKI Postoperative: 0.74 (0.71–0.76) AKI 0.60 (0.58–0.68) no AKI
Boddi, 2016 [47]	1, 10 beds	125 of 1512	AKI, no urinary infection	NR	100%	NR	NR	83 AKI on admission 42 AKI during stay	0.85 (0.73–0.92) persistent 0.78 (0.70–0.85) transient
Qin, 2017 [33]	1	61 of 72	Surgery for acute type A aortic dissection	NR	NR	NR	NR	39 AKI 22 no AKI	Preoperative: 0.63 ± 0.04 AKI 0.65 ± 0.06 no AKI
Regolisti, 2017 [48]	1	60	Major heart surgery	NR	NR	NR	NR	38% AKI <72 h	High association Doppler RRI and AKI

AKI: acute kidney injury; *LR+*: positive likelihood ratio; *MV*: mechanical ventilation; *NE*: norepinephrine; *Pts*: patients; [a]: total number of included patients or patients included out of evaluated patients; *ICC*: intraclass correlation coefficient; *NR*: not reported; *MAP*: mean arterial pressure

measurements do not reflect the variability within patients, suggesting that repeated measurements might yield a better reflection of a patient's hemodynamic status.

Finally, additional information on hemodynamics in critically ill patients, including cardiac function, collapsibility of the IVC and measures of renal blood flow (with Doppler RRI), can provide insight into underlying pathophysiology and therewith guide clinical management. Insight into the effects of individual components of diagnostics and interventions might unravel whether some components or combinations of components could be beneficial. The recent results of a pilot study in patients with septic shock suggest that restrictive filling might be one of those components [34]. In conclusion, critical care ultrasonography of the heart, IVC and kidneys may assist in a more optimal balance between restrictive and over-restrictive fluid therapy.

Conclusion

The possibilities of critical care ultrasonography are infinite and as new measurements and approaches continue to be investigated our diagnostic accuracy will improve. The whole-body and system focus is important. We have illustrated that for renal failure, the value of critical care ultrasonography of the right heart, IVC and the kidney itself may be beneficial. Measurements should be validated in different cohorts, as they are currently being studied in specific populations. As for renal failure, venous congestion seems to be one of the pathophysiological pathways that may be detected early by critical care ultrasonography. Measurements like Doppler RRI and IVCCI may provide information of paramount importance concerning the hemodynamic status of patients and their possible risk of developing AKI, one of the major problems in critical care today.

Critically ill patients are known to have complex, multifactorial etiologies that predict outcome. We think that a mono-organ focus in unravelling disease states, like ultrasonography of only the heart or the kidney, results in a less clear understanding of the pathophysiologic state as compared to a wide, open focus.

Acknowledgements

We thank Kim Boerma, Madelon Vos, Ruben Eck, Geert Koster, Frederik Keus, members of the Simple Intensive Care Studies (SICS) Investigators for their review of the literature embedded in this overview.

References

1. Narasimhan M, Koenig SJ, Mayo PH (2016) A whole-body approach to point of care ultrasound. Chest 150:772–776
2. Pickkers P, Ostermann M, Joannidis M et al (2017) The intensive care medicine agenda on acute kidney injury. Intensive Care Med 43:1198–1209

3. Koster G, van der Horst ICC (2017) Critical care ultrasonography in circulatory shock. Curr Opin Crit Care 23:326–333
4. Vincent J-L, De Backer D (2013) Circulatory shock. N Engl J Med 369:1726–1734
5. Kotecha A, Vallabhajosyula S, Coville HH, Kashani K (2017) Cardiorenal syndrome in sepsis: a narrative review. J Crit Care 43:122–127
6. Hoste EA, Bagshaw SM, Bellomo R et al (2015) Epidemiology of acute kidney injury in critically ill patients: the multinational AKI-EPI study. Intensive Care Med 41:1411–1423
7. Perner A, Prowle J, Joannidis M, Young P, Hjortrup PB, Pettila V (2017) Fluid management in acute kidney injury. Intensive Care Med 43:807–815
8. Bouchard J, Acharya A, Cerda J et al (2015) A prospective international Multicenter study of AKI in the intensive care unit. Clin J Am Soc Nephrol 10:1324–1331
9. Perinel S, Vincent F, Lautrette A et al (2015) Transient and persistent acute kidney injury and the risk of hospital mortality in critically ill patients: results of a multicenter cohort study. Crit Care Med 43:e269–e275
10. Parikh CR, Mansour SG (2017) Perspective on clinical application of biomarkers in AKI. J Am Soc Nephrol 28:1677–1685
11. Chen KP, Cavender S, Lee J et al (2016) Peripheral edema, central venous pressure, and risk of AKI in critical illness. Clin J Am Soc Nephrol 11:602–608
12. Wei J, Song J, Jiang S et al (2017) Role of intratubular pressure during the ischemic phase in acute kidney injury. Am J Physiol Renal Physiol 312:F1158–F1165
13. Marik PE, Baram M, Vahid B (2008) Does central venous pressure predict fluid responsiveness? A systematic review of the literature and the tale of seven mares. Chest 134:172–178
14. Magder SS (2016) Volume and its relationship to cardiac output and venous return. Crit Care 20:271
15. Aronson D, Abassi Z, Allon E, Burger AJ (2013) Fluid loss, venous congestion, and worsening renal function in acute decompensated heart failure. Eur J Heart Fail 15:637–643
16. Gambardella I, Gaudino M, Ronco C, Lau C, Ivascu N, Girardi LN (2016) Congestive kidney failure in cardiac surgery: the relationship between central venous pressure and acute kidney injury. Interact Cardiovasc Thorac Surg 23:800–805
17. Mullens W, Abrahams Z, Francis GS et al (2009) Importance of venous congestion for worsening of renal function in advanced decompensated heart failure. J Am Coll Cardiol 53:589–596
18. Mao MA, Thongprayoon C, Wu Y et al (2015) Incidence, severity, and outcomes of acute kidney injury in octogenarians following heart valve replacement surgery. Int J Nephrol 2015:237951
19. Haase-Fielitz A, Haase M, Bellomo R et al (2017) Perioperative hemodynamic instability and fluid overload are associated with increasing acute kidney injury severity and worse outcome after cardiac surgery. Blood Purif 43:298–308
20. Raimundo M, Crichton S, Martin JR et al (2015) Increased fluid administration after early acute kidney injury is associated with less renal recovery. Shock 44:431–437
21. Rudski LG, Lai WW, Afilalo J et al (2010) Guidelines for the echocardiographic assessment of the right heart in adults: a report from the American Society of Echocardiography endorsed by the European Association of Echocardiography, a registered branch of the European Society of Cardiology, and the Canadian Society of Echocardiography. J Am Soc Echocardiogr 23:685–713
22. Nohria A, Hasselblad V, Stebbins A et al (2008) Cardiorenal interactions: insights from the ESCAPE trial. J Am Coll Cardiol 51:1268–1274
23. Haddad F, Fuh E, Peterson T et al (2011) Incidence, correlates, and consequences of acute kidney injury in patients with pulmonary arterial hypertension hospitalized with acute right-side heart failure. J Card Fail 17:533–539
24. Mukherjee M, Sharma K, Madrazo JA, Tedford RJ, Russell SD, Hays AG (2017) Right-sided cardiac dysfunction in heart failure with preserved ejection fraction and worsening renal function. Am J Cardiol 120:274–278

25. Guinot PG, Abou-Arab O, Longrois D, Dupont H (2015) Right ventricular systolic dysfunction and vena cava dilatation precede alteration of renal function in adult patients undergoing cardiac surgery: an observational study. Eur J Anaesthesiol 32:535–542

26. Ferrada P, Anand RJ, Whelan J et al (2012) Qualitative assessment of the inferior vena cava: useful tool for the evaluation of fluid status in critically ill patients. Am Surg 78:468–470

27. Muniz Pazeli J, Fagundes Vidigal D, Cestari Grossi T et al (2014) Can nephrologists use ultrasound to evaluate the inferior vena cava? a cross-sectional study of the agreement between a nephrologist and a cardiologist. Nephron Extra 4:82–88

28. De Vecchis R, Ariano C, Fusco A et al (2012) Ultrasound evaluation of the inferior vena cava collapsibility index in congestive heart failure patients treated with intravenous diuretics: new insights about its relationship with renal function: an observational study. Anadolu Kardiyol Derg 12:391–400

29. Kaptein MJ, Kaptein EM (2017) Focused Real-time ultrasonography for nephrologists. Int J Nephrol 2017:3756857

30. Youngrock H, Hongchuen T (2016) The SAFER Lasso; a novel approach using point-of-care ultrasound to evaluate patients with abdominal complaints in the emergency department. Crit Ultrasound J 8(Suppl 1):A12–A22

31. Wilson JG, Breyer KE (2016) Critical care ultrasound: a review for practicing nephrologists. Adv Chronic Kidney Dis 23:141–145

32. Ninet S, Schnell D, Dewitte A, Zeni F, Meziani F, Darmon M (2015) Doppler-based renal resistive index for prediction of renal dysfunction reversibility: A systematic review and meta-analysis. J Crit Care 30:629–635

33. Qin H, Wu H, Chen Y, Zhang N, Fan Z (2017) Early detection of postoperative acute kidney injury in acute stanford type a aortic dissection with Doppler renal resistive index. J Ultrasound Med 36:2105–2111

34. Hjortrup PB, Haase N, Wetterslev J et al (2017) Effects of fluid restriction on measures of circulatory efficacy in adults with septic shock. Acta Anaesthesiol Scand 61:390–398

35. Stevens PE, Gwyther SJ, Hanson ME, Boultbee JE, Kox WJ, Phillips ME (1990) Noninvasive monitoring of renal blood flow characteristics during acute renal failure in man. Intensive Care Med 16:153–158

36. Lerolle N, Guerot E, Faisy C, Bornstain C, Diehl JL, Fagon JY (2006) Renal failure in septic shock: predictive value of Doppler-based renal arterial resistive index. Intensive Care Med 32:1553–1559

37. Lauschke A, Teichgraber UK, Frei U, Eckardt KU (2006) 'Low-dose' dopamine worsens renal perfusion in patients with acute renal failure. Kidney Int 69:1669–1674

38. Deruddre S, Cheisson G, Mazoit JX, Vicaut E, Benhamou D, Duranteau J (2007) Renal arterial resistance in septic shock: effects of increasing mean arterial pressure with norepinephrine on the renal resistive index assessed with Doppler ultrasonography. Intensive Care Med 33:1557–1562

39. Darmon M, Schortgen F, Vargas F et al (2011) Diagnostic accuracy of Doppler renal resistive index for reversibility of acute kidney injury in critically ill patients. Intensive Care Med 37:68–76

40. Bossard G, Bourgoin P, Corbeau JJ, Huntzinger J, Beydon L (2011) Early detection of postoperative acute kidney injury by Doppler renal resistive index in cardiac surgery with cardiopulmonary bypass. Br J Anaesth 107:891–898

41. Schnell D, Deruddre S, Harrois A et al (2012) Renal resistive index better predicts the occurrence of acute kidney injury than cystatin C. Shock 38:592–597

42. Dewitte A, Coquin J, Meyssignac B et al (2012) Doppler resistive index to reflect regulation of renal vascular tone during sepsis and acute kidney injury. Crit Care 16:R165

43. Schnell D, Camous L, Guyomarc'h S et al (2013) Renal perfusion assessment by renal Doppler during fluid challenge in sepsis. Crit Care Med 41:1214–1220

44. Schnell D, Reynaud M, Venot M et al (2014) Resistive Index or color-Doppler semiquantitative evaluation of renal perfusion by inexperienced physicians: results of a pilot study. Minerva Anestesiol 80:1273–1281

45. Lahmer T, Rasch S, Schnappauf C, Schmid RM, Huber W (2016) Influence of volume administration on Doppler-based renal resistive index, renal hemodynamics and renal function in medical intensive care unit patients with septic-induced acute kidney injury: a pilot study. Int Urol Nephrol 48:1327–1334

46. Marty P, Ferre F, Labaste F et al (2016) The Doppler renal resistive index for early detection of acute kidney injury after hip fracture. Anaesth Crit Care Pain Med 35:377–382

47. Boddi M, Bonizzoli M, Chiostri M et al (2016) Renal Resistive Index and mortality in critical patients with acute kidney injury. Eur J Clin Invest 46:242–251

48. Regolisti G, Maggiore U, Cademartiri C et al (2017) Renal resistive index by transesophageal and transparietal echo-doppler imaging for the prediction of acute kidney injury in patients undergoing major heart surgery. J Nephrol 30:243–253

Acute Kidney Injury Risk Prediction

K. Kashani

Introduction

Acute kidney injury (AKI) is considered one of the most common complications of acute illness, with a substantial impact on patient outcome and hospital costs [1–3]. It has been reported that higher severity of AKI is associated with more severe short- and long-term mortality and morbidities. In many cases, AKI is a preventable disease. In a recent study, protocolized intervention after cardiac surgery was associated with a considerable reduction in the incidence of AKI [4]. Appropriate preventive measures need to be given in a time-sensitive manner. A delay in recognition and intervention may result in progression of injury and increase the risk of death, the need for renal replacement therapy (RRT), and likelihood of chronic kidney disease [5].

Currently, the diagnosis of AKI is based on two functional biomarkers of the kidney: serum creatinine and urinary output [6]. Unfortunately, both of these biomarkers have substantial shortcomings in the timely recognition of AKI. Serum creatinine levels can demonstrate a decrease in glomerular filtration, but only after 24 to 48 h. Given the considerable volume resuscitation and reduced serum creatinine production during critical illness, this delay is even more pronounced in patients who are admitted to the intensive care unit (ICU) [7]. Disadvantages of using urinary output as an effective AKI biomarker include a lack of specificity to AKI etiology, the widespread use of diuretics among hospitalized patients, and the unreliability of monitoring strategies.

As AKI management is very time-sensitive, finding strategies to identify high-risk patients seems the next natural step in improving AKI outcome. To achieve this goal, not only should traditional and novel risk factors be considered and identi-

K. Kashani (✉)
Division of Pulmonary and Critical Care Medicine, Mayo Clinic
Rochester, MN, USA
Division of Nephrology and Hypertension, Mayo Clinic
Rochester, MN, USA
e-mail: kashani.kianoush@mayo.edu

© Springer International Publishing AG 2018   321
J.-L. Vincent (ed.), *Annual Update in Intensive Care and Emergency Medicine 2018*,
Annual Update in Intensive Care and Emergency Medicine,
https://doi.org/10.1007/978-3-319-73670-9_25

fied, but use of forecasting tools (e.g., AKI stress test, early functional and injury biomarkers, prediction models) should also be considered. In this chapter, I describe a 3-phase strategy for clinically effective AKI risk stratification in the ICU and general hospital wards.

Phase I: Identification of AKI Risk Factors

Fig. 1 summarizes the five dimensions of AKI risk factors that need to be identified prior to an efficient prediction strategy [8, 9]. These dimensions include inherent, acute exposure/disease, process of care, socioeconomic and/or cultural, and environmental factors.

Traditional and Known AKI Risk Factors

Inherent Risk Factors
Inherent risk factors include susceptibilities of each individual patient. Age, for example, is one of the most important risk factors for AKI. In a study by Kane-Gill et al. [10], the impact of age was found to be so substantial that other risk factors (e.g., sepsis, hypertension, nephrotoxins) lost their ability to predict AKI among patients older than 75 years. The role of sex as an AKI risk factor has not been persistent in the literature, and its reliability varies with different disease entities.

Other inherent risk factors for AKI are those associated with decreased kidney reserve or failure of other organs with known cross-talk with the kidneys (e.g., heart, liver, respiratory system) [11]. For example, patients who suffer from diabetes mellitus, hypertension, or chronic kidney disease have less kidney reserve and, therefore, a greater risk of developing AKI. Genetic predisposition also should be considered as one of the inherent risk factors for AKI [12]. In one report, for example, impaired ability of the kidney to deal with hemodynamic stress was noted in individuals who had lower genotype II of the angiotensin converting enzyme (ACE) gene [13].

Acute Exposure/Disease-related AKI Risk Factors
Exposure to nephrotoxins is a known risk factor for AKI. Some of these exposures are before hospitalization (e.g., non-steroidal anti-inflammatory drugs) and some happen after patients are admitted to the hospital (e.g., contrast administration, antibiotics). The risk of AKI depends on the length and dose of exposure, as well as the number of nephrotoxic agents that a patient is exposed to. Recently, exposures to hydroxyethyl starch and high-chloride content solution, warfarin, and mechanical ventilators have been speculated as AKI risk factors among hospitalized patients [12].

Aside from the traditional and known risk factors for AKI, there are some recognized disease-specific risk factors. Many disease entities are investigated individually to evaluate the AKI risk factors specific to them. Among procedures and

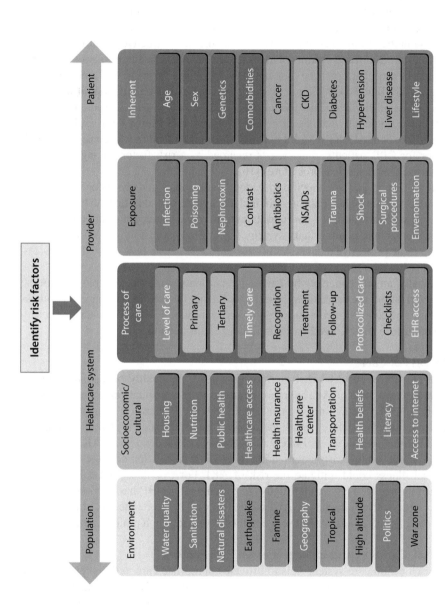

Fig. 1 Acute kidney injury (AKI) risk stratification steps – Phase 1: Identification of risk factors. *CKD*: chronic kidney disease; *NSAID*: non-steroidal anti-inflammatory drug; *EHR*: electronic health record. Adapted from [8, 9]

diseases, cardiopulmonary bypass (CPB) surgery, coronary angiography and sepsis are the most studied.

Concerning CPB surgery, several perioperative factors are considered risk factors for AKI. Among susceptibilities that are unique to CPB, congestive heart failure with left ventricular ejection fraction less than 35%, emergent procedure, severe disease in the left main coronary artery, and chronic obstructive pulmonary disease (COPD) are the more prominent risk factors for AKI. There are also procedure-related factors that could be associated with a higher risk of AKI, including the length of CPB and cross-clamp, on-pump surgery (vs off-pump), nonpulsatile flow, hemolysis and euvolemic hemodilution [14]. Prediction models based on these factors could potentially enable clinicians to risk stratify patients for cardiovascular surgery-associated AKI [15]. Interestingly, although female sex is considered a risk factor for CPB patients, male sex is regarded as a risk factor among those who undergo general surgical procedures [16].

Risk factors that are specific to patients with sepsis and are independently associated with a higher risk of AKI include female sex, duration of hypotension, delayed administration of appropriate antimicrobial therapy and infection site in the abdomen and genitourinary system. Interestingly, a history of COPD has been found to be protective against AKI in patients with sepsis (OR 0.4; 95% CI, 0.21–0.75) [17].

Finally, among patients who have acute coronary syndrome and require cardiac catheterization, the procedure-specific risk factors for AKI include amount and osmolarity of contrast media, undergoing left ventriculography, hypotension during the procedure and the need for an intra-aortic balloon pump [18].

Process of Care
One risk factor for AKI that is often ignored is the quality of care for patients with a greater risk of AKI who are admitted to the hospital for acute illness. In the community setting, increasing awareness about diseases (e.g., peripheral vasculopathy, diabetes mellitus and hypertension) and optimization of care for patients with chronic conditions will likely decrease the risk of developing AKI. Similarly, in the acute setting, early intervention to avoid the escalation of acute disease into critical illness could mitigate the risk of AKI. For example, protocolized hemodynamic management among high-risk patients after CBP has been shown to be associated with a reduction in AKI incidence [4]. Therefore, the risk of AKI would be lower at institutions that have the ability to provide such protocolized care.

Social, Cultural, and Environmental Risk Factors
When a health care system fails to provide appropriate care to the population, the risk of AKI in that population increases; therefore, both the location and the societal norms of a given population should be considered in determining such a risk. For example, in one report, the number of crush injuries reported to the Renal Disaster Relief Task Force for dialysis in Port-au-Prince, Haiti, was only 19 out of 230,000 to 300,000—well below the average reported in similar incidences [19]. This could be due to poor communication and a lack of medical infrastructure in Haiti.

A population's cultural norms can also affect AKI risk, as noted during an Ebola virus outbreak in West Africa in 2014, where burial practices greatly increased the spread of disease in rural areas [20]. In addition, the risk of AKI may be higher in populations with only limited trust in modern medical care providers.

Novel AKI Risk Factors

In recent years, there have been several reports regarding novel and previously unknown risk factors for AKI. Some of these risk factors are outlined below.

Hyperuricemia is considered to be associated with AKI due to its effect on renal vasoconstriction, pro-inflammatory effects and oxidative stress, as seen in patients who have undergone CPB surgery or cardiac angiography [21, 22]. Following observations that indicated an independent association between low albumin levels and AKI in multiple settings (particularly in surgical patients) in a systematic analysis of 3,917 patients, hypoalbuminemia was found to be an independent risk factor for AKI (OR 2.34; 95% CI 1.74–3.14), and for a higher mortality rate among those who already had AKI (OR 2.47; 95% CI 1.51–4.05) [23]. Despite these findings, albumin replacement does not seem to be associated with an improvement in outcome in patients with sepsis [24].

Another potential risk factor for AKI is obesity. A high amount of adipose tissue is known to be associated not only with hypertension, peripheral vasculopathy and diabetes, but is also related to oxidative stress and higher inflammatory cytokines [12]. Obstructive sleep apnea has been reported to have a strong association with chronic kidney disease [25]. In a recent report, its relationship with AKI was also highlighted [26]. The risk of AKI also increases for patients who have baseline hypochloremia or develop hyperchloremia during hospitalization [27, 28].

Phase II: Assign Each Individual Patient to a Risk Category

Fig. 2 describes how the collection of risk factors could be merged into an AKI prediction strategy, to assign a risk category to each patient admitted to the ICU.

Prognostic Tests

Although it is an important and necessary step in the prediction of AKI development, clinical risk stratification is not the only tool at the clinician's disposal. In clinical practice, patients who have a very low or very high risk of AKI may not need additional testing for a risk category assignment. However, further testing could help to clarify which patients are at greater risk for further prophylactic and management measures. Among these tools, biomarkers for kidney function and injury, along with furosemide stress tests (FSTs), are worth mentioning.

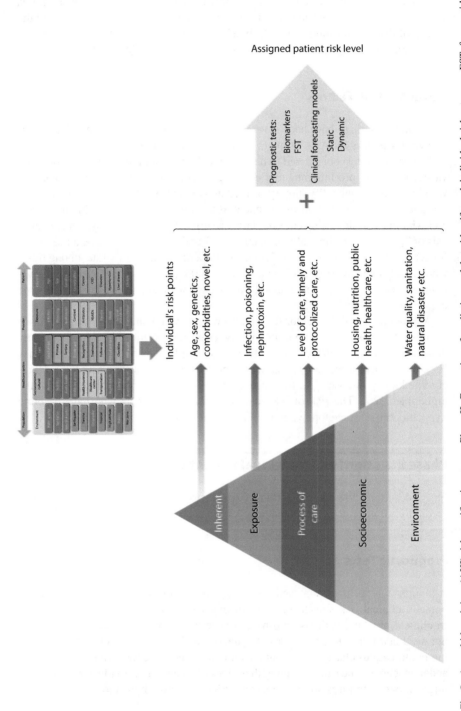

Fig. 2 Acute kidney injury (AKI) risk stratification steps – Phase II: Generation of predictive models to identify each individual risk category. *FST*: furosemide stress test. Adapted from [8, 9]

Biomarkers

In the past two decades, there has been substantial development and research in the field of AKI concerning early recognition biomarkers, which provide clinicians and investigators with the ability to risk stratify patients or enrich research populations. These markers could even be divided into groups to indicate early change in kidney function and stress of injury.

Among the early functional biomarkers of the kidney, cystatin C and proenkephalin can potentially identify changes in glomerular filtration rate (GFR) earlier than serum creatinine can [29–31]. In addition, the use of a fluorescent tracer to measure the real-time point-of-care in GFR has been recently described, which could potentially play a role in determining rapidly changing GFR during critical illness. Measuring renal reserve before a major surgical procedure could provide further information regarding the risk of AKI [32].

The main focus in AKI detection has been placed on research and development of AKI stress and injury biomarkers. Cell cycle arrest biomarkers (insulin-like growth factor-binding protein 7 [IGFBP-7] and tissue inhibitor of metalloproteinase 2 [TIMP-2]) were first introduced in 2013, and are currently available for clinical use in Europe and North America [33]. These proteins increase in urine when tubular cells are under stress and can predict moderate to severe AKI up to 12 h before its development. In plasma or urine, elevated levels of neutrophil gelatinase-associated lipocalin (NGAL)—one of the most studied kidney injury biomarkers—not only can predict AKI development, but may also be able to provide information regarding the intensity and location of the injury [34, 35]. Other injury biomarkers, including urinary kidney injury molecule-1 (KIM-1), urinary interleukin 18 (IL-18) and liver fatty acid-binding protein (L-FABP), are potentially associated with risk of AKI in different settings and could be used for risk stratification. It is critical to know that most kidney injury biomarkers have limited performance in the adult patient population and are associated with multiple comorbidities, particularly when the time of injury onset is not known. It is also important to understand that the use of biomarkers could add considerable cost and lead to insufficient results if the clinical risk of AKI and the context in which these biomarkers are measured are not considered [36].

Furosemide Stress Test

Healthy proximal tubular cells are critical in the transportation of furosemide into the tubular space; therefore, if there is an inadequate response to a preset dose of furosemide, the risk of developing AKI is dramatically higher. Chawla and colleagues [37] showed that if individuals who are well hydrated and have a high risk of AKI (or already have stage I AKI) do not excrete 200 ml of urine within 2 h in response to 1 mg/kg of furosemide (1.5 mg/kg in those who received loop diuretics within the past 7 days), their risk of progression to stage II or III AKI is greatly increased (sensitivity 87% and specificity 84%). In an independent study, Koyner et al. [38] compared FST with other kidney injury biomarkers and found FST performance to be superior to all other biomarkers.

Predictive Models

AKI forecasting models using many of the above-mentioned risk factors have been used in several settings. These models are generally divided into two distinct categories: static and dynamic.

1. Static. The static model is the most common AKI forecasting model. It is developed and validated based on a series of data that is available usually at the beginning of the medical encounter, and provides an estimated risk of AKI throughout the rest of the hospitalization period. Most static models are designed for specific diseases (e.g., CPB surgery [15], general surgery [16], coronary angiography [18]). Other static models are designed for a wide array of patients in the ICU [39] or hospital [40]. These models are computed at the bedside by clinicians or computers to provide an estimate of AKI risk on the index encounter. Although most of the developed models have a very reasonable performance, utilization has not become widespread due to difficulties gathering appropriate data and calculations.
2. Dynamic. A dynamic model is able to change its prediction score based on a continuous collection of new information. It can provide a real-time estimation of AKI risk and is more efficient for use with a computer, which then provides the processed estimation of AKI risk to the provider. As the complexity of these models is substantial, the number of available dynamic models for AKI forecasting is extremely limited. In a recent effort to generate a semidynamic model by using the random Forest technique, Flechet et al. [41] designed a series of models able to estimate AKI risk at a different timeline in comparison with ICU admission time, including availability of data. They showed that their model had excellent performance (area under the receiver operating characteristic curve was 0.82 for prediction of all AKI stages). Given the dynamic model's ability to provide real-time risk estimates and recommendations, future development should address its limited ability to adapt to any data set and provide information at point-of-care.

Phase III: Provide Early Management and Preventive Interventions

Following the development of the appropriate risk stratification strategies, merging the assigned risk category with current management or preventive interventions (e.g, Kidney Disease: Improving Global Outcomes [KDIGO] guidelines for AKI management) or future novel therapeutic interventions would have the potential to improve the care of patients with AKI (Fig. 3). This approach not only could allow clinicians to provide earlier and thus more effective interventions, but also could play a substantial role in the search for new therapeutic options in the future.

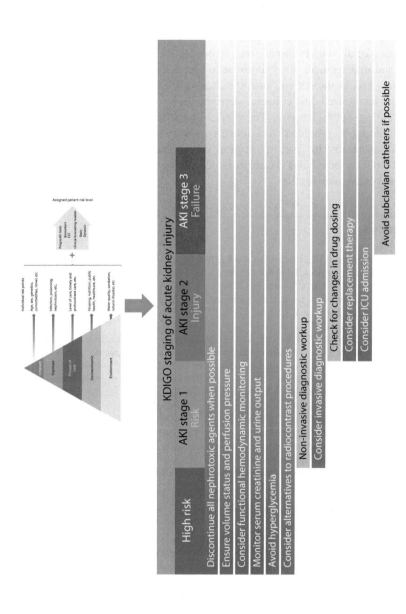

Fig. 3 Acute kidney injury (AKI) risk stratification steps – Phase III: Providing prophylactic and management strategies. Adapted from [8, 9]

Conclusion

AKI is a daunting complication of critical illness, with substantial mortality and morbidities. However, in many situations, AKI is preventable if it is found early. Diagnosis is often delayed due to the limitations of current diagnostic criteria, which enables the injury to become more intense with considerably higher sequelae. Risk stratification of all acutely ill patients enables clinicians to design appropriate prevention and management plans. In order to successfully risk stratify patients, risk factors for AKI at the patient, provider, healthcare system and population levels need to be recognized, and collected data should be used in forecasting models to identify patients at higher risk. The prediction models could be merely static, or complex enough to provide risk estimate on a continuous basis. Regardless of the methods that are used for risk stratification, surveillance of patients throughout their stay in the ICU or hospital is crucial to avoid missing the opportunity to provide effective preventive intervention.

References

1. Hsu RK, McCulloch CE, Dudley RA, Lo LJ, Hsu CY (2013) Temporal changes in incidence of dialysis-requiring AKI. J Am Soc Nephrol 24:37–42
2. Lowell L, Kathleen DL, Chi-yuan H (2009) Long-term outcomes after acute kidney injury: where we stand and how we can move forward. Am J Kidney Dis 53:928–931
3. Silver SA, Long J, Zheng Y, Chertow GM (2017) Cost of acute kidney injury in hospitalized patients. J Hosp Med 12:70–76
4. Meersch M, Schmidt C, Hoffmeier A et al (2017) Prevention of cardiac surgery-associated AKI by implementing the KDIGO guidelines in high-risk patients identified by biomarkers: the PrevAKI randomized controlled trial. Intensive Care Med 43:1551–1561
5. Himmelfarb J, Joannidis M, Molitoris B et al (2008) Evaluation and initial management of acute kidney injury. Clin J Am Soc Nephrol 3:962–967
6. KDIGO (2012) Section 2: AKI definition. Kidney Int Suppl 2:19–36
7. De Rosa S, Samoni S, Ronco C (2016) Creatinine-based definitions: from baseline creatinine to serum creatinine adjustment in intensive care. Crit Care 20:1–5
8. KDIGO (2012) Summary of recommendation statements: AKI. Kid Int Suppl 2:8–12
9. Kashani K, Macedo E, Burdmann EA et al (2017) Acute kidney injury risk assessment: differences and similarities between resource-limited and resource-rich countries. Kidney Int Rep 2:519–529
10. Kane-Gill SL, Sileanu FE, Murugan R, Trietley GS, Handler SM, Kellum JA (2014) Risk factors for acute kidney injury in older adults with critical illness: a retrospective cohort study. Am J Kidney Dis 65:860–869
11. Leblanc M, Kellum JA, Gibney RT, Lieberthal W, Tumlin J, Mehta R (2005) Risk factors for acute renal failure: inherent and modifiable risks. Curr Opin Crit Care 11:533–536
12. Varrier M, Ostermann M (2014) Novel risk factors for acute kidney injury. Curr Opin Nephrol Hypertens 23:560–569
13. du Cheyron D, Fradin S, Ramakers M et al (2008) Angiotensin converting enzyme insertion/deletion genetic polymorphism: its impact on renal function in critically ill patients. Crit Care Med 36:3178–3183
14. Rosner MH, Okusa MD (2006) Acute kidney injury associated with cardiac surgery. Clin J Am Soc Nephrol 1:19–32
15.

Thakar CV, Arrigain S, Worley S, Yared JP, Paganini EP (2005) A clinical score to predict acute renal failure after cardiac surgery. J Am Soc Nephrol 16:162–168

16. Kheterpal S, Tremper KK, Heung M et al (2009) Development and validation of an acute kidney injury risk index for patients undergoing general surgery: results from a national data set. Anesthesiology 110:505–515

17. Bagshaw S, Lapinsky S, Dial S et al (2009) Acute kidney injury in septic shock: clinical outcomes and impact of duration of hypotension prior to initiation of antimicrobial therapy. Intensive Care Med 35:871–881

18. Mehran R, Aymong ED, Nikolsky E et al (2004) A simple risk score for prediction of contrast-induced nephropathy after percutaneous coronary intervention: development and initial validation. J Am Coll Cardiol 44:1393–1399

19. Remillard BD, Buteau JH, Cleophat P (2015) Kidney care in Haiti—the role of partnerships. Nat Rev Nephrol 11:183–188

20. Nielsen CF, Kidd S, Sillah AR et al (2015) Improving burial practices and cemetery management during an Ebola virus disease epidemic – Sierra Leone, 2014. MMWR Morb Mortal Wkly Rep 64:20–27

21. Park SH, Shin WY, Lee EY et al (2011) The impact of hyperuricemia on in-hospital mortality and incidence of acute kidney injury in patients undergoing percutaneous coronary intervention. Circ J 75:692–697

22. Ejaz AA, Kambhampati G, Ejaz NI et al (2012) Post-operative serum uric acid and acute kidney injury. J Nephrol 25:497–505

23. Wiedermann CJ, Wiedermann W, Joannidis M (2010) Hypoalbuminemia and acute kidney injury: a meta-analysis of observational clinical studies. Intensive Care Med 36:1657–1665

24. Caironi P, Tognoni G, Masson S et al (2014) Albumin replacement in patients with severe sepsis or septic shock. N Engl J Med 370:1412–1421

25. Adeseun GA, Rosas SE (2010) The impact of obstructive sleep apnea on chronic kidney disease. Curr Hypertens Rep 12:378–383

26. Dou L, Lan H, Reynolds DJ et al (2017) Association between obstructive sleep apnea and acute kidney injury in critically ill patients: a propensity-matched study. Nephron 135:137–146

27. Shao M, Li G, Sarvottam K et al (2016) Dyschloremia is a risk factor for the development of acute kidney injury in critically ill patients. PLoS One 11:e160322

28. Thongprayoon C, Cheungpasitporn W, Cheng Z, Qian Q (2017) Chloride alterations in hospitalized patients: prevalence and outcome significance. PLoS One 12:e174430

29. Ng LL, Sandhu JK, Narayan H et al (2014) Proenkephalin and prognosis after acute myocardial infarction. J Am Coll Cardiol 63:280–289

30. Shah KS, Taub P, Patel M et al (2015) Proenkephalin predicts acute kidney injury in cardiac surgery patients. Clin Nephrol 83:29–35

31. Roos JF, Doust J, Tett SE, Kirkpatrick CMJ (2007) Diagnostic accuracy of cystatin C compared to serum creatinine for the estimation of renal dysfunction in adults and children—a meta-analysis. Clin Biochem 40:383–391

32. Sharma A, Mucino MJ, Ronco C (2014) Renal functional reserve and renal recovery after acute kidney injury. Nephron Clin Pract 127:94–100

33. Kashani K, Al-Khafaji A, Ardiles T et al (2013) Discovery and validation of cell cycle arrest biomarkers in human acute kidney injury. Crit Care 17:R25

34. de Geus HRH, Ronco C, Haase M, Jacob L, Lewington A, Vincent J-L (2016) The cardiac surgery-associated neutrophil gelatinase-associated lipocalin (CSA-NGAL) score: A potential tool to monitor acute tubular damage. J Thorac Cardiovasc Surg 151:1476–1481

35. Hunsicker O, Feldheiser A, Weimann A et al (2017) Diagnostic value of plasma NGAL and intraoperative diuresis for AKI after major gynecological surgery in patients treated within an intraoperative goal-directed hemodynamic algorithm: A substudy of a randomized controlled trial. Medicine (Baltimore) 96:e7357

36. Vanmassenhove J, Vanholder R, Nagler E, Van Biesen W (2013) Urinary and serum biomarkers for the diagnosis of acute kidney injury: an in-depth review of the literature. Nephrol Dial Transplant 28:254–273
37. Chawla LS, Davison DL, Brasha-Mitchell E et al (2013) Development and standardization of a furosemide stress test to predict the severity of acute kidney injury. Crit Care 17:R207
38. Koyner JL, Davison DL, Brasha-Mitchell E et al (2015) Furosemide stress test and biomarkers for the prediction of AKI severity. J Am Soc Nephrol 26:2023–2031
39. Malhotra R, Kashani KB, Macedo E et al (2017) A risk prediction score for acute kidney injury in the intensive care unit. Nephrol Dial Transplant 32:814–822
40. Koyner JL, Adhikari R, Edelson DP, Churpek MM (2016) Development of a multicenter ward-based AKI prediction model. Clin J Am Soc Nephrol 11:1935–1943
41. Flechet M, Güiza F, Schetz M et al (2017) AKIpredictor, an online prognostic calculator for acute kidney injury in adult critically ill patients: development, validation and comparison to serum neutrophil gelatinase-associated lipocalin. Intensive Care Med 43:764–773

Early Detection of Acute Kidney Injury after Cardiac Surgery: A Problem Solved?

M. Heringlake, C. Schmidt, and A. E. Berggreen

Introduction

Acute kidney injury (AKI) is a frequent complication in patients undergoing cardiac surgery and associated with increased morbidity as well as short- and long-term mortality [1]. Unfortunately, although the number of patients with severe AKI after major surgery is steadily increasing, mortality has not changed substantially for decades [2]. This contrasts sharply with other fields of critical care medicine – like the treatment of myocardial infarction – in which the development of sensitive markers of myocardial injury has fostered earlier diagnosis, rapid interventions, and thereby ultimately has led to improved outcomes [3].

It has thus been argued that the lack of medical progress in preventing and treating cardiac surgery-associated AKI as well as the poor prognosis may, at least in part, be related to the fact that the diagnosis of AKI is often delayed until kidney function is severely reduced and renal replacement becomes necessary, and that measures allowing earlier detection of kidney injury may be pivotal to develop treatments to prevent further deterioration of organ function [4].

Over recent years, a steadily increasing number of 'kidney-specific' biomarkers has been developed that have been shown to be associated with the development of AKI and/or a poor prognosis in critically ill patients and patients undergoing cardiac surgery [5–7]. Based on these observations, a paradigm shift has occurred, expanding the classical concept of AKI to a pathophysiological entity of increased renal excretion or plasma levels of renal biomarkers despite preserved glomerular filtration rate (GFR), the latter being entitled "subclinical renal injury" or "increased risk" [4, 8].

However, from the clinical perspective, the question remains whether kidney-specific biomarkers do indeed allow an earlier detection of cardiac surgery-associ-

M. Heringlake (✉) · C. Schmidt · A. E. Berggreen
Department of Anesthesiology and Intensive Care Medicine, University of Lübeck
Lübeck, Germany
e-mail: Heringlake@t-online.de

© Springer International Publishing AG 2018   333
J.-L. Vincent (ed.), *Annual Update in Intensive Care and Emergency Medicine 2018*,
Annual Update in Intensive Care and Emergency Medicine,
https://doi.org/10.1007/978-3-319-73670-9_26

ated AKI than urine flow and changes in plasma creatinine or whether alternative methods to immediately detect changes in renal function are available. In the present chapter, we summarize available knowledge on the clinical role of relevant renal biomarkers for the early detection of AKI in cardiac surgical patients and describe alternative measures for the clinical monitoring of kidney function in this field.

KDIGO AKI: Definition

According to the Kidney Disease Improving Global Outcomes Initiative (KDIGO), AKI may be defined as an abrupt decrease in kidney function that includes, but may not necessarily be limited to acute renal failure [9]. AKI may be triggered by various etiologies, among them specific kidney diseases, extrarenal pathology, toxic injury, and ischemia.

The KDIGO classification of AKI is based on urine output and serum creatinine criteria (Table 1). Although the consensus guideline acknowledges that these criteria may have limitations for the early detection and accurate estimation of renal injury, they are the current basis for all diagnostic criteria for AKI [9].

Pathophysiological Aspects

The pathophysiological mechanisms mediating AKI in cardiac surgical patients are complex [10–13]. In addition to other factors, increased activity of the renin-angiotensin-aldosteron system (RAAS), the renal sympathetic nervous system, and the tubuloglomerular feedback system plays an important role in mediating this complication [10–13].

Table 1 KDIGO staging system for the severity of Acute Kidney Injury [9]

Stage	Serum creatinine	Urine output
1	1.5–1.9 times baseline or ≥ 0.3 mg/dl (≥ 26.5 µmol/l) increase	<0.5 ml/kg/h for 6–12 h
2	2.0–2.9 times baseline	<0.5 ml/kg/h for ≥ 12 h
3	3.0 times baseline or increase in serum creatinine to ≥ 4.0 mg/dl (≥ 353.6 µmol/l) or initiation of renal replacement therapy or, in patients < 18 years, decrease in eGFR to <35 ml/min per 1.73 m^2	<0.3 ml/kg/h for ≥ 24 h or anuria for ≥ 12 h

eGFR: estimated glomerular filtration rate

Unfortunately, it is far from easy to elucidate which factors contribute to the development of cardiac surgery-associated AKI in an individual patient: patient-specific risk factors like chronic kidney disease and diabetes mellitus; prolonged duration of cardiopulmonary bypass (CPB) and perioperative ischemia/reperfusion injury; increased production of endogeneous nephrotoxins such as hemoglobin; hemodynamic disturbances; a mismatch between oxygen delivery and demand; increased production of pro-inflammatory cytokines; and prolonged postoperative respirator support have all been associated with an increased risk of AKI [10–13].

Despite being interrelated, the leading mechanism may have implications for the diagnosis of AKI in an individual patient, since, for example, inflammation has been shown to decrease renal function by different pathophysiological mechanisms [14] than changes in intratubular pressure upon experimental variation in renal blood flow or venous congestion [15]. Additionally, the effects of surgical insult – independent from what happens at the level of the kidney – need to be taken into account [16].

Biomarkers for Predicting AKI After Cardiac Surgery

Tremendous scientific effort has been made in recent years to develop specific biomarkers for the prediction of AKI. Many of these markers have been derived from renal ischemia/reperfusion animal models. The most frequently studied biomarkers are cystatin C (Cys-C), neutrophil gelatinase-associated lipocalin (NGAL), kidney-injury molecule-1 (KIM-1), and the product of tissue inhibitor of metalloproteinase-2 (TIMP-2) and insulin-like growth factor binding protein 7 (IGFBP-7).

Cystatin C

Cys-C is a low molecular weight protease inhibitor that is freely filtered by the glomeruli, completely reabsorbed by tubules but not secreted. Cys-C is produced at a constant rate by all nucleated cells and minimally bound to proteins. During normal conditions, only minimal concentrations of Cys-C are found in the urine [17]. Changes in the plasma levels of Cys-C have been shown to correlate with the GFR, thus this marker may be used to determine acute change in glomerular function. The blood levels of Cys-C are less affected by age, sex, race or overall muscle mass than creatinine [11, 17].

Urinary levels of Cys-C increase when the reabsorptive capacity of proximal tubular cells is impaired. The urinary excretion of this peptide may therefore also be used as an endogenous marker for the severity of acute tubular damage [17]. As an important confounder, the reabsorption of Cys-C (by receptor-mediated endocytosis) competes with excess albumin in urine. Since glomerular damage after cardiac surgery is often associated with albuminuria (see below), changes in glomerular function may also lead to a decrease in the tubular uptake of Cys-C [17].

Increased plasma Cys-C levels immediately after surgery identified patients with renal complications [18]. However, despite immediate normalization of plasma creatinine levels after surgery, postoperative plasma Cys-C levels have been shown to increase up to the third postoperative day in parallel with C-reactive protein (CRP) [19], suggesting that Cys-C levels may also increase as an acute phase inflammatory response.

As part of a large observational trial, Koyner and colleagues analyzed the predictive capacity of urinary Cys-C for mild and severe AKI in more than 1,200 adult cardiac surgical patients. Mild correlations between urinary Cys-C were observed within the first 12 h after surgery; however, after adjustment for potential confounders, this effect was no longer statistically significant [20]. In the same cohort of patients, the role of Cys-C for preoperative prediction and early postoperative detection of AKI was analyzed [21, 22]. These analyses showed that preoperative Cys-C enabled improved prediction of AKI in comparison with serum creatinine [21]; however, postoperative Cys-C had a lower predictability for AKI than plasma creatinine level [22].

A recent meta-analysis revealed only a moderate composite area under the curve (AUC) of Cys-C for predicting AKI: 0.69 (0.63–0.74) in five studies analyzing serum or plasma, and 0.63 (95% CI: 0.37 to 0.89) in three studies using urine [7].

Neutrophil Gelatinase-Associated Lipocalin

NGAL was originally identified as a 25 kDa protein of the family of lipocalins covalently bound to gelatinase from human neutrophils and is stored in neutrophil granules [23]. Physiologically, NGAL has the capacity to bind iron-siderophore complexes as a bacteriostatic function and additionally provides anti-apoptotic effects, is important for local defense against infection, and enhances proliferation of renal tubular cells. In addition to the distal tubule and the collecting duct of the kidney, NGAL is expressed on various cell types such as bone marrow, lung, trachea and colon [23]. NGAL transcription is upregulated after ischemic, septic or toxic AKI, suggesting that this peptide may be used as an early marker of structural renal tubular damage. Additionally, reabsorption of glomerular filtered NGAL by proximal tubular cells may be disturbed during AKI [17, 23]. Typically there is an initial increase in NGAL in the urine, followed by a rise in the plasma concentration [23]. The diagnostic performance of NGAL is significantly influenced by baseline renal function [24] and the duration of CPB [25, 26].

A recent meta-analysis showed that the predictive capacity of postoperative NGAL levels for AKI is only moderate with an AUC of 0.72 (0.66–0.79) for urinary samples (16 studies) and 0.71 (0.64–0.77) for plasma or serum samples (6 studies) [7].

Kidney-Injury Molecule-1

KIM-1 is a 38.7 kDa type I transmembrane glycoprotein. It is expressed in the proximal tubule of the kidney as well as in other organs and is upregulated after ischemia/reperfusion injury or drug-induced injury of the kidney. Therefore, it is a marker of proliferation and regeneration of proximal tubular cells and mediates phagocytosis of apoptotic cells in post-ischemic kidney [23]. It has been suggested that KIM-1 could be helpful to distinguish between ischemic AKI and prerenal azotemia or chronic kidney disease and predict adverse clinical outcomes [23]. However, comparable to Cys-C and NGAL, the capacity of urinary KIM-1 to predict cardiac surgery-associated AKI is only moderate (AUC: 0.72 (0.59–0.84); 6 studies) [7]. Of note, again similar to Cys-C and NGAL, in some studies, pre-operative KIM-1 had a comparable or even better predictive capacity for cardiac surgery-associated AKI than the immediate postoperative urinary levels [27].

Tissue Inhibitor of Metalloproteinase-2 and Insulin-Like Growth Factor Binding Protein-7

TIMP-2 and IGFBP-7 are among the most promising biomarkers for AKI. TIMP-2 is expressed and secreted from distal tubular cells, whereas IGFBP-7 is secreted mostly from proximal tubule cells [23]. Both peptides induce G1 cell cycle arrest to prevent tubular cells with damaged DNA from dividing. Recent *in vitro* data show that acute reduction of oxygen and/or nutrients suppressed basal secretion, while restoration of oxygen or nutritive supplementation led to a rapid increase in the excretion of both peptides [28].

In an observational trial analyzing the association between plasma levels and urinary excretion of almost 300 peptides and moderate or severe AKI in critically ill patients, the product of the urinary excretion of TIMP-2 and IGFBP-7 showed predictive capacity with an AUC of 0.8, which was significantly higher than the AUC of all other tested peptides, including NGAL, KIM-1 and liver-type fatty acid-binding protein (L-FABP) [29]. A recent meta-analysis in critically ill patients supports these findings with a pooled AUC of 0.846 ± 0.027 [30].

However, the results of studies of patients undergoing cardiac surgery are inconclusive. Although some studies showed that the postoperative time-course of urinary TIMP-2 and IGFBP-7 – determined with a commercially available bed-side test (Nephrocheck®) – may be used for early detection of AKI and renal risk stratification in the cardiac surgical setting [31, 32], Finge et al. recently observed that in two thirds of patients, AKI could not be accurately predicted by [TIMP-2] × [IGFBP-7] [33].

Although TIMP-2 and IGFBP-7 are among the most promising biomarkers for early detection of AKI, clinical data on potential confounders are still sparse. For example, no data are available on whether the duration of CPB has a comparable influence on the urinary excretion of these markers, as has been shown for NGAL and KIM-1 [25, 26]. Another limitation is that most studies investigating the predictive capacity of TIMP-2 and IGFBP-7 for AKI (usually employing the Nephrocheck® system) did not adjust the urinary peptide levels for creatinine excretion; although such adjustments may impact on the postoperative time course of TIMP-2 and IGFBP-7 excretion [31] and may lead to variable associations with outcomes [34].

Taken together, current evidence does not support the suggestion that currently used renal biomarkers are a clinically reliable method for early detection of AKI in the cardiac surgical setting. Some authors have suggested that a combination of biomarkers may increase the accuracy for early detection of this complication [35]. However, adequately powered studies supporting this concept are still missing.

Other Biomarkers

The field of renal biomarker research is rapidly expanding and there are many new markers undergoing research for early detection of AKI. However, most peptides have only been investigated in relatively small samples and thus most findings need to be replicated in larger populations.

Biochemical Methods for Early Detection of AKI

Repetitive Determination of Creatinine Concentrations

Although changes in serum creatinine are the basis for grading AKI according to the KDIGO criteria and for calculating GFR (from additional measurements of urinary creatinine excretion), this variable has frequently been criticized as being a far from optimal functional biomarker of AKI, because serum creatinine concentrations are influenced by various potential confounders, e.g., hemodilution due to fluid resuscitation. However, Lassnigg and coworkers have shown that perioperative changes in creatinine – expressed as delta creatinine based on preoperative baseline and the highest postoperative creatinine values within 48 h after surgery – have important prognostic implications [36]. Similarly, De Loor et al. recently reported that delta-creatinine within the first 4 h after surgery had excellent predictive value for cardiac surgery-associated AKI grade 2 [37].

Urinary Albumin Concentration

Increased urinary albumin excretion is a pathophysiological mediator of glomerular sclerosis and a hallmark of chronic kidney disease. Sugimoto et al. demonstrated that elevated urinary albumin measured on admission to the ICU correlated significantly with the development of AKI in pediatric patients [38]; findings that have been replicated by several other groups in pediatric cardiac surgical populations.

Unfortunately, only sparse data on the use of urinary albumin excretion for predicting AKI after adult cardiac surgery are available. Outside the cardiac surgical setting, but in a population with a comparable risk profile – patients with acute myocardial infarction – Tziakas et al. showed that a urinary albumin/creatinine ratio of > 66.7 µg/mg had a predictive accuracy for AKI better than urinary NGAL and urinary or serum cystatin C in [39]. The Translational Research Investigating Biomarker Endpoints (TRIBE)-AKI consortium analyzed the association of urinary biomarkers (including urinary albumin) and AKI in 1,198 adult cardiac surgical patients and showed that increased albuminuria immediately after surgery was associated with an increased risk for AKI. Interestingly, in this study, the albumin/creatinine ratio was not predictive of AKI [40].

Very recently, Levey and coworkers systematically analyzed the use of GFR and albumin excretion for detection and grading of acute as well as chronic kidney disease in adults and concluded that estimated GFR (eGFR) and the urine albumin/creatinine ratio in a spot urine specimen enabled an initial assessment of the presence or absence of kidney disease and its severity [41].

Technical Methods for Early Detection of AKI

Ultrasound Techniques

Doppler estimates of renal blood flow, such as maximal systolic blood flow velocity, renal resistive index (RRI) and the renal pulsatility index, are established parameters for the evaluation of renal perfusion [42]. These variables may be determined by transesophageal echocardiography (TEE) or conventional renal ultrasonography. Repeated measurements could thus be easily performed throughout the perioperative period.

The RRI is calculated as the ratio between delta velocity (renal peak systolic velocity minus end-diastolic velocity) and peak systolic velocity. The pulsatility index is the ratio between delta velocity (peak systolic velocity minus end-diastolic velocity) and mean renal blood flow velocity. Bossard and colleagues showed that the immediate postoperative RRI predicted a postoperative increase in serum creatinine and the need for renal replacement therapy in a cohort of 65 cardiac surgical patients at risk for cardiac surgery-associated AKI [43]. Comparable findings were reported in patients undergoing transcutaneous aortic valve implantation and in patients with aortic dissection. A recent meta-analysis (9 studies) concluded that "elevated RRI or pulsatility index was associated with an increased risk of persistent AKI with an odds ratio of 29.8" [44]. However, taking into account that no multicenter data are available and it is presently unclear to which extent renal ultrasound parameters are influenced by hemodynamics and the individual characteristics of the arterial vascular tree, this technology needs to be studied more rigorously before implementation into clinical routine.

Tissue Oxygenation Monitoring

Regional tissue oxygenation monitoring using near-infrared spectroscopy (NIRS) – rimarily developed for the monitoring of cerebral blood flow and cerebral oxygen saturation – is increasingly used 'extracerebrally' for monitoring systemic and organ perfusion. Several studies in pediatric patients undergoing cardiac surgery suggest that renal oxygenation determined by NIRS may be used to determine renal perfusion and that low renal oxygenation is associated with an increased risk of AKI. Comparable observations were made intraoperatively in adult patients [45]. Unfortunately, no data on the use of renal NIRS for the early detection of AKI in adult patients after cardiac surgery are available. Although this monitoring approach is rather attractive due its continuous and non-invasive nature and could be easily employed for monitoring of kidney function in the perioperative period, obvious technology-specific limitations, such as the depth of tissue penetration in lean versus obese patients, need to be addressed ahead of larger studies.

Direct Monitoring of Glomerular Filtration Rate

As outlined above, the lack of precise tools for direct monitoring of GFR is still an important limitation in critical care nephrology, since the available bedside clearance techniques (either based on creatinine or Cys-C) lack reliability during short sampling periods and are often difficult to integrate into clinical practice. Thus, in recent years, there has been an increasing interest in developing methods for direct monitoring of GFR, e.g., by fluorescent technology [46]. Although these technologies show promising results compared with established radio-labelled clearing techniques during experimental conditions, they will not be readily available for clinical use within the next few years.

Pharmacological Methods for Early Detection of AKI

The furosemide stress test (FST) is a novel means of assessing tubular function. During the test, patients receive a standardized high-dose of 1 mg/kg of furosemide in naive patients or 1.5 mg/kg furosemide in patients with prior exposure to furosemide. The urine output 2 h after the administration of furosemide has a predictive capacity to identify clinically euvolemic patients with severe and progressive AKI. A 2 h urinary output of less than 200 ml after a FST has a sensitivity of 87.1% and a specificity of 84.1% for AKI progression [47]. Unfortunately, no specific data on the use of the FST in cardiac surgical patients are available. Thus it is presently unknown whether this test has comparable predictability in this specific population. Additionally, one has to remember that the use of furosemide may itself trigger AKI after cardiac surgery [48] and thus the safety of this diagnostic approach in these patients remains to be determined ahead of larger studies.

Conclusion

Taken together, early detection of AKI after cardiac surgery is a problem that is far from being solved. Despite considerable effort to find biomarkers that may serve as 'troponins' for the kidney, the predictive capacity is at best moderate. This may be an expression of potential confounders and the complex pathophysiology, but may also reflect the lack of a precise gold standard to determine the severity of acute kidney disease. Without doubt, functional grading systems, like the KDIGO criteria have been a huge step forward towards a better understanding of acute renal disease. Nonetheless, the variables behind these grading systems – creatinine and urine flow – may be clinically influenced in many ways.

Consequently, future developments will depend on bedside techniques to grade kidney function with high reliability, e.g., technologies for the continuous monitoring of glomerular filtration and tubular function. While point-of-care GFR monitoring will hopefully be available in the future [49], no tools for continuous online monitoring of tubular function are currently on the horizon.

Until then, as depicted in Fig. 1, the available evidence suggests that the most reliable method for early detection of AKI in the immediate postoperative period after cardiac surgery is currently the immediate and repeated postoperative determination of serum creatinine for calculation of delta-creatinine [40].

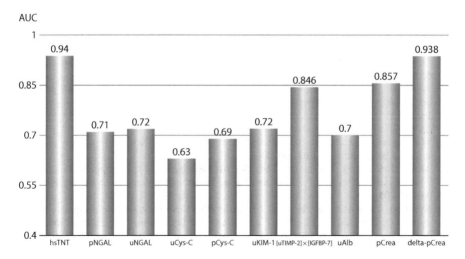

Fig. 1 Predictive capacity (presented as areas under the curve [AUC]) of frequently used biomarkers for acute kidney injury (AKI), derived from recent meta-analyses (neutrophil gelatinase-associated lipocalin [NGAL], cystatin C [Cys-C], kidney injury molecule [KIM]-1, tissue inhibitor of metalloproteinase 2 × insulin-like growth factor-binding protein 7 [TIMP-2] × [IGFBP-7]) or larger trials (albumin [Alb], creatinine [Crea], change in plasma creatinine [delta-pCrea]) compared to the predictive capacity of high-sensitive troponin-T (hsTNT) [49] for acute myocardial infarction. *p*: plasma; *u*: urinary

References

1. Hu J, Chen R, Liu S, Xu X, Zou J, Ding X (2016) Global incidence and outcomes of adult patients with acute kidney injury after cardiac surgery: a systematic review and meta-analysis. J Cardiothorac Vasc Anesth 30:82–89
2. Siddiqui NF, Coca SG, Devereaux PJ et al (2012) Secular trends in acute dialysis after elective major surgery 1995 to 2009. CMAJ 184:1237–1245
3. Dégano IR, Salomaa V, Veronesi G et al (2015) Twenty-five-year trends in myocardial infarction attack and mortality rates, and case-fatality, in six European populations. Heart 101:1413–1421
4. Soares DM, Pessanha JF, Sharma A, Brocca A, Ronco C (2017) Delayed nephrology consultation and high mortality on acute kidney injury: a meta-analysis. Blood Purif 43:57–67
5. Lombi F, Muryan A, Canzonieri R, Trimarchi H (2016) Biomarkers in acute kidney injury: evidence or paradigm? Nefrologia 36:339–346
6. Vandenberghe W, De Loor J, Hoste EAJ (2017) Diagnosis of cardiac-surgery associated acute kidney injury from functional to damage biomarkers. Curr Opin Anaesthesiol 30:66–75
7. Ho J, Tangri N, Komenda P et al (2015) Urinary, plasma, and serum biomarkers' utility for predicting acute kidney injury associated with cardiac surgery in adults: a meta-analysis. Am J Kidney Dis 66:993–1005
8. Huen SC, Parikh CR (2015) Molecular phenotyping of clinical AKI with novel urinary biomarkers. Am J Physiol Renal Physiol 309:F406–F413
9. KDIGO (2012) Clinical practice guideline for acute kidney injury. Kidney Int 2(Suppl 2):1–149
10. Fuhrman DY, Kellum JA (2017) Epidemiology and pathophysiology of cardiac surgery-associated acute kidney injury. Curr Opin Anaesthesiol 30:60–65
11. Ortega-Loubon C, Fernández-Molina M, Carrascal-Hinojal Y, Fulquet-Carreras E (2016) Cardiac surgery-associated acute kidney injury. Ann Card Anaesth 19:687–698
12. Moore EM, Bellomo R, Nichol AD (2012) The meaning of acute kidney injury and its relevance to intensive care and anaesthesia. Anaesth Intensive Care 40:929–948
13. Wang Y, Bellomo R (2017) Cardiac surgery-associated acute kidney injury: risk factors, pathophysiology and treatment. Nat Rev Nephrol 13:697–711
14. Gómez H, Kellum JA (2016) Sepsis-induced acute kidney injury. Curr Opin Crit Care 22:546–553
15. Wei J, Song J, Jiang S et al (2017) Role of intratubular pressure during the ischemic phase in acute kidney injury. Am J Physiol Renal Physiol 312:F1158–F1165
16. Parissis H, Mbarushimana S, Ramesh BC et al (2015) The impact of off-pump surgery in end-organ function: practical end-points. J Cardiothorac Surg 10:159
17. Mårtensson J, Martling CR, Bell M (2012) Novel biomarkers of acute kidney injury and failure: clinical applicability. Br J Anaesth 109:843–850
18. Mosa OF, Skitek M, Kalisnik JM, Jerin A (2016) Evaluation of serum cysteine-rich protein 61 and cystatin C levels for assessment of acute kidney injury after cardiac surgery. Ren Fail 38:699–705
19. Svensson AS, Kvitting JP, Kovesdy CP, Cederholm I, Szabó Z (2016) Changes in serum cystatin C, creatinine, and C-reactive protein after cardiopulmonary bypass in patients with normal preoperative kidney function. Nephrology (Carlton) 21:519–525
20. Koyner JL, Garg AX, Shlipak MG et al (2013) Urinary cystatin C and acute kidney injury after cardiac surgery. Am J Kidney Dis 61:730–738
21. Shlipak MG, Coca SG, Wang Z et al (2011) Presurgical serum cystatin C and risk of acute kidney injury after cardiac surgery. Am J Kidney Dis 58:366–373
22. Spahillari A, Parik CR, Sint K et al (2012) Serum cystatin C – versus creatinine-based definitions of acute kidney injury following cardiac surgery: a prospective cohort study. Am J Kidney Dis 60:922–929

23. Kashani K, Cheungpasitporn W, Ronco C (2017) Biomarkers of acute kidney injury: the pathway from discovery to clinical adoption. Clin Chem Lab Med 55:1074–1089
24. McIlroy DR, Wagener G, Lee HT (2010) Neutrophil gelatinase-associated lipocalin and acute kidney injury after cardiac surgery: the effect of baseline renal function on diagnostic performance. Clin J Am Soc Nephrol 5:211–219
25. Wagener G, Jan M, Kim M et al (2006) Association between increases in urinary neutrophil gelatinase-associated lipocalin and acute renal dysfunction after adult cardiac surgery. Anesthesiology 105:485–491
26. Paarmann H, Charitos EI, Beilharz A et al (2013) Duration of cardiopulmonary bypass is an important confounder when using biomarkers for early diagnosis of acute kidney injury in cardiac surgical patients. Appl Cardiopulm Pathophysiol 17:284–297
27. Koyner JL, Vaidya VS, Bennett MR et al (2010) Urinary biomarkers in the clinical prognosis and early detection of acute kidney injury. Clin J Am Soc Nephrol 5:2154–2165
28. Emlet DR, Pastor-Soler N, Marciszyn A et al (2017) Insulin-like growth factor binding protein 7 and tissue inhibitor of metalloproteinases-2: differential expression and secretion in human kidney tubule cells. Am J Physiol Renal Physiol 312:F284–F296
29. Kashani K, Al-Khafaji A, Ardiles T et al (2013) Discovery and validation of cell cycle arrest biomarkers in human acute kidney injury. Crit Care 17:R25
30. Jia HM, Huang LF, Zheng Y, Li WX (2017) Diagnostic value of urinary tissue inhibitor of metalloproteinase-2 and insulin-like growth factor binding protein 7 for acute kidney injury: a meta-analysis. Crit Care 21:77
31. Meersch M, Schmidt C, Van Aken H et al (2014) Urinary TIMP-2 and IGFBP7 as early biomarkers of acute kidney injury and renal recovery following cardiac surgery. PLoS One 9:e93460
32. Pilarczyk K, Edayadiyil-Dudasova M, Wendt D et al (2015) Urinary [TIMP-2]*[IGFBP7] for early prediction of acute kidney injury after coronary artery bypass surgery. Ann Intensive Care 5:50
33. Finge T, Bertran S, Roger C et al (2017) Interest of urinary [TIMP-2] × [IGFBP-7] for predicting the occurrence of acute kidney injury after cardiac surgery: a gray zone approach. Anesth Analg 125:762–769
34. Ralib AM, Pickering JW, Shaw GM et al (2012) Test characteristics of urinary biomarkers depend on quantitation method in acute kidney injury. J Am Soc Nephrol 23:322–333
35. Elmedany SM, Naga SS, Elsharkawy R, Mahrous RS, Elnaggar AI (2017) Novel urinary biomarkers and the early detection of acute kidney injury after open cardiac surgeries. J Crit Care 40:171–177
36. Lassnigg A, Schmidlin D, Mouhieddine M et al (2004) Minimal changes of serum creatinine predict prognosis in patients after cardiothoracic surgery: a prospective cohort study. J Am Soc Nephrol 15:1597–1605
37. De Loor J, Herck I, Francois K et al (2017) Diagnosis of cardiac surgery-associated acute kidney injury: differential roles of creatinine, chitinase 3-like protein 1 and neutrophil gelatinase-associated lipocalin: a prospective cohort study. Ann Intensive Care 7:24
38. Sugimoto K, Toda Y, Iwasaki T et al (2016) Urinary albumin levels predict development of acute kidney injury after pediatric cardiac surgery: a prospective observational study. J Cardiothorac Vasc Anesth 30:64–68
39. Tziakas D, Chalikias G, Kareli D et al (2015) Spot urine albumin to creatinine ratio outperforms novel acute kidney injury biomarkers in patients with acute myocardial infarction. Int J Cardiol 197:48–55
40. Molnar AO, Parikh CR, Sint K et al (2012) Association of postoperative proteinuria with AKI after cardiac surgery among patients at high risk. Clin J Am Soc Nephrol 7:1749–1760
41. Levey AS, Becker C, Inker LA (2015) Glomerular filtration rate and albuminuria for detection and staging of acute and chronic kidney disease in adults: a systematic review. JAMA 313:837–846

42. Momen A, Thomas K, Blaha C et al (2006) Renal vasoconstrictor responses to static exercise during orthostatic stress in humans: effects of the muscle mechano- and the baroreflexes. J Physiol 573:819–825

43. Bossard G, Bourgoin P, Corbeau JJ, Huntzinger J, Beydon L (2011) Early detection of postoperative acute kidney injury by Doppler renal resistive index in cardiac surgery with cardiopulmonary bypass. Br J Anaesth 107:891–898

44. Ninet S, Schnell D, Dewitte A, Zeni F, Meziani F, Darmon M (2015) Doppler-based renal resistive index for prediction of renal dysfunction reversibility: A systematic review and meta-analysis. J Crit Care 30:629–635

45. Choi DK, Kim WJ, Chin JH et al (2014) Intraoperative renal regional oxygen desaturation can be a predictor for acute kidney injury after Cardiac Surgery. J Cardiothorac Vasc Anesth 28:564–571

46. Molitoris BA, Reilly E (2016) Quantifying glomerular filtration rates in acute kidney injury: a requirement for translational success. Semin Nephrol 36:31–41

47. Chawla LS, Danielle L et al (2013) Development and standardization of a furosemide stress test to predict the severity of acute kidney injury. Crit Care 17:R207

48. Lassnigg A, Schmid ER, Hiesmayr M et al (2008) Impact of minimal increases in serum creatinine on outcome in patients after cardiothoracic surgery: do we have to revise current definitions of acute renal failure? Crit Care Med 36:1129–1137

49. Rubini Gimenez M, Twerenbold R, Reichlin T et al (2014) Direct comparison of high-sensitivity-cardiac troponin I vs. T for the early diagnosis of acute myocardial infarction. Eur Heart J 35:2303–2323

Biomarker-guided Care Bundles for Acute Kidney Injury: The Time has Come

J. A. Kellum, A. Zarbock, and I. Göcze

Introduction

Although acute kidney injury (AKI) is not a single disease but rather a loose collection of syndromes [1] brought on by a wide array of insults (e.g., sepsis, drugs, toxins, surgery, cardiac dysfunction), there are some general principles that can be applied to its prevention and management. For example, the 2012 Kidney Disease Improving Global Outcomes (KDIGO) clinical practice guideline recommends a series of prevention and stage-based management steps (Fig. 1; [2]). Although general consensus exists around these interventions, they have only recently come under evaluation in clinical trials [3, 4].

Three major challenges exist for operationalizing these actions in clinical trial protocols. First, the effect size from each individual step is expected to be small so investigators have generally combined multiple steps into a 'care bundle'. Bundles have advantages for adoption and for generating a positive effect through combined efficacy of the individual interventions. However, they complicate the interpretation of the studies that use them. We cannot know, for example, which components of

J. A. Kellum (✉)
The Center for Critical Care Nephrology, Department of Critical Care Medicine, University of Pittsburgh School of Medicine, and University of Pittsburgh Medical Center
Pittsburgh, USA
e-mail: kellumja@upmc.edu

A. Zarbock
The Center for Critical Care Nephrology, Department of Critical Care Medicine, University of Pittsburgh School of Medicine, and University of Pittsburgh Medical Center
Pittsburgh, USA
Department of Anesthesiology, Intensive Care Medicine and Pain Medicine, University Hospital Münster
Münster, Germany

I. Göcze
Department of Surgery, University Hospital Regensburg
Regensburg, Germany

© Springer International Publishing AG 2018   345
J.-L. Vincent (ed.), *Annual Update in Intensive Care and Emergency Medicine 2018*,
Annual Update in Intensive Care and Emergency Medicine,
https://doi.org/10.1007/978-3-319-73670-9_27

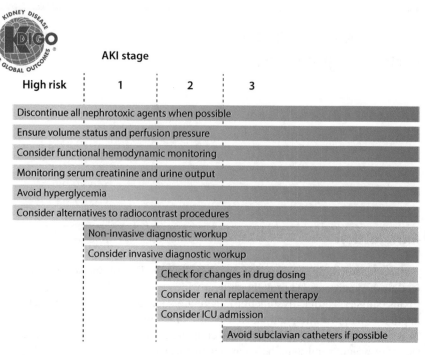

Fig. 1 Stage-based management of acute kidney injury (AKI). Shading of boxes indicates priority of action—solid shading indicates actions that are equally appropriate at all stages whereas graded shading indicates increasing priority as intensity increases. From [2] with permission

a care bundle are most critical to the success of the 'package' or, when a bundle fails, whether certain components actually caused harm while others were beneficial. Second, interventions for AKI will also need to be specific to the patient population being studied. Even care bundles will need to be tailored because the interventions differ in terms of specific medications to avoid or hemodynamic targets. For example, in two recent trials, the implementation of KDIGO bundles differed according to the patients. In a trial in cardiac surgery, inotropes, vasopressors and fluids were managed according to a hemodynamic support algorithm based on stroke volume variation [3]. Conversely, in a trial in elective, non-cardiac surgery patients, fluid use was controlled in the intervention arm using fluid challenge, passive leg raise or ultrasound evaluation of the inferior vena cava [4]. This latter trial did not control inotropes or vasopressors. Both trials addressed nephrotoxic drug use, but in different ways. In the end, the KDIGO bundle will likely look different for different patients and in different settings. Third, there is a deficient adherence to applying bundles. Most physicians believe that they adequately apply guidelines and bundles to their patients. However, it has been shown in other fields of medicine (e.g., sepsis) that the compliance to adhere to guidelines is low [5]. The application of all measures of the bundle is important as the pathophysiology of AKI is very complex and consists of renal ischemia, reperfusion, inflammation, oxidative stress, hemolysis and toxins. Applying the KDIGO bundle is a multifactorial approach that may improve renal perfusion and reduces inflammation and oxidative stress.

Cardiac Surgery: The PrevAKI Study

In the PrevAKI study, Meersch and colleagues studied the effect of a "KDIGO bundle" consisting of optimization of volume status and hemodynamics, avoidance of nephrotoxic drugs (mainly angiotensin-converting enzyme [ACE] inhibitors, angiotensin II receptor blockers, and non-steroidal anti-inflammatory drugs [NSAIDs]) and preventing hyperglycemia in cardiac surgery patients at high risk of AKI [3]. High-risk patients were identified using urinary insulin-like growth factor-binding protein 7 (IGFBP-7) and tissue inhibitor of metalloproteinases-2 (TIMP-2). This bundle reduced the rate of AKI compared to controls (55.1 vs. 71.7%; absolute risk reduction [ARR] 16.6% [95 CI 5.5–27.9%]; p = 0.004). Even moderate-to-severe AKI was reduced with this intervention (29.7 vs. 44.9%; ARR 15.2% [95% CI, 4.0–26.5%]; p = 0.009).

The implementation of the bundle resulted in significantly improved hemodynamics, less hyperglycemia and less use of ACE inhibitors or angiotensin II receptor blockers compared to controls. Although mortality rates (about 5% at 30-days and 7% at 90-days) and dialysis rates were not impacted by the bundle, a 23% relative risk reduction was attained for the primary endpoint, AKI (34% for stage 2–3 AKI). Even the same proportional effect on mortality (a 23 or 34% relative risk reduction) would have translated into a 1.6 or 2.4% ARR and would have required more than 10 times the sample size to evaluate.

Efforts to increase renal blood flow using fluids and vasodilators have failed to prevent or treat AKI. By contrast, nephrotoxins and cardiac dysfunction are probably the two major pathogenic factors in cardiac surgery-associated AKI. During the study by Meersch et al., significantly more patients in the intervention group (31.2%) received dobutamine compared to the control group (9.4%; p < 0.001) resulting in significantly increased mean arterial and central venous pressures [3]. Together with the reduction in nephrotoxins, inotropic support may well have been a decisive intervention.

As the KDIGO bundle may contradict other guidelines, it might be better to apply this bundle only to a selected group of patients, especially to patients at high risk for AKI. For example, the American College of Cardiology/American Heart Association (ACC/AHA) guidelines for cardiac surgery recommend initiating (or resuming) ACE inhibitors/angiotensin II receptor blockers after cardiac surgery in patients without contraindications [6]. Thus, withholding these agents in patients without a high risk for AKI would be unnecessary and potentially dangerous.

Non-Cardiac Surgery: The BigpAK Study

In the Biomarker Guided Intervention for Prevention of Acute Kidney Injury (Big-pAK) study, Göcze et al. implemented a care bundle consisting of functional hemo-dynamic monitoring, increased fluid administration for fluid responsive patients and nephrology consultation for adjustment of potential nephrotoxic medication and additional advice on managing the hemodynamic, acid-base and electrolyte status [4]. This version of the KDIGO bundle was applied to patients undergoing major elective non-cardiac surgery and who had at least one additional risk factor for AKI, such as age > 75, critical illness, pre-existing chronic kidney disease (estimated glomerular filtration rate [eGFR] < 60 ml/min) or intraoperative use of an intravenous radio-contrast agent. The intervention resulted in marginally lower rates of AKI (odds ratio [OR] 0.51 [95% CI, 0.24, 1.08]; p = 0.076) (the primary endpoint), and significantly lower rates of moderate-to-severe AKI (OR 0.29 [0.09, 0.96] p = 0.04), a key secondary endpoint. Moreover, ICU length of stay decreased by a day with the intervention (p = 0.035) and hospital length of stay decreased by 5 days (p = 0.04). Interestingly, despite additional fluid infusion during the intervention, the intervention group did not have increased fluid administration. Daily fluid balance for day 1 did not differ between the 2 groups, and fluid balance was lower on day 2 in the intervention group (864 vs. 1,342 ml; p = 0.023). Although additional fluid administration in patients with already established AKI has detrimental effects on renal recovery [7], appropriate fluid resuscitation and kidney protection in patients with tubular cellular stress in the "pre-AKI phase" was associated with a significant decrease in postoperative creatinine and biomarker values in the BigpAK study.

Sepsis and Nephrotoxic Drugs

Care bundles have also been developed for septic AKI but to our knowledge have not been studied. The use of strategies to limit AKI in the setting of multiple nephrotoxic drugs should also be noted, especially in pediatrics [8]. Opportunities to reduce the incidence or consequences of AKI in these patients are considerable. Sepsis is the most common cause of AKI in the critically ill [9] and drugs represent a common and underappreciated etiology. Indeed, reducing nephrotoxicity is a priority in any KDIGO bundle.

For sepsis, an important starting point is to realize that AKI is often the sepsis-defining organ failure in a patient with infection. For example, in patients with community-acquired pneumonia (CAP), AKI occurred in 631 of 1,836 patients (34%) [10]. However, even in patients without other organ failures (n = 1,264), AKI occurred in 302 patients (24%) and was associated with a similar impact on 1-year mortality (15 vs. 25% compared to 20 vs. 36% for the overall cohort—odds ratios of 1.89 and 2.25 respectively). Furthermore, when AKI was the only organ failure present, mortality was similar to other cases of single-organ failure. Thus, any care bundles for patients with infection need to first consider early identification of AKI and hence, sepsis.

Next, because septic AKI is a disease of tubular epithelial cell injury, possibly with superimposed microvascular dysfunction [11], and is characterized by increased inflammation [12], it is important to limit further inflammatory and oxidative injury. Despite being life-saving, antibiotics worsen AKI in experimental models [13] and numerous association studies and even some interventional trials have confirmed this risk in humans [8]. Certain drug combinations appear to be particularly problematic. For example, the concomitant use of piperacillin/tazobactam and vancomycin appears to be strongly associated with AKI even when confounding variables (e.g., indication) are controlled for [14]. Efforts to reduce exposure to certain nephrotoxic antibiotics/combinations in high-risk patients are underway from multiple sources.

Another contributor to AKI in sepsis is the composition of fluids used for resuscitation. Perner and colleagues reported that using Ringer's acetate solution instead of hydroxyethyl starch (HES) resulted in less AKI, less use of renal replacement therapy (RRT) and improved 90-day survival [15]. Although, the benefit of this single intervention was small in absolute terms—the risk of stage 2–3 AKI decreased by 7% (p = 0.04) and mortality decreased by 8% (p = 0.03)—the relative risk reduction was 16% for both. Therefore, from a patient point of view, avoiding this one nephrotoxin prevented AKI and death in nearly 1 in 6. Considerable pre-clinical [16], observational [17] and interventional [18] evidence points to a worsening of AKI with saline compared to balanced electrolyte solutions. However, evidence is lacking in low-risk patients [19, 20] especially when exposure to saline is limited to 1–3 l. Still, for high risk patients, especially those with sepsis, avoiding starch or saline is prudent.

Hypovolemia

The most life-saving treatment for the world's most common infections is not antibiotics but rather fluids. Cholera, for example, was once a near-fatal disease. Even as recently as the 1950s, case fatality rates for cholera exceeded 70% in epidemics in India and parts of Africa. In 2015, the overall case fatality rate for cholera was 0.8% (www.who.int). With this kind of response to therapy, it is easy to see how fluids are viewed as an essential part of patient management across a whole range of acute illness. Even given the concerns about certain fluids discussed above, the risk-benefit ratio in the setting of life-threatening dehydration is overwhelmingly positive. In cases where volume depletion is less severe or even less certain, some fluid may still be helpful. However, medical science has long understood that just because something is good does not mean that more of it is better. An important lesson of the Fluids and Catheters Treatment Trial (FACTT) was that not only did liberal fluid use in acute lung injury patients increase ventilator days, it actually resulted in more severe AKI. Indeed, there was a near-significant increase in patients receiving dialysis over the first 60 days (10 vs. 14% p = 0.06) [21]. Similarly, in the Protocolized Care for Early Septic Shock (ProCESS) trial, two fluid protocols were compared to standard care. Dialysis rates over the first week were greatest with the treatment arm providing the most fluids (6 vs. 3.1%/2.8% p = 0.04) [22]. We examined this issue further in subsequent analyses that have shown that neither AKI severity nor duration was different between study arms. Among patients with severe AKI, complete and partial recovery were 50.7 and 13.2% for protocolized patients and 49.1 and 13.4% for usual care patients (p = 0.93) [23]. Thus, giving more fluids in well-resuscitated patients, even with septic shock, does not attenuate kidney injury nor improve recovery. Conversely, positive fluid balance is well recognized to be associated with decreased hospital survival [24, 25]. Patients with AKI are obviously at increased risk for fluid overload and, therefore, fluids should be used with caution in such patients. While oliguria should prompt resuscitation in patients with hypovolemia it should signal caution in patients without. Indeed, when oliguria is due to AKI, fluids cause harm.

Risk Assessment: The Role of Biomarkers

Until recently, there was another major limitation to adopting KDIGO recommendations for high-risk patients—there was no reliable way to determine high risk. On the one hand, all patients admitted to the ICU are at high risk for AKI. On the other hand, not all patients are at the same level of risk or at risk for the same thing. Furthermore, risk varies with time. Patients are also at risk for other conditions besides AKI and this may lead to contradictory recommendations for management. For example, narcotic use should be limited in patients because of well-known short- and long-term hazards. NSAIDs can be very effective in reducing narcotic use and yet they can also increase the risk for AKI. Patients at high risk for narcotic use but low risk for AKI should be treated differently than patients at low risk for narcotic use but high risk for AKI. Until recently, there were few tools available to clinicians to help sort out the risk for AKI. However, with the introduction of AKI biomarkers, risk assessment for AKI is now much more feasible.

In both the PrevAKI study by Meersch et al. [3] and the BigpAK Study by Göcze and coworkers [4], high risk patients were identified using urinary TIMP-2 and IGFBP-7 using the Nephrocheck test™ (Astute Medical, San Diego, USA). Selecting patients for even benign interventions is important for two reasons. First, providing therapy for patients with little-to-no chance of benefit is a waste of resources. In several large studies, the negative predictive value for [TIMP-2] × [IGFBP-7] ≤ 0.3 is 97% [26]. Therefore, providing a KDIGO bundle for patients with a negative biomarker would result in an enormous expense for very little benefit. Especially in prevention studies, where the number needed to treat (NNT) to prevent one case of AKI may be very high (e.g., 30–40), the use of a biomarker to select high risk patients will result in an intervention that has a much lower NNT [27]. The NNT in the PrevAKI was only 6 for any AKI and 7 for moderate-to severe AKI. Similar results were found in the BigpAK trial with an NNT of 6 and 8 for any and moderate-to-severe AKI respectively.

Fig. 2 Early detection of tubular cellular stress and mechanism of action to prevent development of acute kidney injury (AKI). Detection of reversible cellular stress by biomarkers and early initiation of a Kidney Disease Improving Global Outcomes (KDIGO) care bundle in biomarker positive patients may prevent progression to AKI. Patients with very high biomarker levels may have irreversible stress. *T2*: tissue inhibitor of metalloproteinases-2 (TIMP-2); *I7*: insulin-like growth factorbinding protein 7 (IGFBP7); *sCR*: serum creatinine

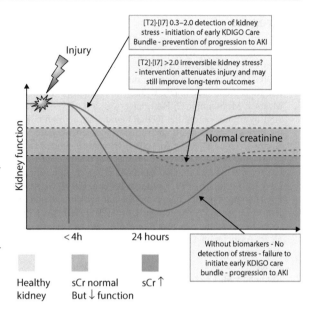

Another reason to apply the KDIGO bundle used in these studies to only a select group of patients is that the bundle may contradict other guidelines as mentioned earlier.

Finally, an intriguing subgroup analysis in the BigpAK trial of patients with different biomarker values of [TIMP-2] × [IGFBP-7] (0.3–2.0 [high risk for AKI] versus > 2.0 [very high risk for AKI]) [26] showed that the effect of the KDIGO care bundle was greatest in the 0.3–2.0 group. This observation may suggest the existence of a 'reversible zone', in which early intervention indeed effectively prevents development of AKI but the intervention is only able to reduce the severity of imminent AKI in the higher group (Fig. 2).

Conclusion

AKI is extremely common in the critically ill and injured and after major surgery. AKI is prevalent across all nations and knows no geographic or socioeconomic boundaries. At its most severe stage, it reduces the odds of survival by 7-fold [9]. However, AKI is not inevitable and it may largely be within our control. Despite years of negative trials for AKI, we can, in fact, do plenty to prevent and manage AKI. Various implementations of a 'KDIGO bundle' can save kidneys. Now that we have evidence that AKI can be prevented, it is our duty to find more ways to do it.

References

1. Kellum JA (2016) Why are patients still getting and dying from acute kidney injury? Curr Opin Crit Care 22:513–519
2. KDIGO (2012) Kidney disease: improving global outcomes (KDIGO) clinical practice guideline for acute kidney injury. Kidney Int 2(Suppl):1–138
3. Meersch M, Schmidt C, Hoffmeier A et al (2017) Prevention of cardiac surgery-associated AKI by implementing the KDIGO guidelines in high risk patients identified by biomarkers: the PrevAKI randomized controlled trial. Intensive Care Med 43:1551–1561
4. Göcze I, Jauch D, Götz M (2017) Biomarker-guided intervention to prevent acute kidney injury after major surgery: the prospective randomized BigpAK Study. Ann Surg. https://doi.org/10.1097/SLA.0000000000002485 (Aug 29, Epub ahead of print)
5. Levy MM, Pronovost PJ, Dellinger RP et al (2004) Sepsis change bundles: converting guidelines into meaningful change in behavior and clinical outcome. Crit Care Med 32:S595–S597
6. Hillis LD, Smith PK, Anderson JL et al (2011) 2011 ACCF/AHA guideline for coronary artery bypass graft surgery. A report of the American College of Cardiology Foundation/American Heart Association task force on practice guidelines. Developed in collaboration with the American association for thoracic surgery, society of cardiovascular anesthesiologists, and society of thoracic surgeons. J Am Coll Cardiol 58:e123–e210
7. Raimundo M, Crichton S, Martin JR et al (2015) Increased fluid administration after early acute kidney injury is associated with less renal recovery. Shock 44:431–437
8. Goldstein SL, Kirkendall E, Nguyen H et al (2013) Electronic health record identification of nephrotoxin exposure and associated acute kidney injury. Pediatrics 132:e756–e767
9. Hoste EAJ, Bagshaw SM, Bellomo R et al (2015) Epidemiology of acute kidney injury in critically ill patients: the multinational AKI-EPI study. Intensive Care Med 41:1411–1423
10. Murugan R, Karajala-Subramanyam V, Lee M et al (2010) Acute kidney injury in non-severe pneumonia is associated with an increased immune response and lower survival. Kidney Int 77:527–535
11. Gomez H, Ince C, De Backer D et al (2014) A unified theory of sepsis-induced acute kidney injury: inflammation, microcirculatory dysfunction, bioenergetics, and the tubular cell adaptation to injury. Shock 41:3–11
12. Murugan R, Wen X, Shah N et al (2014) Plasma inflammatory and apoptosis markers are associated with dialysis dependence and death among critically ill patients receiving renal replacement therapy. Nephrol Dial Transplant 29:1854–1864
13. Peng Z-Y, Wang HZ, Srisawat N et al (2012) Bactericidal antibiotics temporarily increase inflammation and worsen acute kidney injury in experimental sepsis. Crit Care Med 40:538–543
14. Hammond DA, Smith MN, Li C, Hayes SM, Lusardi K, Bookstaver PB (2017) Systematic review and meta-analysis of acute kidney injury associated with concomitant vancomycin and piperacillin/tazobactam. Clin Infect Dis 64:666–674
15. Perner A, Haase N, Guttormsen AB et al (2012) Hydroxyethyl starch 130/0.42 versus Ringer's acetate in severe sepsis. N Engl J Med 367:124–134
16. Zhou F, Peng ZY, Bishop JV, Cove ME, Singbartl K, Kellum JA (2013) Effects of Fluid resuscitation with 0.9 % saline versus a balanced electrolyte solution on acute kidney injury in a rat model of sepsis. Crit Care Med 42:e270–e278
17. Shaw AD, Bagshaw SM, Goldstein SL et al (2012) Major complications, mortality, and resource utilization after open abdominal surgery. Ann Surg 255:821–829
18. Yunos NM, Bellomo R, Hegarty C, Story D, Ho L, Bailey M (2012) Association between a chloride-liberal vs chloride-restrictive intravenous fluid administration strategy and kidney injury in critically ill adults. JAMA 308:1566–1572
19. Raghunathan K, Shaw AD, Nathanson B et al (2014) Association between the choice of iv crystalloid and in-hospital mortality among critically ill adults with sepsis. Crit Care Med 42:1585–1591

20. Young P, Bailey M, Beasley R et al (2015) Effect of a buffered crystalloid solution vs saline on acute kidney injury among patients in the intensive care unit: The SPLIT randomized clinical trial. JAMA 314:1701–1710

21. Wiedemann HP, Wheeler AP, Bernard GR et al (2006) Comparison of two fluid-management strategies in acute lung injury. N Engl J Med 354:2564–2575

22. Yealy DM, Kellum JA, Huang DT et al (2014) A randomized trial of protocol-based care for early septic shock. N Engl J Med 370:1683–1693

23. Kellum JA, Chawla LS, Keener C et al (2016) The effects of alternative resuscitation strategies on acute kidney injury in patients with septic shock. Am J Respir Crit Care Med 193:281–287

24. Boyd JH, Forbes J, Nakada TA, Walley KR, Russell JA (2011) Fluid resuscitation in septic shock: a positive fluid balance and elevated central venous pressure are associated with increased mortality. Crit Care Med 39:259–565

25. Balakumar V, Murugan R, Sileanu FE, Palevsky P, Clermont G, Kellum JA (2017) Both positive and negative fluid balance may be associated with reduced long-term survival in the critically ill. Crit Care Med 45:e749–e757

26. Bihorac A, Chawla LS, Shaw AD et al (2014) Validation of cell-cycle arrest biomarkers for acute kidney injury using clinical adjudication. Am J Respir Crit Care Med 189:932–939

27. Kellum JA (2017) Acute kidney injury: AKI: the myth of inevitability is finally shattered. Nat Rev Nephrol 13:140–141

Part VIII
Renal Replacement Therapy

High Cut-off Membranes for Continuous Renal Replacement Therapy

Z. Ricci, S. Romagnoli, and C. Ronco

Introduction

The technology of continuous renal replacement therapy (CRRT) has rapidly evolved over the last 30 years [1], in all aspects of CRRT set-up: monitor, circuit, roller pumps, anticoagulation, alarms, available modalities and accuracy of flow rates [2]. Filter type, size and material quality have paralleled this general improvement [3] and highly water permeable (high-flux), biocompatible membranes are now routinely used for CRRT delivery. Traditionally, such evolution in the field of acute dialysis has followed (and rarely preceded) similar achievements obtained in the field of chronic dialysis. Current monitors for intermittent hemodialysis (IHD) for several reasons (including the need for online water preparation, the presence of several biofeedback mechanisms and the need for extreme net ultrafiltration accuracy) can be considered jewels of modern bioengineering. By contrast with CRRT, the choice of filter membrane for IHD is more specific and tailored to patient needs. In this context, use of the so-called high cut-off (HCO) membrane is well established in selected chronic dialysis patients (e.g., those with cast nephropathy secondary to myeloma). An extended use of such membranes has recently been proposed (so-called expanded hemodialysis) [4]. Their use has also been recently

Z. Ricci (✉)
Department of Cardiology and Cardiac Surgery, Pediatric Cardiac Intensive Care Unit, Bambino Gesù Children's Hospital, IRCCS
Rome, Italy
e-mail: zaccaria.ricci@gmail.com

S. Romagnoli
Department of Anesthesiology and Intensive Care, Azienda Ospedaliero-Universitaria Careggi
Florence, Italy

C. Ronco
Department of Nephrology, Dialysis and Transplantation, San Bortolo Hospital
Vicenza, Italy
International Renal Research Institute of Vicenza (IRRIV)
Vicenza, Italy

© Springer International Publishing AG 2018   357
J.-L. Vincent (ed.), *Annual Update in Intensive Care and Emergency Medicine 2018*,
Annual Update in Intensive Care and Emergency Medicine,
https://doi.org/10.1007/978-3-319-73670-9_28

proposed for CRRT in septic patients and in patients with other indications (e.g., hypermyoglobinemia, hypercytokinemia), but, as commonly happens in critical illness, no unequivocal high level evidence of clinical benefit has been published so far. In a recent systematic review of human studies on techniques of extracorporeal cytokine removal, Atan and coworkers [5] showed that HCO techniques may be most consistent for moderate to high cytokine removal regardless of operating characteristics. Other techniques, such as extracorporeal liver support and plasma filtration-adsorption, may also be effective but their complexity is greater and the number of studies less.

The present chapter will detail technical aspects of HCO membranes and their clinical application, including all published human studies and the major practical aspects (indications, prescription, anticoagulation). Future evolution of HCO therapies will also be discussed in the conclusion of the paper.

Basic Concepts

According to a recent attempt to standardize nomenclature of acute renal replacement therapies, for a specific membrane, the cut-off represents the molecular weight of the smallest solute retained by the membrane. Clinically, the expression "high cut-off membrane" describes membranes with a cut-off value that approximates the molecular weight of albumin (before exposure to blood or plasma) [6]. Also recently, a classification method [7] exactly characterized HCO membranes based on their molecular weight retention onset (MWRO) and molecular weight cut-off (MWCO). MWRO is the molecular weight of a given solute at which the membrane sieving coefficient is 0.9 and describes when the sieving coefficient starts to fall from 1 to 0. MWCO is defined as the molecular weight at which the sieving coefficient is 0.1. With these general aspects in mind, we now define HCO membranes as having, *in vitro*, a water permeability of $1100 \, ml/(m_2/h/mmHg)$ – almost thrice the value of a high flux membrane –, and beta2 microglobulin and albumin sieving coefficients of 1 and 0.2, respectively. Albumin loss with HCO membranes, when measured during conventional hemodialysis after a 4-h session with blood flow of $250 \, ml/min$ and dialysate flow of $500 \, ml/min$ for membrane areas between $1.7 \, m^2$ and $2.1 \, m^2$, is about 28 g (with standard high flux filters, with the same experimental conditions, albumin loss is negligible). HCO filters have a MWRO and a MWCO of 15–20 and 170–320 kDa, respectively (these values are respectively double and 5-fold those of standard filters). Pore radius is increased to 8–12 nm which is about twice that of standard high flux filters for CRRT.

The issue of membrane classification is very important because the incorrect choice of membrane material might imply a significant bias in trial results. A recent, interesting review on treatments using HCO membranes [8] highlighted that among eligible studies describing HCO use, about 15% (4 of 28) incorrectly described the applied technology as HCO.

Currently available membranes are HCO 1100, Septex and Theralite, all marketed by Gambro, and composed of a polyarylethersulfone/polyvinylpyrrolidone blend. Such membranes achieve effective removal of substances in the range of 20 to 60 kDa *in vivo*: larger molecules are retained, although pore size ranges nominally reach larger values, due to quick protein layer formation and membrane fouling. However, interestingly, these membrane characteristics outperform the glomerular filtration barrier, which is barely capable of filtering solutes up to 60 KDa (only through high convection rates) [7]. The final practical and important aspects regarding HCO membranes [9] are that they are apparently able to remove free light chains up to 4 h after session start, although clearance is reduced at this point; furthermore, in a continuous session, although protein fouling affects the clearance of molecules approaching the MWCO of the membrane, the removal capability for small molecules (MWRO) is maintained throughout the treatment whereas it decreases with time for middle molecules: HCO membranes tend to lose their large pore sieving coefficient capacity but they remain effective high flux filters in long session runs.

Available Clinical Evidence

Publications related to HCO membranes are currently limited. Excluding case reports, studies on animals, and *in vitro/ex vivo* studies, 10 clinical studies [10–19] have been published so far (Table 1). A randomized clinical trial "Comparing High Cut-off Haemofiltration With Standard Haemofiltration in Acute Renal Failure" (NCT00912184) has been completed but results have not yet been published.

The first clinical experiences with HCO membranes were entirely conducted by the group of Stanislao Morgera and Michael Haase in sepsis patients with severe acute kidney injury (AKI) requiring CRRT. In all these studies, the biological effects of HCO therapies during sepsis, rather than their clinical relevance on hard outcomes, was addressed. The main relevant finding of an initial pivotal study was the efficacy of HCO hemofiltration (1 l/h in all 28 enrolled patients) to induce, compared to standard hemofiltration, a restoration of proliferation of anti-CD3-stimulated peripheral blood mononuclear cells (PBMCs) (similar to healthy controls) [10]. Although the authors did not directly address which mediator was removed by HCO treatment, they speculated that at the basis of septic PBMC function suppression is an increased release of inflammatory and anti-inflammatory mediators, such as prostaglandin E2 (PGE2), transforming growth factor-beta (TGF-β), interleukin (IL)-6, IL-4 and IL-10 [20]. In a second small study, the authors explored intermittent HCO hemofiltration (12 h) performed over 5 days and alternated with conventional hemofiltration (1 l/h was the dose of both treatments) in 16 septic patients [11]. They clearly showed a significant effect on IL-6 removal with the HCO filter and a tendency of IL-6 serum levels to reduce over the 12-h HCO session. The effect on IL-6 levels was consistent over the five studied days with average final values being significantly lower than at baseline (although there was significant interindividual variability). The authors also interestingly confirmed that HCO effectively removed albumin and total proteins and they needed to repeatedly replace them throughout the study: despite the low prescribed dose, during the study

Table 1 List of human studies on high cut-off (HCO) membrane renal replacement therapy

Study first author, year [ref]	Study type (severity of illness)	Modalities	Prescription	HCO membrane	Number of patients	Endpoint	Clinical data
Morgera, 2003 [10]	RCT, single center (APACHE II 21–34)	HCO-CVVH (12 h) alternated with C-HF (12 h) vs. C-HF for 60 h (vs. short HCO and C-HF in 3 healthy volunteers)	1 l/h, post-dilution (both methods)	High-flux polyamide hemofilter (P2SH, surface area 0.6 m²)	28 (14:14:3)	PBMC function restoration by HCO	None
Morgera, 2003 [11]	Observational, single center (APACHE II 24–29)	HCO-CVVH (12 h) alternated with C-HF (12 h) for 5 days	1 l/h, post-dilution (both methods)	High-flux polyamide hemofilter (P2SH, surface area 0.6 m²)	16	IL-6 K: 12–17 ml/min TNF-α K: negligible	Non-significant improvement of SOFA score
Morgera, 2004 [12]	Block randomization to group 1, 2, 3, 4 (APACHE II 19–38)	Group 1: CVVH 1 l/h Group 2: CVVH 2.5 l/h Group 3: CVVHD 1 l/h Group 3: CVVHD 2.5 l/h	1 or 2.5 l/h post dilution hemofiltration vs. 1 or 2.5 l/h hemodialysis for 72 h	High-flux polyamide hemofilter (P2SH, surface area 1.1 m²)	24 (6:6:6:6)	IL-1ra K: 18–26 ml/min IL-6 K: 16–20 ml/min	No differences between groups in different severity scores
Morgera, 2004 [13]	RCT, single center (APACHE II 26–28)	HCO-CVVH (12 h) alternated with C-HF (12 h) vs. C-HF for 60 h (vs. short HCO and C-HF in 2 healthy volunteers)	1 l/h, post-dilution (both methods)	High-flux polyamide hemofilter (P2SH, surface area 0.6 m²)	28 (14:14:2)	PML phagocytosis rate measured at the end of the third HCO session significantly decreased compared with baseline values	None

Table 1 (Continued)

Study first author, year [ref]	Study type (severity of illness)	Modalities	Prescription	HCO Membrane	Number of patients	Endpoint	Clinical data
Morgera, 2006 [14]	RCT, single center (APACHE II 22–34)	HCO-CVVH vs. C-HF for 48 h	2.5 l/h, post-dilution (both methods)	High-flux polyamide hemofilter (P2SH, surface area 1.1 m²)	30 (20:10) – 2 HCO patients subsequently excluded	IL-1ra K: 39 ml/min IL-6 K: 36–40 ml/min	Slight reduction in SAPS score in the HCO group; significant reduction in adjusted norepinephrine dose
Haase, 2007 [15]	Double-blind, crossover, randomized, controlled, phase 1 (APACHE II 20–34)	4 h of HCO-IHD and 4 h of standard HF-IHD in random order with a 4-h wash-out (no treatment)	Blood flow at 200 ml/min and dialysate flow at 300 ml/min in both groups	Polyflux filters (polyarylether-sulfone) surface area of 1.1 m²; custom-made	10	IL-6 K: 9.6–14.1 mL/min; reduction in plasma levels of IL-6, IL-8 and IL-10	Non-significant greater reduction in norepinephrine dose in HCO group
Kade, 2016 [16]	Retrospective, single center (SOFA 14)	HCO-CVVHDF	Blood flow 150 ml/min, the dialysis flow 1200 ml/h. Predilution fluid 250 ml/h	Polyarylether-sulfone (PAES) membrane (Sep-tex)	28	IL-6 K: 59–75 ml/min	None

Table 1 (Continued)

Study first author, year [ref]	Study type (severity of illness)	Modalities	Prescription	HCO Membrane	Number of patients	Endpoint	Clinical data
Chelazzi, 2013 [17]	Retrospective, case-control, single center (SOFA 10–14)	HCO-CVVHD vs. CVVHDF	HCO: 35 ml/kg/h vs. CVVHDF 45 ml/kg/h	Polyarylethersulfone (PAES) membrane (Septex)	24 (16:8)	None	HCO group lower ICU-LOS, ventilation days/ICU-LOS, vasopressor days/ICU-LOS, ICU mortality
Atan, 2016 [18]	Double blind RCT (APACHE II 12–27)	HCO-CVVH vs. CVVH	Blood flow 250 ml/min, 25 ml/kg/h pre-dilution both groups	Polyethersulfone filters, surface area of 1.1 m²	14 (6:8)	IL-6 K: 36 ml/min IL-8 K: 26 ml/min IL-10 K: 9.66 ml/min	None
Villa, 2017 [19]	Prospective, multi-center (APACHE II 37)	HCO-CVVHD	35 ml/kg/h for 72 h (any KDIGO stage >0)	Polyarylethersulfone (PAES) membrane (Septex)	38	Decrease in IL-6, IL-10 and TNF-α especially in survivors	Survivors quick SOFA decrease. KDIGO stage and lactate associated with mortality

CVVHD: continuous veno-venous hemodialysis; *CVVHDF*: continuous veno-venous hemodiafiltration; *SOFA*: sequential organ failure assessment; *IL*: interleukin; *TNF*: tumor necrosis factor; *ICU*: intensive care unit; *LOS*: length of stay; *PML*: polymorphonuclear leukocyte; *ra*: receptor antagonist; *RCT*: randomized controlled trial; *PBMC*: peripheral blood mononuclear cell; *K*: clearance; *C-HF*: conventional HF; *IL-1ra*: interleukin-1 receptor antagonist

they estimated a cumulative protein loss of 8 g/day (in large part due to the first treatment hours). The clinical relevance of this adverse effect should not be overlooked. With a similar protocol in a further 28 patients, the authors showed that 12 h of HCO hemofiltration (followed by conventional hemofiltration) was also able to decrease polymorphonuclear leukocyte phagocytosis activity, restoring it to a level close to that of healthy volunteers. The same effect was not shown with continuous conventional treatments [12]. As a further evolution of previous studies, these authors tried to compare different HCO dialysis vs. hemofiltration flows in terms of cytokine clearance and protein losses [13]. In brief, the authors compared HCO continuous veno-venous hemodialysis (HCO-CVVHD) at 1 and at 2.5 l/h vs. similar prescriptions during HCO continuous veno-venous post-dilution hemofiltration (HCO-CVVH) in four groups composed of six patients with sepsis and AKI, during the first 50 h of continuous treatment (filters were changed daily). The authors detailed very clearly that the 2.5 l/h hemofiltration mode was associated with greater protein and albumin loss compared to dialysis. By contrast, no differences were found between the 1 l/h HCO-CVVH and HCO-CVVHD as far as protein and albumin losses were concerned. Measured cytokines during this study were not always detectable in enrolled sepsis patients. The authors also reported data on IL-1 receptor antagonist (IL-1ra) and IL-6. Not surprisingly, the most significant decline in cytokine plasma values over time was present in patients with the highest baseline levels. By contrast with what happened with proteins and albumin, RRT dose, more than modality, increased the clearance of target molecules. Membrane fouling tended to decrease cytokine clearances but significant removal was still achieved by HCO after 24 h. The messages that can be drawn from this study are very important. First, a substantial effect on circulating cytokines is especially present in patients with the highest levels: although it is possible that a positive evolution of the septic syndrome might induce a normalization of mediator levels, especially in patients with the most significant initial expression of these molecules, it is also a fact that the greatest benefits of this therapy could potentially be tailored based on specific plasma markers. Second, increasing effluent flow during HCO-CVVHD consistently increases cytokine clearance but not protein losses. Finally, changing the filter every 24 h is safe and feasible in terms of achieving optimal solute clearance throughout the whole session.

Hence, the same author group conducted a randomized clinical trial to explore the clinical effects of HCO therapy [14]. Thirty patients, diagnosed with sepsis and AKI and receiving norepinephrine for hemodynamic instability, were allocated with a 2:1 ratio to HCO-CVVH or conventional CVVH (2.5 l/h post-dilution hemofiltration). The median norepinephrine dose at baseline was 0.30 in the HCO group and 0.21 mcg/kg/min in the conventional hemofiltration group. Only the HCO group showed a significant 48-h decline in norepinephrine dose over time, after adjustment to baseline levels. The authors further confirmed that clearance rates for IL-6 and IL-1ra were significantly higher in the HCO-CVVH group, which translated into a significant decline in corresponding plasma levels. This further exploration of HCO modality finally enabled correlation of some biological modifications induced by the treatment and clinical effects. The last (double-blind, crossover, randomized, controlled, phase 1) trial of this initial series, conducted on 10 patients, was able to confirm previous results on cytokine clearance even when HCO membranes were compared to standard high flux filters during intermittent therapies (4 h, 200 ml/min blood flow, 300 ml/min dialysate) [15]. HCO intermittent hemodialysis achieved substantially greater diffusive cytokine clearances than standard hemodialysis and a greater relative decrease in IL-8 and IL-10 plasma concentrations.

With this initial body of literature available, Kade and co-authors [16] conducted a retrospective study on a relatively large sample of 28 septic patients who were "routinely" treated with HCO-CVVHD (dialysate flow rate 1200 ml/h). From their observations, the authors provided two interesting aspects: HCO-CVVHD sessions can be administered at the bedside, as simple and safe as standard treatments, even outside the edges of a strict research protocol. Then, they acknowledged that although cytokine clearances were averagely high and HCO treatment effective in this aspect, they were not able, in all cases, to control mediator plasma levels. In particular, low baseline IL-6 levels were correlated with a subsequent increase, regardless of extracorporeal treatment. By contrast, elevated IL-6 levels were easily controlled by HCO. The inability to normalize IL-6 levels was associated with a bad outcome. Indeed, it is still unknown what the exact molecular target of HCO treatments is and whether the pharmacokinetics of inflammatory mediators and immunomodulatory mechanisms can actually be impacted by any extracorporeal removal [21]. However, the concept of modifying, day by day, RRT doses and modalities in order to precisely tailor the treatment and to optimize patient outcomes is currently the object of intense debate [22]. With a similar retrospective approach, and a pragmatic target, Chelazzi and coworkers [17] conducted a case-control (16:8) study in order to evaluate whether HCO-CVVHD was superior to standard hemodiafiltration for decreasing vasopressor requirements and mechanical ventilation duration in patients with septic shock caused by multidrug resistant Gram-negative bacteria. HCO modality was prescribed with an effluent dose of 35 ml/kg/h whereas hemodiafiltration was delivered at about 40 ml/kg/h. The authors were able to show that HCO therapy enabled them to decrease vasopressor support significantly: this aspect was strictly related to an improvement in ICU mortality. The authors hypothesized that the main beneficial immunomodulatory effect of HCO was to enable time for antibiotic action and source control to become effective. For the first time, a clinical study, conducted in an appropriately selected cohort of septic patients, demonstrated clear clinical results.

In the last 2 years, two important studies have been published [18, 19]. The first study, in a nested cohort of a larger (still unpublished) randomized controlled trial (NCT00912184), enrolled critically ill patients with AKI and shock, and compared HCO-CVVH to standard hemofiltration [18]. The prescribed dose in all patients was 25 ml/kg/h of predilution bicarbonate buffered replacement with a blood flow of 250 ml/min. The authors analyzed a large panel of cytokines in 14 patients with a complete set of blood samples (from baseline, 12 h after hemofiltration start, to 72–96 h) and confirmed good clearances for IL-6 and IL-8. Interestingly, all the other analyzed mediators displayed either low sieving coefficients or negligible plasma levels. Because of the small sample size, only by combining all cytokines together was it possible to determine a statistically significant difference between the HCO and standard groups' sieving coefficients. Also, surprisingly, the percentage modification at 72 h with respect to baseline of all cytokines was significant in both groups (slightly superior in the HCO group). The authors also tried to analyze the kinetics of mediator removal but found that only IL-1β and IL-10 actually decreased their plasma concentration across the filter. The key messages of this first (nested) double-blind randomized trial are several: although conducted in a very small sample, once again previous insights into cytokine clearances were confirmed – therapy should be targeted at specific goals; not all inflammatory mediators are present in all patients; not all are cleared; standard hemofiltration already provides clearances of some of these molecules; large interindividual variability exists and potentially affects the results of this kind of treatments. It is possible that we will have to wait for the results of the full study to understand whether HCO is actually associated with clinically relevant improvements compared to standard hemofiltration and whether further research has to be dedicated to understanding the mechanisms and the kinetics of inflammatory mediators.

The only clinical multicenter prospective study published so far was conducted in Italy [19]. Thirty-eight patients with septic shock were enrolled for HCO-CVVHD treatment with the aim of identifying baseline clinical and biochemical parameters statistically associated with 72-h mortality in order to delineate the best timing and indications for extracorporeal treatment. The authors exclusively included patients with sepsis diagnosed within 12 h and AKI diagnosed within 24 h. The HCO treatment was early both in terms of time elapsed after AKI diagnosis and severity (16% of patients were Kidney Disease: Improving Global Outcomes [KDIGO] stage 1, 34% stage 2 and the remaining 50% KDIGO 3). The subgroup of non-surviving patients had a higher baseline lactate level and KDIGO severity, whereas those who survived had a rapid (within 6 h) improvement in sequential organ failure assessment (SOFA) score. Again, interestingly, the authors confirmed what was previously shown: a more significant improvement in IL-6 and tumor necrosis factor (TNF)-α levels was present in survivors, who were also those who tended to have the highest baseline levels. Although these findings are clearly hampered by the absence of a control group, this study represents, so far, the largest multicenter prospective application of HCO-CVVHD in selected patients: the overall cohort mortality was relatively low (40%) and about half of what was expected based on APACHE scores. This experience, once again, showed that this technique is feasible and safe, applicable also in a multicenter experience (first example of good external validity), and potentially effective in reducing patient mortality. It is possible that, similarly to what was targeted in the recent Euphrates study of polymyxin-B hemoperfusion [NCT01046669], one of the main aspects to implement in the near future in order to optimize clinical results with application of HCO techniques will be to find a target molecule (or molecules) and, possibly, their threshold plasma level to indicate when treatment should be started.

Current Indications and Prescription Issues

Current guidelines on sepsis and septic shock do not provide any recommendation regarding the choice of blood purification technique because publications are currently limited [23]. At the same time, the board suggests further research to clarify the clinical benefit of the different available blood purification modalities. Therefore, although the HCO technique cannot currently be recommended for routine clinical application due to the absence of high quality studies, what has clearly emerged from initial experiences is that HCO techniques are easily implemented in centers with adequate experience of standard RRT. HCO filters are currently available on the market and allowed for human use, outside clinical research. The circuits and machines needed to use HCO membranes do not change with respect to what is already commonly used. Anticoagulation methodology can also be left unchanged, although, possibly, citrate infusion may optimize fiber patency and pore cut-offs. Currently, indications for HCO-CVVHD are sepsis with AKI and hypercytokinemia. Several case reports have also described effective HCO treatments in patients with increased plasma myoglobin levels (crush syndromes, etc.) [24]. The optimal modality for HCO application is probably dialysis, in order to cope for albumin loss, while achieving adequate cytokine clearances. Another important aspect to consider is unwanted antibiotic clearance and altered pharmacokinetics: linezolid clearance [25] and other antiblastic drugs [26] have been evaluated during HCO dialysis and the authors found significant drug removal with this modality, suggesting that drug levels should be monitored when possible or unwanted losses estimated by mathematical simulation.

In this context, the HCO-CVVHD dose should be prescribed in the range of 25 to 40 ml/kg/h (similar to currently recommended by the KDIGO guidelines) [27], also depending on patient condition, filter lifespan and center policies for membrane substitution. Considering that the sieving coefficients of target cytokines (IL-6, IL-8, IL-10, as the most studied) range from about 0.5 to 0.9, a 60 kg patient should obtain a mediator clearance of about 10–40 ml/min. As clearly showed in previous studies though, cytokine reduction from patient plasma may be unpredictable and should be checked repeatedly for precise treatment monitoring and dose tailoring.

Potential Indications and Future Development

The current era of HCO dialysis is probably at its dawn. HCO technology will probably develop further in order to improve MWRO/MWCO values and optimize solute clearances with respect to albumin loss [4]. Diagnostic tools and biomarkers for initiation of HCO treatment will also be likely available in the next few years with the hope of tailoring treatments, similar to what is currently done with creatinine during standard CRRT [16]. The potential for this relatively easy technique to rapidly and effectively impact patient immune status also needs to be further explored and analyzed. It is possible that purification of cytokines is simply the tip of the iceberg and we need to discover other mechanisms at the basis of sepsis and inflammation-related organ dysfunction. As also already attempted by Morgera and coworkers, for example, it is possible that lymphocyte and white blood cell activity modulation can be (or should be) one of the targets of HCO therapy. In the same line, cases of immune regulation disturbances leading to direct organ dysfunction are increasing and, in most cases, these patients are admitted and treated as critically ill. Some of the clearest examples are myocarditis, heart transplant rejection and unknown origin dilated cardiomyopathy that may require extracorporeal assistance (e.g., extracorporeal membrane oxygenation, ventricular assist devices) and may lead to the need for (urgent) heart transplantation. In these patients, auto-immune pathophysiology has been hypothesized and shown in some cases [28]. It is possible that HCO therapy may act as an ancillary continuous therapy to blunt inflammation cascades between intermittent sessions of plasma exchange or immune-adsorption that directly target immunoglobulins. Several other complex pathogenetic pathways of multiple organ dysfunction (e.g., AKI [29], acute pancreatitis [30], acute liver failure [31], acute respiratory distress syndrome (ARDS) [32]) likely have cytokine-driven mechanisms and may benefit from properly targeted and timely HCO treatment.

Conclusion

The available literature suggests that HCO technology is promising but still inadequate. HCO-CVVHD is effective in enhancing clearance of specific cytokines and other substances with a molecular weight between 20 and 60 Kda. HCO has also been shown to be effective in reducing plasma concentrations of target molecules. It is possible that HCO hemodialysis technology may develop further with improved range of cleared molecules, thus reducing adverse effects such as consistent albumin loss. Whether this dialytic modality is effective in improving hard outcomes has not been unequivocally demonstrated and the results of the first adequately powered double-blind randomized clinical trial are eagerly awaited. In the meanwhile, research trying to explain the immune pathogenesis of several critical illnesses will be helpful in order to better understand the role, the indications and the timing of HCO therapy.

References

1. Bartlett RH (2017) A moment in history: the origins of continuous renal replacement therapy. ASAIO J. https://doi.org/10.1097/MAT.0000000000000573 (March 22, Epub ahead of print)
2. Ronco C, Ricci Z, De Backer D, Kellum JA et al (2015) Renal replacement therapy in acute kidney injury: controversy and consensus. Crit Care 19:146
3. Bellomo R, Ronco C (2009) Continuous renal replacement therapy: hemofiltration, hemodiafiltration or hemodialysis. In: Ronco C, Bellomo R, Kellum JA (eds) Critical Care Nephrology, 2nd edn. Elsevier Saunders, Philadelphia, pp 1354–1358
4. Ronco C, La Manna G (2017) Expanded hemodialysis: a new therapy for a new class of membranes. Contrib Nephrol 190:124–133

5. Atan R, Crosbie D, Bellomo R (2013) Techniques of extracorporeal cytokine removal: a systematic review of the literature on animal experimental studies. Int J Artif Organs 36:149–158

6. Neri M, Villa G, Garzotto F, Bagshaw S et al (2016) Nomenclature for renal replacement therapy in acute kidney injury: basic principles. Crit Care 20:318

7. Boschetti-de-Fierro A, Voigt M, Storr M, Krause B (2013) Extended characterization of a new class of membranes for blood purification: the high cut-off membranes. Int J Artif Organs 36:455–463

8. Villa G, Zaragoza JJ, Sharma A, Neri M, De Gaudio AR, Ronco C (2014) Cytokine removal with high cut-off membrane: review of literature. Blood Purif 38:167–173

9. Hutchison CA, Harding S, Mead G et al (2008) Serum free-light chain removal by high cut-off hemodialysis: optimizing removal and supportive care. Artif Organs 32:910–917

10. Morgera S, Haase M, Rocktäschel J et al (2003) High permeability haemofiltration improves peripheral blood mononuclear cell proliferation in septic patients with acute renal failure. Nephrol Dial Transplant 18:2570–2576

11. Morgera S, Rocktäschel J, Haase M et al (2003) Intermittent high permeability hemofiltration in septic patients with acute renal failure. Intensive Care Med 29:1989–1995

12. Morgera S, Haase M, Rocktäschel J et al (2003) Intermittent high-permeability hemofiltration modulates inflammatory response in septic patients with multiorgan failure. Nephron Clin Pract 94:c75–c80

13. Morgera S, Slowinski T, Melzer C et al (2004) Renal re-placement therapy with high-cutoff hemofilters: impact of convection and diffusion on cytokine clearances and protein status. Am J Kidney Dis 43:444–453

14. Morgera S, Haase M, Kuss T et al (2006) Pilot study on the effects of high cutoff hemofiltration on the need for norepinephrine in septic patients with acute renal failure. Crit Care Med 34:2099–2104

15. Haase M, Bellomo R, Baldwin I et al (2007) Hemodialysis membrane with a high-molecular-weight cutoff and cytokine levels in sepsis complicated by acute renal failure: a phase 1 randomized trial. Am J Kidney Dis 50:296–304

16. Kade G, Lubas A, Rzeszotarska A, Korsak J, Niemczyk S (2016) Effectiveness of high cut-off hemofilters in the removal of selected cytokines in patients during septic shock accompanied by acute kidney injury-preliminary study. Med Sci Monit 22:4338–4344

17. Chelazzi C, Villa G, D'Alfonso MG et al (2016) Hemodialysis with high cut-off hemodialyzers in patients with multi-drug resistant gram-negative sepsis and acute kidney injury: a retrospective, case-control study. Blood Purif 42:186–193

18. Atan R, Peck L, Visvanathan K et al (2016) High cut-off hemofiltration versus standard hemofiltration: effect on plasma cytokines. Int J Artif Organs 39:479–486

19. Villa G, Chelazzi C, Morettini E et al (2017) Organ dysfunction during continuous venovenous high cut-off hemodialysis in patients with septic acute kidney injury: a prospective observational study. PLoS One 12:e172039

20. O'Sullivan ST, Lederer JA, Horgan AF, Chin DH, Mannick JA, Rodrick ML (1995) Major injury leads to predominance of the T helper-2 lymphocyte phenotype and diminished interleukin-12 production associated with decreased resistance to infection. Ann Surg 222:482–484

21. De Vriese AS, Vanholder RC, Pascual M, Lameire NH, Colardyn FA (1999) Can inflammatory cytokines be removed efficiently by continuous renal replacement therapies? Intensive Care Med 25:903–910

22. Bagshaw SM, Chakravarthi MR, Ricci Z et al (2016) Precision continuous renal replacement therapy and solute control. Blood Purif 42:238–247

23. Rhodes A, Evans LE, Alhazzani W et al (2017) Surviving sepsis campaign: international guidelines for management of sepsis and septic shock: 2016. Crit Care Med 45:486–552

24. Zhang L, Kang Y, Fu P et al (2012) Myoglobin clearance by continuous venous-venous haemofiltration in rhabdomyolysis with acute kidney injury: a case series. Injury 43:619–623

25. Villa G, Cassetta MI, Tofani L et al (2015) Linezolid extracorporeal removal during haemodialysis with high cut-off membrane in critically ill patients. Int J Antimicrob Agents 46:465–468
26. Krieter DH, Devine E, Wanner C, Storr M, Krause B, Lemke HD (2014) Clearance of drugs for multiple myeloma therapy during in vitro high-cutoff hemodialysis. Artif Organs 38:888–893
27. Kidney Disease Improving Global Outcomes (2012) KDIGO clinical practice guideline for acute kidney injury. Kidney Int Suppl 2:1–138
28. Shankar-Hari M, Fear D, Lavender P et al (2017) Activation-associated accelerated apoptosis of memory B cells in critically ill patients with sepsis. Crit Care Med 45:875–882
29. Bonavia A, Singbartl K (2017) A review of the role of immune cells in acute kidney injury. Pediatr Nephrol. https://doi.org/10.1007/s00467-017-3774-5 (Aug 11, Epub ahead of print)
30. Pupelis G, Plaudis H, Zeiza K, Drozdova N, Mukans M, Kazaka I (2012) Early continuous veno-venous haemofiltration in the management of severe acute pancreatitis complicated with intra-abdominal hypertension: retrospective review of 10 years' experience. Ann Intensive Care 2(Suppl 1):S21
31. Larsen FS, Schmidt LE, Bernsmeier C, Rasmussen A, Isoniemi H, Patel VC (2016) High-volume plasma exchange in patients with acute liver failure: An open randomised controlled trial. J Hepatol 64:69–78
32. Fanelli V, Ranieri VM (2015) Mechanisms and clinical consequences of acute lung injury. Ann Am Thorac Soc 12(Suppl 1):S3–S8

The Role of Intraoperative Renal Replacement Therapy in Liver Transplantation

C. J. Karvellas and S. M. Bagshaw

Introduction

Acute kidney injury (AKI) is a frequent complication of cirrhosis (or acute-on-chronic liver failure [ACLF]), occurring in up to 50% of hospitalized patients with cirrhosis [1–4]. The majority of patients with cirrhosis (~ 70%) have AKI without structural changes to the kidney [5]. The main causes of AKI include hypovolemia, intrinsic renal/parenchymal disorders (e.g., interstitial nephritis, glomerulonephritis/nephropathy), obstructive nephropathy and hepatorenal syndrome (HRS) [6]. HRS, a diagnosis of exclusion, is a severe complication of advanced cirrhosis and is a consequence of intense renal vasoconstriction due to a decrease in overall systemic vascular resistance. The result of the kidney limiting excretion of sodium and free water in response to the upregulation of compensatory mechanisms (renin-angiotensin system, antidiuretic hormone) is a reduction in renal perfusion and glomerular filtration without histological changes.

Patients with cirrhosis and HRS have a worse prognosis compared to patients with cirrhosis with other causes of AKI in the absence of liver transplant [7]. For almost 20 years, AKI in patients with cirrhosis was defined, according to the International Club of Ascites (ICA) criteria, as an increase in serum creatinine (sCr) of 50% from baseline to a final value > 1.5 mg/dl (133 μmol/l) [8, 9]. More recently, the Kidney Disease Improving Global Outcomes (KDIGO) criteria, which are based on changes in sCr, to define AKI have been widely adopted (Table 1; [10]). The newer ICA definition of AKI in patients with cirrhosis includes either an absolute increase

C. J. Karvellas (✉)
Department of Critical Care Medicine, Faculty of Medicine and Dentistry, University of Alberta
Edmonton, Canada
Division of Gastroenterology (Liver Unit), University of Alberta
Edmonton, Canada
e-mail: dean.karvellas@ualberta.ca

S. M. Bagshaw
Department of Critical Care Medicine, Faculty of Medicine and Dentistry, University of Alberta
Edmonton, Canada

© Springer International Publishing AG 2018   371
J.-L. Vincent (ed.), *Annual Update in Intensive Care and Emergency Medicine 2018*,
Annual Update in Intensive Care and Emergency Medicine,
https://doi.org/10.1007/978-3-319-73670-9_29

Table 1 Diagnostic criteria for acute kidney injury (AKI) in cirrhosis. Modified from [11]

	RIFLE Criteria [26]	AKIN Criteria [28]	KDIGO Criteria [10]	ICA: AKI in cirrhosis [29]
Diagnostic Criteria	Increase in SCr to ≥ 1.5 times baseline, within 7 days; or GFR decrease > 25%; or urine volume < 0.5 ml/kg/h for 6 h	Increase in sCr by ≥ 0.3 mg/dl (26.5 µmol/l) within 48 h; or increase in sCr ≥ 1.5 times baseline within 48 h; or urine volume < 0.5 ml/kg/h for 6 h	Increase in sCr by ≥ 0.3 mg/dl (26.5 µmol/l) within 48 h; or increase in SCr to ≥ 1.5 times baseline, which is known or presumed to have occurred within the prior 7 days; or urine volume < 0.5 ml/kg/h for 6 h	A percentage increase in sCr of 50% or more to a final value of sCr > 1.5 mg/dl (133 µmol/l)
Staging	*Risk:* sCr increase 1.5–1.9 times baseline; or GFR decrease 25–50%; or urine output < 0.5 ml/kg/h for 6 h	*Stage 1:* sCr increase 1.5–1.9 times baseline; or sCr increase ≥ 0.3 mg/dl (26.5 µmol/l); or urine output < 0.5 ml/kg/h for 6 h	*Stage 1:* sCr increase 1.5–1.9 times baseline; or Cr increase ≥ 0.3 mg/dl (26.5 µmol/l); or urine output < 0.5 ml/kg/h for 6–12 h	
	Injury: sCr increase 2.0–2.9 times baseline; or GFR decrease 50–75%; or urine output < 0.5 ml/kg/h for 12 h	*Stage 2:* sCr increase 2.0–2.9 times baseline; or urine output < 0.5 ml/kg/h for 12 h	*Stage 2:* sCr increase 2.0–2.9 times baseline; or urine output < 0.5 ml/kg/h for ≥ 12 h	
	Failure: sCr increase ≥ 3.0 times baseline; or GFR decrease 50–75%; or sCr increase ≥ 4.0 mg/dl (353.6 µmol/l) with an acute increase of at least 0.5 mg/dl (44 µmol/l); or urine output < 0.3 ml/kg/h for ≥ 24 h; or anuria for ≥ 12 h	*Stage 3:* sCr increase 3.0 times baseline; or sCr increase ≥ 4.0 mg/dl (353.6 µmol/l) with an acute increase of at least 0.5 mg/dl (44 µmol/l); or urine output < 0.3 ml/kg/h for ≥ 24 h; or anuria for ≥ 12 h	*Stage 3:* sCr increase 3.0 times baseline; or sCr increase to ≥ 4.0 mg/dl (353.6 µmol/l); or initiation of RRT; or urine output < 0.3 ml/kg/h for ≥ 24 h; or anuria for ≥ 12 h	

AKIN: Acute Kidney Injury Network; *GFR*: glomerular filtration rate; *KDIGO*: Kidney Disease Improving Global Outcome; *RIFLE*: Risk, Injury, Failure, Loss, End stage renal disease; *sCr*: serum creatinine; *ICA*: the International Club of Ascites

in sCr of at least 0.3 mg/dl ($\geq$ 26.4 µmol/l) in less than 48 h or a percentage increase in sCr of at least 50% (a minimum increase of 1.5 from baseline) in less than seven days [11]. AKI has been associated with worse clinical outcomes in patients with cirrhosis [4]. While vasopressors (e.g., terlipressin) may improve HRS specifically in some patients, the only treatment associated with a survival benefit in cirrhotic patients with AKI is liver transplantation [12].

Transplantation in the Patient with Cirrhosis and AKI

Preoperative AKI presents significant challenges in the perioperative management of patients with cirrhosis or acute liver failure (ALF) undergoing liver transplant and has been demonstrated to be associated with worse patient survival post-transplant [13]. Prior to liver transplant, renal replacement therapy (RRT) is often used to support patients with cirrhosis or ALF, particularly continuous RRT (CRRT). This modality provides enhanced hemodynamic tolerance, reduced risk of exacerbation of cerebral edema (in ALF patients), along with improved metabolic, acid-base and azotemic control. CRRT has being used as intraoperative renal support for critically ill patients undergoing liver transplantation; however most of these studies have been retrospective and observational [14–16]. Despite the purported benefits, intraoperative CRRT may have added risk and resource implications including patient exposure to an extracorporeal circuit; intraoperative filter/circuit disruption; need for additional consultants/specialized personnel to prime, operate and adjust the RRT machine; and added costs.

Physiological Challenges of Liver Transplantation in AKI

Liver transplantation in patients with AKI poses significant challenges [17]. The intraoperative course can be complicated by periods of hemodynamic instability, acid-base and electrolyte abnormalities, and intraoperative blood loss/coagulation failure often necessitating the use of vasoactive therapy and large resuscitation with transfused blood products. AKI/oliguria may compound these challenges by provoking rapid intravascular fluid accumulation, rapid shifts in acid-base balance and electrolytes (potassium) that may not response to conventional measures (i.e., diuretics) [18].

Specific metabolic complications are dependent on different aspects of the liver transplantation procedure. Lactic acidosis usually occurs and can become more severe during the anhepatic phase because of the clamping of large vessels [19]. The presence of AKI adds to the degree of metabolic acidosis and makes it more challenging to correct and reverse the problem. Relative hyperkalemia commonly occurs during liver transplantation, especially during the reperfusion of the donor liver/graft and release of inferior vena cava (IVC) cross-clamp, which in some cases can provoke cardiac arrhythmias, hemodynamic instability and cardiac arrest [20]. After unclamping of the portal vein, this can lead to bradycardia and hypotension followed by dysrhythmias. Although the severity of hemodynamic changes that accompany reperfusion depends on several factors, such as the cross-clamp time, medical comorbidity of the recipient, and the quality of the donor graft (e.g., deceased cardiac donor), hyperkalemia remains one of the main causes of hemodynamic compromise during this phase. Intraoperative CRRT can theoretically prevent complications from acute hyperkalemia and maintain acceptable potassium levels throughout the procedure. Patients with cirrhosis and ALF frequently suffer from coagulopathy and hemodynamic instability. In a patient with co-existent AKI, the correction of this with infusions of large amounts of blood products, crystalloids, and colloids makes management of intravascular volume challenging. During the clamping of the IVC, a large volume of crystalloid is often required to maintain the filling pressure on the right side of the heart, but immediately after the unclamping of the IVC, this volume can become a burden on the right ventricle and lead to right ventricular failure if rapid removal of the excess volume is not achieved. In a recipient with pre-liver transplantation AKI, where patients are often fluid overloaded going into liver transplantation in the absence of RRT, this could potentially be managed with intraoperative CRRT/ultrafiltration [21].

Patient Selection for Intraoperative RRT

Given the paucity of data in this field and equipoise regarding timing of CRRT in critically ill patients, one of the challenges in evaluating retrospective studies is the heterogeneity of indications for intraoperative CRRT [22]. In a retrospective study from the University of Wisconsin, Zimmerman and colleagues made the decision to initiate intraoperative CRRT based on local consensus policy developed by the transplant surgical, anesthesiology and nephrology teams. In their cohort (see results later), indications included severe acid/base derangement (base deficit > 6), electrolyte abnormalities (potassium > 5.5 mmol/l), significant fluid disturbances (volume overload, pulmonary edema), creatinine level > 2.0 mg/dl (177 μmol/l), oliguria/anuria, high acuity of illness (Model for End-Stage Liver Disease [MELD] score [23] > 30, patient requiring pre-liver transplantation intensive care unit (ICU) management and two or more vasopressor agents), and the anticipated need for a large volume of intraoperative blood products (> 8 units of fresh frozen plasma/packed cells) due to an international normalized ratio [INR] > 3, platelet count < 30,000/ul and fibrinogen < 100 mg/dl [24]. Most other cohort studies similarly followed institutional consensus due to a lack of evidence [16].

Evidence to Date

Studies to date have all been retrospective, where the decision to initiate intraoperative RRT was made by the clinical teams. Townsend and colleagues demonstrated in a retrospective cohort analysis, that 41 (6% out of 636) liver transplantation recipients at a single center between 1996–2005 received intraoperative CRRT [14].

This cohort had a high burden of organ failure (median MELD 38, 63% receiving RRT prior to liver transplantation). Other indications for use of intraoperative CRRT included perceived need for large volume transfusion in operating room, hyperkalemia, dysnatremia (Na < 130) and lactic acidosis. The median duration of intraoperative CRRT was 258 min (~ 57% of total operative time). Filter circuit clotting occurred in 40% but was not associated with a shorter CRRT duration. Intraoperative CRRT permitted an even or negative intraoperative fluid balance in 93% of liver transplant recipients. CRRT was continued after liver transplantation in 78% of patients for a median of 5 days. Twenty-four patients were subsequently transitioned to intermittent hemodialysis (IHD). Survival was 76% at 1 year (expected survival for ambulatory liver transplant recipients ~ 85–90% at one year). Renal recovery to RRT independence occurred in 100% of survivors by 1 year. While intraoperative CRRT appeared to be well tolerated with good post-liver transplantation outcomes, this study did not have a control group.

In a subsequent study from the same institution, Parmar and colleagues [25] performed a retrospective matched case-control study of liver transplantation recipients receiving intraoperative CRRT between 2006–2009 (n = 36) with 1:1 controls matched for demographics and MELD on the day of liver transplantation (n = 36). Despite the effort to match by MELD, intraoperative CRRT cases still had significantly higher MELD scores (35 vs. 30, p = 0.01), received more vasopressors (p = 0.006), and more pre-liver transplantation RRT (94 vs. 26%, p < 0.0001). There was no difference in complications between patients who did and did not receive intraoperative CRRT, nor was there a difference in in-hospital mortality (p = 0.6). Hence, despite higher illness severity for intraoperative CRRT patients, there were no differences in complications or mortality.

More recently, Zimmerman and colleagues evaluated a cohort of 96 liver transplantation recipients for ACLF/cirrhosis in a single center study between 2012–2016 [24]. Groups were stratified into: (1) patients with pre-liver transplantation AKI who underwent intraoperative CRRT (Group I, n = 30); (2) patients with pre-liver transplantation AKI who did not receive intraoperative CRRT (Group II, n = 9); and (3) liver transplant patients without pre-liver transplantation AKI (Group III, n = 37). MELD scores were significantly higher in Groups 1 (mean 43), and II (39) compared to Group 3 (18). Despite being sicker, there were no differences in 12-month survival between Group I (intraoperative CRRT) vs. patients without AKI at the time of liver transplantation (78 vs. 88%, p = 0.2). In patients with AKI, patients who received intraoperative CRRT had significantly shorter stays in hospital post-liver transplantation (25 vs. 38 days, p = 0.02).

In a single center cohort study, Agopian and colleagues examined the use of intraoperative RRT in 500 patients (cirrhosis n = 448; ALF n = 52) undergoing liver transplantation with AKI prior to liver transplantation between 2004–2012, with mean MELD scores > 35 [16]. The decision to initiate intraoperative RRT was based on an institutional consensus policy. Of this group, 401 patients did not receive intraoperative RRT, 70 patients received planned intraoperative RRT and 29 patients received emergent intraoperative RRT due to complications during the procedure. In patients with cirrhosis and AKI (n = 448), independent predictors for the receipt of intraoperative RRT were re-transplant, hyperkalemia, vasopressor use, CRRT use prior to operating room, increasing bilirubin (MELD) and receipt from a donor after cardiac death (DCD). They derived a risk score based on these variables (area under the receiver operating characteristic curve [AUROC] 0.83) [16].

Nadim and colleagues evaluated their 10-year experience (2002–2012) of 238 transplants (liver only n = 155, liver-kidney n = 83) where patients were treated with intraoperative IHD [21]. The choice of intraoperative IHD was made for preference for rapid correction of metabolic acidosis and hyperkalemia post-unclamping. Eighty percent (n = 191) of these patients were receiving RRT prior to liver transplantation (CRRT n = 103, IHD n = 88) and 61% (n = 145) were in the ICU prior to liver transplantation. Overall, 74% (n = 175) achieved a negative fluid balance during the transplant procedure. Among patients receiving liver transplantation only (n = 155), 1 year survival was 79% with no difference irrespective of whether pre-liver transplantation MELD was < 40 or ≥ 40 or whether recipients received RRT prior to liver transplantation.

Limitations/impact on Outcomes

The limitations of current observational studies are that they are retrospective and are limited by selection bias, confounding by indication, single center experiences and a lack of standardized criteria for receipt of intraoperative RRT. In general, sicker potential liver transplantation recipients (e.g., MELD > 40) were more likely to receive more interventions, such as intraoperative CRRT [25]. Overall, these retrospective observational studies have demonstrated that intraoperative RRT is safe and feasible (intraoperative CRRT or IHD) with acceptable patient (~ 80% survival at 1 year post-liver transplantation) and renal (> 90% RRT-free at 1 year) outcomes [16, 21, 25]. However due to the limitations of retrospective/matched case control study designs, previous studies have not conclusively demonstrated the benefit of intraoperative CRRT to justify additional costs and potential risks to the patient. Higher quality clinical investigations, ideally in the form of well-designed randomized studies aimed at minimizing the bias introduced in observational studies are needed to definitely determine the role and benefit of intraoperative CRRT. Higher quality evidence will translate into safer and more standardized practice for intraoperative application of this technology with evidence-based clinical/biochemical indications for intraoperative CRRT *a priori* [16].

Phase II Randomized Study: Intraoperative CRRT in Liver Transplantation

Recently, Bagshaw and colleagues completed the INCEPTION study (NCT01575015) evaluating the use of intraoperative CRRT in liver transplantation recipients. This was a phase II, randomized, non-blinded, controlled trial with allocation concealment, of patients undergoing liver transplantation stratified by preoperative RRT. Patients were included if their preoperative unadjusted (natural) MELD [23] score was greater than 25 and they had evidence of preoperative AKI, defined by a minimum RIFLE-RISK [26], and/or preoperative estimated glomerular filtration rate (eGFR) < 60 ml/min/1.73 m^2, calculated by the Modification of Diet in Renal Disease (MDRD) equation [27]. Patients were excluded if they had overt hyperkalemia or acidosis (preoperative pH < 7.3) where patients were placed on intraoperative CRRT outside of the study. The primary outcomes of this study were feasibility (ability to enroll 50 subjects) and safety; adverse events included complications of dialysis catheter insertion (bleeding, vascular injury), bleeding attributable to intraoperative CRRT, complications/unplanned interruption of CRRT and major metabolic complications. Results of this study are pending.

Conclusion

Liver transplantation in patients with preoperative AKI can be challenging and associated with significant perioperative morbidity. Although CRRT is being used for intraoperative support, evidence-based recommendations are lacking. While current retrospective observational studies have demonstrated that intraoperative CRRT is safe and feasible with acceptable patient, graft and renal outcomes, these studies are limited, due to selection bias, in their ability to definitively determine efficacy, safety and resource implications for the role of intraoperative CRRT in liver transplantation. Higher quality clinical investigations, ideally in the form of well-designed randomized studies aimed at minimizing the bias introduced in observational studies are needed to definitely determine the role and benefit of intraoperative CRRT in liver transplantation patients.

Acknowledgements

Dr. Bagshaw is supported by a Canada Research Chair in Critical Care Nephrology.

References

1. Tsien CD, Rabie R, Wong F (2013) Acute kidney injury in decompensated cirrhosis. Gut 62:131–137
2. Barreto R, Fagundes C, Guevara M et al (2014) Type-1 hepatorenal syndrome associated with infections in cirrhosis: natural history, outcome of kidney function, and survival. Hepatology 59:1505–1513
3. Piano S, Rosi S, Maresio G et al (2013) Evaluation of the Acute Kidney Injury Network criteria in hospitalized patients with cirrhosis and ascites. J Hepatol 59:482–489
4. Wong F, O'Leary JG, Reddy KR et al (2013) New consensus definition of acute kidney injury accurately predicts 30-day mortality in patients with cirrhosis and infection. Gastroenterology 145:1280–1288
5. Warner NS, Cuthbert JA, Bhore R, Rockey DC (2011) Acute kidney injury and chronic kidney disease in hospitalized patients with cirrhosis. J Invest Med 59:1244–1251

6. Garcia-Tsao G, Parikh CR, Viola A (2008) Acute kidney injury in cirrhosis. Hepatology 48:2064–2077
7. Martin-Llahi M, Guevara M, Torre A et al (2011) Prognostic importance of the cause of renal failure in patients with cirrhosis. Gastroenterology 140:488–496
8. Salerno F, Gerbes A, Gines P, Wong F, Arroyo V (2007) Diagnosis, prevention and treatment of hepatorenal syndrome in cirrhosis. Gut 56:1310–1318
9. Arroyo V, Gines P, Gerbes AL et al (1996) Definition and diagnostic criteria of refractory ascites and hepatorenal syndrome in cirrhosis. International Ascites Club. Hepatology 23:164–176
10. KDIGO (2012) Clinical practice guideline for acute kidney injury. Kidney Int Suppl 2:1–138
11. Angeli P, Gines P, Wong F et al (2015) Diagnosis and management of acute kidney injury in patients with cirrhosis: revised consensus recommendations of the International Club of Ascites. J Hepatol 64:531–537
12. Sanyal AJ, Boyer T, Garcia-Tsao G et al (2008) A randomized, prospective, double-blind, placebo-controlled trial of terlipressin for type 1 hepatorenal syndrome. Gastroenterology 134:1360–1368
13. Nair S, Verma S, Thuluvath PJ (2002) Pretransplant renal function predicts survival in patients undergoing orthotopic liver transplantation. Hepatology 35:1179–1185
14. Townsend DR, Bagshaw SM, Jacka MJ, Bigam D, Cave D, Gibney RT (2009) Intraoperative renal support during liver transplantation. Liver Transpl 15:73–78
15. LaMattina JC, Kelly PJ, Hanish SI et al (2015) Intraoperative continuous veno-venous hemofiltration facilitates surgery in liver transplant patients with acute renal failure. Transplant Proc 47:1901–1904
16. Agopian VG, Dhillon A, Baber J et al (2014) Liver transplantation in recipients receiving renal replacement therapy: outcomes analysis and the role of intraoperative hemodialysis. Am J Transplant 14:1638–1647
17. Wiklund RA (2004) Preoperative preparation of patients with advanced liver disease. Crit Care Med 32(4 Suppl):S106–S115
18. Angeli P, Bezinover D, Biancofiore G et al (2017) Acute kidney injury in liver transplant candidates: a position paper on behalf of the Liver Intensive Care Group of Europe. Minerva Anestesiol 83:88–101
19. Vitin A, Muczynski K, Bakthavatsalam R, Martay K, Dembo G, Metzner J (2010) Treatment of severe lactic acidosis during the pre-anhepatic stage of liver transplant surgery with intraoperative hemodialysis. J Clin Anesth 22:466–472
20. Xia VW, Ghobrial RM, Du B et al (2007) Predictors of hyperkalemia in the prereperfusion, early postreperfusion, and late postreperfusion periods during adult liver transplantation. Anesth Analg 105:780–785
21. Nadim MK, Ananthapanyasut W, Matsuoka L et al (2014) Intraoperative hemodialysis during liver transplantation: a decade of experience. Liver Transpl 20:756–764
22. Karvellas CJ, Farhat MR, Sajjad I et al (2011) A comparison of early versus late initiation of renal replacement therapy in critically ill patients with acute kidney injury: a systematic review and meta-analysis. Crit Care 15:R72
23. Kamath PS, Wiesner RH, Malinchoc M et al (2001) A model to predict survival in patients with end-stage liver disease. Hepatology 33:464–470
24. Zimmerman MA, Selim M, Kim J et al (2017) Outcome analysis of continuous intraoperative renal replacement therapy in the highest acuity liver transplant recipients: a single-center experience. Surgery 161:1279–1286
25. Parmar A, Bigam D, Meeberg G et al (2011) An evaluation of intraoperative renal support during liver transplantation: a matched cohort study. Blood Purif 32:238–248
26. Bellomo R, Ronco C, Kellum JA, Mehta RL, Palevsky P (2004) Acute Dialysis Quality Initiative w: Acute renal failure – definition, outcome measures, animal models, fluid therapy and information technology needs: the Second International Consensus Conference of the Acute Dialysis Quality Initiative (ADQI) Group. Crit Care 8:R204–R212

27. Levey AS, Stevens LA, Schmid CH et al (2009) A new equation to estimate glomerular filtration rate. Ann Intern Med 150:604–612
28. Mehta RL, Kellum JA, Shah SV et al (2007) Acute Kidney Injury Network: report of an initiative to improve outcomes in acute kidney injury. Crit Care 11:R31
29. Wong F, Nadim MK, Kellum JA et al (2011) Working Party proposal for a revised classification system of renal dysfunction in patients with cirrhosis. Gut 60:702–709

Part IX
Fluid Administration

Effects of Fluids on the Macro- and Microcirculations

V. A. Bennett, A. Vidouris, and M. Cecconi

Introduction

Intravenous fluid administration is one of the most frequently performed interventions in the intensive care unit (ICU) and in hospital in general. In fact, most inpatients will receive fluids at some point during their hospital stay [1]. In critically ill patients, fluid resuscitation is a vital component of patient management. It has been shown that both too little and too much fluid can be detrimental. A positive cumulative fluid balance on day four of a critical care admission has been associated with increased morbidity [2, 3]. Both perioperatively and during sepsis, a U-shaped curve has been described for volume of fluid administered and morbidity. Higher mortality is observed at both extremes of volume of fluid given [4, 5].

However, despite extensive research in the field, controversy remains regarding the best approach to fluid therapy. The FENICE study focused on the fluid challenge and found wide disparity in practice; from fluid choice to method of administration and clinician response to the result [6]. To help guide decision making around fluid administration, the effects, both desirable and potentially detrimental ones, need to be considered. This can be considered at both the macrocirculatory and the microcirculatory level. Whilst in health coherence between the macrocirculation and microcirculation can be assumed, this is lost in some disease states. This overview explores the effects of the fluid on the macro- and microcirculations and how we can monitor these effects.

Indications for Fluid

Classically, the need for fluid therapy is identified using information from the clinical history, examination, measurement of hemodynamic variables and markers of

V. A. Bennett (✉) · A. Vidouris · M. Cecconi
Department of Intensive Care Medicine, St George's University Hospital NHS Foundation Trust
London, UK
e-mail: v.bennett1@nhs.net

© Springer International Publishing AG 2018
J.-L. Vincent (ed.), *Annual Update in Intensive Care and Emergency Medicine 2018*,
Annual Update in Intensive Care and Emergency Medicine,
https://doi.org/10.1007/978-3-319-73670-9_30

tissue hypoperfusion [7]. Markers of hypoperfusion may include lactate, prolonged capillary refill time and skin mottling [6]. A fluid challenge is given when tissue hypoperfusion is suspected [7]. Fluid is given to optimize cardiovascular status with the aim of ensuring adequate end-organ perfusion and improving oxygen delivery to the tissues. Fluid is given as a fluid challenge so that response can be assessed and the need for ongoing fluid therapy ascertained. To mitigate against the risk of fluid overload in those who do not require additional intravascular volume, the smallest volume that provides an effective challenge of the cardiovascular system should be used [8].

Most often, measures of the macrocirculation are used to assess and treat hemodynamic compromise in the critically ill patient and measures of the microcirculation are not routinely used at the bedside. Resuscitation based on macrocirculatory endpoints is expected to result in parallel improvement in the microcirculation [9].

Macrocirculation

The macrocirculatory response to intravenous fluid administration is based on the principles of the Frank-Starling law of the heart. Venous return is always equal to cardiac output. The Frank-Starling principle describes how the heart is able to accommodate increased venous return and then eject the increased volume from the heart, with an increase in stroke volume. Increased venous return increases ventricular filling, which results in increased stretch of the cardiac myocyctes. This increased stretch results in increased contractility, or in other words, the increased diastolic expansion results in increased systolic contraction [10, 11]. Administration of fluid aims to challenge this and assess whether a patient can accommodate an increased preload with an increased stroke volume.

The hemodynamic response to a fluid challenge can be understood by considering the effects at different points on the cardiovascular system. The first change seen is an expansion of the intravascular volume. Intravascular volume can be divided into stressed and unstressed volumes. The unstressed volume fills the vessels but does not generate any pressure. The stressed volume causes stretch of the vessel walls and increases the pressure within the vessels. Mean systemic filling pressure (Pmsf) is the measurement of the pressure when there is no flow in the vessels, or in circulatory arrest. Whilst Pmsf cannot be measured under the circumstances with which it was initially described, alternative techniques have been validated [12]. If an effective fluid challenge is given, it will, at least transiently, increase the stressed volume and cause a rise in Pmsf. This increases cardiac preload, which ultimately increases cardiac output in preload-responsive patients. The response to the increase in cardiac preload can be explained by the Frank-Starling principle.

In a patient who is fluid responsive, an effective fluid challenge will result in a significant increase, of more than 10%, in the stroke volume or cardiac output. If a fluid challenge is given, which is effective in significantly increasing Pmsf, but no subsequent increase in cardiac output is seen, the patient is labeled as non-responsive [13]. This is demonstrated in Fig. 1: an adequate fluid challenge administered

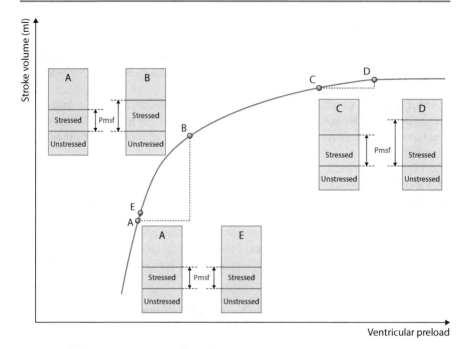

Fig. 1 Assessment of fluid responsiveness using a fluid challenge; effects on mean systemic filling pressure (Pmsf) and stroke volume, explained using the Frank Starling Curve. See text for explanation

at point A, increases Pmsf and a significant increase in stroke volume is seen at point B – this patient is fluid responsive. At C, although an adequate fluid challenge is given, as demonstrated by an increase in Pmsf, no significant increase in stroke volume is seen at point D – this patient is not fluid responsive. If an inadequate fluid challenge, of too small a volume to increase Pmsf, is given at point A, an increase in stroke volume is not seen at point E and the patient would incorrectly be labeled as non-responsive to fluid.

Cecconi et al. demonstrated that a change in the pressure gradient of venous return, defined as the difference between the Pmsf and central venous pressure (CVP), following a fluid challenge was seen in responders but not in non-responders. In the non-responders, the increase in Pmsf was mirrored by an increase in CVP [14]. In those that respond, the maximal change in cardiac output is seen one minute after completion of the fluid challenge. The increase in cardiac output is a transient response; a return to baseline values is seen ten minutes post-fluid administration [13].

The decision to give fluids should be based on whether an increase in cardiac output is likely to occur with fluid loading and whether it would be likely to improve tissue perfusion. These are clinical questions that the clinician should ask before considering giving fluids. A patient who is non-responsive is unlikely to benefit from further fluid loading. Not all patients who are responsive to fluid require the additional volume [8]. For example, in a study of healthy volunteers, by definition not in shock, a significant increase in stroke volume was seen following a head down tilt (mimicking a fluid challenge). Despite being fluid responsive these healthy volunteers were unlikely to need fluid resuscitation or have evidence of tissue hypoperfusion [15].

Other hemodynamic parameters, used more historically, include static endpoints, such as heart rate. However, a change in heart rate in response to fluid administration is not a sensitive marker of fluid responsiveness and can be influenced by numerous other factors [13].

CVP has historically also been used to guide fluid administration. Targeting a CVP of 8–12 cmH$_2$O was part of several optimization protocols in the past [16, 17]. The role of CVP in predicting fluid responsiveness has since been refuted. Use of the CVP as an indicator of fluid responsiveness has been shown to be unreliable [18, 19]. It does not provide accurate information about blood volume [20]. Monitoring trends in CVP over time may provide information about cardiovascular function but should not be used alone to guide fluid resuscitation [21].

Microcirculation and Hemodynamic Coherence

In health, hemodynamic coherence is assumed to exist. This means changes within the macrocirculation are reflective of changes in the microcirculation. As described earlier, the macrocirculation is generally used to guide fluid resuscitation, although ultimately the target is normalization of the microcirculation and maintenance of end-organ perfusion. However, although optimization of fluid status may result in normalization of macrocirculatory hemodynamics, such as blood pressure, this does not always translate to paralleled improvements or normalization of the microcirculation, or guarantee adequate tissue perfusion. In these conditions, a lack of hemodynamic coherence is described. This means that targeting the normalization of macrocirculatory variables may not be effective in restoring perfusion of end organs and tissues [22].

Under normal physiological conditions, the macrocirculation regulates the distribution of blood and thus end-organ perfusion. Systemic responses occur to alter macrovascular factors in order to compensate for hypovolemia, hypoxia or other nutrient delivery insufficiencies and to ensure removal of waste products. The macrocirculation is controlled by the central nervous system via the sympathoadrenomedullary axis and the parasympathetic nervous system. The renin-angiotensin-aldosterone axis, vasopressin, natriuretic peptides and adipocytokines are also important in the control of blood volume and blood pressure [23]. These pathways and hormones affect the blood supply to the microcirculation via modulation of the function of the heart, the tone of the vasculature and the volume, viscosity and composition of the blood.

The microcirculation has a hugely important role in maintaining homeostasis of end organs and regulating tissue perfusion and also in thermoregulation by controlling cutaneous blood flow. Local mechanisms regulate vascular tone at the microcirculatory level by acting upon smooth muscle. They respond to physical stimuli in the microcirculation, such as increased blood pressure, causing constriction in the arterioles of the microcirculation. Some of the molecules that are active in the vasculature of the microcirculation are released from the endothelial wall including prostaglandins, nitric oxide (NO) and endothelin, which are released as a result of shear stress on the vessels. NO release can also be stimulated by other vasoactive peptides. Metabolic stimuli, such as adenosine, hydrogen ions, carbon dioxide and oxygen tension, generated in tissues also control blood flow in the microcirculation via dilation of the vessels [9]. The function of the microcirculation is also controlled by the permeability of the capillaries, their structure, the osmotic and diffusion gradients across the cell membranes and the transport systems across the vessel walls.

There may be a lack of hemodynamic coherence in disease states. States of shock, inflammation and infection can interfere with the sensing and homeostatic control mechanisms of the microcirculation [22]. Coherence is often altered in states of hemorrhagic shock or septic shock [24]. The loss of hemodynamic coherence can be the result of physiological changes in the environment resulting in nitrosative and oxidative mechanisms affecting regulation of the vasculature, changes in cell function or through changes in barrier mechanisms and concentration gradients, all of which will inhibit normal tissue perfusion. Hemodynamic coherence has been shown to vary in different tissue types dependent upon the disease state present [25].

Coherence can be lost between different tissues in a single organ system. In a pig model, resuscitation with fluids was successful in improving perfusion of the microcirculation in the mucosa of the gut, but not effective in the villi [26]. It was observed that the NO synthase (NOS) enzyme was not homogenously distributed, which caused variable and abnormal blood flow regulation in the microcirculation [27]. NOS enzymes form NO from L-arginine, which acts to decrease response to vasoactive agents. One such enzyme, NOS 3 is also utilized in the maintenance of vascular tone. NO is pivotal in the formation of cyclic guanosine monophosphate (cGMP), which induces smooth muscle relaxation through various mechanisms. These include activation of potassium ion channels in the cell membrane and reduction in the intracellular concentration of calcium ions. These enzymes are activated in disease states with high cytokine and endotoxin release, such as sepsis. This results in increased NO production, and subsequent dilation of the vasculature and both macrocirculatory and microcirculatory dysfunction, to varying degrees in different tissues [28]. Inappropriate vasodilation, vasoconstriction or microcirculatory tamponade induced by increased venous pressure can result in decreased oxygenation of the tissues.

In sepsis, neutrophil adhesion and a hypercoagulable state may lead to capillary occlusion, alongside other capillaries with normal blood flow. This results in heterogeneous blood flow through the microcirculation, with subsequent hypoperfusion and tissue hypoxia. Oxidative stress also occurs, in which endothelial dysfunction and capillary fluid and protein leaks occur. There is a loss of cellular barriers and tight junctions leading to worsening tissue edema [29].

Another area in which hemodynamic coherence may be affected is in hemor-rhagic shock. Permissive hypotension and low volume fluid resuscitation are some-times used in the initial stages of treatment and over time these can lead to insid-ious microcirculatory hypoperfusion. This may disrupt both coherence and cause a reperfusion injury. If this occurs, then monitoring and restoring the macrocircu-lation will not result in benefit to the microcirculation [30]. Loss of hemodynamic coherence has been associated with poor outcomes [24, 31].

As previously discussed, intravenous fluids are given to improve end-organ per-fusion and oxygen delivery. Macrocirculatory parameters are used to deduce infor-mation about what is occurring at the microcirculatory level. However, as a lack of coherence may exist between the macro- and the microcirculation there is increas-ing evidence in favor of monitoring the effects of fluid at the microcirculatory level [22].

The microcirculation can be observed using a handheld camera at the patient's bedside. There are currently four generations of technology available. Through recording short video sequences of the microcirculation, information regarding fluid status can be ascertained. The images obtained can be scored and a number of mea-surements made. The microcirculation consensus meeting of 2007 described the following scoring systems: vessel density measurement including total vessel den-sity and perfused vessel density and vessel perfusion assessment using proportion of perfused vessels and microcirculatory flow index (MFI). These parameters can be used to monitor the effects of fluid on the microcirculation [32]. Due to the limited availability of monitoring equipment and the need for offline analysis of images ac-quired, at present microcirculation measurement remains primarily a research tool [33].

The effect of intravenous fluid on the microcirculation varies depending on the underlying disease state. Shock can be broadly divided into four different classes: hypovolemic, distributive, cardiogenic and obstructive shock. Hypovolemic, cardio-genic and obstructive shock are associated with a low cardiac output. However, in sepsis, a form of distributive shock, cardiac output may be either low or high. In cardiogenic and obstructive shock there is increased afterload, with an expansion of the volume of the microcirculation. Hypovolemic and distributive shock are both characterized by impaired flow in the microcirculation [34]. However, the changes seen in the microcirculation in distributive shock are the most marked. Disruption occurs, with adjacent small vessels often exhibiting markedly different patterns of flow. Much of the research on the effects of fluids on the microcirculation has there-fore focused on patients with sepsis [29]. The changes within the microcirculation that pre-date fluid administration must be considered to help predict the possible consequences of fluid administration.

Several mechanisms by which fluids exert their effects on the microcirculation have been described. The first, and arguably most important, is via increased flow. The effect of a fluid challenge on the macrocirculation, as previously described, increases filling within the system. In the volume-responsive patient this increases flow, which will increase microcirculatory perfusion by increasing pressure at the level of the capillaries.

Secondary effects relate to decreased viscosity secondary to hemodilution from fluid administration. The decreased viscosity will promote flow. In the hemoconcentrated patient this desirable feature will likely predominate; however, it may be that the hemodilution decreases oxygen carriage and cause shunting within the microcirculation [34].

Other adverse effects of fluid administration can be clearly demonstrated through direct vision of the microcirculation. Leakage of fluid extravascularly with increased tissue edema can be visualized and objectively monitored, as the vessel density will decrease. This results in increased diffusion distance from red blood cells to the tissues and decreased efficiency of oxygen delivery with subsequent hypoxia [29].

Measurement of flow within the microcirculation, at baseline, can be used to predict those that may benefit from a fluid challenge. Optimization of fluid status using macrocirculatory parameters does not always equate to improvement in clinical markers of hypoperfusion. Pranskunas et al. demonstrated that, in those with normal microcirculatory flow, no clinical benefit was gained by a fluid challenge, neither from the perspective of improvement in clinical markers of hypoperfusion nor an increase in MFI. In those with a low MFI, a significant improvement in MFI and clinical signs of hypoperfusion were seen following a fluid challenge [35]. Perioperatively, patients who develop postoperative complications have been shown to be more likely to have had microvascular flow abnormalities [36]. Those patients with a low MFI could not be identified by observing macrocirculatory parameters. Additionally, an increase in MFI did not correlate well with those who responded with an increase in stroke volume. The authors hypothesized this may be related to the fact that not all those who respond to a fluid challenge need the additional volume [35].

The effect of fluid administration on the microcirculation has been shown to vary dependent on the stage of the illness. In early sepsis, total vessel density, small vessel density and MFI all increased with fluid administration. The same effect was not seen in patients in the later stages of sepsis, defined as patients more than 48 h after diagnosis. These changes are not mirrored in the macrocirculation [37].

Predicting Response to Fluids

There are a number of different methods that can be used to try and predict which patients will be fluid responsive, prior to administering any fluid. Pulse pressure variation (PPV) and stroke volume variation (SVV) compare beat-to-beat variations, with a variation of more than 12% used as a marker of fluid responsiveness [38, 39]. These methods are only validated for use in ventilated patients, with tidal volumes of more than 8 ml/kg and with no significant alteration in chest wall compliance. They can also only be used in patients in sinus rhythm [40].

Another predictor is vena cava collapsibility index. Variation in the diameter of the inferior vena cava (IVC) on transthoracic echocardiography is reasonably predictive of fluid responsiveness; however, measurement of the collapsibility of the superior vena cava on transesophageal echocardiography is more reliable. Measurement of the vena cava has the same limitations related to ventilation as PPV or SVV. It can, however, be used in patients with arrhythmias [40].

The end-expiratory occlusion test can also be used in patients receiving mechanical ventilation. Interruption of ventilation at end-expiration for at least 15 s causes an increase in preload. If cardiac output increases by more than 5% in response then this is predictive of fluid responsiveness [41].

Passive leg raise has gained increasing popularity as a method of assessing fluid responsiveness. It provides approximately 300 ml of fluid as a challenge, increasing preload, from which fluid responsiveness can be determined. The technique can be reliably used in both ventilated and spontaneously ventilating patients. It provides a challenge of preload without the need to give intravenous fluids in patients who are then shown to be non-responsive. However, it has its own limitations: for practical reasons it may not always be possible to perform and its reliability in the presence of intraabdominal hypertension has also been questioned [42].

As previously discussed it is important to try and predict the likely response to fluid administration prior to actually giving fluids. Figure 2 provides a simple flow chart of the possible decision pathway that a clinician may follow when considering fluid prescription for a patient in shock.

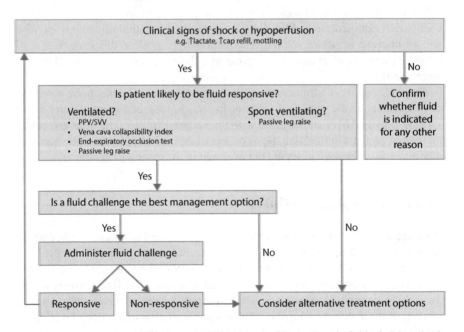

Fig. 2 Flow chart to demonstrate the possible decision-making process in fluid administration in shock. *PPV*: pulse pressure variation; *SVV*: stroke volume variation

Conclusion

The decision to give intravenous fluid to a patient is a clinical one. The clinical assessment of each patient should include a prediction of whether it is likely that he/she will respond to additional volume and whether he/she requires and will benefit from it. Fluid administration is in general guided by the changes seen within the macrocirculation. Historically, this was presumed to represent the microcirculation; however, in illness, it has been shown that coherence may not exist. There are still many uncertainties regarding the effects of fluids on the microcirculation. The effects vary depending on the disease process and indeed the stage of the disease. At this stage, the effects of fluids on the microcirculation remain a focus of ongoing study and research.

References

1. Padhi S, Bullock I, Li L, Stroud M, National Institute for Health and Care Excellence (NICE) Guideline Development Group (2013) Intravenous fluid therapy for adults in hospital: summary of NICE guidance. BMJ 347:f7073
2. Boyd JH, Forbes J, Nakada T, Walley KR, Russell JA (2011) Fluid resuscitation in septic shock: a positive fluid balance and elevated central venous pressure are associated with increased mortality. Crit Care Med 39:259–265
3. Vaara ST, Korhonen AM, Kaukonen K-M et al (2012) Fluid overload is associated with an increased risk for 90-day mortality in critically ill patients with renal replacement therapy: data from the prospective FINNAKI study. Crit Care 16:R197
4. Liu V, Morehouse JW, Soule J, Whippy A, Escobar GJ (2013) Fluid volume, lactate values, and mortality in sepsis patients with intermediate lactate values. Ann Am Thorac Soc 10:466–473
5. Bellamy MC (2006) Wet, dry or something else? Br J Anaesth 97:755–757
6. Cecconi M, Hofer C, Teboul JL et al (2015) Fluid challenges in intensive care: the FENICE study: a global inception cohort study. Intensive Care Med 41:1529–1537
7. Gruartmoner G, Mesquida J, Ince C (2015) Fluid therapy and the hypovolemic microcirculation. Curr Opin Crit Care 21:276–284
8. Cecconi M, Parsons AK, Rhodes A (2011) What is a fluid challenge? Curr Opin Crit Care 17:290–295
9. Charlton M, Sims M, Coats T, Thompson JP (2016) The microcirculation and its measurement in sepsis. J Intensive Care Soc 18:221–227
10. Patterson SW, Piper H, Starling EH (1914) The regulation of the heart beat. J Physiol 48:465–513
11. Patterson SW, Starling EH (1914) On the mechanical factors which determine the output of the ventricles. J Physiol 48:357–379
12. Aya HD, Rhodes A, Fletcher N, Grounds RM, Cecconi M (2016) Transient stop-flow arm arterial-venous equilibrium pressure measurement: determination of precision of the technique. J Clin Monit Comput 30:55–61
13. Aya HD, Ster IC, Fletcher N, Grounds RM, Rhodes A, Cecconi M (2015) Pharmacodynamic analysis of a fluid challenge. Crit Care Med 44:880–891
14. Cecconi M, Aya HD, Geisen M et al (2013) Changes in the mean systemic filling pressure during a fluid challenge in postsurgical intensive care patients. Intensive Care Med 39:1299–1305

15. Nixon JV, Murray RG, Leonard PD, Mitchell JH, Blomqvist CG (1982) Effect of large variations in preload on left ventricular performance characteristics in normal subjects. Circulation 65:698–703
16. Rivers E, Nguyen B, Havstad S et al (2001) Early goal directed therapy in the treatment of severe sepsis and septic shock. N Engl J Med 345:1368–1377
17. Dellinger RP, Levy MM, Carlet JM et al (2008) Surviving Sepsis Campaign: international guidelines for management of severe sepsis and septic shock: 2008. Intensive Care Med 34:17–60
18. Bentzer P, Griesdale DE, Boyd J, MacLean K, Sirounis D, Ayas NT (2016) Will this hemodynamically unstable patient respond to a bolus of intravenous fluids? JAMA 316:1298–1309
19. Marik PE, Cavallazzi R (2013) Does the central venous pressure predict fluid responsiveness? An updated meta-analysis and a plea for some common sense. Crit Care Med 41:1774–1781
20. Marik PE, Baram M, Vahid B (2008) Does central venous pressure predict fluid responsiveness? Chest 134:172–178
21. Magdar S (2010) Fluid status and fluid responsiveness. Curr Opin Crit Care 16:289–296
22. Ince C (2015) Hemodynamic coherence and the rationale for monitoring the microcirculation. Crit Care 19(Suppl 3):S8
23. Thiriet M (2014) Macrocirculation. In: Lanzer P (ed) PanVascular Medicine. Springer, Berlin, pp 1–54
24. Arnemann P, Seidel L, Ertmer C (2016) Haemodynamic coherence – the relevance of fluid therapy. Best Pract Res Clin Anaesthesiol 30:419–427
25. Van Iterson M, Bezemer R, Heger M, Siegemund M, Ince C (2012) Microcirculation follows macrocirculation in heart and gut in the acute phase of hemorrhagic shock and isovolemic autologous whole blood resuscitation in pigs. Transfusion 52:1552–1559
26. Siegemund M, Van Bommel J, Sinaasappel M et al (2007) The NO donor SIN-1 improves intestinal-arterial Pco2 gap in experimental endotoxemia: an animal study. Acta Anaesthesiol Scand 51:693–700
27. Almac E, Siegemund M, Demirci C, Ince C (2006) Microcirculatory recruitment maneuvers correct tissue CO2 abnormalities in sepsis. Minerva Anestesiol 72:509–519
28. Lush CW, Kvietys PR (2000) Microvascular dysfunction in sepsis. Microcirculation 7:83–101
29. Elbers PWG, Ince C (2006) Mechanisms of critical illness – classifying microcirculatory flow abnormalities in distributive shock. Crit Care 10:221
30. Libert N, Harrois A, Duranteau J (2016) Haemodynamic coherence in haemorrhagic shock. Best Pract Res Clin Anaesthesiol 30:429–435
31. Vellinga NA, Ince C, Boerma EC (2013) Elevated central venous pressure is associated with impairment of microcirculatory blood flow in sepsis: a hypothesis generating post hoc analysis. BMC Anesthesiol 13:17
32. De Backer D, Hollenberg S, Boerma C et al (2007) How to evaluate the microcirculation: report of a round table conference. Crit Care 11:R101
33. Tafner PFDA, Chen FK, Filho RR, Corrêa TD, Chaves RCF, Neto SA (2017) Recent advances in bedside microcirculation assessment in critically ill patients. Rev Bras Ter Intensiva 29(2):238–247
34. Boldt J, Ince C (2010) The impact of fluid therapy on microcirculation and tissue oxygenation in hypovolemic patients: a review. Intensive Care Med 36:1299–1308
35. Pranskunas A, Koopmans M, Koetsier PM, Pilvinis V, Boerma EC (2013) Microcirculatory blood flow as a tool to select ICU patients eligible for fluid therapy. Intensive Care Med 39:612–619
36. Jhanji S, Lee C, Watson D, Hinds C, Pearse RM (2009) Microvascular flow and tissue oxygenation after major abdominal surgery: Association with post-operative complications. Intensive Care Med 35:671–677
37. Ospina-Tascon G, Neves AP, Occhipinti G et al (2010) Effects of fluids on microvascular perfusion in patients with severe sepsis. Intensive Care Med 36:949–955

38. De Backer D, Heenen S, Piagnerelli M, Koch M, Vincent JL (2005) Pulse pressure variations to predict fluid responsiveness: influence of tidal volume. Intensive Care Med 31:517–523
39. Marik PE, Cavallazzi R, Vasu T, Hirani A (2009) Dynamic changes in arterial waveform derived variables and fluid responsiveness in mechanically ventilated patients: a systematic review of the literature. Crit Care Med 37:2642–2647
40. Monnet X, Marik PE, Teboul JL (2016) Prediction of fluid responsiveness: an update. Ann Intensive Care 6:111
41. Monnet X, Osman D, Ridel C, Lamia B, Richard C, Teboul JL (2009) Predicting volume responsiveness by using the end-expiratory occlusion in mechanically ventilated intensive care unit patients. Crit Care Med 37:951–956
42. Monnet X, Marik P, Teboul JL (2016) Passive leg raising for predicting fluid responsiveness: a systematic review and meta-analysis. Intensive Care Med 42:1935–1947

Regulation of Cardiac Output and Manipulation with Fluids

H. D. Aya, M. Cecconi, and M. I. Monge García

Introduction

The normal acute physiological response to critical illness is to increase oxygen consumption (VO_2) and oxygen delivery (DO_2) by increasing cardiac output to meet the augmented metabolic demands. In that situation, normal values are inadequate. This concept is the basis of hemodynamic optimization, also called early goal-directed therapy (EGDT), which consists of a sequence of therapeutic interventions on the cardiovascular system using hemodynamic monitoring and well-defined interventions to increase DO_2. This approach has been shown to improve tissue oxygenation, prevent postoperative complications and decrease mortality in high-risk patients undergoing major surgery [1–12]. This concept was extrapolated to patients with septic shock in a clinical trial published by Rivers and colleagues [13]. However, three multicenter clinical trials [14–16] showed no benefit of this intervention in this population of critically ill patients. Hence, it is important to know the physiology of the regulation of cardiac output to understand when and how some interventions may result in better clinical outcomes.

Cardiac Output Regulation

The main function of the heart is to continuously pump blood volume from the venous system without increasing intracardiac pressures and with the lowest energy expenditure. Cardiac output varies widely depending mainly on metabolic demand, age, and body size.

H. D. Aya · M. Cecconi
Department of Intensive Care Medicine, St. George's University Hospital, NHS Foundation Trust
London, UK

M. I. Monge García (✉)
Unidad de Cuidados Intensivos, Hospital SAS de Jerez
Jerez de la Frontera, Spain
e-mail: ignaciomonge@gmail.com

© Springer International Publishing AG 2018   395
J.-L. Vincent (ed.), *Annual Update in Intensive Care and Emergency Medicine 2018*,
Annual Update in Intensive Care and Emergency Medicine,
https://doi.org/10.1007/978-3-319-73670-9_31

In a steady and healthy situation, the amount of blood coming from the venous system to the right atrium must equal the volume ejected by the heart into the arterial system. Accordingly, cardiac output and venous return are considered synonymous terms. To maintain this equilibrium, the heart has the Frank-Starling mechanism: when the blood flow to the heart increases, the enlarged stretch of the cardiac muscle fibers (i.e., cardiac preload) increases their force of contraction to empty the cardiac ventricles. The relationship between preload and cardiac output is called the cardiac function curve (Fig. 1).

It is noteworthy that this curve was initially described as the relationship between right atrial pressure (RAP), instead of preload, and cardiac output. Preload is defined as the end-diastolic myocardial stretching (sarcomere tension), which is determined by the diastolic properties of the ventricle and the end-diastolic volume. Moreover, the relationship between myocardial tension and myocardial volume is neither linear nor unique: compliance decreases as end-diastolic volume increases and some pathological situations (e.g., myocardial ischemia, ventricular hypertrophy) may alter this relationship.

By contrast, under isovolemic conditions (no changes in intravascular volume), the relationship between RAP and blood flow defines a different curve: the venous return curve. In this case, if we decrease the heart's ability to pump, the blood will progressively accumulate in the venous system, and RAP will increase until a certain point when the heart stops. At this moment, when the circulatory flow is zero, the pressure is equal in every point of the circulatory system. This pressure is created by the stressed volume filling the cardiovascular system and is known as the mean circulatory filling pressure (Pmcf). If the pulmonary circulation is excluded, it is called the mean systemic filling pressure (Pmsf). These variables are relevant to define the venous return curves described by Guyton (Fig. 2).

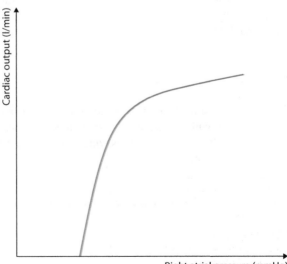

Fig. 1 Normal cardiac function curve: relationship between right atrial pressure and cardiac output with increasing values of blood volume

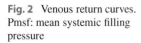
Fig. 2 Venous return curves.
Pmsf: mean systemic filling
pressure

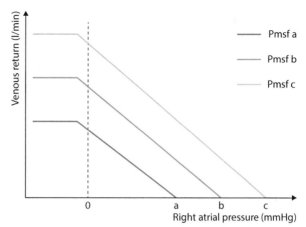

Some important concepts to remember from these curves are that: for any given RAP, the greater the Pmsf, the greater the venous return; and, in contrast to the Frank-Starling curves, under isovolemic conditions, the greater the RAP, the lower the venous return. It is easy to understand now, why a healthy heart will try to keep RAP as low as possible to facilitate venous return, and why Pmsf plays an important role in the regulation of cardiac output.

Cardiac output or venous return is just the sum of the volumes flowing through all the organs and tissues. Organ blood flow is finely regulated by local chemical, neurological and hormonal signals to keep the balance between VO_2 and DO_2. Under normal conditions, most of the capillary sphincters are closed and a minimal number of capillaries supply enough oxygen. An increase in metabolic demand will induce an increase in perfused capillaries and a certain level of venoconstriction to increase the effective circulating blood volume. Therefore, the regulation of cardiac output depends on the metabolic demands of the organs and tissues.

Manipulation of Cardiac Output and Fluid Therapy

The aim of intravenous fluid administration is to increase intravascular volume, cardiac preload and eventually stroke volume. This is based on Frank-Starling's law, which states that the energy of contraction is proportional to the length of the muscle fiber before contraction [17].

The best heart performance under a given contractile state is achieved by using consecutive fluid challenges until the initial flat portion of the Frank-Starling curve is reached. This pragmatic approach (stroke volume maximization) was proposed by Mythen et al. [18], and has been used as a fundamental aspect of most EGDT protocols. A positive response is usually defined as an increase in stroke volume by 10 or 15%.

However, there is increasing concern about fluid overload in critically ill patients. Several studies have suggested that a positive fluid balance is associated with acute lung injury (ALI) [19]. Patients with fluid overload had greater risk of respiratory failure and sepsis and longer duration of mechanical ventilation. Wiedemann et al. [20] reported a clinical trial comparing two fluid management strategies (conservative and liberal) in 1000 patients with ALI. Mortality at 60 days (primary outcome) was similar between the groups, but the conservative strategy improved the oxygenation index, the lung injury score, the number of days free of mechanical ventilation (14.6 vs 12.1 days, $p < 0.001$) and the length of stay in the intensive care unit (ICU; 13.4 vs 11.2 days, $p < 0.001$) without increasing non-pulmonary organ failures.

Fluid overload is also associated with higher mortality in patients with acute kidney injury (AKI), even after adjustment for severity of illness [21], modality of dialysis [22] fluid-strategy or mean daily central venous pressure (CVP) [23]

Fluid balance also has an impact in patients with sepsis. Boyd et al. [24] conducted a retrospective review of the use of intravenous fluids during the first 4 days of care in 778 patients enrolled in the Vasopressin and Septic Shock Trial (VASST) with septic shock and receiving at least 5 µg/min of norepinephrine. After correcting for age and APACHE II score, a more positive fluid balance both at 12 h and at day 4 correlated significantly with increased mortality.

The evidence, therefore, suggests that positive fluid balance is associated with higher mortality and, although association does not necessarily mean causality, this relationship has triggered a therapeutic initiative to manage critically ill patients with minimal fluids, regardless of the underlying disease. In a sub-study of the study by Wiedemann et al. [20], Mikkelsen et al. [25] assessed neuropsychological function at 2 and 12 months post-hospital discharge in survivors of ALI. Lower PaO_2 was associated with cognitive impairment at 12 months ($p = 0.02$) in the conservative fluid group. Lower PaO_2 values ($p = 0.05$), lower CVP ($p = 0.02$) and enrolment in the conservative fluid group ($p < 0.001$) were correlated with worse executive function. After adjustment for potential covariates, lower PaO_2 and enrolment in the conservative fluid group were independently associated with cognitive impairment at 12 months. In a *post hoc* study of patients with traumatic brain injury (TBI) recruited into the SAFE (Saline versus Albumin Fluid Evaluation) trial [26], fluid resuscitation with albumin was associated with higher mortality rates than was resuscitation with saline. During the first 48 h in the ICU, patients in the albumin group received significantly less fluid than did patients in the saline group and the fluid balance was less positive than in the saline group. Recently, Hjortrup et al. [27] assessed the effects of restricting resuscitation fluid (fluid challenges) after initial resuscitation. They randomized 151 adult patients with septic shock who had received initial fluid resuscitation. In the fluid restriction group, fluid boluses were permitted only if signs of severe hypoperfusion occurred, whereas in the standard care group, fluid boluses were permitted as long as circulation continued to improve. Although the amount of fluid used for resuscitation was significantly reduced in the restriction group, there were no differences in terms of total fluid input or cumulative fluid balance. Similarly, patient-centered outcomes (such as death by day 90, ischemic events in the ICU or worsening AKI) all pointed towards benefit with fluid restriction, but none achieved statistical significance. Malbrain et al.

[28] conducted a systematic review of the association between positive fluid balance and outcomes of critically ill patients. A restrictive fluid management strategy was associated with a lower mortality compared to patients treated with a more liberal fluid management strategy (24.7 vs. 33.2%; OR 0.42; 95% CI 0.32–0.55; p < 0.0001). However, the results of this meta-analysis are difficult to interpret, because the selected studies were a combination of randomized controlled trials, other interventional designs and observational studies. Overall, there is no clear evidence that therapeutic interventions to reduce fluid balance are effective in improving clinical outcomes.

As a result, in the intensive care community, there is increasing awareness of the concept that intravenous fluids are drugs with undesirable adverse effects. Thus, as with any other drug, it is necessary to understand their pharmacodynamics, dosage and methods of administration and monitoring. Nonetheless, fluid therapy is essential in the resuscitation of critically ill patients. It is a surprise then, that the dosing of intravenous fluids remains empirical and heterogeneous, even in the case of a fluid challenge. The Pmsf is an old concept, but its estimation in critically ill patients could lead to a better understanding of cardiovascular physiology and the effects of fluid therapy at the bedside. This parameter may also help to standardize the fluid challenge technique.

From the current data available, several concepts can be summarized about the fluid challenge technique:

1) The Pmsf should increase in both responders and non-responders [29, 30]. If Pmsf remains unchanged, then the fluid challenge has failed to increase the driving pressure of the venous return. This phenomenon can be attributed to a low dose of fluid, a simultaneous change in vasopressor dose or concomitant vasodilation. A lack of change in Pmsf reveals that the fluid challenge has been not effective, thus, not valid to draw any hemodynamic conclusions.

2) Mean arterial pressure (MAP) increases in responders, although these changes appear to be dose-dependent and related to changes in arterial load [31].

3) CVP increases similarly in both groups, although the overall impact appears to be greater in non-responders [32]. At the bedside, it is not easy to calculate the overall impact of the fluid challenge on CVP, and no other single CVP value seems to be a good index of fluid responsiveness. CVP remains a complex signal, difficult to interpret in isolation from other clinical and hemodynamic variables.

4) Maximal hemodynamic changes occur within one minute after the end of fluid infusion [32]. This immediate change mainly reflects the ventricular response, and provides the appropriate answer for defining fluid responsiveness. However, these changes are not long-lasting (no more than 10 min), particularly if small volumes are used. This delayed effect may reflect a vascular response, although its interpretation needs further investigation.

5) The dose required for an effective fluid challenge is around 4 ml/kg in postoperative patients [29]. This is the conclusion of a recent clinical trial testing the minimal dose for a fluid challenge and observing the changes in the Pmsf and

the rate of responders in four groups (1, 2, 3 and 4 ml/kg). There are some studies that suggest a lower dose (a mini-fluid challenge technique) [33–35] with different predictive values compared with volumes of 250 or 500 ml. In a recent study, Biais et al. [33] concluded that changes in stroke volume index induced by rapid infusion of 100 ml crystalloid predicted the effects of 250 ml crystalloid in patients who were ventilated mechanically in the operating room. This information could be useful in clinical practice, although there are some uncertainties about the effectiveness of a small volume fluid challenge: if a patient responds positively to 100 ml, it is very likely that he/she will still respond to 250 or 500 ml. However, if there is a negative response, the picture is not so clear: even after a bolus of 250 ml, there is the possibility that the lack of response is related to insufficient volume. In addition, no data are currently available regarding the minimal volume required in septic patients, a group of patients that usually requires a greater amount of fluids and in whom fluid overload has been associated with significant complications.

6) Finally, if we agree that the main purpose of the cardiovascular system is to maintain peripheral perfusion, we need to examine the effect of the fluid challenge on tissue perfusion. It has been shown that an impaired microcirculation may persist, despite restored macrohemodynamics [36, 37]. The microcirculation can be affected by several factors, such as endothelial cell inflammation, circulating inflammatory biomarkers [38], increased leukocyte adhesion [39], microthrombi and rheologic abnormalities [40]. Therefore, as previously suggested [41], it is very difficult to know the state of the microcirculation only by examining macrohemodynamic variables. The main determinant of tissue perfusion is the local metabolic demand of each particular tissue. This process involves at least three mechanisms: perivascular sympathetic innervation [42], which will mediate in the control of arterioles; red blood cells, which are also O_2 sensors and regulators of arteriole tone [43]; and the activation of the K_{ATP} channels by a decrease in cellular ATP concentration, coupled with an increase in cellular concentrations of hydrogen ion and lactate. Activation of K_{ATP} channels causes vasodilation by allowing an efflux of potassium. This hyperpolarizes the plasma membrane and prevents the entry of calcium into the cell [44]. Previous studies of tissue perfusion in hemorrhagic models have reported a good correlation between hemodynamic changes and measures of tissue perfusion. For example, Gottrup et al. [45] observed that subcutaneous ($PscO_2$), conjunctival ($PcjO_2$) and transcutaneous ($PtcO_2$) oxygen tension values mirrored changes in arterial pressure and cardiac output during hemorrhage and resuscitation in eight dogs. Singer et al. [46] observed, in a rat model of hemorrhage, that resuscitation of bladder epithelial oxygen tension (BEOT) closely mirrored both systemic (blood pressure and aortic blood flow) and regional (renal blood flow) hemodynamic changes. Whitehouse et al. [47] demonstrated, in a rat model of hemorrhage reperfusion, that tissue oxygen tension (PtO_2) was maintained in the three regions of the kidney (cortical, cortical-medullar junction and medullar), despite significant falls in blood pressure and total renal blood flow. Dyson et al. [48] observed that progressive hemorrhage produced proportional decreases in

liver, muscular and bladder PtO_2, although not in the renal cortex PtO_2, until severe blood loss had occurred. These studies suggest that in the context of frank hypovolemia (hemorrhagic model), resuscitation with intravenous fluids can improve tissue perfusion and systemic hemodynamics. In humans, Ospina-Tascon et al. [49] evaluated the effect of 1 l of Ringer's lactate solution (or 400 ml of 4% albumin) in 60 patients with severe sepsis: 37 in the "early" stage (within 24 h of diagnosis) and 23 in the "late" stage (more than 48 h). There was no correlation between the changes in microcirculation and changes in hemodynamics. They observed that microvascular perfusion indexes (perfused vessel density [PVD], proportion of perfused vessels and microvascular flow index [MFI]) increased only in the "early" group. Pranskunas et al. [50] reported results from a study in which a fluid challenge was given to 50 patients with clinical signs of impaired organ perfusion (mixed population of sepsis, post-cardiac surgery and post-cardiac arrest). Microvascular perfusion indexes improved only in the group of patients with prior microcirculatory derangement, regardless of changes in macrohemodynamics. Edul et al. [37] also reported a significant correlation between baseline values of sublingual red blood cell velocity (RBCV) and the changes in RBCV, and baseline PVD and the changes in PVD 20 minutes after a 10 ml/kg infusion of colloids in septic patients. Animal studies [51, 52] assessing tissue perfusion using other techniques have also reported that systemic and local hemodynamics are uncoupled in sepsis, and that restoration of macrohemodynamic variables does not usually translate into an improvement in tissue perfusion. Hence, impaired microcirculatory changes may represent an adaptive response to a low metabolic state in multiorgan failure states, responding to a programmed bio-energetic shutdown rather than cellular necrosis [53]. Further studies are required to elucidate whether normal tissue perfusion at baseline in postoperative patients indicates that additional fluid administration could be useless or harmful, despite the apparent improvement in systemic hemodynamics.

In summary, the current evidence suggests that manipulation of hemodynamics only has a significant impact on tissue perfusion when this is already impaired. In a cardio-centric model of the human circulation, where the heart governs the blood flow based on the principles of preload, contractility and afterload, manipulation of systemic hemodynamics (with fluids, inotropes, etc.) should consistently have an impact on tissue perfusion. In this model, the microcirculation is seen as a completely passive area that follows the orders coming from the hemodynamic level in terms of flow and pressure. However, if we accept that blood flow is finely governed at the microcirculatory level, and the hemodynamics are just a reflection of all those different territories in the body, manipulation of hemodynamics should then be performed in the context of the tissue perfusion state. However, discovering feasible ways to assess and monitor tissue perfusion and defining clinical goals that can be easily applied at the bedside still remains a challenge.

Clinical Implications

The concept of goal-directed therapy has been shown to improve outcomes after surgery, but given the adverse effects of fluid overload, the maximization of preload is currently being challenged by new approaches [54, 55]. A better understanding of fluid administration constitutes the first step to move toward a more refined and individualized treatment of high-risk surgical patients.

The administration of intravenous fluids in the absence of tissue hypoperfusion seems, at the least, questionable in postoperative patients. The maximization of cardiac output or stroke volume as a first step of EGDT puts the prediction and assessment of fluid responsiveness at the center of hemodynamic management. Current evidence suggests that this should be replaced by the assessment of tissue perfusion before any other intervention. The goals of EGDT should probably be reformulated, moving from the hemodynamic level to the tissue perfusion level. The question would then be how to assess and monitor tissue perfusion reliably in critically ill patients. On the other hand, tissue hypoperfusion does not necessarily indicate the requirement for intravenous fluids in other contexts, such as septic shock, as suggested by other studies [48, 51]. This could be one of the reasons why recent trials of EGDT failed to demonstrate improved outcomes in patients with septic shock [14–16]. And, even in postoperative patients, the inflammatory response to the critical illness may generate a mixed picture, which could be difficult to interpret.

The short-lived hemodynamic effect of the fluid challenge is one of the most controversial results of recent studies. It could be argued that if the effects of the intravenous fluids are almost completely dissipated in about ten minutes, why should we use fluids at all? The answer might come again from the microcirculatory level of the cardiovascular system: as long as the tissue perfusion abnormalities are corrected, the short-lived hemodynamic effect of the fluid challenge should not represent a problem. However, there are still some methodological questions that will require an answer: when should we assess the effect of a fluid challenge in the microcirculation? Or how long should that effect last? These questions require further investigation.

Once an effective fluid challenge is performed, there are two-time points that require attention: the immediate response (one minute after fluid infusion), which will indicate ventricular performance; and the delayed response (10–15 min after the fluid infusion), which will probably indicate a vascular response. At this moment, reassessment of tissue perfusion appears very important and there are at least two possibilities: (1) intravenous fluids are redistributed into the cardiovascular system, improving tissue perfusion or (2) intravenous fluid leaks out of the capillaries, generating edema in the interstitial space and worsening oxygen diffusion.

Conclusion

Because of the pragmatic approach of maximization of stroke volume, many hemodynamic studies published so far have been focused on prediction of fluid responsiveness. This approach is now more questionable, given that fluid responsiveness does not necessarily mean fluid requirement. In addition, impaired tissue perfusion does not necessarily mean that additional fluids are required. Therefore, there is an important gap in information, which can potentially be filled by observing the Pmsf. Manipulation of hemodynamics should be tissue-perfusion orientated.

References

1. Kern JW, Shoemaker WC (2002) Meta-analysis of hemodynamic optimization in high-risk patients. Crit Care Med 30:1686–1692
2. Poeze M, Greve JW, Ramsay G (2005) Meta-analysis of hemodynamic optimization: relationship to methodological quality. Crit Care 9:R771–R779
3. Giglio MT, Marucci M, Testini M, Brienza N (2009) Goal-directed haemodynamic therapy and gastrointestinal complications in major surgery: a meta-analysis of randomized controlled trials. Br J Anaesth 103:637–646
4. Brienza N, Giglio MT, Marucci M, Fiore T (2009) Does perioperative hemodynamic optimization protect renal function in surgical patients? A meta-analytic study. Crit Care Med 37:2079–2090
5. Rahbari NN, Zimmermann JB, Schmidt T, Koch M, Weigand MA, Weitz J (2009) Meta-analysis of standard, restrictive and supplemental fluid administration in colorectal surgery. Br J Surg 96:331–341
6. Dalfino L, Giglio MT, Puntillo F, Marucci M, Brienza N (2011) Haemodynamic goal-directed therapy and postoperative infections: earlier is better. A systematic review and meta-analysis. Crit Care 15:R154
7. Gurgel ST, do Nascimento P Jr (2011) Maintaining tissue perfusion in high-risk surgical patients: a systematic review of randomized clinical trials. Anesth Analg 112:1384–1391
8. Hamilton MA, Cecconi M, Rhodes A (2011) A systematic review and meta-analysis on the use of preemptive hemodynamic intervention to improve postoperative outcomes in moderate and high-risk surgical patients. Anesth Analg 112:1392–1402
9. Corcoran T, Rhodes JE, Clarke S, Myles PS, Ho KM (2012) Perioperative fluid management strategies in major surgery: a stratified meta-analysis. Anesth Analg 114:640–651
10. Aya HD, Cecconi M, Hamilton M, Rhodes A (2013) Goal-directed therapy in cardiac surgery: a systematic review and meta-analysis. Br J Anaesth 110:510–517
11. Arulkumaran N, Corredor C, Hamilton MA et al (2014) Cardiac complications associated with goal-directed therapy in high-risk surgical patients: a meta-analysis. Br J Anaesth 112:648–659
12. Cecconi M, Corredor C, Arulkumaran N et al (2013) Clinical review: goal-directed therapy-what is the evidence in surgical patients? The effect on different risk groups. Crit Care 17:209
13. Rivers E, Nguyen B, Havstad S et al (2001) Early goal-directed therapy in the treatment of severe sepsis and septic shock. N Engl J Med 345:1368–1377
14. Peake SL, Delaney A, Bailey M et al (2014) Goal-directed resuscitation for patients with early septic shock. N Engl J Med 371:1496–1506
15. Yealy DM, Kellum JA, Huang DT et al (2014) A randomized trial of protocol-based care for early septic shock. N Engl J Med 370:1683–1693
16. Mouncey PR, Osborn TM, Power GS et al (2015) Trial of early, goal-directed resuscitation for septic shock. N Engl J Med 372:1301–1311
17. Starling EH, Visscher MB (1927) The regulation of the energy output of the heart. J Physiol 62:243–261
18. Mythen MG, Webb AR (1995) Perioperative plasma volume expansion reduces the incidence of gut mucosal hypoperfusion during cardiac surgery. Arch Surg 130:423–429

19. Rosenberg AL, Dechert RE, Park PK, Bartlett RH, NIH NHLBI ARDS Network (2009) Review of a large clinical series: association of cumulative fluid balance on outcome in acute lung injury: a retrospective review of the ARDSnet tidal volume study cohort. J Intensive Care Med 24:35–46

20. Wiedemann HP, Wheeler AP, Bernard GR et al (2006) Comparison of two fluid-management strategies in acute lung injury. N Engl J Med 354:2564–2575

21. Bellomo R, Cass A, Cole L et al (2012) An observational study fluid balance and patient outcomes in the Randomized Evaluation of Normal vs. Augmented Level of Replacement Therapy trial. Crit Care Med 40:1753–1760

22. Bouchard J, Soroko SB, Chertow GM et al (2009) Fluid accumulation, survival and recovery of kidney function in critically ill patients with acute kidney injury. Kidney Int 76:422–427

23. Grams ME, Estrella MM, Coresh J et al (2011) Fluid balance, diuretic use, and mortality in acute kidney injury. Clin J Am Soc Nephrol 6:966–973

24. Boyd JH, Forbes J, Nakada TA, Walley KR, Russell JA (2011) Fluid resuscitation in septic shock: a positive fluid balance and elevated central venous pressure are associated with increased mortality. Crit Care Med 39:259–265

25. Mikkelsen ME, Christie JD, Lanken PN et al (2012) The adult respiratory distress syndrome cognitive outcomes study: long-term neuropsychological function in survivors of acute lung injury. Am J Respir Crit Care Med 185:1307–1315

26. Finfer S, Bellomo R, Boyce N et al (2004) A comparison of albumin and saline for fluid resuscitation in the intensive care unit. N Engl J Med 350:2247–2256

27. Hjortrup PB, Haase N, Bundgaard H et al (2016) Restricting volumes of resuscitation fluid in adults with septic shock after initial management: the CLASSIC randomised, parallel-group, multicentre feasibility trial. Intensive Care Med 42:1695–1705

28. Malbrain ML, Marik PE, Witters I et al (2014) Fluid overload, de-resuscitation, and outcomes in critically ill or injured patients: a systematic review with suggestions for clinical practice. Anaesthesiol Intensive Ther 46:361–380

29. Aya HD, Rhodes A, Ster IC, Fletcher N, Grounds RM, Cecconi M (2017) Hemodynamic effect of different doses of fluids for a fluid challenge: a quasi-randomized controlled study. Crit Care Med 45:e161–e168

30. Cecconi M, Aya HD, Geisen M et al (2013) Changes in the mean systemic filling pressure during a fluid challenge in postsurgical intensive care patients. Intensive Care Med 39:1299–1305

31. Monge Garcia MI, Guijo Gonzalez P, Gracia Romero M et al (2015) Effects of fluid administration on arterial load in septic shock patients. Intensive Care Med 41:1247–1255

32. Aya HD, Ster IC, Fletcher N, Grounds RM, Rhodes A, Cecconi M (2016) Pharmacodynamic analysis of a fluid challenge. Crit Care Med 44:880–891

33. Biais M, de Courson H, Lanchon R et al (2017) Mini-fluid challenge of 100 ml of crystalloid predicts fluid responsiveness in the operating room. Anesthesiology 127:450–456

34. Mallat J, Meddour M, Durville E et al (2015) Decrease in pulse pressure and stroke volume variations after mini-fluid challenge accurately predicts fluid responsiveness. Br J Anaesth 115:449–456

35. Muller L, Toumi M, Bousquet PJ et al (2011) An increase in aortic blood flow after an infusion of 100 ml colloid over 1 minute can predict fluid responsiveness: the mini-fluid challenge study. Anesthesiology 115:541–547

36. Sakr Y, Dubois MJ, De Backer D, Creteur J, Vincent JL (2004) Persistent microcirculatory alterations are associated with organ failure and death in patients with septic shock. Crit Care Med 32:1825–1831

37. Edul VS, Ince C, Navarro N et al (2014) Dissociation between sublingual and gut microcirculation in the response to a fluid challenge in postoperative patients with abdominal sepsis. Ann Intensive Care 4:39

38. Gardner AW, Parker DE, Montgomery PS et al (2015) Endothelial cell inflammation and antioxidant capacity are associated with exercise performance and microcirculation in patients with symptomatic peripheral artery disease. Angiology 66:867–874

39. Roller J, Wang Y, Rahman M et al (2013) Direct in vivo observations of P-selectin glycoprotein ligand-1-mediated leukocyte-endothelial cell interactions in the pulmonary microvasculature in abdominal sepsis in mice. Inflamm Res 62:275–282
40. Chesnutt JK, Marshall JS (2009) Effect of particle collisions and aggregation on red blood cell passage through a bifurcation. Microvasc Res 78:301–313
41. Harrois A, Dupic L, Duranteau J (2011) Targeting the microcirculation in resuscitation of acutely unwell patients. Curr Opin Crit Care 17:303–307
42. Hungerford JE, Sessa WC, Segal SS (2000) Vasomotor control in arterioles of the mouse cremaster muscle. FASEB J 14:197–207
43. Ellsworth ML, Forrester T, Ellis CG, Dietrich HH (1995) The erythrocyte as a regulator of vascular tone. Am J Physiol 269:H2155–H2161
44. Jackson WF (2000) Ion channels and vascular tone. Hypertension 35:173–178
45. Gottrup F, Gellett S, Kirkegaard L, Hansen ES, Johansen G (1989) Effect of hemorrhage and resuscitation on subcutaneous, conjunctival, and transcutaneous oxygen tension in relation to hemodynamic variables. Crit Care Med 17:904–907
46. Singer M, Millar C, Stidwill R, Unwin R (1996) Bladder epithelial oxygen tension – a new means of monitoring regional perfusion? Preliminary study in a model of exsanguination/fluid repletion. Intensive Care Med 22:324–328
47. Whitehouse T, Stotz M, Taylor V, Stidwill R, Singer M (2006) Tissue oxygen and hemodynamics in renal medulla, cortex, and corticomedullary junction during hemorrhage-reperfusion. Am J Physiol Renal Physiol 291:F647–F653
48. Dyson A, Stidwill R, Taylor V, Singer M (2007) Tissue oxygen monitoring in rodent models of shock. Am J Physiol Heart Circ Physiol 293:H526–H533
49. Ospina-Tascon G, Neves AP, Occhipinti G et al (2010) Effects of fluids on microvascular perfusion in patients with severe sepsis. Intensive Care Med 36:949–955
50. Pranskunas A, Koopmans M, Koetsier PM, Pilvinis V, Boerma EC (2013) Microcirculatory blood flow as a tool to select ICU patients eligible for fluid therapy. Intensive Care Med 39:612–619
51. Dyson A, Rudiger A, Singer M (2011) Temporal changes in tissue cardiorespiratory function during faecal peritonitis. Intensive Care Med 37:1192–1200
52. Ince C (2015) Hemodynamic coherence and the rationale for monitoring the microcirculation. Crit Care 19(Suppl 3):S8
53. Brealey D, Karyampudi S, Jacques TS et al (2004) Mitochondrial dysfunction in a long-term rodent model of sepsis and organ failure. Am J Physiol Regul Integr Comp Physiol 286:R491–R497
54. Wodack KH, Poppe AM, Tomkotter L et al (2014) Individualized early goal-directed therapy in systemic inflammation: is full utilization of preload reserve the optimal strategy? Crit Care Med 42:e741–e751
55. Ackland GL, Iqbal S, Paredes LG et al (2015) Individualised oxygen delivery targeted haemodynamic therapy in high-risk surgical patients: a multicentre, randomised, double-blind, controlled, mechanistic trial. Lancet Respir Med 3:33–41

Assessment of Fluid Responsiveness in Patients with Intraabdominal Hypertension

A. Beurton, X. Monnet, and J.-L. Teboul

Introduction

During the last 20 years, the issue of predicting fluid responsiveness has become one of the main topics of clinical research in intensive care medicine. In practice, clinicians are increasingly getting used to asking the question whether cardiac output will increase or not as a result of fluid administration. Of course, this is based on evidence that not all patients respond to fluid administration because of basic cardiovascular physiology. But this practice has been stimulated even more by the growing evidence that excessive fluid administration is definitely harmful, in the perioperative setting as well as in the intensive care unit (ICU). To detect the presence of fluid responsiveness at the bedside, many tests have been developed in recent years.

At the same time, the issue of intraabdominal hypertension (IAH) has gained interest. This pathologic condition, which has various deleterious effects, the main being to worsen hemodynamic status, may worsen the prognosis of critically ill patients. As IAH is one of the numerous consequences of fluid overload, predicting fluid responsiveness becomes even more crucial in patients with this pathologic condition than in others. However, the hemodynamic changes induced by IAH may change the effects and the reliability of the tests that are used to test preload responsiveness at the bedside.

The first printed copies of the book were unfortunately printed with an incorrect version of Fig. 1. An erratum sheet with the correct version was placed in the affected copies. This copy has been printed with the correct version.

A. Beurton
Service de réanimation médicale, Hôpitaux universitaires Paris-Sud, Hôpital de Bicêtre
Le Kremlin-Bicêtre, France

X. Monnet · J.-L. Teboul (✉)
Service de réanimation médicale, Hôpitaux universitaires Paris-Sud, Hôpital de Bicêtre
Le Kremlin-Bicêtre, France
INSERM UMR S_999, Univ Paris-Sud
Le Kremlin-Bicêtre, France
e-mail: jean-louis.teboul@aphp.fr

© Springer International Publishing AG 2018   407
J.-L. Vincent (ed.), *Annual Update in Intensive Care and Emergency Medicine 2018*,
Annual Update in Intensive Care and Emergency Medicine,
https://doi.org/10.1007/978-3-319-73670-9_32

What are the hemodynamic changes induced by IAH? How does IAH affect the mechanisms underlying the tests of preload responsiveness? Are these tests still relevant in patients with IAH? These are the questions we will attempt to answer in this chapter.

Fluid Responsiveness: Concept and Relevance in Critically Ill Patients

Fluid responsiveness describes a condition in which increasing cardiac preload by fluid administration will result in a significant increase in stroke volume. Fluid responsiveness is conventionally defined as an increase of at least 10 to 15% in stroke volume or in cardiac output in response to a fluid challenge [1, 2]. Intravenous fluid, the first-line treatment of acute circulatory failure, has the potential to restore tissue perfusion to vital organs by increasing cardiac output. Depending on the slope of the Frank-Starling curve (cardiac systolic function curve), the same volume of fluid could induce either a significant or a negligible effect in cardiac output [1].

It has been shown that administration of fluid induces an increase in cardiac output in only half of ICU patients [3]. It has also been demonstrated that fluid overload has detrimental consequences, by prolonging mechanical ventilation, and increasing the mortality rate in patients with sepsis [4, 5], acute kidney injury (AKI) [6, 7] or acute respiratory distress syndrome (ARDS) [8, 9]. The potentially beneficial effect of this treatment, related to an increase in cardiac output and oxygen delivery (DO_2), may become particularly deleterious by aggravating lung and tissue edema.

Predicting fluid responsiveness may help ICU physicians to decide whether or not to administer intravenous fluids but also whether or not to stop fluid infusion. It thus allows clinicians to better individualize their treatment by selecting patients who can benefit from volume expansion and preventing fluid infusion in those who would be fluid unresponsive and who may experience harmful effects, such as development or worsening tissue edema.

Static measures of cardiac preload, such as central venous pressure (CVP) and pulmonary artery occlusion pressure (PAOP), are unreliable to predict fluid responsiveness [10, 11]. By contrast, dynamic methods have been developed to predict fluid responsiveness more accurately [1]. These methods consist in observing short-term changes in cardiac output or stroke volume induced by either postural changes (passive leg raising test [PLR]) or mechanical ventilation (pulse pressure variation [PPV], stroke volume variation [SVV], respiratory variation of the vena cava diameter).

IAH and Fluid Responsiveness: Concept and Relevance in Critically Ill Patients

Intra-abdominal pressure (IAP) levels up to 5 mmHg are considered physiological in adults. IAP values between 5 and 7 mmHg are commonly encountered in critically ill patients [12]. IAH is defined as a sustained increase in IAP ≥ 12 mmHg and abdominal compartment syndrome (ACS) is defined as a persistent elevation of IAP >20 mmHg with new onset of organ failure [13]. IAH may have deleterious consequences on all organs leading to multi-visceral failure. IAH is an independent risk factor for increased mortality [12]. The World Society of the Abdominal Compartment Syndrome has updated its clinical practice guidelines and recommends optimizing fluid administration [14]. A positive fluid balance is probably the most important risk factor for promoting or worsening IAH [14]. As a consequence, assessment of fluid responsiveness is of major importance. However, the applicability of the indices and tests of fluid responsiveness to patients with IAH is unclear. To address this issue, it is important to understand the impact of IAH on hemodynamics and then on fluid responsiveness indices.

Impact of IAH on Hemodynamics

An experimental study in pigs nicely illustrated the effects of increased IAP on hemodynamics [15]. The acute increase in IAP from 0 to 30 mmHg was associated with an increase in intrathoracic pressure related to an abdomino-thoracic pressure transmission of 47% on average. This should eventually result in increases in the pressures of all the intrathoracic structures and thus in an increase in the intramural right atrial pressure (RAP). At the same time, the increased IAP limits the diaphragmatic descent during inspiration and thus reduces the compliance of the respiratory system. As a consequence, the transpulmonary pressure (plateau pressure minus intrathoracic pressure) should increase with an inherent increase in the pulmonary vascular resistance as the intraalveolar vessels are particularly sensitive to the transpulmonary pressure. Accordingly, in the experimental study by Jacques et al. [15], the increase in IAP from 0 to 30 mmHg resulted in large increases in transpulmonary pressure and pulmonary vascular resistance, which in turn can increase pulmonary artery pressure and RAP (Fig. 1). Accordingly the RAP was observed to increase markedly with increased IAP [15]. One part of this increase was due to the influence of the increased intrathoracic pressure (see above) and the other part was due to the increased afterload of the right ventricle secondary to the increase in transpulmonary pressure. It is noteworthy that in this study by Jacques et al. [15], not only the intramural RAP, but also the transmural RAP increased confirming that the two mechanisms described above co-exist. The marked increase in the intramural RAP – considered the backpressure of venous return – should decrease venous return and thus cardiac output, in spite of the increase in the forward pressure of venous return induced by the direct effect of IAP on the extrathoracic veins (Fig. 1). It is noteworthy that stroke volume and cardiac output decreased when IAP was increased from 0 to 30 mmHg [15]. In addition, the increase in IAP should increase the left ventricular (LV) afterload by increasing the resistance of the extrathoracic arteries and this can contribute – along with the increased intramural RAP and the increased right ventricular afterload – to decrease cardiac output.

The respective importance of each of these three mechanisms of cardiac output decrease depends on the baseline cardiovascular status:

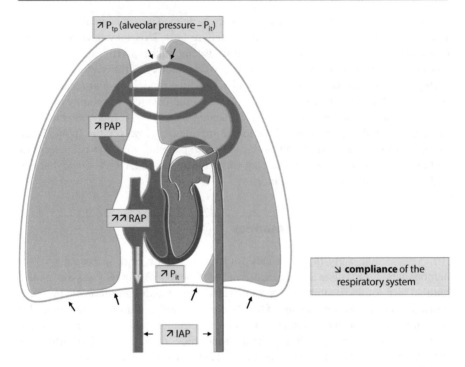

Fig. 1 Schematic representation of the effects of increased abdominal pressure on the cardiovascular system. Increase in intraabdominal pressure (IAP) increases the intrathoracic pressure (P_{it}), which in turn increases the right atrial pressure (RAP). At the same time, the increase in IAP decreases the compliance of the respiratory system – especially the chest wall compliance – and thus increases the transpulmonary pressure (P_{tp} = alveolar pressure − P_{it}) for a given tidal volume. This will increase the resistance of the pulmonary vessels and hence the pulmonary artery pressure (PAP), which eventually results in a further increase in the RAP. The increased RAP – resulting from the two above-mentioned mechanisms – will be responsible for a decrease in venous return. In addition, the increase in IAP will increase the afterload of the left ventricle with a potential further decrease in cardiac output in patients with left heart dysfunction

- In case of volume depletion, the role of the increased intramural RAP on venous return is probably predominant. Moreover, volume depletion could favor the abdominal vascular zones 2 conditions (waterfall effect), according to the model described by Takata et al. [16] by analogy with West's pulmonary vascular zone conditions. Indeed, when abdominal zone 2 conditions are favored (e.g., in case of volume depletion), the increased IAP no longer increases the forward pressure of venous return so that the decrease in venous return – due to the increased backpressure (RAP) – should be particularly marked.
- In case of prior right ventricular (RV) dysfunction, the main mechanism responsible for the decrease in cardiac output is likely to be the increased RV afterload due to the increased transpulmonary pressure.
- In case of prior LV dysfunction, the increased LV afterload secondary to the increased IAP can be the predominant mechanism responsible for the decrease in

cardiac output. Indeed, in conditions where its contractility is impaired, the left ventricle is particularly sensitive to any increase in its afterload, which eventually results in a decrease in cardiac output. Alfonsi et al. [17] investigated the influence of an acute increase in IAP during peritoneal carbon dioxide insufflation in patients scheduled for laparoscopic aortic surgery. The authors performed transesophageal echocardiography and found that the increase in IAP (up to 14 mmHg) was associated with increased afterload of the two ventricles.

How can IAH alter Markers of Cardiac Preload and of Fluid Responsiveness?

Influence of IAH on Markers of Cardiac Preload

Since IAH increased the intrathoracic pressure during both inspiration and expiration, RAP and PAOP, even measured at end-expiration, should overestimate the transmural RAP and PAOP, which reflect the RV and LV filling pressures, respectively. To estimate the transmural RAP and PAOP values and thus the cardiac filling pressure in cases of IAH, it is better to subtract approximately 50% of the IAP from the measured RAP and PAOP. Nevertheless, it should be stressed that even reliably estimated, the cardiac filling pressures are poor predictors of fluid responsiveness [10].

It is generally admitted that volumetric markers of cardiac preload such as global end-diastolic volume (GEDV) are better estimates of cardiac preload than cardiac filling pressures especially in case of IAH [18]. Nevertheless, GEDV is a static marker of preload and as such is an unreliable predictor of fluid responsiveness [19].

Influence of IAH on the Dynamic Indices of Fluid Responsiveness

PPV and SVV

As mentioned above, a PPV (or SVV) value of ≥ 12% has been shown to be a specific and sensitive indicator of preload responsiveness in patients receiving mechanical ventilation with relative large tidal volumes (≥ 8 ml/kg), in the absence of cardiac arrhythmias and of spontaneous breathing activity [20].

In case of IAH, not only the absolute value of intrathoracic pressure but also the respiratory swings of intrathoracic pressure should increase for a given tidal volume [15, 21]. This is certainly due to the decrease in chest wall compliance induced by the increased IAP [15, 22]. Since SVV and PPV are highly dependent on the respiratory changes in intrathoracic pressure, SVV and PPV could thus increase with increased IAP, independently of any change of volume status. In experimental studies in which IAP was acutely increased up to 25 or 30 mmHg, increases in PPV and SVV were constantly observed before any induced change in volume status (blood withdrawal or fluid loading) [15, 21, 22]. However, it cannot be concluded that PPV and SVV are poor markers of fluid responsiveness during IAH. First, since increased IAP also increased the mean intrathoracic pressure due to the high abdomino-thoracic pressure transmission, venous return should be lower than in normal IAP conditions. It is thus likely that the cardiac preload is also lower during IAH (compared to normal IAP conditions) and the heart more preload responsive during IAH (compared to normal IAP conditions). In line with this hypothesis, Duperret et al. [21] reported a decrease in the mean inferior vena cava blood flow and in the mean LV end-diastolic area (a marker of the LV preload) when IAP was increased up to 30 mmHg in animals. Second, in two other animal studies in which hypovolemia was experimentally induced, PPV and SVV increased with hypovolemia during IAH [15, 22] suggesting that these variables are still sensitive to change in volume status during IAH. Third, in one of these animal studies, fluid was administered in normovolemic as well as hypovolemic conditions after IAP was elevated to 30 mmHg [15]. PPV and SVV (measured with an aortic ultrasound transit-time flow probe) predicted fluid responsiveness well with threshold values of 41 and 67%, respectively. These latter values are high compared to those found in clinical studies [20]. These findings can be attributed not only to the high IAP but also to the experimental model (very high tidal volume and low chest wall compliance). In another porcine study [22], PPV was accurate to predict fluid responsiveness at normal as well as at high IAP (25 mmHg) with threshold values of 11.5 and 20.5%, respectively. It is noteworthy that in that study [22], SVV (measured using a pulse contour method) predicted fluid responsiveness well, only in cases of normal IAP. The message of these two animal studies [15, 22] was that PPV can still predict fluid responsiveness in cases of high IAP, but that the threshold value could be higher than in normal IAP conditions. However, the applicability of these findings to clinical conditions should be made with caution. Indeed, the experimental conditions (acute increase in IAP, very high values of IAP achieved, high tidal volume and low chest compliance) were far from those encountered in ICU patients. In a clinical study in which moderate IAH (IAP = 12 mmHg) was induced by carbon dioxide insufflation before laparoscopic surgery, Liu et al. reported that PPV and SVV were still accurate predictors of fluid responsiveness during IAH with threshold values of 10.5% for both variables [23]. These values are close to those usually found in patients with no IAH. However, in that study [23]: i) fluid responsiveness was defined by an increase in pulse contour stroke volume $\geq 10\%$ and not $> 15\%$ as in most of the previous studies; ii) tidal volume was set at 7 ml/kg, which is generally considered a condition of poor reliability for PPV and SVV; iii) IAP was set at 12 mmHg, which represents only a moderate increase. Finally, in another experimental study in which 11 rabbits were submitted to pneumoperitoneum, there was no change in the value of PPV when IAP was increased [24]. In addition, during IAH, PPV increased significantly after hemorrhage and returned to its baseline value after blood re-infusion. From all these experimental and clinical studies, it seems that PPV and SVV still keep their reliability to predict fluid responsiveness but it is hard to definitively conclude on the threshold values. Experts in this field consider that these dynamic variables can be reliably used but the threshold values should be higher [25]. It is intuitive that the higher the IAP, the higher the PPV (or SVV) threshold, although no magic number can be proposed [26].

The PLR Test

Among the methods that are currently available to identify preload responsiveness, the PLR test is one of the most applicable to ICU patients. The test consists of moving the patient's bed from the semi-recumbent position to a position in which the patient's trunk is horizontal and the inferior limbs are passively elevated at 45° [27]. This postural maneuver can transfer venous blood from the inferior limbs and abdominal compartments toward the cardiac cavities and as such mimics a volume challenge. The test has been demonstrated to be reliable in many studies [28, 29].

The way PLR is performed is important because it fundamentally affects the hemodynamic effects. Five rules should be respected [27]:

- PLR should start from the semi-recumbent position and not from the supine position.
- The effects of PLR should be assessed by directly measuring the cardiac output and not by simply measuring blood pressure.
- A real-time measurement of cardiac output (pulse contour analysis, echocardiography, esophageal Doppler, contour analysis of the volume clamp-derived arterial pressure, end-tidal exhaled carbon dioxide) should be used, because the effects are very transient and can disappear within less than one minute.
- The cardiac output should be measured before, during and after the PLR test.
- To avoid any misinterpretation of the test, confounding factors (pain, cough, awakening, and discomfort) should be avoided.

A clinical study investigated the reliability of PLR in patients with IAH [30]. In this study, which included 31 fluid-responsive patients, 15 patients (48%) were non-responders to PLR (no increase in CO by more than 12%) [30]. At baseline, the median IAP was significantly higher in the non-responders to PLR than in the responders to PLR [30]. An IAP cut-off value of 16 mmHg discriminated between responders and non-responders to PLR with a sensitivity of 100% (confidence interval, 78–100) and a specificity of 87.5% (confidence interval, 61.6–98.1) [30]. An IAP ≥ 16 mmHg was the only independent predictor of non-response to PLR in a multivariate analysis [30]. In a recent study including 29 patients with IAP > 12 mmHg (mean IAP $= 20 \pm 6$ mmHg), we also found that IAH was responsible for false negatives to the PLR test, although we found that the PLR maneuver itself was able to reduce IAP by around 30% [31]. The area under the receiver operating characteristic (ROC) curve for the prediction of fluid responsiveness with PLR was only 0.58 ± 0.11, largely due to low sensitivity (40%). The unreliability of the PLR test during IAH has been attributed to compression of the inferior vena cava during the postural maneuver leading to an increase in resistance to venous return [32].

Conclusion

Volume expansion is the first-line therapy in cases of shock but fluid overload may have deleterious effects and worsen outcome, especially in patients with IAH. Hemodynamic monitoring is essential to test fluid responsiveness and thus to prevent administration of fluid in preload unresponsive patients. In patients with IAH, dynamic heart-lung interaction indices such as PPV and SVV still seem to be valid (in the absence of low tidal volume, cardiac arrhythmias, spontaneous breathing activity). It is likely however that threshold values higher than those found in patients with no IAH should be considered in the case of IAH, although no definite values can be recommended. The PLR test, which is generally applicable in most conditions, including low tidal volume, arrhythmias, spontaneous breathing activity, seems not to predict fluid responsiveness well in patients with IAH.

References

1. Monnet X, Marik PE, Teboul JL (2016) Prediction of fluid responsiveness: an update. Ann Intensive Care 6:111
2. Toscani L, Aya HD, Antonakaki D et al (2017) What is the impact of the fluid challenge technique on diagnosis of fluid responsiveness? A systematic review and meta-analysis. Crit Care 21:207
3. Michard F, Teboul JL (2002) Predicting fluid responsiveness in ICU patients: a critical analysis of the evidence. Chest 121:2000–2008
4. Vincent J-L, Sakr Y, Sprung CL et al (2006) Sepsis in European intensive care units: results of the SOAP study. Crit Care Med 34:344–353
5. Sakr Y, Rubatto Birri PN, Kotfis K et al (2017) Higher fluid balance increases the risk of death from sepsis: results from a large international audit. Crit Care Med 45:386–394
6. Payen D, de Pont AC, Sakr Y, Spies C, Reinhart K, Vincent JL, Sepsis Occurrence in Acutely Ill Patients (SOAP) Investigators (2008) A positive fluid balance is associated with a worse outcome in patients with acute renal failure. Crit Care 12:R74
7. Bouchard J, Soroko SB, Chertow GM et al (2009) Fluid accumulation, survival and recovery of kidney function in critically ill patients with acute kidney injury. Kidney Int 76:422–427
8. Rosenberg AL, Dechert RE, Park PK, Bartlett RH (2009) Review of a large clinical series: association of cumulative fluid balance on outcome in acute lung injury: a retrospective review of the ARDSnet tidal volume study cohort. J Intensive Care Med 24:35–46
9. Jozwiak M, Silva S, Persichini R et al (2013) Extravascular lung water is an independent prognostic factor in patients with acute respiratory distress syndrome. Crit Care Med 41:472–480
10. Osman D, Ridel C, Ray P et al (2007) Cardiac filling pressures are not appropriate to predict hemodynamic response to volume challenge. Crit Care Med 35:64–68
11. Marik PE, Cavallazzi R (2013) Does the central venous pressure predict fluid responsiveness? An updated meta-analysis and a plea for some common sense. Crit Care Med 41:1774–1781
12. Malbrain ML, Cheatham ML, Kirkpatrick A et al (2006) Results from the international conference of experts on intra-abdominal hypertension and abdominal compartment syndrome. I. Definitions. Intensive Care Med 32:1722–1732
13. Regli A, Keulenaer BD, Laet ID, Roberts D, Dabrowski W, Malbrain ML (2015) Fluid therapy and perfusional considerations during resuscitation in critically ill patients with intra-abdominal hypertension. Anaesthesiol Intensive Ther 47:45–53

14. Kirkpatrick AW, Roberts DJ, De Waele J et al (2013) Intra-abdominal hypertension and the abdominal compartment syndrome: updated consensus definitions and clinical practice guidelines from the World Society of the Abdominal Compartment Syndrome. Intensive Care Med 39:1190–1206
15. Jacques D, Bendjelid K, Duperret S, Colling J, Piriou V, Viale JP (2011) Pulse pressure variation and stroke volume variation during increased intra-abdominal pressure: an experimental study. Crit Care 15:R33
16. Takata M, Wise RA, Robotham JL (1985) Effects of abdominal pressure on venous return: abdominal vascular zone conditions. J Appl Physiol 69:1961–1972
17. Alfonsi P, Vieillard-Baron A, Coggia M et al (2006) Cardiac function during intraperitoneal CO_2 insufflation for aortic surgery: a transesophageal echocardiographic study. Anesth Analg 102:1304–1310
18. Malbrain ML, De Waele JJ, De Keulenaer BL (2015) What every ICU clinician needs to know about the cardiovascular effects caused by abdominal hypertension. Anaesthesiol Intensive Ther 47:388–399
19. Marik PE, Cavallazzi R, Vasu T, Hirani A (2009) Dynamic changes in arterial waveform derived variables and fluid responsiveness in mechanically ventilated patients. A systematic review of the literature. Crit Care Med 37:2642–2647
20. Yang X, Du B (2014) Does pulse pressure variation predicts fluid responsiveness in critically ill patients: a critical review and meta-analysis. Crit Care 18:650
21. Duperret S, Lhuillier F, Piriou V et al (2007) Increased intra-abdominal pressure affects respiratory variations in arterial pressure in normovolaemic and hypovolaemic mechanically ventilated healthy pigs. Intensive Care Med 33:163–171
22. Renner J, Gruenewald M, Quaden R et al (2009) Influence of increased intra-abdominal pressure on fluid responsiveness predicted by pulse pressure variation and stroke volume variation in a porcine model. Crit Care Med 37:650–658
23. Liu X, Fu Q, Mi W, Liu H, Zhang H, Wang P (2013) Pulse pressure variation and stroke volume variation predict fluid responsiveness in mechanically ventilated patients experiencing intra-abdominal hypertension. Biosci Trends 7:101–108
24. Bliacheriene F, Machado SB, Fonseca EB, Otsuke D, Auler JOC, Michard F (2007) Pulse pressure variation as a tool to detect hypovolaemia during pneumoperitoneum. Acta Anaesthesiol Scand 51:1268–1272
25. Malbrain ML, de Laet I (2009) Functional hemodynamics and increased intra-abdominal pressure: same thresholds for different conditions . . . ? Crit Care Med 37:781–783
26. Tavernier B, Robin E (2011) Assessment of fluid responsiveness during increased intra-abdominal pressure: keep the indices, but change the thresholds. Crit Care 15:134
27. Monnet X, Teboul JL (2015) Passive leg raising: five rules, not a drop of fluid! Crit Care 19:18
28. Monnet X, Marik P, Teboul JL (2016) Passive leg raising for predicting fluid responsiveness: a systematic review and meta-analysis. Intensive Care Med 42:1935–1947
29. Cherpanath TGV, Hirsch A, Geerts BF et al (2016) Predicting fluid responsiveness by passive leg raising: a systematic review and meta-analysis of 23 clinical trials. Crit Care Med 44:981–991
30. Mahjoub Y, Touzeau J, Airapetian N et al (2010) The passive leg-raising maneuver cannot accurately predict fluid responsiveness in patients with intra-abdominal hypertension. Crit Care Med 38:1824–1829
31. Beurton A, Teboul JL, Girotto V, Galarza L, Richard C, Monnet X (2016) Accuracy of the passing leg raising test in patients with intraabdominal hypertension. Crit Care 21(Supp 1):P130
32. Malbrain ML, Reuter DA (2010) Assessing fluid responsiveness with the passive leg raising maneuver in patients with increased intra-abdominal pressure: be aware that not all blood returns! Crit Care Med 38:1912–1915

Assessment of Fluid Overload in Critically Ill Patients: Role of Bioelectrical Impedance Analysis

M. L. N. G. Malbrain, E. De Waele, and P. M. Honoré

Introduction

The association of a positive fluid balance and increased morbidity and mortality has been well documented [1–5]. However, little is known about the best method to assess fluid status and fluid overload. Fluid overload is defined by a cut-off value of 10% fluid accumulation above baseline body weight [5–7]. The human body consists of around 60% of water, 18% protein, 16% fat and 6% minerals [8]. Intracellular water (ICW) counts for two-thirds of total body water (TBW) while one-third is extracellular water (ECW). ECW contains 75% interstitial fluid and 25% intravascular fluid. Thus, the plasma accounts for only 5.5% of TBW. In critically ill patients, fluid overload results mainly from excessive fluid administration. After 1 h, infusion of 1 l of isotonic fluid (e.g., so-called normal saline) will increase the intravascular volume by 250 ml and the interstitial fluid volume by 750 ml. On the other hand, infusion of 1 l of hypotonic fluid (e.g., glucose or dextrose 5% in water) will increase the intravascular volume after 1 h by 100 ml and the interstitial fluid volume by 900 ml. Therefore, hypotonic solutions should not be used during the resuscitation phase but only for maintenance. Fluid overload is usually accompanied by some degree of pulmonary edema (especially in sepsis and capillary leak) and can be assessed by clinical signs (anasarca, pitting edema, body weight), biomarkers, assessment of daily and cumulative fluid balance, and hemodynamic monitoring (e.g., extravascular lung water [EVLW] measurement via transpulmonary thermodilution). Biomarkers include beta type natriuretic peptide (BNP), low albumin and

M. L. N. G. Malbrain (✉)
Dept of Intensive Care, University Hospital Brussels
Brussels, Belgium
Intensive Care Unit and High Care Burn Unit, Ziekenhuis Netwerk Antwerpen, ZNA Stuivenberg
Antwerp, Belgium
e-mail: manu.malbrain@telenet.be

E. De Waele · P. M. Honoré
Dept of Intensive Care, University Hospital Brussels
Brussels, Belgium

© Springer International Publishing AG 2018   417
J.-L. Vincent (ed.), *Annual Update in Intensive Care and Emergency Medicine 2018*,
Annual Update in Intensive Care and Emergency Medicine,
https://doi.org/10.1007/978-3-319-73670-9_33

total protein levels (hemodilution), increased urine albumin to creatinine ratio, and increased serum C-reactive protein (CRP) to albumin ratio. Finally, fluid overload can also be assessed using bioelectrical impedance analysis (BIA). BIA uses an electric current transmitted at different frequencies to measure regional, segmental or whole body impedance, phase angle, resistance, reactance and capacitance [8, 9]. New multifrequency and multipolar techniques allow measurement of TBW with separation into ECW and ICW and provide an estimate of volume excess (VE) and thus fluid overload [8]. BIA may provide useful information not only in patients with chronic kidney disease (CKD) on hemodialysis but also in critically ill patients with burns, trauma and sepsis undergoing fluid resuscitation or goal-directed therapy [10–13]. After a brief overview of relevant definitions, this book chapter summarizes the recent literature on how to assess fluid overload with a focus on BIA, and its role to guide fluid management in critically ill patients.

Definitions

- Fluid balance: Daily fluid balance is the daily difference between all intakes and outputs. Daily fluid balance can be negative, neutral or positive. Usually, the daily fluid balance does not include insensible losses [5, 6, 14, 15].
- Cumulative fluid balance: The cumulative fluid balance is the total sum of fluid accumulation over a set period. Usually the first week of intensive care unit (ICU) stay is taken into account [5, 14, 15].
- Fluid accumulation: Fluid accumulation (sometimes also called hyperhydration) is defined as a positive fluid balance, with or without associated fluid overload [6].
- Fluid overload: The percentage of fluid accumulation is defined by dividing the cumulative fluid balance in liters by the patient's baseline body weight and multiplying by 100%. Fluid overload is defined as a cut-off value of 10% fluid accumulation, as this is associated with worse outcomes [5, 7, 15]. Fluid overload is usually associated with a degree of pulmonary edema or peripheral edema and is usually associated with the absence of fluid responsiveness.
- Fluid responsiveness: A test to predict fluid responsiveness assesses whether or not a patient will respond to a fluid bolus in a given situation. Fluid responsiveness is defined by an increase in the cardiac index by 15% or more after administration of a fluid bolus or challenge [16]. Functional hemodynamic monitoring tests, such as stroke volume variation (SVV), pulse pressure variation (PPV) or systolic pressure variation (SPV) are useful to assess fluid responsiveness.
- Early adequate fluid management: The recently updated Surviving Sepsis Campaign guidelines define early adequate fluid management as 30 ml/kg, given within the first 6 h of resuscitation [17]. Although this amount may be insufficient in some patients (e.g., severe burns), others have argued that such "large" volumes may lead to "iatrogenic salt water drowning" [18]. In any case, fluids

should only be given in patients with intravascular hypovolemia who are fluid responsive.

- Late conservative fluid management: Late conservative fluid management is defined as two consecutive days of negative fluid balance within the first week of ICU stay. Recent data have demonstrated that achievement of late conservative fluid management is a strong and independent predictor of survival [2–5, 19, 20].
- Late goal-directed fluid removal: Late goal-directed fluid removal is the active mobilization of excess second and third space fluids in patients with fluid overload. Late goal-directed fluid removal can be performed either using diuretics or renal replacement therapy (RRT) with net ultrafiltration [20]. This is referred to as de-resuscitation or de-escalation [5, 20].
- Classification of fluid dynamics: Four distinct groups can be identified with respect to the dynamics of fluid therapy by combining early adequate (EA) or early conservative (EC) with either late conservative (LC) or late liberal (LL) fluid management: EALC, EALL, ECLC and ECLL. Murphy et al. performed a landmark study (albeit retrospective) in septic patients and showed that EALC and ECLC groups had the best prognosis [2].

Etiology of Fluid Overload

In this chapter, we will not discuss fluid overload associated with CKD, acute kidney injury (AKI) or congestive heart failure. We will only address so-called iatrogenic fluid overload after administration of excessive intravenous fluids (mainly crystalloids), or blood transfusions. However, the ICU physician must take into account that the risk of fluid overload is higher in elderly patients especially if there is pre-existing cardiac or renal impairment, sepsis, major injury (burns or trauma) or major surgery. Some other important issues are listed below:

- Postoperative patients may receive inappropriately large amounts of intravenous fluid and/or sodium leading to fluid overload [21, 22], especially since some studies advocated goal-directed therapy with administration of more than 6 l of fluids in elective hip surgery [23].
- In the setting of capillary leak, fluid overload will result in bowel edema, intestinal swelling, increased intraabdominal pressure (IAP), mesenteric vein compression and venous hypertension, hence triggering a vicious cycle leading to more fluid resuscitation and intraabdominal hypertension (IAH). IAH is defined as a sustained increase in IAP equal to or greater than 12 mmHg [24]. Therefore IAH and fluid overload, unfortunately, go hand-in-hand resulting in polycompartment syndrome [24].
- The presence of IAH, traumatic brain or head injury (TBI), or major surgery may all result in increased antidiuretic hormone secretion leading to fluid overload.
- As the result of various physiological responses, the excretion of excess sodium and water is more difficult for injured or surgical patients [21, 22].

- Recently, complex interactions between heart, abdomen, and kidneys affecting body fluid and sodium regulation have been identified. This is known as the cardio-abdominal-renal syndrome (CARS) [25]. Within this concept, IAP has been identified as the missing link explaining why some patients with congestive heart failure may go into worsening renal failure with the need for RRT [25].

Impact of Fluid Overload on Organ Function

Fluid overload has a tremendous impact on organ function. Peripheral edema is not only of cosmetic concern but reflects organ edema and organ function [5]. For example, fluid overload results in bowel edema, and this will result in diminished bowel contractility [5]. Numerous studies have been performed looking at the impact of fluid overload on kidney function [5]. Since the kidneys are an encapsulated organ, kidney edema following fluid overload will result in increased renal (intracapsular) pressure and renal compartment syndrome, while the increased renal venous pressure will result in diminished renal perfusion pressure and hormonal changes within the renin-angiotensin-aldosterone system that will result in further salt and water retention. It is beyond the scope of this chapter to discuss in detail the effects of fluid overload on end-organ function. The effects of fluid overload are summarized in Fig. 1.

Assessment of Fluid Overload

Accurate volume status evaluation is essential for appropriate therapy; therefore inadequate assessment of volume status can be associated with increased mortality [6]. Most of the available methods to assess volume status are quite inaccurate. We will describe the most commonly used methods.

Clinical Examination

This should include ideally measurement of daily body weight. If the patient is cooperative ask for the last known weight. If the patient is unconscious or sedated and receiving mechanical ventilation, ask the relatives or check previous charts. As a surrogate, daily fluid balance and cumulative fluid balance can be calculated. However, although this seems easy, correct measurement of daily fluid balance is difficult. Furthermore, there exists no ideal formula to take into account insensible losses, especially in severe burns. Albeit the fact that determination of body weight measurement is feasible and reproducible in critically ill patients, great variance exists between daily body weight and fluid balance [26, 27]. The patient with fluid overload will often present with second space fluid accumulation and pitting edema or anasarca (to be differentiated from lymph edema, hypothyroidism, preeclampsia, hypoproteinemia or venous obstruction) and some form of pulmonary

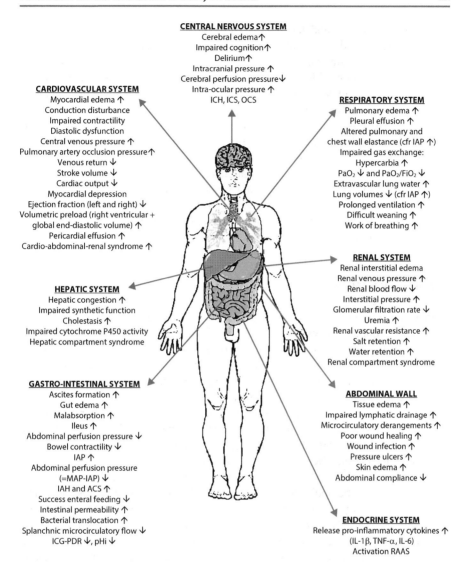

CENTRAL NERVOUS SYSTEM
Cerebral edema↑
Impaired cognition↑
Delirium↑
Intracranial pressure ↑
Cerebral perfusion pressure↓
Intra-ocular pressure ↑
ICH, ICS, OCS

CARDIOVASCULAR SYSTEM
Myocardial edema ↑
Conduction disturbance
Impaired contractility
Diastolic dysfunction
Central venous pressure ↑
Pulmonary artery occlusion pressure↑
Venous return ↓
Stroke volume ↓
Cardiac output ↓
Myocardial depression
Ejection fraction (left and right) ↓
Volumetric preload (right ventricular +
global end-diastolic volume) ↑
Pericardial effusion ↑
Cardio-abdominal-renal syndrome ↑

RESPIRATORY SYSTEM
Pulmonary edema ↑
Pleural effusion ↑
Altered pulmonary and
chest wall elastance (cfr IAP ↑)
Impaired gas exchange:
Hypercarbia ↑
PaO_2 ↓ and PaO_2/FiO_2 ↓
Extravascular lung water ↑
Lung volumes ↓ (cfr IAP ↑)
Prolonged ventilation ↑
Difficult weaning ↑
Work of breathing ↑

HEPATIC SYSTEM
Hepatic congestion ↑
Impaired synthetic function
Cholestasis ↑
Impaired cytochrome P450 activity
Hepatic compartment syndrome

RENAL SYSTEM
Renal interstitial edema
Renal venous pressure ↑
Renal blood flow ↓
Interstitial pressure ↑
Glomerular filtration rate ↓
Uremia ↑
Renal vascular resistance ↑
Salt retention ↑
Water retention ↑
Renal compartment syndrome

GASTRO-INTESTINAL SYSTEM
Ascites formation ↑
Gut edema ↑
Malabsorption ↑
Ileus ↑
Abdominal perfusion pressure ↓
Bowel contractility ↓
IAP ↑
Abdominal perfusion pressure
(=MAP-IAP) ↓
IAH and ACS ↑
Success enteral feeding ↓
Intestinal permeability ↑
Bacterial translocation ↑
Splanchnic microcirculatory flow ↓
ICG-PDR ↓, pHi ↓

ABDOMINAL WALL
Tissue edema ↑
Impaired lymphatic drainage ↑
Microcirculatory derangements ↑
Poor wound healing ↑
Wound infection ↑
Pressure ulcers ↑
Skin edema ↑
Abdominal compliance ↓

ENDOCRINE SYSTEM
Release pro-inflammatory cytokines ↑
(IL-1β, TNF-α, IL-6)
Activation RAAS

Fig. 1 Impact of fluid overload on organ function. *ICH*: intracranial hypertension; *IAP*: intraabdominal pressure; *IL*: interleukin; *TNF*: tumor necrosis factor; *ICG-PDR*: indocyanine green plasma disappearance rate; *MAP*: mean arterial pressure; *ACS*: abdominal compartment syndrome; *IAH*: intraabdominal hypertension; *ICS*: intracranial compartment syndrome; *OCS*: ocular compartment syndrome; *pHi*: intramucosal pH (tonometry); *RAAS*: renin–angiotensin–aldosterone system. Adapted from [5] with permission

edema (with orthopnea and desaturation in supine position). Third space fluid accumulation (ascites and pleural effusions) should also be looked for. Jugular venous pressure and distention can be assessed clinically. Ideally, the patient needs to be in the supine position with the head at an angle of 45°. When pulsations are not visible, fluid overload is less likely. When pulsations are visible up to the mandibular bone, the patient most likely has elevated right atrial pressure (RAP). The RAP can be estimated as the distance from the maximal jugular vein distension to the level of the sternal junction augmented by 5 cmH$_2$O. However, it must be stated that previous studies have shown that, in general, clinical assessment of volume status remains difficult in critically ill patients as physical signs or symptoms (with assessment of skin turgor, skin temperature, inspection of external jugular vein, auscultation and percussion of thorax, inspection of legs and abdomen) do not correlate well with transpulmonary thermodilution assessment of volume status, preload, or pulmonary hydration [28, 29].

Laboratory Results

Kidney function analysis can show increased serum urea, creatinine, and altered electrolytes, although the values may be diluted initially. AKI is often one of the first signs of organ impairment following fluid overload. Therefore, one should always check if there are contributing electrolyte imbalances and perform a urinalysis. Full blood count often shows dilutional anemia together with signs of infection. Due to capillary leak and hemodilution, albumin and protein levels are often decreased. Dilutional hypoproteinemia needs to be differentiated from hypoproteinemia resulting from nephrotic syndrome, malnutrition, malabsorption or liver disease. The urinary albumin to creatinine ratio can be increased [30], together with an increased capillary leak index (serum CRP to serum albumin ratio) [19].

Decreased serum osmolarity and colloid oncotic pressure are the hallmarks of fluid overload with hemodilution and capillary leak. Arterial blood gases are altered in case of pulmonary edema and can give a clue to diagnosis if the cause of dyspnea is unclear. BNP and N-terminal (NT)-pro-BNP levels can be increased. Some patients have chronically elevated levels, especially when systolic function is poor and when CKD is present. Patients with obesity, on the other hand, can have decreased levels. The greatest utility of BNP levels is when they are not elevated, because low BNP levels have a high negative predictive value for excluding a diagnosis of heart failure [6].

Imaging

Chest X-ray
Chest x-ray has been one of the most used tests to evaluate hypervolemia. Radiographic signs of fluid overload include cardiomegaly, congestive vascular hili, Kerley B-lines and signs of pulmonary edema or pleural effusions. However, in

critically ill patients in general and in patients with congestive heart failure in particular, radiographic signs have poor predictive value for identifying patients with fluid overload [6, 28].

Ultrasound
Bedside transthoracic echocardiography enables assessment of filling status and fluid responsiveness (diastolic function and tissue Doppler imaging with E/e', left ventricular outflow tract [LVOT] velocity time integral [VTI] variations) and may help to identify the cause of cardiac dysfunction e.g., ventricular failure, cardiac tamponade or large pulmonary embolus [31, 32]. Ultrasound of the inferior vena cava (IVC) diameter in monodimensional (M)-mode can help to differentiate between volume depletion (IVC diameter < 1.5 cm) and fluid overload (IVC diameter > 2.5 cm). The IVC collapsibility index can also be calculated [32]. In general, fluid overload is usually associated with the absence of fluid responsiveness, except for some extreme cases associated with intravascular underfilling (e.g., severe burns). The presence of Kerley B-lines and comet-tail artifacts on lung ultrasound is associated with increased pulmonary artery occlusion pressure (PAOP) and EVLW [33]. Abdominal ultrasound can identify the presence of bowel edema and ascites. Other causes for ascites must be excluded like cirrhosis, portal hypertension or malignancy.

Hemodynamic Monitoring

Increased central venous pressure (CVP) has been shown to be a poor predictor of fluid overload especially in the setting of increased intrathoracic pressure as seen with high positive end-expiratory pressure (PEEP) ventilation, dynamic hyperinflation with auto-PEEP, IAH or polycompartment syndrome, obesity, etc. The same holds true for increased PAOP [34]. Moreover in order to obtain the PAOP value an invasive right heart catheterization procedure needs to be performed. The use of transmural filling pressures may have some benefit, however clinical data in critically ill patients are lacking [34]. A volumetric right heart catheterization can be used to estimate right ventricular end-diastolic volume (RVEDV) and RV ejection fraction (RVEF) while transpulmonary thermodilution (with PiCCO or Volumeview) allows measurement of global end-diastolic volume (GEDV), EVLW and pulmonary vascular permeability index (PVPI) [35].

The Role for Bioelectric Impedance Analysis

BIA will be discussed more in detail as this is a promising non-invasive method to assess not only TBW but also EVW, ICW, the ECW/ICW ratio and volume excess (Table 1; [8]).

Table 1 Some of the parameters that can be obtained with BIA. Adapted from [8] with permission

ABSOLUTE MEASUREMENTS
- Impedance (Z)
- Phase angle
- Resistance (R)
- Reactance (X)
- Capacitance (C)

DRY WEIGHT
- Dry weight (kg)

BODY COMPOSITION
- Fat %
- Fat mass
- Fat free mass (FFM, L or %)
- Fat free mass hydration (FFMH, %)
- Body volume
- Body density
- Body mass index (BMI)
- Target fat (min/max) %
- Target weight (min/max)
- Target water (min/max) %

KIDNEY FUNCTION
- Glomerular filtration rate (GFR)

MINERALS AND PROTEIN
- Total body potassium (TBK)
- Total body calcium
- Protein mass
- Mineral mass

GLYCOGEN
- Glycogen mass

FLUID STATUS
- Extracellular fluid
- Intracellular water volume (ICW, l or %)
- Extracellular water volume (ECW, l or %)
- Total body water volume (TBW, l or %)
- Extracellular/intracellular water, ECW/ICW ratio
- Extracellular water/total body water
- Intracellular water/total body water
- Interstitial-fluid extravascular
- Plasma-fluid (intravascular)
- Intracellular water/total body water
- Volume excess (l)

NUTRITIONAL STATUS
- Body cell mass (BCM)
- Muscle mass
- Extracellular mass
- Extracellular solids
- Resting metabolic rate

Definitions

Definitions of electrical parameters generated by BIA are briefly listed below [8]. More detailed information on this topic and the BIA principles can be found elsewhere [9, 36].

- Conductor: A conductor is tissue that allows electricity to flow easily. Examples are muscles or tissues that consist mainly of water with low resistance and low impedance.
- Insulator: An insulator is a tissue that consists of cells that are not conducting electrical signals. Examples are fat cells with high resistance and high impedance.
- Capacitance (C): In electrical terms, the capacitance is the storage of an electrical charge by a condenser for a short moment in time. The capacitance measurement in a human being is related to the amount and health status of cell membranes (the more and the healthier the cells, the higher the capacitance value).
- Resistance (R): The resistance of an electrical conductor is the opposition to the passage of an electric current through that conductor and is inversely related to the water content.
- Reactance (X): The opposition of an electrical circuit element (due to that element's capacitance) to a change of electric current is called reactance and is related to the cell mass.
- Impedance (Z): Impedance represents the ratio of insulation tissue to conductive tissue, or thus the resistance divided by the conductance.

BIA Principle

BIA allows calculation of body composition and volumes using an electric current going through the body (Fig. 2). Five assumptions are made to obtain a reproducible measurement: the human body is considered as a cylinder; this cylinder consists of five smaller cylinders (one central, two for the arms and two for the legs); body composition is assumed to be homogenous; body composition has no individual variations; and, finally, there is no impact from the environment (temperature, stress, fluid infusions ...). Five factors are indispensable to obtain a good BIA-measurement: the absolute impedance value, the patient's height, weight, sex and age. Of these five factors, sex and age are the most important [8].

BIA Measurement

The use of tetrapolar electrodes is preferred with two current electrodes to drive electricity into the human body and two electrodes to detect impedance placed on hands and feet to obtain reproducible measurements [8]. Although some studies looked at separate measurements of the arm, leg, and trunk, segmental BIA should

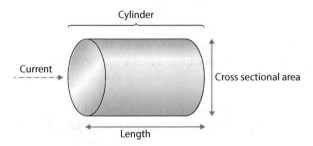

Fig. 2 The principle of volumetric monitoring with bioelectrical impedance analysis. When electric current goes through a cylinder shaped body, the impedance (Z) is related to the length (L) and specific resistivity (ρ) of the tissue and inversely related to the cross-sectional area (A) of the cylinder. The volume of a cylinder (V) can be calculated as L multiplied by A. Bioelectrical impedance analysis calculates volumes as follows: $Z = \rho \cdot \frac{L}{A}$, $Z = \rho \cdot \frac{L}{A} \cdot \frac{L}{L}$, $Z = \rho \cdot \frac{L^2}{V}$. Extrapolated to a critically ill patient, L stands for the patient's height (in cm) so that the body composition and the specific volume (V) can be calculated as follows: $V = \rho \cdot \frac{L^2}{Z}$ where $\frac{L^2}{Z}$ corresponds to the impedance index that can be calculated with bioelectrical impedance analysis. Adapted from [8] with permission

at present be considered as purely experimental [9]. Modern devices also use multiple frequencies that may further improve the accuracy and reproducibility of the values obtained with BIA. The frequency is the number of repetitions per second of a complete electric waveform (one repetition per second is 1 Hz) [37]. A current with a frequency below 100 Hz will not pass the cell membranes and will only measure ECW. Currents with frequencies greater than 100 Hz will go through cells and measure TBW [9]. The ICW can be calculated by subtracting ECW from TBW. The phase angle is the time delay that occurs when electric current passes the cell membrane. The phase angle reflects the relationship between resistance and reactance. A phase angle of 0° is an indicator of absence of cell membranes whereas 90° represents a capacitive circuit which consists of only membranes without fluid [9]. The presence of cell membranes causes time delays compared to the time current takes when passing through extracellular water. Hence, the greater the number of cell membranes the signal has to pass through, the longer the time delay and, therefore, the greater the phase angle and the greater the proportion of ICW compared to ECW [36]. A high phase angle is consistent with high reactance and a preserved body cell mass as seen in healthy individuals [9]. Critically ill patients, on the other hand, usually have a lower phase angle [12, 38].

BIA Obtained Parameters (Table 1)

Body composition and nutritional assessment is important in order to identify malnutrition [8]. Body cell mass assesses a healthy subject's nutritional status or a patient's degree of malnutrition and is used for calculation of energy expenditure. The glomerular filtration rate (GFR) is an important indicator of kidney function.

Some studies showed reasonable correlation between BIA and other GFR estimation techniques, avoiding the necessity of 24-hour urine collection. BIA can
obtain information on both mineral (bone, soft tissue) and protein content of the
body. Glycogen mass is the primary storage form of carbohydrates. Absolute measurements of impedance, reactance, resistance and capacitance have been highly
correlated to changes in the human body and are good prognostic indicators for morbidity and mortality [8]. Most importantly, BIA can be used in critically ill patients
to assess intracellular and extracellular body fluid status. ECW increases in different disease states (especially septic shock with capillary leak and fluid overload)
and peripheral edema is the most common sign of ECW expansion. Monitoring
these changes over time in patients can be important to guide fluid therapy. Correct
estimation of dry weight has been shown to affect the survival and quality of life of
patients on renal replacement therapy [8]. Furthermore, the assessment of volume
excess can help to identify patients that may be eligible for de-resuscitation.

Validation

Although BIA is a simple, non-invasive, rapid, portable, reproducible and convenient method for measuring fluid distribution and body composition, it is still
unclear whether it is sufficiently accurate for clinical use in critically ill patients
[8]. As BIA measures TBW, it needs to be validated with other methods (such as
densitometry) used to derive TBW, fat-free mass (FFM), and body fat. Because
BIA disproportionately takes the extremities into account, the relationship between
impedance and TBW is assumed to be empirical. This places an important con-
straint on the derived value, because TBW must change in a fixed relationship in
the torso and extremities in healthy as well as in critically ill individuals to retain
its predictive value [9]. This relationship probably exists in most normal subjects,
in those with mild-to-moderate obesity and other chronic illnesses without fluid
overload. The gold standard techniques for measuring body composition and TBW,
such as isotope dilution (labeled deuterium), dual energy X-ray absorptiometry
(DEXA), underwater weighing, and air-displacement plethysmography are not applicable in the critically ill [8]. Abdominal and visceral fat can also be measured
with computed tomography (CT) and magnetic resonance imaging (MRI) but are
again not useful for monitoring. Portable methods consist of infrared analysis, skin-
fold caliper measurement and BIA. Different studies comparing BIA with a gold
standard (e.g., DEXA) showed good correlation [8]. For clinical purposes, three devices are available to be used in (critically ill) patients: the Fresenius Medical Care
(BCM) Body Composition Monitor (Fresenius Medical Care, Bad Homburg, Germany), the SECA medical body composition analyzer mBCA 525 (SECA, Chino,
CA, USA) and the Maltron BioScan 920 (Maltron International Ltd, Rayleigh, Es-
sex, UK)[9]. However, so far, no large study with head-to-head comparison has been
performed in critically ill patients.

Clinical Applications

Traditional BIA Applications

Historically, BIA has been used in CKD where it can detect changes in body composition even in the early stages of kidney disease and in patients with cardio-(abdominal)-renal syndromes, showing lower resistance, abnormal bioelectrical impedance vector analysis (BIVA), reduced phase angle, and higher TBW together with lower body cell mass [9]. However, patients need to have overt signs of fluid overload or malnutrition for BIA to detect these alterations [8]. In chronic hemodialysis patients, multifrequency whole body BIA can give an objective measure of fluid status and can calculate volume excess with an accuracy of one liter [39]. As such it seems an appropriate and non-invasive method for determination and targeting of dry weight, resulting in an improved fluid status and better control of blood pressure in CKD [8]. The use of BIA measurements has also been advocated by the European Society for Clinical Nutrition and Metabolism (ESPEN) guidelines as a clinical tool for evaluation of the metabolic status in critically ill patients [40]. BIA is inexpensive and non-invasive and provides useful information concerning fluid imbalance as well as altered body composition at the tissue level measured by the phase angle [8]. From a theoretical point of view, BIA can be useful in burn patients, cardiovascular disease, peripheral edema, gastroenteritis, hemodialysis, continuous venovenous hemofiltration (CVVH), peritoneal dialysis, liver disease, second and third fluid spacing (segmental analysis), lung disease (such as acute respiratory distress syndrome [ARDS] with capillary leak), malnutrition, bariatric surgery, postoperative fluid status, renal failure, stroke, etc.

Critical Care

For the ICU clinician, it is important to be aware that the normal ECW/ICW ratio is usually less than 1 (around 0.8). Increase in ICW is seen in patients with heart failure, liver cirrhosis and CKD (especially in early stage). A decrease in ICW is related to osmotic factors, whereas increases in ECW are mostly due to shift from the intra- to extracellular space as seen with second and third space edema, and in the late stages of heart, liver or kidney failure. Critically ill patients, especially those with sepsis or septic shock easily develop changes in distribution of body fluids with the migration of fluid from the intravascular to the extravascular space. A previous study showed that, although changes in TBW were similar, patients with blunt trauma (n = 18) had lower ECW values compared to those with peritonitis and sepsis (n = 12) [11]. Others found that in cardiac patients presenting with dyspnea, increasing fluid volume was associated with increased CVP [41].

A retrospective study comparing BIA data in critically ill patients (n = 101) and healthy volunteers (n = 101) showed significant differences in body water composition [38]. In this study patients had higher values for TBW (46.1 ± 10.8 vs. 38.5 ± 8 liters, $p < 0.001$), ECW (23.4 ± 7 vs. 16.7 ± 4 liters, $p < 0.001$) and ECW/ICW ratio (1 ± 0.2 vs. 0.8 ± 0.1, $p < 0.001$) whereas ICW remained unchanged (22.7 ± 4.8 vs. 21.8 ± 4.3 liters, $p = 0.158$) (Fig. 3). Also ECW% ($50.4 \pm 5\%$ vs. $43.2 \pm 2.4\%$, $p < 0.001$), ICW% ($49.6 \pm 5\%$ vs. $56.8 \pm 2.4\%$, $p < 0.001$) and TBW%

$(57.3 \pm 11.3\%$ vs. $53.2 \pm 5.8\%$, $p < 0.001$) showed significant differences [38]. Patients had a volume excess of 6.2 ± 6.4 vs. -0.2 ± 0.9 liters in healthy volunteers ($p < 0.001$). Patients who died in the hospital ($n = 40$) had similar values of ECW and TBW, but significantly lower values for ICW (21.5 ± 4.6 vs. 23.5 ± 4.9 liters, $p = 0.017$), resulting in an increased ECW/ICW ratio (1.1 ± 0.2 vs. 1 ± 0.2, $p = 0.002$). Non-survivors also had a significantly higher ECW% ($52.1 \pm 5.3\%$ vs. $49.3 \pm 4.8\%$, $p = 0.002$), lower ICW% ($47.9 \pm 5.3\%$ vs. $50.7 \pm 4.8\%$, $p = 0.002$) and higher TBW% ($60.1 \pm 11.3\%$ vs. $55.6 \pm 10.7\%$, $p = 0.024$) compared to ICU survivors (Fig. 4). Non-survivors had a volume excess of 7.5 ± 5.8 vs. 4.6 ± 9.1 liters in survivors ($p = 0.029$). Another study showed that fluid overload measured by BIVA was present in 70% of critically ill patients ($n = 64$) and a significant predictor of mortality regardless of continuous renal replacement therapy (CRRT) [42]. Recently, similar results were observed in a larger dual center study ($n = 125$) in which fluid overload measured by BIVA was the only variable significantly associated with ICU mortality (OR 22.91; 95% CI 2.38–220.07; $p < 0.01$) [43].

Fig. 3 Fluid status monitoring with bioelectrical impedance analysis in healthy subjects and critically ill patients. **a** Bar graph showing mean values (in l) for total body water (TBW), intracellular water (ICW) and extracellular water (ECW) in 101 intensive care unit (ICU) patients compared to 101 healthy volunteers. *denotes p value < 0.05. **b** Bar graph showing mean values (in l) for volume excess (VE), and the extracellular water (ECW) to intracellular water (ICW) ratio (ECW/ICW) in 101 ICU patients compared to 101 healthy volunteers. *denotes p value < 0.05. Adapted from [38] with permission

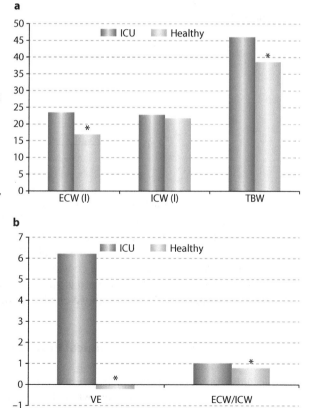

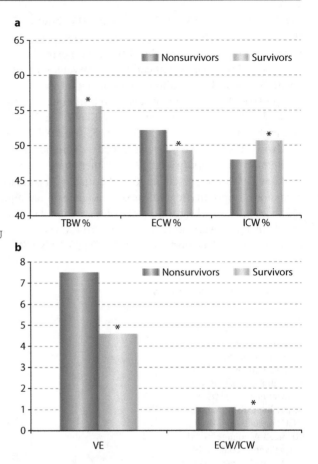

Fig. 4 Fluid status monitoring with bioelectrical impedance analysis in 101 critically ill patients. **a** Bar graph showing mean values (in %) for total body water (TBW), intracellular water (ICW) and extracellular water (ECW) in 101 ICU patients comparing survivors (n = 61) vs non-survivors (n = 40). **b** Bar graph showing mean values (in l) for volume excess (VE), and the extracellular water (ECW) to intracellular water (ICW) ratio (ECW/ICW) in 101 ICU patients comparing survivors (n = 61) vs non-survivors (n = 40). *denotes p value < 0.05. Adapted from [38] with permission

However, many conditions exist in critical illness (ascites, anasarca, severe peripheral edema, pleural effusions, massive fluid overload as well as other clinical conditions in which there are disturbances in fluid and electrolyte distribution) where conventional BIA may be a poor measure of TBW [8]. Therefore, until more data become available, BIA can only be considered as a research tool in critically ill patients because the TBW-to-FFM ratio is variable and the body impedance-to-TBW ratio may often vary during the above-cited conditions [8].

BIA Pitfalls and Limitations in Clinical Practice

BIA has numerous advantages as it is non-invasive and relatively inexpensive and can be performed easily at the bedside, while it does not expose to ionizing radiation compared to other techniques to assess TBW. Modern BIA devices have very limited between-observer variation. However, the use of BIA has some limitations in ICU patients. First, the five BIA assumptions only occur in an ideal situation, which may differ from real life conditions, especially in the critically ill. Second, critically ill patients can have significant body asymmetry (amputations), unilateral hemiparesis (tissue atrophy) or other neuromuscular conditions that may produce localized changes in conductance [9]. Third, there may be differences between men and women and old and young patients in terms of cylindrical body shape. Fourth, other not well-understood factors may interfere with BIA measurements, such as increased body mass index (BMI) $> 34 \, kg/m^2$, use of intravenous infusions with large amounts of (ab)normal saline, presence of peripheral edema and fluid overload, administration of parenteral and enteral nutrition or oral feeding, altered nutritional status, changes in ambient air and skin temperature or fever, sweating, changes in sodium and potassium content, specific conductance of metal hospital bed, etc. ... Fifth, body position and position of the arms (should be next to the body) may interfere with BIA measurements with the best position being supine, whereas most patients and especially those with TBI or raised intracranial pressure are kept with the head of bed at the $30°–45°$ position. Changes in body position may also lead to incorrect contact with electrodes or contact with another person or object during measurement. Sixth, whole-body BIA measures the bioelectrical properties between the wrist and the ankle under the assumption of a steady body fluid distribution [9]. This divides the body into three independent electrical segments with different lengths and cross-sectional areas: the trunk, the arms, and the legs. The geometrical differences of these three segments influence their contribution to overall whole-body bioimpedance substantially [8]. Moreover, as water is not evenly distributed in the human body, the same volume of ECW in the legs may lead to different results in whole-body bioimpedance measurements than a similar volume of ECW in the trunk [9]. An increase in abdominal water content as seen in patients with intraperitoneal inflammation or ascites also significantly disturbs whole-body bioimpedance findings. Therefore, whole-body bioimpedance is much more sensitive to volume changes in the extremities compared to volume changes in the trunk [8]. Seventh, an increase in IAP also affects whole-body bioimpedance findings especially in third ($> 20 \, mmHg$) or fourth ($> 25 \, mmHg$) grade IAH. Increased IAP significantly congests abdominal vessels reducing venous return from the limbs [8]. An increase in intravenous splanchnic mesenteric volume and decrease in venous compliance further lead to interstitial edema in the limbs, which increases the electrical conductivity, hence disturbing whole body bioimpedance findings [8]. Therefore, the measurement of body water distribution should always be interpreted in relation to IAP values. Finally, the presence of a (temporary) pacemaker or implanted defibrillator is a formal contraindication for BIA measurements as even the small electric currents used during BIA evaluations can disturb the devices and thus need to be avoided until more data are available [9].

Prevention of Fluid Overload

In patients with pre-existing heart or kidney failure, treatment should focus on optimization of heart and kidney function. The clinician should be aware that caution is needed with intravenous fluid replacement, including blood transfusion, and hypotonic solutions should be avoided for resuscitation. The National Institute for Health and Care Excellence (NICE) has published guidance on intravenous fluid therapy in adults in the hospital with algorithms covering assessment, fluid resuscitation, routine maintenance and replacement and resuscitation [44]. For surgical patients, guidelines on appropriate postoperative fluid replacement are now available [21]. For patients with severe sepsis or septic shock, the Surviving Sepsis Campaign guidelines include details of appropriate fluid therapy [17].

Treatment of Fluid Overload

Fluid overload is mainly an issue in septic patients with AKI. Sepsis and septic shock together with AKI is associated with a high mortality rate of around 40–50% [45]. Several studies have shown the beneficial impact of conservative (late) fluid management with early negative fluid balance upon mortality [5]. Therefore, avoidance and correction of fluid overload are mandatory. Diuretics and especially loop diuretics represent the first line of fluid removal therapy; indapamide can be associated in case of hypernatremia. Patients with fluid overload and AKI unfortunately have a poor response to diuretics even given in high doses. CRRT, including the modality of CVVH, is now recognized in the critical care nephrology community and also indicated in the recent Kidney Disease: Improving Global Outcomes (KDIGO) guidelines as a true indication when fluid overload is present even in the absence of AKI or any other metabolic disturbances [46]. CRRT has the enormous advantage compared to diuretics in that it can dissociate the removal of free water and sodium and therefore avoid the hyper- or hyponatremia that can be seen with the excessive use of diuretics. Those electrolyte disturbances may increase mortality and morbidity in severely ill patients [45]. Early use of CRRT when the patient is resistant to diuretics is increasingly used in the ICU despite the lack of good evidence regarding improvement in mortality and better data are eagerly awaited. A recent study showed that mean and maximum hydration levels measured by BIA had a stronger correlation with mortality in patients undergoing de-resuscitation with CRRT than with mean and maximum cumulative fluid balance reached during the observation period, thus shedding light on the possible advantage of BIA as a better guide for active fluid removal when using CRRT during the de-resuscitation phase of management of patients with septic shock and AKI [42]. In a study on the use of CVVH to adjust fluid volume excess in 30 septic shock patients with AKI, sustained increases in TBW, ECW and ECW/ICW ratio were observed in non-survivors [47]. In this study, volume excess was also associated with increased IAP and worse outcomes. The use of CVVH with net ultrafiltration successfully reduced TBW, ECW, ICW and IAP in those patients who survived 96 h of CVVH.

Very often, fluid removal may be quite difficult to realize with CRRT even in hemodynamically stable patients. The concomitant use of an oncotic agent, such as concentrated albumin (20–25%), or an osmotic agent, such as hypertonic saline (3 or 6%), to improve the rate of fluid removal during CRRT is under investigation but shows promising results [48]. In patients with fluid overload and acute lung injury or ARDS, studies have shown that PEEP application facilitates alveolar fluid clearance [49]. The addition of hyperoncotic albumin 20% to furosemide further enhances interstitial fluid clearance [50]. Recently, the combination of PEEP, set equal to IAP, followed by hyperoncotic albumin 20% and furosemide resulted in a less positive cumulative fluid balance after 1 week, a decrease in IAP and EVLW, improvement in the P/F ratio, faster weaning and better survival in a pilot study of 114 patients with ALI [20].

Conclusion

Fluid overload is defined by a cut-off value of 10% of fluid accumulation and is associated with increased morbidity and mortality. Different tools are available for the clinician to assess fluid overload. BIA seems to find its place amongst other tools, including clinical assessment, biomarkers, imaging and hemodynamic monitoring. BIA enables assessment of different parameters related to the patient's fluid status, including TBW, ICW, ECW, ECW/ICW ratio and volume excess and, as such, it can help guide resuscitation and de-resuscitation (which may be even of greater importance). However, although BIA seems to be a promising tool, the recommendations for fluid monitoring using BIA are still conceptual and at an infant stage. They can at best be described as open for discussion and debate, awaiting confirmation in clinical practice. More research on the deleterious effects of fluid overload and the role of BIA to guide fluid therapy is needed in critically ill patients, especially those with AKI.

References

1. Vincent JL, Sakr Y, Sprung CL et al (2006) Sepsis in European intensive care units: results of the SOAP study. Crit Care Med 34:344–353
2. Murphy CV, Schramm GE, Doherty JA et al (2009) The importance of fluid management in acute lung injury secondary to septic shock. Chest 136:102–109
3. Acheampong A, Vincent JL (2015) A positive fluid balance is an independent prognostic factor in patients with sepsis. Crit Care 19:251
4. Silversides JA, Major E, Ferguson AJ et al (2017) Conservative fluid management or deresuscitation for patients with sepsis or acute respiratory distress syndrome following the resuscitation phase of critical illness: a systematic review and meta-analysis. Intensive Care Med 43:155–170

5. Malbrain ML, Marik PE, Witters I et al (2014) Fluid overload, de-resuscitation, and outcomes in critically ill or injured patients: a systematic review with suggestions for clinical practice. Anaesthesiol Intensive Ther 46:361–380

6. Claure-Del Granado R, Mehta RL (2016) Fluid overload in the ICU: evaluation and management. BMC Nephrol 17:109

7. Vaara ST, Korhonen AM, Kaukonen KM et al (2012) Fluid overload is associated with an increased risk for 90-day mortality in critically ill patients with renal replacement therapy: data from the prospective FINNAKI study. Crit Care 16:R197

8. Malbrain MLNG, Huygh J, Dabrowski W, De Waele J, Wauters J (2014) The use of bio-electrical impedance analysis (BIA) to guide fluid management, resuscitation and dere-suscitation in critically ill patients: a bench-to-bedside review. Anaesthesiol Intensive Ther 46:381–391

9. National Institute of Health (1994) Bioelectrical Impedance Analysis in Body Composition Measurement. NIH Technol Assess Statement Dec 12–14:1–35

10. Wabel P, Chamney P, Moissl U, Jirka T (2009) Importance of whole-body bioimpedance spectroscopy for the management of fluid balance. Blood Purif 27:75–80

11. Plank LD, Hill GL (2000) Similarity of changes in body composition in intensive care patients following severe sepsis or major blunt injury. Ann N Y Acad Sci 904:592–602

12. Savalle M, Gillaizeau F, Maruani G et al (2012) Assessment of body cell mass at bedside in critically ill patients. Am J Physiol Endocrinol Metab 303:E389–E396

13. Streat SJ, Beddoe AH, Hill GL (1985) Measurement of total body water in intensive care patients with fluid overload. Metabolism 34:688–694

14. Macedo E, Bouchard J, Soroko SH et al (2010) Fluid accumulation, recognition and staging of acute kidney injury in critically-ill patients. Crit Care 14:R82

15. Hoste EA, Maitland K, Brudney CS et al (2014) Four phases of intravenous fluid therapy: a conceptual model. Br J Anaesth 113:740–747

16. Marik PE, Monnet X, Teboul JL (2011) Hemodynamic parameters to guide fluid therapy. Ann Intensive Care 1:1

17. Rhodes A, Evans LE, Alhazzani W et al (2017) Surviving sepsis campaign: international guidelines for management of sepsis and septic shock: 2016. Intensive Care Med 43:304–377

18. Marik PE (2014) Iatrogenic salt water drowning and the hazards of a high central venous pressure. Ann Intensive Care 4:21

19. Cordemans C, De Laet I, Van Regenmortel N et al (2012) Fluid management in critically ill patients: the role of extravascular lung water, abdominal hypertension, capillary leak and fluid balance. Ann Intensive Care 2(Suppl 1):S1

20. Cordemans C, De Laet I, Van Regenmortel N et al (2012) Aiming for a negative fluid balance in patients with acute lung injury and increased intra-abdominal pressure: a pilot study looking at the effects of PAL-treatment. Ann Intensive Care 2(Suppl 1):S15

21. Powell-Tuck J, Gosling P, Lobo D et al (2009) Summary of the British consensus guidelines on intravenous fluid therapy for adult surgical patients (GIFTASUP). J Intensive Care Soc 10:13–15

22. Soni N (2009) British consensus guidelines on intravenous fluid therapy for adult surgical patients (GIFTASUP): cassandra's view. Anaesthesia 64:235–238

23. Cecconi M, Fasano N, Langiano N et al (2011) Goal-directed haemodynamic therapy during elective total hip arthroplasty under regional anaesthesia. Crit Care 15:R132

24. Kirkpatrick AW, Roberts DJ, De Waele J et al (2013) Intra-abdominal hypertension and the abdominal compartment syndrome: updated consensus definitions and clinical practice guidelines from the World Society of the Abdominal Compartment Syndrome. Intensive Care Med 39:1190–1206

25. Verbrugge FH, Dupont M, Steels P et al (2013) Abdominal contributions to cardiorenal dysfunction in congestive heart failure. J Am Coll Cardiol 62:485–495

26. Freitag E, Edgecombe G, Baldwin I, Cottier B, Heland M (2010) Determination of body weight and height measurement for critically ill patients admitted to the intensive care unit: A quality improvement project. Aust Crit Care 23:197–207

27. Schneider AG, Baldwin I, Freitag E, Glassford N, Bellomo R (2012) Estimation of fluid status changes in critically ill patients: fluid balance chart or electronic bed weight? J Crit Care 27(745):e747–e712

28. Saugel B, Ringmaier S, Holzapfel K et al (2011) Physical examination, central venous pressure, and chest radiography for the prediction of transpulmonary thermodilution-derived hemodynamic parameters in critically ill patients: a prospective trial. J Crit Care 26:402–410

29. Perel A, Saugel B, Teboul JL et al (2015) The effects of advanced monitoring on hemodynamic management in critically ill patients: a pre and post questionnaire study. J Clin Monit Comput 30:511–518

30. Vlachou E, Gosling P, Moiemen NS (2006) Microalbuminuria: a marker of endothelial dysfunction in thermal injury. Burns 32:1009–1016

31. Lichtenstein D, Malbrain ML (2015) Critical care ultrasound in cardiac arrest. Technological requirements for performing the SESAME-protocol – a holistic approach. Anaesthesiol Intensive Ther 47:471–481

32. Vermeiren GL, Malbrain ML, Walpot JM (2015) Cardiac Ultrasonography in the critical care setting: a practical approach to asses cardiac function and preload for the "non-cardiologist". Anaesthesiol Intensive Ther 47:89–104

33. Agricola E, Bove T, Oppizzi M et al (2005) "Ultrasound comet-tail images": a marker of pulmonary edema: a comparative study with wedge pressure and extravascular lung water. Chest 127:1690–1695

34. Vandervelden S, Malbrain ML (2015) Initial resuscitation from severe sepsis: one size does not fit all. Anaesthesiol Intensive Ther 47:44–55

35. Hofkens PJ, Verrijcken A, Merveille K et al (2015) Common pitfalls and tips and tricks to get the most out of your transpulmonary thermodilution device: results of a survey and state-of-the-art review. Anaesthesiol Intensive Ther 47:89–116

36. Foster KR, Lukaski HC (1996) Whole-body impedance – what does it measure? Am J Clin Nutr 64(3 Suppl):388S–396S

37. Streat SJ, Plank LD, Hill GL (2000) Overview of modern management of patients with critical injury and severe sepsis. World J Surg 24:655–663

38. Vandervelden S, Teering S, Hoffman B et al (2015) Prognostic value of bioelectrical impedance analysis (BIA) derived parameters in critically ill patients. Anaesth Intensive Ther 47(Suppl 2):14–16

39. Tattersall J (2009) Bioimpedance analysis in dialysis: state of the art and what we can expect. Blood Purif 27:70–74

40. Kyle UG, Bosaeus I, De Lorenzo AD et al (2004) Bioelectrical impedance analysis-part II: utilization in clinical practice. Clin Nutr 23:1430–1453

41. Piccoli A, Codognotto M, Cianci V et al (2012) Differentiation of cardiac and noncardiac dyspnea using bioelectrical impedance vector analysis (BIVA). J Card Fail 18:226–232

42. Basso F, Berdin G, Virzi GM et al (2013) Fluid management in the intensive care unit: bioelectrical impedance vector analysis as a tool to assess hydration status and optimal fluid balance in critically ill patients. Blood Purif 36:192–199

43. Samoni S, Vigo V, Resendiz LI et al (2016) Impact of hyperhydration on the mortality risk in critically ill patients admitted in intensive care units: comparison between bioelectrical impedance vector analysis and cumulative fluid balance recording. Crit Care 20:95

44. Padhi S, Bullock I, Li L et al (2013) Intravenous fluid therapy for adults in hospital: summary of NICE guidance. BMJ 347:f7073

45. Joannes-Boyau O, Honore PM, Perez P et al (2013) High-volume versus standard-volume haemofiltration for septic shock patients with acute kidney injury (IVOIRE study): a multicentre randomized controlled trial. Intensive Care Med 39:1535–1546

46. Lameire N, Kellum JA, Group KAGW (2013) Contrast-induced acute kidney injury and renal support for acute kidney injury: a KDIGO summary (Part 2). Crit Care 17:205
47. Dabrowski W, Kotlinska-Hasiec E, Schneditz D et al (2014) Continuous veno-venous hemofiltration to adjust fluid volume excess in septic shock patients reduces intra-abdominal pressure. Clin Nephrol 82:41–50
48. Paterna S, Di Gaudio F, La Rocca V et al (2015) Hypertonic saline in conjunction with high-dose furosemide improves dose-response curves in worsening refractory congestive heart failure. Adv Ther 32:971–982
49. Luecke T, Roth H, Herrmann P et al (2003) PEEP decreases atelectasis and extravascular lung water but not lung tissue volume in surfactant-washout lung injury. Intensive Care Med 29:2026–2033
50. Martin GS, Moss M, Wheeler AP et al (2005) A randomized, controlled trial of furosemide with or without albumin in hypoproteinemic patients with acute lung injury. Crit Care Med 33:1681–1687

Part X
Coagulopathy and Blood Products

Prothrombin Complex Concentrate: Anticoagulation Reversal and Beyond

O. Grottke and H. Schöchl

Introduction

Prothrombin complex concentrates (PCCs) are plasma-derived coagulation factor concentrates. All PCCs contain factors II, IX and X, and four-factor PCCs also contain factor VII. Most PCCs contain coagulation factors that are not activated, but activated PCC contains activated factor VII (FVII). The ratio of quantities of coagulation factor concentrations varies from one PCC to another [1]. Further differences between PCCs relate to constituents other than coagulation factors: they contain different amounts of inhibitors, such as heparin, antithrombin and proteins C, S and Z. Despite this variability, however, levels of inhibitors are always much lower than those of the coagulation factors.

PCCs are mainly used for emergency reversal of the effects of vitamin K antagonists (VKAs). Circumstances demanding rapid anticoagulation reversal include unplanned, urgent surgery and trauma-related bleeding. VKAs, such as warfarin, function by preventing synthesis of the vitamin K-dependent coagulation factors (factors II, VII, IX and X). Four-factor PCCs provide all four of these factors, enabling the restoration of hemostasis. Three-factor PCCs have also been shown to reverse the effects of VKAs, but there is evidence that four-factor products are more effective.

In Europe, PCCs have broad approval for use in acquired deficiency of the PCC factors [2]. Accordingly, PCCs have been explored as hemostatic therapy for

O. Grottke (✉)
Department of Anesthesiology, RWTH Aachen University Hospital
Aachen, Germany
e-mail: ogrottke@ukaachen.de

H. Schöchl
Ludwig Boltzmann Institute for Experimental and Clinical Traumatology, AUVA Research Centre
Vienna, Austria
Department of Anaesthesiology and Intensive Care, AUVA Trauma Centre
Salzburg, Austria

© Springer International Publishing AG 2018   439
J.-L. Vincent (ed.), *Annual Update in Intensive Care and Emergency Medicine 2018*,
Annual Update in Intensive Care and Emergency Medicine,
https://doi.org/10.1007/978-3-319-73670-9_34

patients with massive blood loss unrelated to anticoagulation (e.g., in trauma or patients undergoing complex surgery). There is also evidence that PCCs may reverse the effects of direct oral anticoagulants (DOACs: direct thrombin inhibitors and factor Xa inhibitors). In these settings, fresh frozen plasma (FFP) may also be considered as an alternative 'conventional' therapy. However, the concentration of coagulation factors in FFP is low (slightly below physiological plasma levels) meaning that large quantities of FFP must be transfused to effect clinically significant increases in the patient's plasma. The time taken to administer FFP is considerably longer than that for coagulation factor concentrates, and treatment cannot be specifically targeted because all coagulation factors and inhibitors are being given. It can also be argued that the safety profile of coagulation factor concentrates is superior to that of FFP. Commercially available PCCs undergo a variety of viral inactivation and removal steps during manufacture, resulting in a very low risk of disease transmission.

In this chapter, we provide an overview of the increasing number of clinical areas in which PCCs might be applied, with consideration of efficacy and key safety data.

Anticoagulation Reversal

Vitamin K Antagonists

VKAs, such as warfarin and phenprocoumon, limit the availability of vitamin K in its active form, thereby preventing synthesis of coagulation factors II, VII, IX and X, as well as the anticoagulant proteins C, S and Z. The international normalized ratio (INR) is the usual test for monitoring the patient's coagulation status, and a value around 2.5 is typically targeted.

Patients who are being treated with VKAs may be at risk of excessive bleeding if they experience trauma, or if they require urgent surgical procedures. In principle, the anticoagulant effects of VKAs can be reversed by stopping treatment and administering oral vitamin K, but patients with severe bleeding require rapid replenishment of prothrombin complex coagulation factors.

Two randomized, controlled, phase III trials compared the efficacy and safety of four-factor PCC with that of therapeutic plasma in patients requiring urgent VKA reversal. In the first of these studies, non-inferiority of PCC was confirmed regarding the percentage of patients in whom effective hemostasis was achieved (PCC 72% vs plasma 65%), and PCC was superior regarding achievement of a rapid reduction in INR (62% vs 10%) [3]. The second study showed effective hemostasis rates of 90% with PCC and 75% with plasma, with rapid INR reduction rates of 55% and 10%; both variables showed PCC to be superior to plasma [4]. PCC was compared with plasma for warfarin reversal in a retrospective cohort study [5]. INR reversal was achieved in 5.7 hours with PCC versus 11.8 h with therapeutic plasma ($p < 0.0001$), and mean transfusion of red blood cells (RBCs) was significantly reduced. In another retrospective study (described as the "evaluation pronostique de l'antagonisation des hémorragies graves sous antivitamin K" [EPAHK] study), urgent reversal of VKAs with vitamin K and PCC in accordance with guidelines was associated with a reduction in 7-day mortality of ~ 50%, compared with treatment that was not guideline-concordant [6]. Based on evidence from these studies and others, four-factor PCCs are strongly recommended in international guidelines for controlling bleeding related to VKA therapy; examples include the European trauma guidelines and the European Society of Anaesthesiology guidelines on treatment of perioperative bleeding [7, 8]. Depending on pre-treatment INR, doses between 25 and 50 IU per kg bodyweight are usually advised.

Direct Oral Anticoagulants

VKAs have been the mainstay of treatment for patients at risk of thromboembolic events, but they have significant limitations, including the narrow therapeutic window and the need for regular coagulation monitoring. DOACs include the direct thrombin inhibitor dabigatran and factor Xa inhibitors (rivaroxaban, apixaban and edoxaban). Compared with VKAs, DOACs produce a more predictable anticoagulant effect with a reduced risk of hemorrhagic complications; they are given in fixed doses and there is no need for routine coagulation monitoring [9]. Despite the favorable properties of DOACs, bleeding complications remain possible, as with all anticoagulants.

Antidotes have been developed to enable specific reversal of DOACs. Idarucizumab is a monoclonal antibody fragment that specifically binds to and reverses the effects of dabigatran. Clinical data show that idarucizumab achieves rapid and complete reversal of dabigatran [10]. Another reversal agent, andexanet alfa, is in development to reverse the effects of direct and indirect factor Xa inhibitors. In an interim analysis of a phase III study, andexanet alfa provided effective hemostasis in patients with major bleeding associated with factor Xa inhibitors [11].

Specific antidotes are considered as the preferred treatment for emergency DOAC reversal – unlike PCC, they do not exert intrinsic effects on the coagulation system. Despite international approval of idarucizumab, specific antidotes are not yet available for patients with factor Xa inhibitor-related bleeding. In cases of severe bleeding, PCC can potentially serve as a non-specific emergency reversal agent for DOACs, by increasing levels of prothrombin complex coagulation factors to the point where circulating DOAC molecules are outnumbered by thrombin or factor Xa. As a result, the DOAC no longer blocks the coagulation process.

In animal models of trauma, PCC has been shown to be effective in reversing the anticoagulant effects of dabigatran, reducing blood loss and mortality [9]. A balance must be achieved because low-dose PCC may not be sufficiently effective, but high doses may result in excessively high thrombin generation potential, suggesting a need for careful dose titration [12]. Further studies have shown that four-factor PCC can reduce blood loss resulting from trauma in animals treated with edoxaban or apixaban [13, 14]. Available clinical data also support the use of PCC for DOAC reversal. Studies in healthy volunteers have shown that PCC is effective in reversing the effects of edoxaban on endogenous thrombin potential and bleeding duration

[15, 16]. Also in healthy volunteers, PCC has been reported to improve thrombin generation parameters following apixaban treatment [17]. In a prospective study of 84 patients with major bleeding events related to rivaroxaban or apixaban, treatment with PCC (median dose 2000 IU) was assessed as effective in 69% of patients [18]. Ischemic stroke was reported in two patients after PCC treatment and the authors concluded that there was a low risk of thromboembolism.

Although the European trauma guidelines recommend that patients requiring emergency reversal of dabigatran are treated with idarucizumab if possible, high doses of PCC (25–50 IU/kg) are suggested as an alternative [8]. With the lack of approved antidotes for factor Xa inhibitors, 25–50 IU/kg PCC is recommended for emergency reversal of these agents. Based on the ability of PCC to reduce or reverse the effects of a range of DOACs, PCC may also be a useful option for reversal when the patient's exact anticoagulant therapy is unknown. However, it should be noted that PCCs are not licensed for DOAC reversal.

Management of Bleeding Unrelated to Anticoagulation

PCCs are increasingly being used for coagulation management in patients not receiving anticoagulation therapy. The rationale for this therapeutic approach is that PCCs provide more effective supplementation of coagulation factors than is possible with therapeutic plasma, reducing patients' exposure to allogeneic blood products and the need for rapid intervention. Thus, PCCs are often included as part of a multimodal, coagulation factor concentrate-based approach to treatment.

The causes of coagulopathy in patients with perioperative or trauma-related bleeding are multifactorial and inter-related. They include consumption and dilution of coagulation factors and platelets, dysfunction of platelets and the wider coagulation system, increased fibrinolysis, hemodilution by the infusion of crystalloids or colloids, and hypocalcemia. Also, it is important to consider that fibrinogen is the first coagulation factor to reach critically low levels during major bleeding [19]. Published algorithms in trauma and cardiac surgery recommend fibrinogen supplementation as first-line hemostatic therapy, with PCCs being given second-line in case of continued bleeding and a confirmed need for increased thrombin generation. Many patients with perioperative or trauma-related bleeding have low levels of anticoagulants, such as antithrombin. Because PCC therapy increases thrombin generation potential while the concentration of anticoagulants remains essentially unchanged, there is a risk of thromboembolic complications. For this reason, PCC should be administered cautiously and the dose should be tailored according to clinical needs.

Trauma

Following trauma, critical bleeding is often accompanied by coagulopathy. Treatment with PCCs may potentially facilitate the restoration of hemostasis, and PCC is

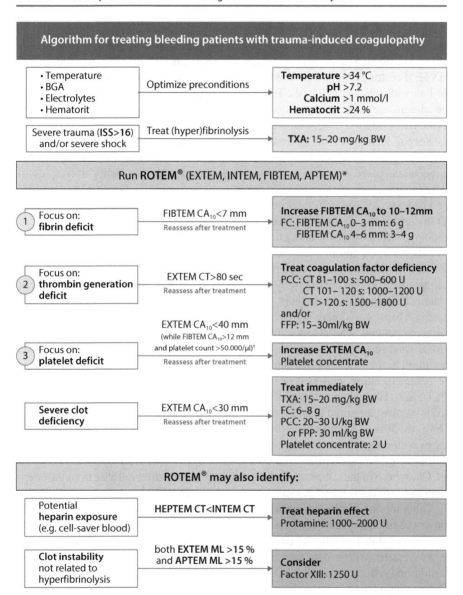

Fig. 1 ROTEM-guided treatment algorithm [43]. ROTEM®-guided treatment algorithm: managing trauma-induced coagulopathy and diffuse microvascular bleeding (AUVA Trauma Hospital, Austria). *For patients who are unconscious or known to be taking a platelet inhibitor medication, multiplate tests (adenosine diphosphate test, arachidonic acid test, and thrombin receptor activating peptide-6 test) are also performed. †Traumatic brain injury: platelet count 80,000–100,000/μl. *APTEM*: extrinsically activated ROTEM® assay with added aprotinin; *BGA*: blood gas analysis; *BW*: body weight; *CA10*: clot amplitude after 10 min; *CT*: clotting time; *EXTEM*: extrinsically activated ROTEM® assay; *FC*: fibrinogen concentrate; *FFP*: fresh-frozen plasma; *FIBTEM*: extrinsically activated ROTEM® assay with inactivation of platelets; *HEPTEM*: intrinsically activated ROTEM® assay with added heparinase; *ISS*: injury severity score; *ML*: maximum lysis; *PCC*: prothrombin complex concentrate; *ROTEM®*: thromboelastometry; *TIC*: trauma-induced coagulopathy; *TXA*: tranexamic acid. Reproduced from [20] and [43] with permission

included in point-of-care guided algorithms designed to facilitate the treatment of bleeding trauma patients. In one such algorithm developed by Schöchl et al., PCCs are administered as a second-line treatment in patients with ongoing bleeding and an EXTEM clotting time (CT) > 80 s after restoration of fibrinogen levels (Fig. 1; [20]). In line with this algorithm, the European trauma guidelines recommend that PCC be administered in bleeding trauma patients with normal fibrinogen levels, based on evidence of delayed coagulation initiation from viscoelastic monitoring [8].

Several studies of PCC treatment of trauma-related bleeding in patients who are not receiving anticoagulants have involved the implementation of coagulation factor concentrate-based management. A retrospective analysis by Schöchl et al. compared trauma patients treated with fibrinogen concentrate and/or PCC and no FFP (80 patients), or with FFP and no fibrinogen concentrate/PCC (601 patients) [21]. Transfusion was significantly reduced with coagulation factor concentrate-based therapy, with RBC and platelet transfusion avoided in 29% and 91%, respectively, of patients in the fibrinogen/PCC group compared with 3% and 56% of patients in the FFP group. Mortality was comparable between the two treatment groups. A subsequent prospective cohort study was conducted in 144 patients with major blunt trauma [22]. Patients treated with fibrinogen concentrate and/or PCC alone showed restored hemostasis, with significantly reduced RBC and platelet transfusion compared to patients who also received FFP. The incidence of multiple organ failure (MOF) and sepsis were also reduced in the group receiving fibrinogen concentrate and/or PCC. In a second prospective study, trauma patients were randomly allocated to treatment either with FFP or coagulation factor concentrate therapy (including PCC) [23]. Higher percentages of patients in the FFP group required rescue therapy (52% vs. 4%), required massive transfusion (30% vs. 12%), and experienced MOF (66% vs. 50%). In both of the prospective studies, PCC was only administered in cases with delayed initial thrombin formation (as shown by prothrombin time [PT] < 50% or < 35% and/or EXTEM CT > 90 s) [22, 23]. The median 24-hour dose of PCC was zero in the cohort study [22], and only eight patients (16%) from the coagulation factor concentrate group were treated with PCC in the randomized trial [23].

Other trauma studies have assessed PCC alone, rather than in combination with other coagulation factor concentrates. A retrospective analysis compared patients who received PCC+FFP with patients who received FFP alone [24]. PCC treatment was associated with a more rapid INR correction, reductions in RBC and FFP transfusion, and reduced mortality. In another retrospective study, treatment with PCC or FFP was compared in injured patients with pelvic and/or lower extremity fractures [25]. PCC was again associated with faster correction of INR and reduced blood product requirements. In both studies, the overall costs of transfusion were lower with PCC.

Cardiac Surgery

Patients undergoing complex cardiac surgery are at risk of major blood loss. Key contributors to this include platelet dysfunction, hemodilution, fibrinolytic activation and anticoagulant medication. The use of cardiopulmonary bypass (CPB) has a major impact on coagulation status.

As in trauma, some research groups have attempted to reduce patient exposure to allogeneic blood products by using coagulation factor concentrates. In one coagulation management algorithm, PCC (20–40 IU/kg) was administered to patients with ongoing bleeding after supplementation of fibrinogen and platelets, and EXTEM CT > 90 s [26]. Görlinger et al. reported that implementation of this algorithm led to a significant reduction in the use of allogeneic blood products, and a decrease in the incidence of thromboembolic events [26]. Similar criteria for PCC therapy were applied in a transfusion algorithm used in a multicenter Canadian study: a dose of 20 IU/kg was given to patients with EXTEM CT > 90 s, following treatment as needed with platelets and fibrinogen [27]. This approach produced significant reductions in transfusion of RBCs and platelets, and a reduced risk of major bleeding [27]. In another study, algorithm-driven administration of hemostatic therapy including PCC was guided by either point-of-care thromboelastometry or by conventional laboratory tests [28]. The use of thromboelastometry was associated with reduced transfusion of allogeneic blood products, a lower rate of adverse events and reduced 6-month mortality.

In the study by Görlinger et al., 8.9% of patients received PCC after implementation of the algorithm compared with 4.4% before [26], whereas Weber et al. reported that 44% of patients receiving treatment guided by thromboelastometry received PCC perioperatively versus 52% when treatment was guided by laboratory testing [28]. In the Canadian study, the algorithm's effect on PCC use was not reported [27].

The impact of PCC monotherapy in cardiovascular surgery has also been reported. Three different treatments (PCC, FFP, and PCC plus FFP) were compared in a retrospective analysis of patients undergoing a variety of cardiac procedures [29]. Mean blood loss during the first hour was lowest in the PCC group, with blood loss of 224, 369 and 434 ml in the three treatment groups, respectively. In another study, PCC was used instead of FFP as first-line treatment of bleeding [30]. Mean 24-hour blood loss was significantly lower with PCC versus FFP, and the likelihood of RBC transfusion was reduced (odds ratio 0.50). PCC has also been investigated for use as rescue therapy for patients with ongoing bleeding after treatment with platelets, FFP and cryoprecipitate [31]. In response to PCC treatment, patients' INR values were significantly reduced as were requirements for transfusion of FFP and platelets.

Liver Disease

Patients with chronic liver disease have reduced levels of most coagulation factors as a result of reduced synthesis. Consequently, coagulation tests such as INR typically suggest hypocoagulability, but such tests do not provide insight into the overall clotting process. Levels of anticoagulants such as antithrombin and protein C are also reduced so that the overall coagulation status is balanced. Nevertheless, patients with liver disease remain at risk of coagulopathic bleeding, for example during surgical procedures.

There have been several reports of PCC being used to treat patients with liver disease. In 2003, Lorenz et al. reported a cohort study of 22 patients requiring correction of hemostatic defects, in which clinical efficacy was rated as "very good" in 76% of cases [32]. More recently, the efficacy of PCC was compared in patients with versus without liver disease [33]. Hemostasis was achieved in a smaller percentage of patients with liver disease, and thromboembolic events were observed in one patient (3.2%) with and eight patients (14.8%) without liver disease (this difference was not statistically significant). In a third study, PCC was evaluated for prevention or control of bleeding in patients with liver coagulopathy [34]. Median INR decreased significantly from 1.6 to 1.3 and no new bleeding events were observed post-PCC.

Other Patient Populations

Several retrospective studies have presented experience of PCC therapy in mixed populations of patients. The first such study included 24 patients undergoing surgical procedures or requiring warfarin reversal [35]. Administration of allogeneic blood products was lower after than before PCC treatment, and partial or complete hemostasis was achieved in 78% of the patients. A second study included 50 general surgery, vascular surgery, trauma and conservative therapy patients, 12 of whom required VKA reversal [36]. Among the bleeding patients, PCC therapy reduced mean INR from 1.7 to 1.4; surgical bleeding was stopped in 36% of cases and diffuse bleeding was stopped in 96% of cases. Patients with liver dysfunction and acute sepsis were included in a third study [37]. Reductions in INR were observed in both of these groups, reaching statistical significance in the sepsis patients but not the liver disease patients.

Risks of PCC

Historically, there have been safety concerns with PCCs, principally in relation to activated coagulation factors within PCCs and a resultant risk of thromboembolic complications [38]. PCCs increase endogenous thrombin potential, which is lacking in patients with deficiency of factors II, VII, IX and X. Most of today's PCCs do not contain activated factors but there is a risk of increasing thrombin potential above the physiologically normal range, raising the possibility of hypercoagulability. The ratio of procoagulants to anticoagulants has been identified as a consideration in this context [38]. Patients requiring VKA reversal have normal levels of antithrombin, meaning that PCC therapy will not necessarily cause an imbalance between pro- and anticoagulants [39]. The situation is different in other indications (e.g., trauma-related bleeding) because levels of anticoagulants, such as antithrombin, as well as coagulation factors are liable to be depleted, in which case PCC therapy is likely to increase thrombin generation to supratherapeutic levels.

The available safety data indicate a low risk of adverse events when using PCCs for VKA reversal. The phase III trials mentioned earlier showed that the incidence of thromboembolic adverse events was no higher with PCC than with therapeutic plasma [3, 4]. Overall adverse event rates were also similar with either PCC or plasma. In the retrospective comparison of PCC with frozen plasma, serious adverse events occurred in a smaller percentage of patients treated with PCC [5]. The EPAHK study reported death related to thromboembolic events in a small percentage of patients (0.6%). Pharmacovigilance data on a four-factor PCC, gathered over a 15-year period during which the principal application was VKA reversal, indicated one thromboembolic event per 31,000 PCC infusions [40]. No cases of virus transmission were attributed to PCC therapy.

In trauma-related bleeding, coagulation inhibitors as well as coagulation factors are likely to be depleted, contributing to concerns regarding the possibility of thromboembolic complications with PCC use. In a porcine model of trauma, thromboembolism was evident in 100% of animals treated with PCC (50 IU/kg), and there were signs of disseminated intravascular coagulation (DIC) in 44% [41]. These data suggest a need for caution with PCCs in trauma, although the applicability of animal data to human patients may be questioned. Schöchl et al. conducted an observational, descriptive study to assess the impact of PCC administration on coagulation status in patients with trauma-induced coagulopathy, comparing patients who received no coagulation therapy, patients who received fibrinogen concentrate only, and patients who received fibrinogen concentrate and PCC [42]. The results demonstrated that patients receiving PCC had low antithrombin concentrations and increased endogenous thrombin potential for several days following treatment, implying a potential prothrombotic state. As such, a cautious approach to the use of PCC in trauma appears to be warranted.

Three of the comparative studies in cardiac surgery described earlier suggested that treatment with PCC did not affect rates of complications including thromboembolic events [27, 29, 30]. Indeed, the study by Görlinger et al. showed a significantly lower incidence of thromboembolic events after implementation of the algorithm [26]. However, it should be noted that the Italian study of PCC as a replacement for FFP reported that PCC increased the risk of postoperative acute kidney injury [30].

PCC Monitoring

No assay for measuring thrombin generation is currently available for routine clinical use, meaning that surrogate markers must be used to guide PCC therapy. Considering the potential risks associated with PCCs, assessment of coagulation status is important for guiding the dose and determining the effectiveness of PCC intervention.

In patients receiving VKA treatment, INR is the usual method for measuring coagulation status. This parameter can also be used to measure the effects of PCC therapy for VKA reversal. Although INR does not provide insight into the whole clotting process, it does appear satisfactory for guiding PCC therapy.

A number of coagulation assays have been explored, including viscoelastic co-agulation tests, thrombin time or activated partial thromboplastin time (aPTT), to monitor the anticoagulant effect of DOACs and their reversal [9]. None of these tests was specifically designed for DOAC-related assessments.

In patients with bleeding related to trauma or cardiovascular surgery, EXTEM clotting time has been recommended as a surrogate marker for thrombin generation in several treatment algorithms for guiding PCC therapy [20, 26, 27]. Viscoelastic coagulation monitoring can be performed at the point of care with short turnaround times. INR, which can also be performed at the point of care, has also been used in these settings to determine the need for PCC therapy. However, it is not validated for this purpose and provides limited specificity; the scope for determining the cause of prolonged clotting times is lower with INR than with viscoelastic testing.

Conclusion

PCC is a well-established and safe treatment for emergency VKA reversal, with strong evidence supporting its use. Another promising area for PCC use would be the treatment of severe bleeding in patients receiving anticoagulant therapy with DOACs. Additionally, PCC is a valuable option to increase thrombin generation when treating severe trauma-related bleeding or in other clinical areas of high-risk hemorrhage (e.g., cardiac surgery) with impaired thrombin generation.

However, in the absence of clinically available thrombin generation measurement, there is a need for improved point-of-care tests to diagnose the need for PCC and monitor the effects of treatment. A cautious approach to PCC dosing is warranted because of the potential for excessively increased thrombin generation. Well-designed, randomized controlled trials are needed to enable recommendations with a robust evidence base.

References

1. Grottke O, Rossaint R, Henskens Y, van Oerle R, Ten Cate H, Spronk HM (2013) Thrombin generation capacity of prothrombin complex concentrate in an in vitro dilutional model. PLoS One 8:e64100
2. Electronic Medicines Compendium (2017) Beriplex P/N 500 summary of product characteristics. https://www.medicines.org.uk/emc/medicine/20797. Accessed 10 January 2018
3. Sarode R, Milling TJ Jr, Refaai MA et al (2013) Efficacy and safety of a 4-factor prothrombin complex concentrate in patients on vitamin K antagonists presenting with major bleeding: a randomized, plasma-controlled, phase IIIb study. Circulation 128:1234–1243
4. Goldstein JN, Refaai MA, Milling TJ Jr et al (2015) Four-factor prothrombin complex concentrate versus plasma for rapid vitamin K antagonist reversal in patients needing urgent surgical or invasive interventions: a phase 3b, open-label, non-inferiority, randomised trial. Lancet 385:2077–2087
5. Hickey M, Gatien M, Taljaard M, Aujnarain A, Giulivi A, Perry JJ (2013) Outcomes of urgent warfarin reversal with frozen plasma versus prothrombin complex concentrate in the emergency department. Circulation 128:360–364

6. Tazarourte K, Riou B, Tremey B, Samama CM, Vicaut E, Vigue B (2014) Guideline-concordant administration of prothrombin complex concentrate and vitamin K is associated with decreased mortality in patients with severe bleeding under vitamin K antagonist treatment (EPAHK study). Crit Care 18:R81

7. Kozek-Langenecker SA, Ahmed AB, Afshari A et al (2017) Management of severe perioperative bleeding: guidelines from the European Society of Anaesthesiology: first update 2016. Eur J Anaesthesiol 34:332–395

8. Rossaint R, Bouillon B, Cerny V et al (2016) The European guideline on management of major bleeding and coagulopathy following trauma: fourth edition. Crit Care 20:1–55

9. Grottke O, Aisenberg J, Bernstein RV et al (2016) Efficacy of prothrombin complex concentrates for the emergency reversal of dabigatran-induced anticoagulation. Crit Care 20:115

10. Pollack CV Jr, Reilly PA, van Ryn J et al (2017) Idarucizumab for dabigatran reversal – full cohort analysis. N Engl J Med 377:431–441

11. Connolly SJ, Milling TJ Jr, Eikelboom JW et al (2016) Andexanet alfa for acute major bleeding associated with Factor Xa inhibitors. N Engl J Med 375:1131–1141

12. Honickel M, Braunschweig T, van Ryn J et al (2015) Prothrombin complex concentrate is effective in treating the anticoagulant effects of dabigatran in a porcine polytrauma model. Anesthesiology 123:1350–1361

13. Herzog E, Kaspereit F, Krege W et al (2015) Effective reversal of edoxaban-associated bleeding with four-factor prothrombin complex concentrate in a rabbit model of acute hemorrhage. Anesthesiology 122:387–398

14. Herzog E, Kaspereit F, Krege W et al (2015) Four-factor prothrombin complex concentrate reverses apixaban-associated bleeding in a rabbit model of acute hemorrhage. J Thromb Haemost 13:2220–2226

15. Brown KS, Wickremasingha P, Parasrampuria DA et al (2015) The impact of a three-factor prothrombin complex concentrate on the anticoagulatory effects of the factor Xa inhibitor edoxaban. Thromb Res 136:825–831

16. Zahir H, Brown KS, Vandell AG et al (2015) Edoxaban effects on bleeding following punch biopsy and reversal by a 4-factor prothrombin complex concentrate. Circulation 131:82–90

17. Nagalla S, Thomson L, Oppong Y, Bachman B, Chervoneva I, Kraft WK (2016) Reversibility of apixaban anticoagulation with a four-factor prothrombin complex concentrate in healthy volunteers. Clin Transl Sci 9:176–180

18. Majeed A, Agren A, Holmstrom M et al (2017) Management of rivaroxaban or apixaban associated major bleeding with prothrombin complex concentrates: a cohort study. Blood 130:1706–1712

19. Hiippala ST, Myllyla GJ, Vahtera EM (1995) Hemostatic factors and replacement of major blood loss with plasma-poor red cell concentrates. Anesth Analg 81:360–365

20. Schöchl H, Voelckel W, Grassetto A, Schlimp CJ (2013) Practical application of point-of-care coagulation testing to guide treatment decisions in trauma. J Trauma Acute Care Surg 74:1587–1598

21. Schöchl H, Nienaber U, Maegele M et al (2011) Transfusion in trauma: thromboelastometry-guided coagulation factor concentrate-based therapy versus standard fresh frozen plasma-based therapy. Crit Care 15:R83

22. Innerhofer P, Westermann I, Tauber H et al (2013) The exclusive use of coagulation factor concentrates enables reversal of coagulopathy and decreases transfusion rates in patients with major blunt trauma. Injury 44:209–216

23. Innerhofer P, Fries D, Mittermayr M et al (2017) Reversal of trauma-induced coagulopathy using first-line coagulation factor concentrates or fresh frozen plasma (RETIC): a single-centre, parallel-group, open-label, randomised trial. Lancet Haematol 4:e258–e271

24. Joseph B, Aziz H, Pandit V et al (2014) Prothrombin complex concentrate versus fresh-frozen plasma for reversal of coagulopathy of trauma: is there a difference? World J Surg 38:1875–1881

25. Joseph B, Khalil M, Harrison C et al (2016) Assessing the efficacy of prothrombin complex concentrate in multiply injured patients with high-energy pelvic and extremity fractures. J Orthop Trauma 30:653–658

26. Görlinger K, Dirkmann D, Hanke AA et al (2011) First-line therapy with coagulation factor concentrates combined with point-of-care coagulation testing is associated with decreased allogeneic blood transfusion in cardiovascular surgery: a retrospective, single-center cohort study. Anesthesiology 115:1179–1191

27. Karkouti K, Callum J, Wijeysundera DN et al (2016) Point-of-care hemostatic testing in cardiac surgery: a stepped-wedge clustered randomized controlled trial. Circulation 134:1152–1162

28. Weber CF, Gorlinger K, Meininger D et al (2012) Point-of-care testing: a prospective, randomized clinical trial of efficacy in coagulopathic cardiac surgery patients. Anesthesiology 117:531–547

29. Arnekian V, Camous J, Fattal S, Rezaiguia-Delclaux S, Nottin R, Stephan F (2012) Use of prothrombin complex concentrate for excessive bleeding after cardiac surgery. Interact Cardiovasc Thorac Surg 15:382–389

30. Cappabianca G, Mariscalco G, Biancari F et al (2016) Safety and efficacy of prothrombin complex concentrate as first-line treatment in bleeding after cardiac surgery. Crit Care 20:5

31. Song HK, Tibayan FA, Kahl EA et al (2014) Safety and efficacy of prothrombin complex concentrates for the treatment of coagulopathy after cardiac surgery. J Thorac Cardiovasc Surg 147:1036–1040

32. Lorenz R, Kienast J, Otto U et al (2003) Efficacy and safety of a prothrombin complex concentrate with two virus-inactivation steps in patients with severe liver damage. Eur J Gastroenterol Hepatol 15:15–20

33. Huang WT, Cang WC, Derry KL, Lane JR, von Drygalski A (2016) Four-factor prothrombin complex concentrate for coagulopathy reversal in patients with liver disease. Clin Appl Thromb Hemost 23:1028–1035

34. Lesmana CR, Cahyadinata L, Pakasi LS, Lesmana LA (2016) Efficacy of prothrombin complex concentrate treatment in patients with liver coagulopathy who underwent various invasive hepatobiliary and gastrointestinal procedures. Case Rep Gastroenterol 10:315–322

35. Bruce D, Nokes TJ (2008) Prothrombin complex concentrate (Beriplex P/N) in severe bleeding: Experience in a large tertiary hospital. Crit Care 12:R105

36. Schick KS, Fertmann JM, Jauch KW, Hoffmann JN (2009) Prothrombin complex concentrate in surgical patients: retrospective evaluation of vitamin K antagonist reversal and treatment of severe bleeding. Crit Care 13:R191

37. Young H, Holzmacher JL, Amdur R, Gondek S, Sarani B, Schroeder ME (2017) Use of four-factor prothrombin complex concentrate in the reversal of warfarin-induced and nonvitamin K antagonist-related coagulopathy. Blood Coagul Fibrinolysis 28:564–569

38. Dusel CH, Grundmann C, Eich S, Seitz R, Konig H (2004) Identification of prothrombin as a major thrombogenic agent in prothrombin complex concentrates. Blood Coagul Fibrinolysis 15:405–411

39. Schöchl H, Grottke O, Sutor K et al (2017) Theoretical modelling of coagulation management with therapeutic plasma or prothrombin complex concentrate. Anesth Analg 125:1471–1474

40. Hanke AA, Joch C, Görlinger K (2013) Long-term safety and efficacy of a pasteurized nanofiltrated prothrombin complex concentrate (Beriplex P/N): a pharmacovigilance study. Br J Anaesth 110:764–772

41. Grottke O, Braunschweig T, Spronk HM et al (2011) Increasing concentrations of prothrombin complex concentrate induce disseminated intravascular coagulation in a pig model of coagulopathy with blunt liver injury. Blood 118:1943–1951

42. Schöchl H, Voelckel W, Maegele M, Kirchmair L, Schlimp CJ (2014) Endogenous thrombin potential following hemostatic therapy with 4-factor prothrombin complex concentrate: a 7-day observational study of trauma patients. Crit Care 18:R147

43. Grottke O, Levy JH (2015) Prothrombin complex concentrates in trauma and perioperative bleeding. Anesthesiology 122:923–931

Advances in Mechanisms, Diagnosis and Treatment of Coagulopathy and Progression of Hemorrhage After Traumatic Brain Injury

M. Maegele

Introduction

Traumatic brain injury (TBI) will surpass many disorders as a principle cause of death and disability by the year 2020 [1]. With approximately 10 million people sustaining a TBI each year, the burden of mortality and morbidity that this entity imposes makes it one of the most challenging health and socioeconomic problems of our times. Recent years have seen changes in the epidemiological pattern of TBI with a shift towards older ages. In these older age groups, falls represent a common cause of TBI, inflicting a higher number of contusional injuries [2]. Although at the moment of impact, disruption of cerebral blood vessels, mainly in the microvasculature, or blood-brain barrier breakdown is common and results in hemorrhagic lesions, TBI-associated factors may then alter the intricate balance between bleeding and thrombosis formation in the later sequelae leading to impaired hemostasis, in the following referred to as coagulopathy, with exacerbation of the initial injury [3, 4].

Prevalence, Definitions and Patterns of Coagulopathy After TBI

The published findings on the reported prevalence of coagulopathy associated with TBI are inevitably dependent on the techniques and definitions used to document coagulopathy [3–5] (Table 1). Most commonly, coagulopathy is defined by abnormalities in conventional coagulation assays, typically the prothrombin time (PT), sometimes reported as a ratio (PT_R). Although this assay is often considered in-

M. Maegele (✉)
Department for Trauma and Orthopaedic Surgery, Cologne-Merheim Medical Center (CMMC), University Witten/Herdecke, Campus Cologne-Merheim
Cologne, Germany
Institute for Research in Operative Medicine (IFOM), University Witten/Herdecke, Campus Cologne-Merheim
Cologne, Germany
e-mail: Marc.Maegele@t-online.de

© Springer International Publishing AG 2018   451
J.-L. Vincent (ed.), *Annual Update in Intensive Care and Emergency Medicine 2018*,
Annual Update in Intensive Care and Emergency Medicine,
https://doi.org/10.1007/978-3-319-73670-9_35

terchangeably with the International Normalized Ratio (INR), strictly the INR is optimized for monitoring anticoagulation therapy. Approximately one out of three patients with TBI displays variable signs of laboratory coagulopathy, based upon conventional coagulation assays on admission, and abnormalities of these tests are almost inevitably associated with increased morbidity and mortality [6, 7] (Table 1). Coagulopathy occurs in over 60% of patients with severe TBI [6], but appears uncommon in mild head injury (< 1%; [8]).

Table 1 Prevalence of coagulopathy after isolated traumatic brain injury (TBI) and outcome. Modified from [4] with permission

First author (year) [ref]	No of patients	Definition of TBI	Definition of coagulopathy	Prevalence of coagulopathy (%)	Mortality with coagulopathy (%)
Meta-analysis					
Harhangi (2008) [6]*	5357	heterogeneous	heterogeneous	32.7 (10–97.5)	51 (25–93)
Epstein (2014) [7]**	7037	heterogeneous	heterogeneous	35.2 (7–86.1)	17–86
Individual studies					
Zehtabchi (2008) [51]	224	AIS$_{head}$ > 2 and/or any intracranial hematoma on CT	INR > 1.3 or aPTT > 34 s	17 (8–30)	–
Talving (2009) [52]	387	AIS$_{head}$ ≥ 3 and extracranial AIS < 3	Platelets < 100,000 mm^3 or INR > 1.1 or aPTT > 36 s	34	34.7
Lustenberger (2010) [16]	278	AIS$_{head}$ ≥ 3 and extracranial AIS < 3	Platelets < 100,000 mm^3 and/or INR > 1.4 and/or aPTT > 36 s	45.7	40.9
Lustenberger (2010) [25]	132	AIS$_{head}$ ≥ 3 and extracranial AIS < 3	Platelets < 100,000 mm^3 or INR > 1.2 or aPTT > 36 s	36.4	32.5
Wafaisade (2010) [53]	3114	AIS$_{head}$ ≥ 3 and extracranial AIS < 3	Quick (PT$_R$) < 70% and/or platelets < 100,000/ml	22.7	50.4
Chhabra (2010) [54]	100	GCS < 13	Fibrinogen < 200 mg/dl	7	–
Greuters (2011) [14]	107	Brain tissue injury on CT and extracranial AIS < 3	aPTT > 40 s and/or INR > 1.2 and/or platelets < 120 × 10^9/l	24 (54#)	41

Table 1 (Continued)

First author (year) [ref]	No of patients	Definition of TBI	Definition of coagulopathy	Prevalence of coagulopathy (%)	Mortality with coagulopathy (%)
Shehata (2011) [55]	101	Isolated TBI on admission brain CT	INR $\geq$ 1.2, PT > 13 s, D-dimer positive, platelets < 100×10^3/ml	63	36
Schöchl (2011) [32]	88	$AIS_{head} \geq 3$ and extracranial AIS < 3	Quick (PT_R) < 70% and/or aPTT > 35 s and/or fibrinogen < 150 mg/dl and/or platelets < 100×10^9/l	15.8	50
Franschman (2012) [56]	226	Isolated TBI on CT and extracranial AIS < 3	aPTT > 40 s and/or PT > 1.2 and/or platelets < 120×10^9/l	25 (44[#])	33
Genet (2013) [57]	23	$AIS_{head} \geq 3$ and extracranial AIS < 3	aPTT > 35 s and/or INR > 1.2	13	22
Alexiou (2014) [58]	149	Isolated TBI with exclusion of multi-system trauma	aPTT > 40 s and/or INR > 1.2 and/or platelets < 120×10^9/l	14.8 (22.8[#])	–
Joseph (2014) [5]	591	$AIS_{head} \geq 3$ and extracranial AIS < 3	INR $\geq$ 1.5 and/or PTT $\geq$ 35 s and/or platelets $\leq 100 \times 10^3$/ml	13.3	23
Epstein (2014) [59]	1718	$AIS_{head} \geq 3$ and extracranial AIS < 3	INR $\geq$ 1.3	7.7	45.1
De Oliveira Manoel (2015) [60]	48	$AIS_{head} \geq 3$ and extracranial AIS < 3	INR $\geq$ 1.5 and/or aPTT $\geq$ 60 s and/or platelets < 100×10^3/mm^{3§}	12.5	66
Dekker (2016) [26]	52	$AIS_{head} \geq 3$	INR > 1.2 and/or aPTT > 40 s and/or platelets < 120×10^9/l	42	45.5

AIS: abbreviated injury scale; *aPTT*: activate partial thromboplastin time; *INR*: International Normalized Ratio; *CT*: computed tomography; *PT*: prothrombin time; *PTR*: Prothrombin ratio/Quick *meta-analysis (1966–2007) with n = 34 studies included; **meta-analysis (1990–2013) with n = 22 studies included; #after 24 hours; §additional abnormal coagulation tests: fibrinogen 1.0 g/L, any clotting factor < 0.5 (<50% activity) and abnormal viscoelastic test results

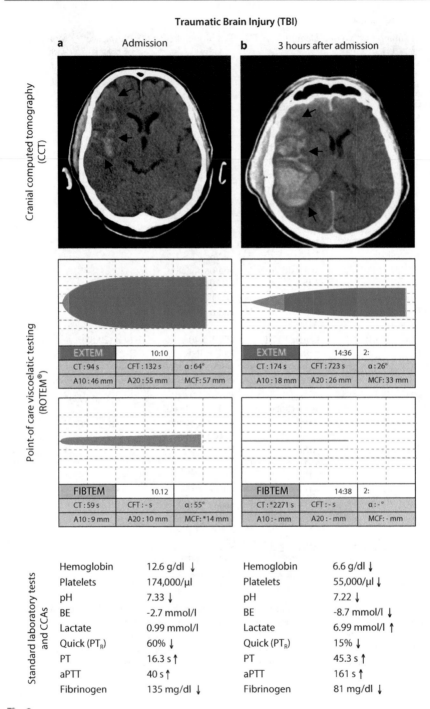

Traumatic Brain Injury (TBI)

Fig. 1

Cranial computed tomography (CCT)

c   **Normal condition**

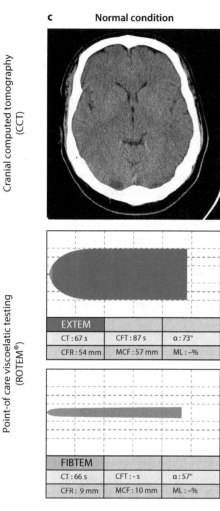

Point-of care viscoelastic testing (ROTEM®)

EXTEM		
CT : 67 s	CFT : 87 s	α : 73°
CFR : 54 mm	MCF : 57 mm	ML : –%

FIBTEM		
CT : 66 s	CFT : – s	α : 57°
CFR : 9 mm	MCF : 10 mm	ML : –%

Standard laboratory tests and CCAs

Hemoglobin	13.3-16.2 g/dl
Platelets	140-360,000/µl
pH	7.37-7.45
BE	-2-3 mmol/l
Lactate	0.5-1.8 mmol/l
Quick (PT$_R$)	70-120%
PT	<12 s
aPTT	26-37 s
Fibrinogen	150-400 mg/dl

Fig. 1 Clinical example of a patient with severe traumatic brain injury (TBI) and initial coagulopathy who developed subsequent hypotensive (multifactorial) coagulopathy with deteriorating intracranial hemorrhage within three hours of hospital admission. Shown are cranial computed tomographies of the brain (CCTs) as well as results from viscoelastic (ROTEM®) and standard laboratory tests and conventional coagulation assays (CCAs) on admission (**a**) and after 3 h of admission (**b**). A reference normal condition (**c**) is displayed for comparison. Viscoelastic assays after 3 h of admission indicate delayed and insufficient clotting as reflected by prolonged initiation times as well as reduced clot amplitudes. The flat line in the FIBTEM channel reflects complete absence of fibrin polymerization. Results from standard laboratory assays and conventional coagulation assays at three hours after admission display signs of shock with deranged coagulation along with hypofibrinogenemia and thrombocytopenia. *aPTT*: activated partial thromboplastin time; *BE*: base excess; *PT*: prothrombin time; PT^R: prothrombin ratio. Modified from [4] with permission

Preinjury Pharmacotherapies

Historically, TBI was predominately seen as a disease of the young. Today, the incidence in the elderly population is increasing worldwide and approximately half, or even more, of the patients are over 50 years old at the time of their injury [2]. Thus, the current demographic change is accompanied by an increased incidence of comorbidities among TBI patients [2] and modern treatment of chronic cerebrovascular/coronary artery disease implies that these patients are often on anticoagulants or antiplatelet drugs, both of which have been explored as causes of increased bleeding and worse outcome after TBI [9]. A meta-analysis estimated a two-fold increase in risk of poor outcome in patients who were on warfarin at the time of TBI [10]; other studies have suggested that preinjury antiplatelet therapy may result in a two-fold increase in traumatic intracranial hemorrhage (ICH) even after mild TBI [11]. Clopidogrel and warfarin medication at the time of TBI are independent predictors of immediate traumatic ICH, disease progression and worse outcome [5]. The newer target specific direct oral anticoagulants (DOACs) confer as yet poorly quantified risks to patients with TBI [12]. Although the risk of spontaneous non-traumatic ICH is lower with these agents, their impact on incidental TBI is poorly quantified, and until recently there were no options available for rapid reversal in the event of bleeding [13].

The Pattern of Coagulopathy After TBI

The number of TBI patients with coagulopathy doubles within 24 h after injury [14] and a similar number display hemorrhagic progression of initial brain contusions or ICH, including coagulopathy, within 6 to 48 h ([15]; Fig. 1). The interval to the onset of coagulopathy is inversely related to injury severity, and alterations in the coagulation system may persist at least until the third day postinjury or longer [16]. Hemorrhagic progression of brain contusions may involve not only the expansion of existing contusions, but also the delayed appearance of non-contiguous hemorrhagic lesions [17].

Coagulopathy as a Prognostic Indicator

Coagulopathy at presentation has been identified a powerful predictor for outcome and overall prognosis in TBI [6, 7] resulting in a nine-fold risk increase in mortality and a 30-fold risk increase of unfavorable outcome [6]. Coagulopathy has been significantly associated with progressive hemorrhagic injury and ICH [15, 18, 19], the latter representing one of the greatest causes of mortality associated with TBI. In elderly patients with coagulopathy and intraparenchymal contusions on admission, progressive hemorrhagic injury was more likely [19]. Signs of clot lysis and systemic presence of fibrinolytic fragments were associated with progressive hemorrhagic injury, outcome and neurosurgical procedures. In addition, patients with abnormal clot formation dynamics had approximately five times the odds of dying from ICH progression than those with normal clot dynamics [15]. Platelet dysfunction and/or decreased platelet numbers further contribute to bleeding complications [3, 5, 20], with platelet counts < 175,000/µl increasing the risk of ICH progression, and counts < 100,000/µl associated with a nine-fold adjusted increased risk of death [5].

Potential Mechanisms Leading to Coagulopathy and Hemorrhagic Progression After TBI

It is often considered that coagulopathy develops as procoagulant tissue factors are released from the damaged brain and coagulation factors are then consecutively consumed leading to ICH expansion, but this is likely to be an oversimplification of a much more complex series of events occurring either simultaneously or sequentially after TBI (Fig. 2). The vast majority of the data supporting the current concept for the development of coagulopathy and hemorrhagic progression after TBI, however, continues to be rather correlative with causative data and links are still lacking. Ongoing inconsistencies in the reported data are primarily due to lack of consensus regarding the mechanism of coagulopathy in isolated TBI as well as to absence of definitions ([18]; Table 1). Coagulopathy itself does not result in hemorrhage within the brain in the absence of (micro)vascular injury or failure including blood-brain barrier breakdown. The incidence of coagulopathy after TBI increases with injury severity and is seen more frequently in penetrating than in blunt trauma [16].

Progressive Microvascular Failure and Hemorrhagic Progression

When kinetic energy is focally delivered to the brain, it typically follows a three-dimensional Gaussian-like distribution pattern with the epicenter of the impact receiving the peak energy and the penumbra and other surrounding regions receiving progressively less energy with distance [17]. In a typical contusion, sufficient energy is deposited in or near the epicenter to induce shear stress and rupture of microvessels, which results in an immediate hemorrhagic contusion. In the penumbra, however, the deposited energy is not strong enough to parallel these events, but may activate mechanosensitive molecular processes, mostly in microvessels, thereby triggering cascades that later will result in the delayed structural failure of microvessels, or better termed hemorrhagic progressive contusions [21]. These processes may also occur in more remote areas of the brain where hemorrhagic contusions are not initially apparent but visible on repeated CT scans. Transcriptional events usually require hours to display their effects and this may be a rational molecular explanation for the interval between the initial impact and the occurrence of delayed hemorrhage.

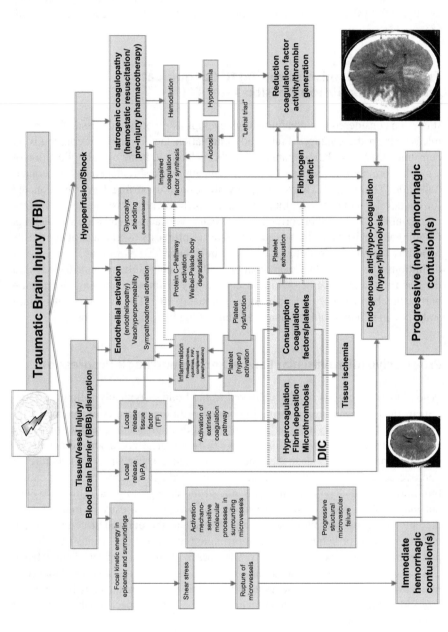
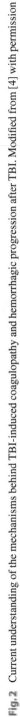

Fig. 2 Current understanding of the mechanisms behind TBI-induced coagulopathy and hemorrhagic progression after TBI. Modified from [4] with permission

Sympathetic Nervous System Activation

Traumatic brain injury induces strong sympathetic nervous system activation with profuse secretion of catecholamines resulting in a hyperadrenergic state that is linked to immunomodulation both locally and systemically [22]. Biomarker profiles in TBI patients with poor outcome display procoagulation, glycocalyx and endothelial damage, vascular activation, inflammation and hyperfibrinolysis with catecholamine levels correlating with endotheliopathy and coagulopathy markers within the first 24 h after TBI [22].

Significant differences in a number of markers have been observed between moderate and severe isolated TBI cohorts providing evidence that exaggerated sympathetic nervous system activation during the acute phase contributes substantially to harmful inflammatory dysregulation. Extensive cross-talk between coagulation and inflammation has been reported, whereby activation of one system may amplify activation of the other, a situation that if unopposed may result in further tissue damage and systemically in multiorgan failure [23].

The Tissue Factor Hypothesis

Direct vessel injury or defragmentation from microvascular failure may lead to blood-brain barrier disruption with the release/activation of tissue factor (TF), which triggers the extrinsic coagulation pathway with consumption of coagulation factors and platelets and disseminated intravascular coagulation (DIC) with further bleeding [5, 17]. Blood-born soluble TF and TF integrated into the surface of activated platelets as well as through microparticles may augment the ongoing amplification of coagulation. The pattern of circulating microparticles is altered after TBI and both platelet-derived and endothelial-derived microparticles exposing TF are generated in the injured brain, whereas leukocyte-derived microparticles exposing TF are accumulated [24]. These microparticles could deliver additional TF to activated platelets thus enhancing coagulation. Platelet-derived microparticles are also enriched in phosphatidylserine, which facilitates the binding of coagulation factors to membranes enabling the formation of procoagulant complexes. Both fibrinogen concentration and platelet counts decrease early after TBI with bleeding reflecting systemic consumption and may underlie a bleeding diasthesis.

Hypoperfusion, Protein C Homeostasis and Hyperfibrinolysis

In TBI, ischemia and hypoperfusion contribute to overall injury and coagulopathy via immediate vasoconstriction/vasospasm, endothelial swelling and systemic hypotension as well as microvascular occlusion by platelet/leucocyte activation, adhesion and aggregation [25]. TBI-related coagulopathy is more profound in patients with acidosis and raised lactate levels with an inverse relationship between hypoperfusion and fibrinolysis [26]. Combined TBI and shock may result in an immediate activation of coagulation and complement systems with subsequent endothelial shedding, protein C pathway activation promoting hyperfibrinolysis and the inhibition of coagulation factors FVa and FVIIIa and inflammation [3]. *Vice versa,* the post-traumatic inflammatory response may result in chronic protein C depletion-mediated enhanced susceptibility to infection and thromboembolism [3]. TBI also initiates fibrinolysis by locally releasing tissue-type (tPA) and urokinase-type (uPA) plasminogen activator from contusional brain tissue [27]. While some authors have suggested an overactivation via TF to drive (hyper)fibrinolysis after TBI, others have proposed alternative mechanisms, such as increased levels of tPA or activated protein C (aPC) and depletion of alpha-2-plasmin inhibitor with an increase in plasmin [3]. Plasmin is the main effector of fibrinolysis, the cleavage product of circulating plasminogen. Both tPA and uPA levels transiently increase in the lesioned brain but with different temporal profiles [27]. The lysine analogue, tranexamic acid (TXA), blocks tPA-mediated fibrinolysis and ICH, but may potentiate uPA-mediated plasminogen activation thereby promoting ICH. The selective uPA increase at later stages may potentially explain why TXA displayed a net benefit when administered within three hours after injury but resulted in more deaths due to bleeding when administered after three hours [28].

Platelet Dysfunction and Platelet-endothelial Interactions

Low platelet counts and platelet dysfunction are central to the early coagulopathy after TBI and disease progression [20, 29]. Even with normal counts there may be clinically significant platelet dysfunction [29]. Platelet dysfunction occurs when platelets do not respond to agonists and a reduced ability of adenosine diphosphate (ADP) to activate platelets is correlated with injury severity and mortality. *Vice versa,* the coincidence of low platelet counts and spontaneous platelet aggregation in the absence of bleeding suggests platelet hyperactivity in TBI. Experimental intravascular microthrombosis resulting in a profound reduction in pericontusional blood flow supports this assumption. Brain-derived platelet-activating factor (PAF) contributes to the hypoxia-induced blood-brain barrier breakdown, which may promote the release of additional PAF and other brain-derived procoagulative molecules. The role of principle platelet ligands, e.g., von Willebrand factor (vWF), which facilitates the capture of platelets to perturbed endothelium or exposed subendothelial matrix at sites of injury resulting in local *in situ* thrombosis and thromboembolism in the downstream microvasculature remains unknown.

Novel Diagnostic Approaches for Coagulopathy

Conventional coagulation assays provide only limited information on platelet count or function, or fibrinogen concentration levels. Furthermore, conventional coagulation assays monitor the initiation of blood coagulation, and characterize only the first 4% of thrombin generation in secondary hemostasis [30]. PT, activated partial thromboplastin time (aPTT) and the INR can measure derangements in individual pathways but do not assess combinations of multiple complex pathways and have not yet been validated for critically ill patients. Standard coagulation screens may appear normal although the overall state of blood hemostasis is abnormal [31]. A meta-analysis reported inconsistent data, in particular for aPTT and PT, in

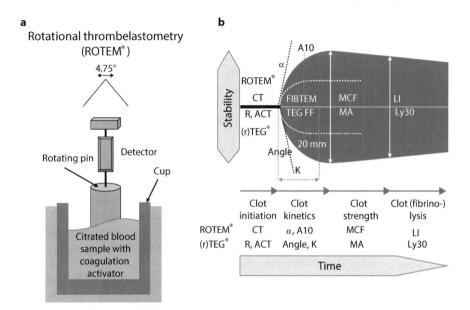

Fig. 3 Viscoelastic test principle as exemplified for rotational thromboelastometry ROTEM® (panel **a**) and overview of test results reflecting the different steps of hemostasis (panel **b**). To perform a viscoelastic test (ROTEM®) a whole citrated blood sample is incubated in a heated cup with a suspended pin connected to a detector. The cup and the pin are rotated relative to each other. The movement is initiated either from the pin (ROTEM®) or the cup (TEG®). A coagulation activator is added and as fibrin strands form between cup and pin, the impedance of the pin rotation (ROTEM®) or the transmitted rotation from the cup to the pin (TEG®) are detected and converted into a trace signal. The trace signal may be subdivided into sections that reflect the different steps of hemostasis such as clot initiation, clot kinetics, clot strength and clot lysis (fibrinolysis). The nomenclature between ROTEM® and TEG® differs slightly and results are not strictly interchangeable due to discrete technical differences and differences in the use of reagents. Panel **b** shows parameters for ROTEM® and TEG® during the different steps of hemostasis. ROTEM®: α: alpha angle reflecting the speed of clot formation (in degrees); *A10*: clot amplitude after 10 min (in mm); CT: clotting time (in seconds); FIBTEM: ROTEM® FIBTEM test amplitude (in mm); *LI*: lysis index (amplitude reduction as an indicator of hyperfibrinolysis (in %)); *MCF*: maximum clot firmness (in mm). *TEG®*: Angle: angle reflecting the speed of clot formation (in degrees); *TEG FF*: TEG functional fibrinogen test maximal amplitude (in mm); *Ly30*: amplitude reduction after 30 min as an indicator of hyperfibrinolysis (in %); *MA*: maximum amplitude (in mm); *R*: reaction time (in minutes). While TEG® uses kaolin activation, rapidTEG® (rTEG®) uses combined kaolin and tissue factor (TF) activation thereby providing faster results. Additional rTEG® parameters are: *ACT*: activated clotting time; *K*: time from end of R until the clot reaches 20 mm amplitude. Modified from [4] with permission

detecting hemocoagulative alterations during monitoring [18]. Therefore, 'global' hemostatic assays, such as viscoelastic (ROTEM® and TEG®) and thrombin generation tests, which can be performed in whole blood, are often considered to provide a better assessment, including information about the overall hemostatic potential, clot formation kinetics and clot stability during dynamic clot formation [32]. The basic principle of viscoelastic testing, as exemplified for rotational thrombelastometry (ROTEM®) including test results reflecting different steps of hemostasis is shown in Fig. 3. 'Global' hemostatic assays have been reported to better predict prognosis and outcome in patients with severe TBI [32] and to provide results in more rapid turn-around times compared to conventional coagulation assays [31], which could lead to more timely correction of hemostatic defects. Fibrinogen is increasingly recognized to play an important role in trauma-related bleeding and is not only the precursor of fibrin but also an important mediator of platelet aggregation. Fibrinogen levels less than 2.0 g/l are a risk factor for the development of progressive hemorrhagic injury and functional deficits in fibrin polymerization can be more rapidly evaluated by 'global' assays.

Point-of-care platelet function tests, such as the Platelet Function Analyzer (PFA-100), Multiplate® and platelet mapping, may have a role in detecting platelet dysfunction and/or therapeutic platelet inhibition. ADP inhibition was strongly correlated with TBI severity and distinguished survivors from non-survivors [33]. One particular role for selected tests may be in detecting and monitoring the effects of antiplatelet agents, which show large interindividual variability. However, these assays are not readily available outside the research setting, quality control protocols are poorly established and the tests are less reliable in the presence of low platelet counts. Experience with monitoring the activity of DOACs is limited and using the above testing approaches for acutely injured patients remains a work in progress.

Treatment Approaches to Coagulopathy After TBI

The most common options for the treatment of TBI-associated coagulopathy remain blood components, including plasma and platelet concentrates, although there is increasing interest in the role of purified or recombinant factors (e.g., factor concentrates) and hemostatic agents such as TXA. In the absence of specific guidelines, TBI treatment strategies for coagulopathy follow those for systemic trauma except for targeting a higher mean arterial pressure (MAP) $\geq$ 80 mmHg and higher platelet counts ($> 100 \times 10^9$/l) [34]. Early correction of coagulopathy in TBI has been independently associated with survival [35]. Table 2 provides a summary of options and current recommendations for the reversal of preinjury anticoagulants and antiplatelet agents in adult patients with ICH in the context of TBI. For the emergency reversal of vitamin K-dependent oral anticoagulants, e.g. warfarin, the early use of prothrombin complex concentrate (PCC) is recommended and effective [34]. The management of TBI patients under DOACs is challenging because of the limited availability of specific antidotes [13]. The emergence of a range of reversal agents is likely to improve the safety profile of these agents and November 2015 saw the

Table 2 Summary of options and current recommendations for the reversal of antithrombotic agents in adult patients with intracranial hemorrhage (ICH) in the context of TBI· The recommendations are in agreement with the guidance document for novel oral anticoagulants from the International Society of Thrombosis and Hemostasis (ISTH)· All antithrombotics (vitamin K antagonists [VKAs], direct factor Xa inhibitors, direct thrombin inhibitors (DTIs), heparins (unfractionated and low molecular weight heparins [LMWHs]), pentasaccharides, thrombolytics and antiplatelet agents) should be discontinued when ICH is present or suspected

Antithrombotic	Options for reversal (reversal agents)	
	Strong recommendation with moderate-to-high quality evidence	*Conditional recommendation with low-to-moderate quality evidence*
Vitamin K antagonists (VKAs)	Vitamin K for INR reversal in VKA-associated ICH as soon as possible or with other reversal agents 3- and 4-factor PCC i. v. preferred to FFP in VKA-associated ICH and INR ≥ 1.4; dosing on weight, INR and type of PCC. Monitoring via repeated INR after PCC administration (15–60 min) and every 6–8 h for 24–48 h; subsequent treatment according to follow-up INR as repeated dosing may increase thrombotic and DIC risk *(Good practice statement)* Treatment with vitamin K and FFP recommended over no treatment!	If INR ≥ 1.4, vitamin K 10 mg i. v. with subsequent treatment according to follow-up INR; if repeated INR ≥ 1.4 within 24–48 h, redosing with vitamin K 10 mg i. v. *(Good practice statement)* or if treated with PCC and repeated INR ≥ 1.4 within first 24–48 h, further correction with FFP FFP (10–15 ml/kg i. v.) along with one dose vitamin K 10 mg i. v. if PCC is not available/contraindicated
Direct factor Xa inhibitors	No recommendation	Four-factor PCC or activated PCC (4-factor PCC 50 U/kg i. v. or aPCC [FEIBA] 50 U/kg i. v.) if ICH occurred within 3–5 terminal half-lives of drug exposure or in context of liver failure Activated charcoal (50 g) within 2 h of drug ingestion to intubated ICH patients with enteral access and/or low risk of aspiration
Direct thrombin inhibitors (DTIs)	Idarucizumab (2 × 2.5 g/50 ml) to ICH associated with dabigatran when administered within 3–5 half-lives and no renal failure and in renal failure with continued drug exposure beyond normal 3–5 half-lives	If idarucizumab not available or in case of overdose consider hemodialysis; consider redosing idarucizumab and repeated hemodialysis if ongoing bleeding Four-factor PCC or activated PCC (4-factor PCC 50 U/kg i. v. or aPCC [FEIBA] 50 U/kg i. v.) if idarucizumab is not available or if ICH with DTIs other than dabigatran and if DTI was administered within 3–5 half-lives and absence of renal failure or in renal failure with continued drug exposure beyond normal 3–5 half-lives Activated charcoal (50 g) within 2 h of drug ingestion to intubated ICH patients with enteral access and/or low risk of aspiration

Table 2 (Continued)

Antithrombotic	Options for reversal (reversal agents)	
	Strong recommendation with moderate-to-high quality evidence	*Conditional recommendation with low-to-moderate quality evidence*
Unfractionated heparin	Protamine sulfate i. v. for heparin reversal with dosing according to heparin dose over the preceding 2–3 h; protamine sulfate 1 mg for every 100 U heparin given over the preceding 2–3 h with maximum single dose 50 mg	If aPTT remains elevated, repeated protamine sulfate at 0.5 mg per 100 U of heparin
Low molecular weight heparin (LMWHs)	Protamine sulfate slowly i. v. over 10 min in the following dosing: if a.) enoxaparin was given within 8 h, 1 mg protamine per 1 mg of enoxaparin administered (maximum single dose 50 mg); if b.) exoxaparin was given within 8–12 h, 0.5 mg protamine per 1 mg enoxaparin (maximum single dose 50 mg). The following dosing applies for dalteparin, nadroparin and tinzaparin: protamine sulfate 1 mg per 100 anti Xa U of LMWH administered during the past 3–5 half-lives with maximum single dose 50 mg. Only minimal effect on reversal > 12 h from dosing!	Redosing protamine sulfate (0.5 mg per 100 anti-Xa U of LMWH or per 1 mg of enoxaparin) if life-threatening bleeding continues or in renal insufficiency. Recombinant factor VIIa (rFVIIa 90 µg/kg i. v.) if protamine is contraindicated. Reversal of danaparoid with rFVIIa in the context of ICH
Pentasaccharides	No recommendation	Activated PCC (aPCC [FEIBA] 20 U/kg i. v.) for pentasaccharide reversal. Recombinant factor VIIa (rFVIIa 90 µg/kg i. v.) if aPCC is contraindicated/not available
Thrombolytic agents (plasminogen activators)	No recommendation	Cryoprecipitate (initial dose 10 U i. v.) in thrombolytic agent-associated symptomatic ICH if administered within the previous 24 h. If contraindicated/not available, antifibrinolytic agent (tranexamic acid 10–15 mg/kg i. v. over 20 min or ε-aminocaproic acid 4–5 g i. v.). If fibrinogen levels < 150 mg/dl, administration of additional cryoprecipitate. Although substitution with fibrinogen concentrate, if available, may be reasonable, there is no recommendation at this time!

Table 2 (Continued)

Antithrombotic	Options for reversal (reversal agents)	
	Strong recommendation with moderate-to-high quality evidence	*Conditional recommendation with low-to-moderate quality evidence*
Antiplatelet agents	Platelet function testing prior to platelet transfusion is recommended; if laboratory-documented platelet function within normal ranges or documented platelet resistance, recommendation against platelet transfusion!	Desmopressin (0.4 µg/kg i. v. × 1) in ICH with aspirin/cyclooxygenase-1 or adenosine diphosphate (ADP) inhibitors Platelet concentrate in aspirin- or ADP inhibitor-associated ICH in case of neurosurgical intervention. Initial dose of one single donor apheresis unit of platelets. Platelet testing suggested prior to repeated platelet transfusion and repeated dosing only if persisting abnormalities!

ADP: adenosine diphosphate; *DIC*: disseminated intravascular coagulation; *FFP*: fresh frozen plasma; *INR*: International Normalized Ratio; *PCC*: prothrombin complex concentrate; *rFVIIa*: activated recombinant factor FVII; *U*: unit

first specific antidote for the acute reversal of factor IIa (thrombin) inhibitor dabigatran, the monoclonal antibody fragment idarucizumab [13]. Factor Xa inhibitor antidotes are in phase II and phase III trials and could be approved in the near future. For acute management and to improve thrombin generation, four-factor PCC may be considered in TBI patients.

Considerable interest in the early empiric use of plasma has been reported in the general (non-TBI) trauma literature, but our understanding of whether these new empiric-based strategies should be equally applied to the TBI population remains unclear. The empirical infusion of fresh frozen plasma (FFP) concentrates in patients with severe TBI [36] or the use of FFP in TBI patients with moderate coagulopathy either alone or combined with packed red blood cell (RBC) concentrates was associated with adverse effects or poorer functional outcomes [37].

Red Blood Cell Transfusions

RBCs, which remain the most commonly transfused blood component, have an important role in hemostasis to rapidly increase hemoglobin levels, but there is no firm consensus yet on hemoglobin targets and transfusion strategies (e.g., restrictive versus liberal) in neurocritically ill and TBI patients [38]. Several clinical studies on optimal transfusion strategy have been performed but are biased by significant confounders [38]. Increasing the hematocrit above 28% during initial surgery following severe TBI was not associated with improved or worsened outcomes and questioned the need for aggressive transfusion management [39]. In randomized trials, neither the administration of erythropoietin nor maintaining hemoglobin levels greater than 10 g/dl resulted in improved neurological outcome at 6 months; the transfusion threshold of 10 g/dl versus 7 g/dl was associated with a higher incidence of adverse events including progressive hemorrhagic injury [40, 41]. The pathophysiology of such complications is complex and even if RBC transfusion produced an improvement in cerebral oxygenation, this was not always associated with changes in brain metabolism. RBC transfusions have been associated with poor long-term functional outcomes in TBI patients with moderate anemia and remain controversial [37]. A restrictive RBC transfusion strategy should be implemented unless poor tolerance to anemia is present [38].

Platelet Transfusions

The role of platelet transfusions is still a topic of controversy. Platelet transfusion in TBI patients with moderate thrombocytopenia did not result in improved outcome [37] and was inferior to standard care for patients taking antiplatelet therapy prior to intracranial hemorrhage [42]. Platelet transfusion in patients with mild TBI, intracranial hemorrhage and preinjury intake of antiplatelet therapy did not improve short-term outcomes and may expose these patients to an unnecessary risk for potential adverse effects associated with platelet transfusions. Five retrospective registry studies provide inadequate evidence to support the routine use of platelet transfusions in patients with traumatic ICH and preinjury antiplatelet use [43]. Prospective evidence may suggest that platelet transfusion in TBI more likely improves aspirin-induced, but not trauma-induced, platelet dysfunction. Although platelet transfusion in TBI patients on antiplatelet therapy is often considered, the current data on the effects of platelet transfusion on platelet function are still conflicting and inconclusive.

Hemostatic Agents

A subgroup analysis of the CRASH-2 trial suggested that TXA might reduce hemorrhage growth [44]. While the overall benefit from TXA in CRASH-2 was limited to patients who were treated within three hours of injury [28], it is presently unclear whether this applies in TBI. The ongoing CRASH-3 study (NCT01402882) should provide further guidance. Pooled data from two randomized controlled trials demonstrated a significant reduction in ICH progression and a statistically non-significant improvement in clinical outcomes with early TXA [45]. One study showed less hematoma progression in TBI rFVIIa-treated patients, but the clinical relevance of this finding is unclear, as the effect size and patient numbers were small and treatment was associated with a higher incidence of thromboses [46]. In patients with preinjury vitamin-K antagonist intake, the use of rFVIIa was associated with a decreased time to normal INR but no difference in mortality. The use of desmopressin (DDAVP) is not recommended routinely in bleeding trauma patients, including those with TBI, because of the risk of aggravating cerebral edema and intracranial hypertension.

Viscoelastic-based Treatment Algorithms

'Global' hemostatic assays, such as viscoelastic assays (ROTEM® and TEG®), may be superior to conventional coagulation assays in the assessment and prognosis of

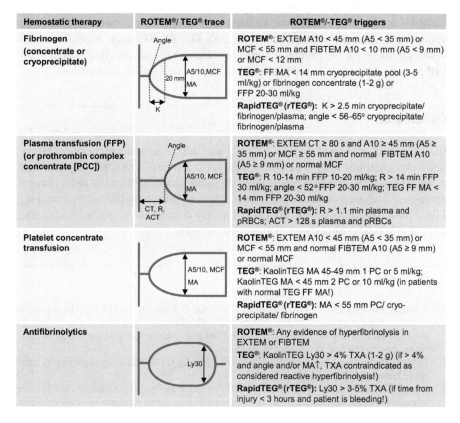

Hemostatic therapy	ROTEM®/ TEG® trace	ROTEM®/-TEG® triggers
Fibrinogen (concentrate or cryoprecipitate)	Angle / 20 mm / A5/10,MCF / MA / K	**ROTEM®**: EXTEM A10 < 45 mm (A5 < 35 mm) or MCF < 55 mm and FIBTEM A10 < 10 mm (A5 < 9 mm) or MCF < 12 mm **TEG®**: FF MA < 14 mm cryoprecipitate pool (3-5 ml/kg) or fibrinogen concentrate (1-2 g) or FFP 20-30 ml/kg **RapidTEG® (rTEG®)**: K > 2.5 min cryoprecipitate/fibrinogen/plasma; angle < 56-65° cryoprecipitate/fibrinogen/plasma
Plasma transfusion (FFP) (or prothrombin complex concentrate [PCC])	Angle / A5/10, MCF / MA / CT, R, ACT	**ROTEM®**: EXTEM CT ≥ 80 s and A10 ≥ 45 mm (A5 ≥ 35 mm) or MCF ≥ 55 mm and normal FIBTEM A10 (A5 ≥ 9 mm) or normal MCF **TEG®**: R 10-14 min FFP 10-20 ml/kg; R > 14 min FFP 30 ml/kg; angle < 52° FFP 20-30 ml/kg; TEG FF MA < 14 mm FFP 20-30 ml/kg **RapidTEG® (rTEG®)**: R > 1.1 min plasma and pRBCs; ACT > 128 s plasma and pRBCs
Platelet concentrate transfusion	A5/10, MCF / MA	**ROTEM®**: EXTEM A10 < 45 mm (A5 < 35 mm) or MCF < 55 mm and normal FIBTEM A10 (A5 ≥ 9 mm) or normal MCF **TEG®**: KaolinTEG MA 45-49 mm 1 PC or 5 ml/kg; KaolinTEG MA < 45 mm 2 PC or 10 ml/kg (in patients with normal TEG FF MA!) **RapidTEG® (rTEG®)**: MA < 55 mm PC/ cryoprecipitate/ fibrinogen
Antifibrinolytics	Ly30	**ROTEM®**: Any evidence of hyperfibrinolysis in EXTEM or FIBTEM **TEG®**: KaolinTEG Ly30 > 4% TXA (1-2 g) (if > 4% and angle and/or MA↑, TXA contraindicated as considered reactive hyperfibrinolysis!) **RapidTEG® (rTEG®)**: Ly30 > 3-5% TXA (if time from injury < 3 hours and patient is bleeding!)

Fig. 4 Algorithm for the use of hemostatic agents and blood products during early care for the bleeding trauma patient based upon viscoelastic test results (ROTEM® and TEG/rTEG®). Overview of viscoelastic triggers for the differential and targeted use of hemostatic agents and blood products currently suggested based upon expert opinion for ROTEM® [50] and TEG/rTEG® [48]. The ROTEM® triggers are based upon ROTEM® subtests EXTEM and FIBTEM where i.) the EXTEM test activates hemostasis via tissue factor (TF) and is used as a screening test for the (extrinsic) hemostasis system, and ii.) the FIBTEM test is an assay for the fibrin part of the clot. FIBTEM eliminates the platelet contribution of clot formation with cytochalasin D and allows for the detection of fibrinogen deficiency or fibrin polymerization disorders. ROTEM®: A5/A10: clot amplitude after 5 and 10 min (in mm); *CT*: clotting time (in seconds); *MCF*: maximum clot firmness (in mm). *TEG®*: angle: angle reflecting the speed of clot formation (in degrees); *TEG FF (MA)*: TEG functional fibrinogen test maximal amplitude (in millimeters); *Ly30*: amplitude reduction after 30 min as an indicator of hyperfibrinolysis (in %); *MA*: maximum amplitude (in millimeters); *R*: reaction time (in minutes). Additional rTEG® parameters are: *ATC*: activated clotting time; *K*: time from end of R until the clot reaches 20 mm amplitude. *FFP*: fresh frozen plasma; *PC*: platelet concentrate; *pRBC*: packed red blood cell; *TXA*: tranexamic acid. Modified from [4] with permission

real-time hemostasis and these attributes might be expected to increase their clinical relevance [47]. Viscoelastic testing has been incorporated into guidelines and vertical algorithms to diagnose and guide hemostatic therapies in high-risk patients with active hemorrhage including trauma related [34, 48, 49]. Thresholds for treatment according to these measures as for all coagulation laboratory parameters are not well defined and require further investigation. A consensus panel has issued recommendations regarding viscoelastic thresholds for triggering the initiation of specific treatments in bleeding trauma patients ([50]; Fig. 4). Although these thresholds were introduced for the general trauma population they may also hold potential for TBI patients with coagulopathy to better target and individualize therapies.

Conclusion

Emerging studies are addressing whether timely and targeted management of hemostatic abnormalities after TBI protect against secondary injury and improve outcome. The increasing use of antiplatelet drugs and anticoagulants in older patients deserves particular consideration in precision medicine approaches to managing TBI. Thresholds for treatment are overall poorly defined, using viscoelastic testing and conventional coagulation laboratory parameters.

References

1. Hyder A, Wunderlich CA, Puvanachandra P, Gururaj G, Kobisingye O (2007) The impact of traumatic brain injuries. NeuroRehabilitation 22:341–353
2. Roozenbeek B, Maas AI, Menon DK (2013) Changing patterns in the epidemiology of traumatic brain injury. Nat Rev Neurol 9:231–236
3. Laroche M, Kutcher ME, Huang MC, Cohen MJ, Manley GT (2012) Coagulopathy after traumatic brain injury. Neurosurgery 70:1334–1345
4. Maegele M, Schöchl H, Menovsky T et al (2017) Coagulopathy and hemorrhagic progression in traumatic brain injury: advances in mechnisms, diagnosis and management. Lancet Neurol 16:630–647
5. Joseph B, Aziz H, Zangbar B et al (2014) Acquired coagulopathy of traumatic brain injury defined by routine laboratory tests: which laboratory values matter? J Trauma Crit Care Surg 76:121–125
6. Harhangi BS, Kompanje EJO, Leebeek FWG, Maas AIR (2008) Coagulation disorders after traumatic brain injury. Acta Neurochir 150:165–175
7. Epstein DS, Mitra B, O'Reilly G, Rosenfeld JV, Cameron PA (2014) Acute traumatic coagulopathy in the setting of isolated traumatic brain injury: a systematic review and meta-analysis. Injury 45:819–824
8. Gomez PA, Lobato RD, Ortega JM, De La Cruz J (1996) Mild head injury: differences in prognosis among patients with a Glasgow Coma Scale score of 13 to 15 and analysis of factors associated with abnormal CT findings. Br J Neurosurg 10:453–460
9. Prinz V, Finger T, Bayerl S et al (2016) High prevalence of pharmacologically induced platelet dysfunction in the acute setting of brain injury. Acta Neurochir (Wien) 158:117–123
10. Batchelor JS, Grayson A (2012) A meta-analysis to determine the effect of anticoagulation on mortality in patients with blunt head trauma. Br J Neurosurg 26:525–530

11. Fabbri A, Servadei F, Marchesini G et al (2013) Antiplatelet therapy and the outcome of subjects with intracranial injury: The Italian SIMEU study. Crit Care 17:R53

12. Miller MP, Trujillo TC, Nordenholz KE (2014) Practical considerations in emergency management of bleeding in the setting of target-specific oral anticoagulants. Am J Emerg Med 32:375–382

13. Maegele M, Grottke O, Schöchl H, Sakowitz OA, Spannagl M, Koscielny J (2016) Direct oral anticoagulants in emergency trauma admissions. Dtsch Arztbl Int 113:575–582

14. Greuters S, van den Berg A, Franschman G et al (2011) Acute and delayed mild coagulopathy are related to outcome in patients with isolated traumatic brain injury. Crit Care 15:R2

15. Rao AJ, Laurie A, Hillard C et al (2016) The utility of thromboelastography for predicting the risk of progression of intracranial hemorrhage in traumatic brain injury patients. Neurosurgery 63(Suppl 1):173–174

16. Lustenberger T, Talvig P, Kobayashi L et al (2010) Time course of coagulopathy is isolated severe traumatic brain injury. Injury 41:924–928

17. Kurland D, Hong C, Arabi B, Gerzanich V, Simard JM (2012) Hemorrhagic progression of a contusion after traumatic brain injury: a review. J Neurotrauma 29:19–31

18. Yuan Q, Sun YR, Wu X et al (2016) Coagulopathy in traumatic brain injury and its correlation with progressive hemorrhage injury: a systematic review and meta-analysis. J Neurotrauma 33:1279–1291

19. Folkerson LE, Sloan D, Cotton BA, Holcomb JB, Tomasek JS, Wade CE (2015) Predicting progressive hemorrhagic injury from isolated traumatic brain injury and coagulation. Surgery 158:655–661

20. Nekludov M, Bellander BM, Blombäck M, Wallen HN (2007) Platelet dysfunction in patients with severe traumatic brain injury. J Neurotrauma 24:1699–1706

21. Simard JM, Kilbourne M, Tsymbalyuk O et al (2009) Key role of sulfonyl urea receptor 1 in progressive secondary hemorrhage after brain contusion. J Neurotrauma 26:2257–2267

22. Di Battista AP, Rizoli SB, Lejnieks B et al (2016) Sympathoadrenal activation is associated with acute traumatic coagulopathy and endotheliopathy in isolated brain injury. Shock 46(3 Suppl 1):96–103

23. Foley JH, Conway EM (2016) Cross talk between coagulation and inflammation. Circ Res 118:1392–1408

24. Nekludoov M, Mobarrez F, Gryth D, Bellander BM, Wallen H (2014) Formation of microparticles in the injured brain of patients with severe isolated traumatic brain injury. J Neurotrauma 31:1927–1933

25. Lustenberger T, Talving P, Kobayashi L et al (2010) Early coagulopathy after isolated severe traumatic brain injury: Relationship with hypoperfusion challenged. J Trauma 69:1410–1414

26. Dekker SE, Duvekot A, De Vries HM et al (2016) Relationship between tissue perfusion and coagulopathy in traumatic brain injury. J Surg Res 205:147–154

27. Hijazi N, Fanne RA, Abramovitch R et al (2016) Endogenous plasminogen activators mediate progressive intracreberal hemorrhage after traumatic brain injury in mice. Blood 125:2558–2567

28. CRASH-2 Collaborators, Shakur H, Roberts I, Bautista R et al (2010) Effects of tranexamic acid on death, vascular occlusive events, and blood transfusion in trauma patients with significant hemorrhage (CRASH-2): A randomised, placebo-controlled trial. Lancet 376:23–32

29. Wohlauer MV, Moore EE, Thomas S et al (2012) Early platelet dysfunction: an unrecognized role in the acute coagulopathy of trauma. J Am Coll Surg 214:739–746

30. Mann KG, Butenas S, Brummel K (2003) The dynamics of thrombin formation. Arter Thromb Vasc Bio 23:17–25

31. Davenport R, Manson J, De'Ath H et al (2011) Functional definition and charaterization of acute traumatic coagulopathy. Crit Care Med 39:2652–2658

32. Schöchl H, Solomon C, Traintinger S et al (2011) Thrombelastometric (ROTEM) findings in patients suffering from isolated severe traumatic brain injury. J Neurotrauma 28:2033–2041

33. Davis P, Musunuru H, Walsh M et al (2012) Platelet dysfunction is an early marker for traumatic brain injury-induced coagulopathy. Neurocrit Care 18:201–208
34. Rossaint R, Bouillon B, Cerny V et al (2016) The European guideline on management of major bleeding and coagulopathy following trauma: fourth edition. Crit Care 20:100
35. Epstein DS, Mitra B, Cameron PA, Fitzgerald M, Rosenfeld JV (2016) Normalization of coagulopathy is associated with improved outcome after isolated traumatic brain injury. J Clin Neurosci 29:64–69
36. Etemadrezaie H, Baharvadat H, Shariati Z, Lari SM, Shakeri MT, Ganjeifar B (2007) The effect of fresh frozen plasma in severe closed head injury. Clin Neurol Neurosurg 109:166–171
37. Anglin CO, Spence J, Warner M et al (2013) Effects of platelet and plasma transfusion on outcome in traumatic brain injury with moderate bleeding diasthesis. J Neurosurg 118:676–686
38. Lelubre C, Bouzat P, Crippa IA, Taccone FS (2016) Anemia management after acute brain injury. Crit Care 20:152
39. Flückinger C, Bechir M, Brenni M et al (2010) Increasing hematocrit above 28% during early resuscitative phase is not associated with decreased mortality following severe traumatic brain injury. Acta Neurochir (Wien) 152:627–636
40. Robertson CS, Hannay HJ, Yamal JM et al (2014) Effect of erythropoietin and transfusion threshold on neurological recovery after traumatic brain injury: A randomized clinical trial. JAMA 312:36–47
41. Veadantam A, Yamal JM, Rubin ML, Robertson CS, Gopinath SP (2016) Progressive hemorrhagic injury after severe traumatic brain injury: effect of hemoglobin transfusion thresholds. J Neurosurg 125:1229–1234
42. Baharoglu MI, Cordonnier C, Al-Shahi Salman R et al (2016) Platelet transfusion versus standard care after acute stroke due to spontaneous cerebral hemorrhage associated with antiplatelet therapy (PATCH): a randomised, open-label, phase 3 trial. Lancet 387:2605–2613
43. Nishijima DK, Zehtabchi S, Berrong J, Legome E (2012) Utility of platelet transfusion in adult patients with traumatic intracranial hemorrhage and preinjury antiplatelet use: a systematic review. J Trauma Acute Care Surg 72:1658–1663
44. Perel P, Al-Shahi Salman R, Kawahara T et al (2012) CRASH-2 (clinical Randomisation of an antifibrinolytic in significant hemorrhage) intracranial bleeding study: the effect of tranexamic acid in traumatic brain injury—a nested randomised controlled trial. Health Technol Assess 16:1–54
45. Zehtabchi S, Baki ASG, Falzon L, Nishijima DK (2014) Tranexamic acid for traumatic brain injury: a systematic review and meta-analysis. Am J Emerg Med 32:1503–1509
46. Narayan RK, Maas AI, Marshall LF et al (2008) Recombinant factor VIIa in traumatic hemorrhage: results of a dose-escalation clinical trial. Neurosurgery 62:776–786
47. Wikkelso A, Wetterslev J, Moller AM, Afshari A (2016) Thromboelastography (TEG) or thromboelastometry (ROTEM) to monitor hemostatic treatment versus usual care in adults or children with bleeding. Cochrane Database Syst Rev CD007871
48. Johansson PI, Stensballe J, Oliveri R, Wade CE, Ostrowksi SR, Holcomb JB (2014) How I treat patients with massive hemorrhage. Blood 124:3052–3058
49. Schöchl H, Maegele M, Solomon C, Görlinger K, Voelckel W (2012) Early and individualized goal-directed therapy for trauma-induced coagulopathy. Scand J Trauma Resusc Emerg Med 20:15
50. Inaba K, Rizoli S, Veigas PV et al (2015) 2014 Consensus conference on viscoelastic test-based transfusion guidelines for early trauma resuscitation: Report of the panel. J Trauma Acute Care Surg 78:1220–1229
51. Zehtabchi S, Soghoian S, Liu Y et al (2008) The association of coagulopathy and traumatic brain injury in patients with isolated head injury. Resuscitation 76:52–56
52. Talving P, Benflield R, Hadjizacharia P, Inaba K, Chan LS, Demetriades D (2009) Coagulopathy in severe traumatic brain injury: a prospective study. J Trauma 66:55–61

53. Wafaisade A, Lefering R, Tjardes T et al (2010) Acute coagulopathy in isolated blunt traumatic brain injury. Neuro Crit Care 12:211–219
54. Chhabra G, Rangarajan K, Subramanian A, Agrawal D, Sharma S, Mukhopadhayay AK (2010) Hypofibrinogenaemia in isolated traumatic brain injury in Indian patients. Neurol India 58:756–757
55. Shehata M, Afify MI, El-Shafie M, Khaled M (2011) Prevalence and clinical implications of coagulopathy in patients with isolated head trauma. Med J Cairo Univ 79:131–137
56. Franschman G, Greuters S, Jansen WH et al (2012) Haemostatic and cranial computed tomography characteristics in patients with acute and delayed coagulopathy after isolated traumatic brain injury. Brain Inj 26:1464–1471
57. Genet GF, Johansson PI, Meyer MA et al (2013) Trauma-induced coagulopathy: Standard coagulation tests, biomarkers of coagulopathy, and endothelial damage in patients with traumatic brain injury. J Neurotrauma 30:301–306
58. Alexiou GA, Lianos G, Fotakopoulos G, Michos E, Pachatouridis D, Voulgaris S (2013) Admission glucose and coagulopathy occurrence in patients with traumatic brain injury. Brain Inj 28:438–441
59. Epstein DS, Mitra B, Cameron PA, Fitzgerald M, Rosenfeld JV (2014) Acute traumatic coagulopathy in the setting of isolated traumatic brain injury: definition, incidence and outcomes. Br J Neurosurg 25:1–5
60. De Oliveira Manoel AL, Neto AC, Veigas PV, Rizoli S (2015) Traumatic brain injury associated coagulopathy. Neurocrit Care 22:34–44

Blood Transfusion in Critically Ill Patients with Traumatic Brain Injury

A. F. Turgeon, F. Lauzier, and D. A. Fergusson

Introduction

Traumatic brain injury (TBI) is the main cause of death in the first half of life and a significant proportion of survivors of severe TBI are left with severe permanent impairment [1, 2]. Not surprisingly, TBI patients also consume the majority of healthcare resources in trauma care [3, 4]. Current management of critically ill patients with TBI focuses on preventing secondary cerebral injuries. Most interventions in the acute phase of care are thus directed at ensuring appropriate brain oxygen delivery (DO_2). However, the majority of these interventions are based on very limited rigorous evidence [5], with highly variable within and between center practice. This variation has led to significant outcome differences being observed across centers [2], including regarding the use of red blood cell (RBC) transfusion. RBC transfusion is a common intervention administered in TBI given the high proportion of anemia in this population. Although there has been a move towards restrictive RBC transfusion strategies (at lower hemoglobin transfusion threshold), concerns have been expressed about the risks of decreased DO_2 to a fragile brain that is vulnerable to secondary permanent hypoxic insults. More liberal use of RBC transfusion (at higher hemoglobin transfusion threshold) has therefore been advocated by some experts. Despite the belief that RBC transfusion may improve DO_2

A. F. Turgeon (✉) · F. Lauzier
Population Health and Optimal Health Practices Unit (Trauma – Emergency – Critical Care Medicine), CHU de Québec-Université Laval Research Centre
Quebec, Canada
Department of Critical Care Medicine, CHU de Québec-Université Laval
Quebec, Canada
e-mail: alexis.turgeon@fmed.ulaval.ca

D. A. Fergusson
Clinical Epidemiology Program, Ottawa Hospital Research Institute Centre for Practice-Changing Research
Ottawa, Canada

© Springer International Publishing AG 2018   473
J.-L. Vincent (ed.), *Annual Update in Intensive Care and Emergency Medicine 2018*,
Annual Update in Intensive Care and Emergency Medicine,
https://doi.org/10.1007/978-3-319-73670-9_36

to the brain, the optimal RBC transfusion strategy to improve clinically-important outcomes in critically ill patients with TBI remains unknown.

Is Anemia Common in Critically Ill Patients and in Traumatic Brain Injury Patients?

Most patients will experience anemia during their stay in the intensive care unit (ICU) and a significant proportion of them will have a hemoglobin level triggering a RBC transfusion on ICU admission [6]. Anemia in critical care is common and multifactorial. Systemic inflammatory response [7, 8], hemodilution, phlebotomy [9] and erythropoietin deficiency [8, 10] are among the numerous causes involved. In critically ill populations, anemia has been consistently associated with increased mortality [11, 12]. In the specific trauma population, including in TBI patients, acute blood loss from extracranial injuries may also play an important role in the etiology of anemia.

A significant proportion of critically ill patients with TBI therefore experience anemia during ICU stay [13–15]. In these patients, an increased risk of death and complications was also observed [13, 14] but, more importantly, there was an association with unfavorable functional outcome at 3 and 6 months, based on the Glasgow Outcome Scale [15]. However, the vast majority of current evidence is derived from retrospective and prospective cohort studies, which suffer from a high risk of selection and information bias. Whether these associations are true independent predictors of unfavorable outcomes or simply markers of disease severity is unclear. Randomized clinical trials are needed to evaluate whether correcting anemia at lower hemoglobin thresholds by administering RBC transfusions is associated with better outcomes.

Are Traumatic Brain Injury Patients Frequently Transfused with Red Blood Cells?

In a recent systematic review of 23 studies (cohort studies and randomized controlled trials) including 7,524 patients, we estimated the frequency of RBC transfusion in TBI patients [16]. More than one-third of patients were transfused at some point during their hospitalization (pooled cumulative incidence of 36%, 95% CI 28–44%). In patients that received at least one transfusion, the mean number of RBC units received ranged from 1.8 to 6.1 per patient. Patients with lower Glasgow Coma Scale (GCS) scores were also more likely to be transfused. Most studies included in our systematic review were published within the last decade and mainly included patients with severe TBI. We observed comparable results in a recent large multicenter cohort study in TBI patients using administrative data from the National Trauma Registry in Canada (n = 7062). In this study, looking at the frequency of RBC transfusion in patients with moderate or severe TBI, 28.2% of patients received at least one RBC transfusion during their hospital stay [17]. RBC transfusion

Table 1 Adjusted* risk ratios for the association between determinants of red blood cell transfusion. Modified from [17]

Potential determinants	Risk ratio (95%CI)
Sex	1.16 (1.10 to 1.23)
Age, years	
18–55	1.00
56–65	1.14 (1.04 to 1.24)
66–75	0.96 (0.84 to 1.09)
≥ 75	0.81 (0.72 to 0.90)
Number of comorbidities	
0	1.00
1	1.11 (1.02 to 1.21)
≥ 2	1.66 (1.40 to 1.97)
Other specific comorbidities	
Ischemic heart disease	1.19 (0.93 to 1.53)
Cerebrovascular disease	1.17 (0.95 to 1.43)
Anemia	2.10 (1.81 to 2.43)
Coagulopathy	1.37 (1.08 to 1.74)
Sepsis	1.57 (1.23 to 2.01)
Hypovolemic shock	1.33 (1.19 to 1.47)
Bleeding/hemorrhage	1.12 (1.03 to 1.22)
TBI severity	
Moderate TBI (GCS 9–12)	0.78 (0.70 to 0.87)
Serious head injury (AIS ≥ 3)	0.93 (0.81 to 1.07)
Extracerebral injury	
Face	1.36 (1.22 to 1.51)
Thorax and abdomen	1.76 (1.55 to 2.00)
Spine	1.24 (1.08 to 1.43)
Upper extremities	1.25 (1.12 to 1.40)
Lower extremities	1.88 (1.75 to 2.02)
Others	1.48 (0.96 to 2.29)

* Adjusted for all covariates in the table
AIS: Abbreviated Injury Severity Score; *GCS*: Glasgow Coma Scale; *TBI*: traumatic brain injury

varied across centers, with greater frequencies in Level I and II trauma centers, accounting for the majority of the variation observed in adjusted analyses for patient risk factors. Extracerebral traumatic injuries and presence of anemia on admission were the most important determinants of RBC transfusion (Table 1). These results show how frequently RBC transfusions are administered in critically ill patients with TBI as well as how variable transfusion practice can be within and across centers and that several determinants affect the decision to transfuse.

Can RBC Transfusions Have Deleterious Effects?

Blood transfusions are the most widely used therapeutic intervention in medicine [18]. Each year, 108 million units of blood are transfused globally. The published evidence suggests that transfused patients have longer lengths of hospital stay, higher infection rates, spend more time in intensive care, and have a higher risk of acute respiratory distress preventing oxygen from getting to the lungs and into the blood. Although often lifesaving, transfusion of blood products is also associated with adverse events and their use has a significant social and economic impact on our health system. The transfusion community is well aware of the infectious and immunological risks associated with transfusion. Over the years, a number of measures have been incorporated into the blood procurement and supply system to improve the safety of transfusions including donor questionnaires that assess risks, improved infectious disease screening, and other quality measures. As such, transfusion-acquired infections are now considered very rare. However, clinical outcome after transfusion is affected by many other transfusion adverse events such as acute and delayed hemolytic reactions, transfusion-related acute lung injury (TRALI), transfusion-associated circulatory overload (TACO), and hypotensive reactions – all associated with higher mortality and morbidity. Other effects, such as transfusion-related immunomodulation, are biologically well documented but their impact on clinical outcomes is less clear.

Why is the Hemoglobin Level Important for the Brain?

For any given tissue, DO_2 to any cell is dependent on the cardiac output, oxygen saturation (SaO_2), arterial partial pressure of oxygen (PaO_2), and hemoglobin concentration (Table 2). Assuming a normal cardiac output and an adequate provision of oxygen in the blood through adequate mechanical ventilation support (normal SaO_2 and PaO_2), the only other way to improve DO_2 to the brain is by optimizing the hemoglobin concentration. However, brain DO_2 may be related to different mechanisms. As for most cells in the body, oxygen is mandatory to allow neuronal metabolism in the brain, as there is no anaerobic pathway. Although the cardiac output is a major determinant in the rest of the body, it does not play an important role in the brain, which has different compensatory mechanisms to improve oxygen delivery. Rather, DO_2 is dependent on cerebral blood flow (CBF) and hemoglobin levels (Table 2; [18]). The CBF is thus one of the key elements in DO_2 to the brain cells and is directly affected by the cerebral perfusion pressure and inversely by the cerebrovascular resistance. Complex autoregulation mechanisms based on metabolic, pressure, chemical and neural changes ensure appropriate DO_2 within a range of non-optimal physiologic conditions [20]. Cerebral DO_2 is thus usually greater than the requirements of the brain for its metabolism. This excess in the total oxygen available is one hypothesis that could explain how hypoxemia and hypoxia are prevented until very low hemoglobin levels are reached.

Table 2 Tissue oxygen delivery (DO_2)

Oxygen delivery to non-cerebral tissue	$DO_2 = (\mathbf{CO} \times Hb \times O_2 \text{ saturation} \times 1.39) + 0.0031 \times PaO_2$
Oxygen delivery to cerebral tissue	$DO_2 = (\mathbf{CBF} \times Hb \times O_2 \text{ saturation} \times 1.39) + 0.0031 \times PaO_2$

CO: cardiac output; Hb: hemoglobin; O_2: oxygen, PaO_2: arterial partial pressure of oxygen

Are These Mechanisms Affected in Critically Ill Patients with Traumatic Brain Injury?

These theoretical physiological mechanisms are however suspected to be altered in critically ill patients with TBI. Several lesions caused by the trauma, such as cerebral contusions, hemorrhage and edema, may impair the integrity of the blood-brain barrier and thus affect the compensatory mechanisms of the brain. The blood-brain barrier keeps the brain protected from many influences from the systemic blood circulation, and the break in its integrity raises concerns on its capacity to adequately compensate and its vulnerability to aggressions such as non-optimal DO_2.

There are some clinical data to support the assumption that transfusion of RBC improves DO_2 to the brain in humans. Studies have assessed DO_2 by using specific surrogate measures of local brain tissue oxygen measurements ($PbtO_2$). In small prospective observational studies in brain injured patients, RBC transfusions were associated with improved $PbtO_2$ [21, 22]. Interestingly, using cerebral microdialysis to measure markers of cerebral metabolism in the same patients, no significant improvement in cerebral metabolism was observed after RBC transfusion [22]. Such mechanistic studies further support the state of clinical equipoise regarding RBC transfusion in TBI, and raise a fundamental concern regarding the significance of such surrogate measures and their association or not with clinically important outcomes in these patients.

What is the Evidence for RBC Transfusion Strategies in Critically Ill Patients?

A landmark study published in 1999, the Transfusion Requirements in Critical Care (TRICC) trial, helped drive the establishment of current transfusion guidelines, not only in critically ill patients, but in the majority of medical and surgical populations. Indeed, the TRICC trial has influenced global transfusion practice and swung the pendulum from the use of more liberal to restrictive transfusion strategies. In this large multicenter trial, patients were randomly allocated to two transfusion strategies: a restrictive strategy (transfusion at low hemoglobin levels [7 g/dl]) and a liberal strategy (transfusion at high hemoglobin levels [9 g/dl]) [23]. The results of this study demonstrated no benefit of aiming at greater hemoglobin thresholds on 28-day mortality and potential harm. However, specific patient populations, such as patients with coronary artery disease or TBI, despite not having been excluded, were underrepresented. A similar study was conducted in the pediatric critical care population by members of our group (TRIP-ICU trial) [24]. The trial evaluated the impact of transfusion thresholds on organ failure and showed no effect of a liberal RBC transfusion strategy as compared to a restrictive RBC transfusion strategy.

More recently, several large-scale trials targeted specific critically ill populations. In a multicenter trial from Scandinavia, no mortality benefit was observed when liberal and restrictive transfusion strategies were compared in patients with septic shock [25]. A trial conducted in patients undergoing non-emergent cardiac surgery in 17 centers in the United Kingdom observed no difference in postoperative morbidities and costs, but a significant increased mortality with the use of a restrictive strategy when comparing 7.5 g/dl to 9 g/dl for triggering a RBC transfusion [26]. Results from a large multicenter randomized controlled trial (RCT) recently completed in high-risk patients having cardiac surgery (TRICS-III, NCT02042898) will help answer remaining evidence gaps in this population. In a recent systematic review published by the Cochrane Collaboration, in which data from 31 trials were pooled representing 12,587 patients, no clinically significant effect of RBC transfusion following restrictive hemoglobin thresholds as opposed to more liberal thresholds was observed [27]. However, the authors explicitly acknowledged that the current evidence for certain specific populations, such as acute coronary syndrome and TBI, was insufficient to inform clinical practice. Interestingly, a recent systematic review targeting the specific population of patients with cardiovascular disease, showed no overall effect of the different strategies, but observed a potential increased risk of acute coronary syndrome with a restrictive strategy [28]. These results thus highlight the importance of carefully evaluating transfusion strategies in these specific patient populations [28].

What is the Evidence for RBC Transfusion Strategies in Traumatic Brain Injury?

Although intensive research has been conducted in the overall critically ill population and other acute care populations, many of the trials had a limited enrolment and representation of patients with cerebral injuries, and even more so with TBI. Analyzing and evaluating the subgroups of TBI patients from such trials can be helpful in exploring associations but is prone to statistical and methodological issues, such as selection bias and inflated type I errors due to multiple testing and low power. We performed a systematic review of comparative studies to evaluate the effect of hemoglobin levels on clinically important outcomes in neurocritically ill patients [29]. Six studies, including the subgroups of patients from the TRICC [23] and TRIP-ICU [24] trials, met inclusion criteria. Half of these studies were considered at high risk of bias and data were not pooled given the heterogeneity observed in study designs and patient populations. Overall, no differential effect between hemoglobin levels was observed in terms of mortality, ICU length of stay, duration of mechanical ventilation and multiorgan failure. Only one RCT was identified. This trial included 44 patients with subarachnoid hemorrhage and failed to detect any difference in outcomes (adverse event and short-term functional outcome) in the two study groups (10 g/dl compared to a threshold of 11.5 g/dl) [30]. Our systematic review highlights the paucity of comparative studies conducted in neurocritically ill populations, particularly in TBI, that have evaluated the effect of transfusion thresholds and anemia in clinically important outcomes.

More recently, a RCT conducted in two trauma centers evaluated the impact of erythropoietin and RBC transfusion in TBI patients using a 2×2 factorial design [31]. In this trial, TBI patients not following commands were enrolled to receive an RBC transfusion triggered by either a hemoglobin level of 7 g/dl or of 10 g/dl. While not confirming their hypothesis (superiority of the liberal arm), the trial was not designed or appropriately powered to look at a reasonable or plausible clinical effect size. The trial was powered to detect a 50% relative risk reduction of unfavorable outcome at 6-months based on the Glasgow outcome scale. Such a sizable effect size in the context of RBC transfusion is unrealistic.

What is the Opinion of Clinicians?

A recent international survey of members of different societies of intensive care medicine evaluated practices and opinions regarding transfusion thresholds in critically ill patients with acute brain injury [32]. The majority of respondents was from Europe and worked in an academic tertiary-care setting. In this survey, although most respondents mentioned targeting a threshold of 7 or 8 g/dl for RBC transfusion in patients with acute brain injury, clinical equipoise could be observed for TBI patients specifically, with comparable proportions of respondents reporting a preferred target of 7, 8, 9 or 10 g/dl. Among all neurocritically ill specific populations, TBI patients were the one population with the broadest level of uncertainty among respondents. A previous survey of transfusion preferences in the United States showed that beliefs on the optimal threshold to target for RBC transfusion in severe acute TBI varied according to the specialty of the respondent [33]. In their survey, neurosurgeons mentioned targeting greater mean hemoglobin thresholds for transfusion (8.9 ± 1.1 g/dl) compared to trauma surgeons (8.0 ± 1.1 g/dl) and critical care physicians (8.3 ± 0.9 g/dl) in severe TBI patients with normal intracranial pressure (ICP). For the three groups of respondents, the threshold for RBC transfusion shifted to higher hemoglobin values in the presence of increased ICP. These results are comparable to those observed in a population of patients with subarachnoid hemorrhage with variation in beliefs and higher thresholds being targeted with greater disease severity by North American intensivists and neurosurgeons [34]. An international self-administered cross-sectional survey of intensivists and neurosurgeons from Canada, Australia and the United Kingdom working in major trauma centers and caring for patients with moderate to severe TBI is currently underway. This survey aims to identify attitudes toward current transfusion practices, but also the determinants of RBC transfusion in critically ill patients with TBI.

What can be Learned from Current Evidence?

While clinical practice is moving towards restrictive transfusion strategies for many critically ill patient populations, many experts have expressed concerns regarding simply adopting similar restrictive strategies in patients with TBI, emphasizing the low level of rigorous evidence driving clinical practice [35–38]. The injured brain is vulnerable to secondary hypoxic insults, and concerns have been raised regarding the safety of restrictive transfusion strategies in acute neurologic conditions [36]. Albeit with little precedent from transfusion trials in other critically ill patient populations, recognized experts in neurocritical care have reasonably communicated plausible concern that low hemoglobin levels in the context of TBI may negatively impact clinical outcomes [35, 36]. RBC transfusion has thus been advocated to increase cerebral DO_2, despite conflicting evidence [39]. Given the heightened inflammation and upregulation of coagulation associated with trauma, especially in TBI, the relative safety of allogenic RBC transfusion is distinctly uncertain. Previous transfusion trials and observational studies have been conducted in general ICU or mixed-trauma populations; none of these studies was well designed to assess patients with TBI [23, 24, 31]. Considering the persistent clinical equipoise and the paucity of data precluding the establishment of evidence-based guidelines in this specific population, a large-scale multicenter RCT is warranted.

What Future Research is Coming?

With the background work and studies conducted so far, along with the persistent clinical equipoise, the next step is the development and conduct of a large-scale pragmatic trial comparing a restrictive to a liberal RBC transfusion strategy in critically ill patients with TBI. Considering the nature of the intervention, this trial will have to be 'open label' due to the impracticality and feasibility of blinding a RBC transfusion. We recently designed the HEMOglobin Transfusion Threshold in Traumatic Brain Injury OptimizatioN Trial (HEMOTION trial), a prospective randomized open blinded end-point (PROBE) trial comparing 7 g/dl to 10 g/dl to trigger RBC transfusion in critically ill adult patients with moderate or severe blunt TBI (NCT03260478). Our primary outcome measure is the Glasgow Outcome Scale extended (GOSe) at 6 months. Secondary outcomes are mortality, the Functional Independence Measure (FIM), quality of life (EQ-5D) and Qolibri, depression (PHQ-9), return to work/study and complications related to transfusion. This multicenter trial of 712 patients is funded by the Canadian Institutes of Health Research (CIHR). The first patient was enrolled in September 2017.

How Will a Large Scale RCT Change Practice?

If, as hypothesized, a liberal RBC transfusion strategy improves clinically important outcomes, it will become standard practice. If a liberal RBC transfusion strategy is not shown to be superior to a restrictive strategy, the use of a restrictive strategy would be justified to preserve scarce resources, rationalize health expenditures and reduce complications related to transfusion. Defining the most effective RBC transfusion strategy in TBI patients will improve patient outcomes while providing the required evidence-base for a precious and scarce resource.

Conclusion

No consensus exists regarding appropriate transfusion strategies in patients with TBI. Unlike other critically ill populations in which restrictive transfusion thresholds prevail, clinicians treating TBI patients appear to favor the continued uncritical use of a liberal transfusion strategy in this vulnerable population, thus exposing patients to the potentially adverse side effects of blood products at an increased cost to the healthcare system. The scientific community has expressed the need for rigorous trials to inform evidence-driven guidelines from high-quality data on RBC transfusion in this population.

References

1. Myburgh JA, Cooper DJ, Finfer SR et al (2008) Australasian Traumatic Brain Injury Study. (traumatic brain injury) Investigators for the Australian and New Zealand Intensive Care Society Clinical Trials Group. Epidemiology and 12-month outcomes from traumatic brain injury in Australia and New Zealand. J Trauma 64:854–862
2. Turgeon AF, Lauzier F, Simard JF et al (2011) Mortality associated with withdrawal of life-sustaining therapy for patients with severe traumatic brain injury: a Canadian multicentre cohort study. CMAJ 183:1581–1588
3. World Health Organization (2012) The WHO strategy on research for health. http://www.who.int/phi/WHO_Strategy_on_research_for_health.pdf. Accessed 10 January 2018
4. SMARTRISK (2009) The economic burden of injury in Canada. http://www.parachutecanada.org/downloads/research/reports/EBI2009-Eng-Final.pdf. Accessed 10 January 2018
5. Carney N, Totten AM, O'Reilly C et al (2016) Guidelines for the management of severe traumatic brain injury, fourth edition. Neurosurgery 80:6–15
6. Walsh TS, Lee RJ, Maciver CR et al (2006) Anemia during and at discharge from intensive care: the impact of restrictive blood transfusion practice. Intensive Care Med 32:100–109
7. Scharte M, Fink MP (2003) Red blood cell physiology in critical illness. Crit Care Med 31:S651–S657
8. Rogiers P, Zhang H, Leeman M et al (1997) Erythropoietin response in blunted in critically ill patients. Intensive Care Med 23:159–162
9. Eyster E, Bernene J (1973) Nosocomial anemia. JAMA 223:73–74
10. Krafte-Jacobs B, Levetown ML, Bray GL et al (1994) Erythropoietin response to critical illness. Crit Care Med 22:821–826
11. Vincent J-L, Baron JF, Reinhart K et al (2002) Anemia and blood transfusion in critically ill patients. JAMA 288:1499–1507
12. Corwin HL, Gettinger A, Pearl RG et al (2004) The CRIT study: anemia and blood transfusion in the critically ill—current clinical practice in the United States. Crit Care Med 32:39–52
13. Carlson AP, Schermer CR, Lu SW (2006) Retrospective evaluation of anemia and transfusion in traumatic brain injury. J Trauma 61:46–56

14. Salim A, Hadjizacharia P, DuBose J et al (2008) Role of anemia in traumatic brain injury. J Am Coll Surg 207:398–406

15. Steyerberg EW, Mushkuidani N, Perel P et al (2008) Predicting outcome after traumatic brain injury: development and validation of international validation of prognostic scores based on admission characteristics. PLoS Med 5:1251–1261

16. Boutin A, Chassé M, Shemilt M et al (2016) Red blood cell transfusion in patients with traumatic brain injury: a systematic review and meta-analysis. Transfus Med Rev 30:15–24

17. Boutin A, Moore L, Lauzier F et al (2017) Transfusion of red blood cells in patients with traumatic brain injuries admitted to Canadian trauma health centres: a multicentre cohort study. BMJ Open 7:e14472

18. Agency for Healthcare Research and Quality (2013) Most Frequent Procedures Performed in U.S. Hospitals, 2011. HCUP Statistical Brief #165. https://www.hcup-us.ahrq.gov/reports/statbriefs/sb165.jsp. Accessed 10 January 2018

19. Rebel A, Ulatowski JA, Kwansa H et al (2003) Cerebrovascular response to decreased hematocrit: effect of cell-free hemoglobin, plasma viscosity, and CO2. Am J Physiol Heart Circ Physiol 285:1600–1608

20. Chodobski A, Zink BJ, Szmydynger-Chodobska J (2011) Blood-brain barrier pathophysiology in traumatic brain injury. Transl Stroke Res 2:492–516

21. Smith MJ, Stiefel MF, Magge S et al (2005) Packed red blood cell transfusion increases local cerebral oxygenation. Crit Care Med 33:1104–1108

22. Zygun DA, Nortje J, Hutchinson PJ et al (2009) The effect of red blood cell transfusion on cerebral oxygenation and metabolism after severe traumatic brain injury. Crit Care Med 37:1074–1078

23. Hébert PC, Wells G, Blajchman MA et al (1999) A multicenter, randomized, controlled clinical trial of transfusion requirements in critical care. Transfusion Requirements in Critical Care Investigators, Canadian Critical Care Trials Group. N Engl J Med 340:409–417

24. Lacroix J, Hébert PC, Hutchison JS et al (2007) Transfusion strategies for patients in pediatric intensive care units. N Engl J Med 356:1609–1619

25. Holst LB, Haase N, Wetterslev J et al (2014) Lower versus higher hemoglobin threshold for transfusion in septic shock. N Engl J Med 371:1381–1391

26. Murphy GJ, Pike K, Rogers CA et al (2015) Liberal or restrictive transfusion after cardiac surgery. N Engl J Med 372:997–1008

27. Carson JL, Stanworth SJ, Roubinian N et al (2016) Transfusion thresholds and other strategies for guiding allogeneic red blood cell transfusion. Cochrane Database Syst Rev 10:CD002042

28. Docherty AB, O'Donnell R, Brunskill S et al (2016) Effect of restrictive versus liberal transfusion strategies on outcomes in patients with cardiovascular disease in a non-cardiac surgery setting: systematic review and meta-analysis. BMJ 352:i1351

29. Desjardins P, Turgeon AF, Tremblay MH et al (2012) Hemoglobin levels and transfusions in neurocritically ill patients: a systematic review of comparative studies. Crit Care 16:R54

30. Naidech AM, Drescher J, Ault ML et al (2006) Higher hemoglobin is associated with less cerebral infarction, poor outcome, and death after subarachnoid hemorrhage. Neurosurgery 59:775–779

31. Robertson CS, Hannay HJ, Yamal JM et al (2014) Effect of erythropoietin and transfusion threshold on neurological recovery after traumatic brain injury: a randomized clinical trial. JAMA 312:36–47

32. Badenes R, Oddo M, Suarez JI et al (2017) Hemoglobin concentrations and RBC transfusion thresholds in patients with acute brain injury: an international survey. Crit Care 21:159

33. Sena MJ, Rivers RM, Muizelaar JP et al (2009) Transfusion practices for acute traumatic brain injury: a survey of physicians at US trauma centers. Intensive Care Med 35:480–488

34. Kramer AH, Diringer MN, Suarez JI et al (2011) Red blood cell transfusion in patients with subarachnoid hemorrhage: a multidisciplinary North American survey. Crit Care 15:R30

35. Kramer AH, Le Roux P (2012) Red blood cell transfusion and transfusion alternatives in traumatic brain injury. Curr Treat Options Neurol 14:150–163

36. Bellapart J, Boots R, Fraser J (2012) Physiopathology of anemia and transfusion thresholds in isolated head injury. J Trauma Acute Care Surg 73:997–1005
37. Roberts DJ, Zygun DA (2012) Anemia, red blood cell transfusion, and outcomes after severe traumatic brain injury. Crit Care 16:154
38. Utter GH, Shahlaie K, Zwienenberg-Lee M et al (2011) Anemia in the setting of traumatic brain injury: the arguments for and against liberal transfusion. J Neurotrauma 28:155–165
39. Kumar MA (2012) Red blood cell transfusion in the neurological ICU. Neurotherapeutics 9:56–64

Part XI
Acute Cerebral Concerns

Systemic Inflammation and Cerebral Dysfunction

A. M. Peters van Ton, P. Pickkers, and W. F. Abdo

Introduction

Advances in patient care over recent decades have resulted in lower mortality rates in the intensive care unit (ICU) despite an aging population and increased disease severity. As a consequence, the expanding group of patients who survive critical illness [1] reveals that surviving critical illness is associated with a wide range of long-lasting negative health outcomes. It is now increasingly recognized that survivors of intensive care may experience physical and cognitive impairment as well as psychological symptoms, which all negatively affect daily functioning and health-related quality of life.

In 2010, the term 'post-intensive care syndrome' (PCIS) was introduced by the Society of Critical Care Medicine to describe the complex of "new or worsening impairments in physical, cognitive or mental health status arising after critical illness and persisting beyond acute care hospitalization" [2]. This term can be applied to both survivors (PICS) and family members of survivors (PICS-F). Individuals with PICS experience symptoms of varying severity and persistence. Although the exact incidence of PICS among ICU survivors is unknown, several studies have shown considerable incidences of impairment in the separate domains (Fig. 1). Especially in elderly patients, a hospitalization may introduce a subsequent downhill course in cognitive abilities. In order to develop neuroprotective interventions it is essential to understand the pathophysiology of cerebral dysfunction following critical illness.

A. M. Peters van Ton · P. Pickkers · W. F. Abdo (✉)
Department of Intensive Care Medicine, Radboud University Medical Center
Nijmegen, Netherlands
e-mail: f.abdo@radboudumc.nl

© Springer International Publishing AG 2018
J.-L. Vincent (ed.), *Annual Update in Intensive Care and Emergency Medicine 2018*,
Annual Update in Intensive Care and Emergency Medicine,
https://doi.org/10.1007/978-3-319-73670-9_37

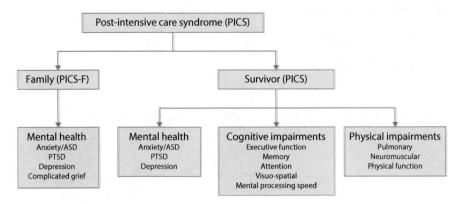

Fig. 1 Domains affected in post-intensive care syndrome (PICS). From [2] with permission. *ASD*: acute stress disorder; *PTSD*: posttraumatic stress disorder

Acute Cerebral Dysfunction

During critical illness, acute cerebral dysfunction often occurs and varies from sickness behavior, mild fluctuating cognitive dysfunction to mental state changes (delirium) to coma. The incidence of delirium in ICU patients ranges from 11 to 89%, depending on ICU admission diagnoses and delirium subtype [3]. In patients with sepsis, in the absence of direct central nervous syndrome (CNS) infection, structural abnormality or other types of encephalopathy, this acute brain dysfunction is called sepsis-associated encephalopathy. Sepsis-associated encephalopathy is reported in up to 70% of patients with sepsis [4]. Surgery is also associated with cerebral dysfunction in the acute postoperative phase which may clinically appear as postoperative delirium. Both delirium and sepsis-associated encephalopathy are associated with increased morbidity and mortality. Although sepsis-associated encephalopathy and postoperative brain dysfunction were long regarded as transient and reversible problems in the acute phase, it has now become clear that serious long-term sequelae can ensue.

Long-term Cerebral Dysfunction

An important long-term complication of critical illness is cognitive impairment. Although elderly patients are especially prone to this, younger and relatively healthy patients are also at risk for cognitive decline following an ICU admission. Studies report that 4–62% of patients develop cognitive impairment after a follow-up of 2–156 months [5]. One out of four patients had cognitive impairment 12 months after critical illness that was similar in severity to that of patients with mild Alzheimer's disease and one out of three had an impairment severity typically associated with moderate traumatic brain injury (TBI). Retrospectively, only 6% of patients had evidence of mild-to-moderate cognitive impairment before ICU admission suggesting that the profound cognitive deficits were new in the majority of patients [6]. Not surprisingly, most studies in this field are limited by the lack of a baseline assessment of cognitive status prior to ICU admission. However, data from a longitudinal study show that patients who experienced acute care hospitalization and critical illness hospitalization had a greater likelihood of cognitive decline compared to those who had no hospitalization [7]. The finding that every hospitalization, not only admission to the ICU, may lead to a substantial cognitive decline in the elderly after controlling for disease severity and prehospital cognitive status was confirmed in another longitudinal study [8]. The negative effect of critical illness on cognition is accompanied by (micro)structural anomalies in brain imaging, such as hippocampal atrophy [9, 10], smaller brain volumes [10] and reduced white matter integrity [11].

Patients who survived severe sepsis were three times more likely to develop cognitive impairment than patients who were hospitalized for reasons other than sepsis [12]. Mild and severe inflammatory events among patients admitted to the ICU (n = 10,348) both independently predicted the risk of developing dementia within 3 years after ICU discharge [13]. Likewise, similar trajectories of global cognitive decline were found in patients hospitalized for severe sepsis, for pneumonia or for other types of infections. Patients from all three infectious groups were twice as likely to develop dementia in the 5–10 years after their disease regardless of the severity of the infection. The mild-to-moderate neurocognitive deficits after an infection may persist for years after hospital discharge and seem to be newly acquired in the majority of patients. Even a higher exposure to simple infections in cohorts of community dwelling people showed a strong association with cognitive decline [14].

Table 1 Incidences of acute and long-term cerebral dysfunction and likelihoods of developing dementia after critical illness, sepsis and surgery

	Incidence	Increased likelihood of developing dementia
Acute brain dysfunction		
– Post-ICU admission	11–89% [3]	
– Post-sepsis	up to 70% [4]	
Long-term brain dysfunction		
– Post-ICU admission	4–62% [5]	Yes, HR 1.6–2.3 [7, 13]
– Post-sepsis		Yes, HR 2.0 [13]
– Post-infection		Yes, HR 1.9 [13]
– Post-cardiac surgery	20–70% in first week postoperatively; 10–40% after six weeks [15]	
– Post-non-cardiac surgery	26–41% in first week postoperatively; 5–13% after 3 months [16, 17]	

HR: hazard ratio

In surgical patients long-term cognitive impairment occurs as well and is described as postoperative cognitive dysfunction or POCD. This is characterized by deterioration in memory, attention and speed of information processing. The incidence of these neurological complications increases with older age and the invasiveness of the surgery. The incidence of postoperative cognitive decline after cardiac surgery ranges from 20–70% in the first week postoperatively. This decreases to 10–40% after six weeks and remains at this level thereafter [15]. In major noncardiac surgery the incidence is, in the majority of studies, slightly lower [16, 17]. Table 1 presents the incidences of cognitive decline and the likelihood of developing dementia in the different study populations mentioned above.

Pathophysiology

Non-inflammatory Causes

Presumed pathophysiological mechanisms related to cerebral dysfunction following critical illness or major surgery include hemodynamic alterations leading to hypoperfusion of the brain, watershed distribution infarcts, leukoencephalopathy, microembolization and microbleeds, along with cellular damage, mitochondrial and endothelial dysfunction, disturbances in neurotransmission and calcium homeostasis and blood-brain barrier disruption.

Sedatives and anesthetics have been presumed to play a role in the etiology of brain dysfunction although animal models have shown that surgery itself rather than anesthetics triggers a neurocognitive decline [18, 19]. Accordingly, clinical research on the relationship between anesthesia and POCD has remained inconclusive [20].

An exaggerated immune system activation is present in practically all ICU patients, irrespective of admission diagnosis or type of major surgery. There has been a surge of research interest in the link between the immune system and brain involvement in the critically ill. This concept has gained more ground as immune system activation has also been found to play an important role in the pathogenesis of neurodegenerative diseases characterized by cognitive decline, such as Alzheimer's disease. Since optimizing hemodynamics is already part of standard critical care and there is presumably not so much more to gain, looking into other pathophysiologic mechanisms, such as an immune-mediated pathway, may help to identify new therapeutic strategies.

Neuroinflammation

Microglia and astrocytes are the main resident innate immune cells in the CNS. The distribution of microglia throughout the brain is heterogeneous, as is the morphology of the cells among and within brain regions [21]. Microglia share common features of myeloid lineage cells and are able to secrete a wide variety of immunomodulatory molecules, which signal neighboring and circulating cells. Microglia exhibit at least four functions: surveillance, neuroprotection, phagocytosis and toxicity. In the healthy brain, resting microglia monitor the brain environment. Microglia and astrocytes are activated upon CNS cell injury or systemic inflammatory stimuli and on activation undergo a transformation into an amoeboid morphology and present upregulation of surface molecules. Depending on the integration of regulatory signals, microglia can acquire either a neurotoxic, pro-inflammatory phenotype (M1-like) upon activation or a neuroprotective, anti-inflammatory phenotype (M2-like). M1-like microglia produce pro-inflammatory cytokines and enzymes that promote sustained tissue inflammation, generating a detrimental microenvironment for neurons. In contrast, M2-like microglia secrete neurotrophic factors and anti-inflammatory mediators and are associated with the resolution of inflammation and tissue repair [22]. However, this division into distinct microglial phenotypes has become more debatable recently [23].

Low-grade chronically activated microglia are present in neurodegenerative diseases, but also in healthy aging. Microglia with a chronic, low-grade activated state have been called primed microglia. Research in animals [24], data from healthy humans [25], and post-mortem brain tissue of patients with severe systemic inflammation [26, 27], show that systemic inflammation is a strong trigger that activates the resident innate immune cells of the brain. Their activation and subsequent inflammatory cascade in the brain tissue, is called 'neuroinflammation' (Fig. 2). During systemic inflammation, systemic inflammatory mediators can enter brain tissue due to a disrupted blood-brain barrier, but also through several parts of the brain that lack a blood-brain barrier. In response to these inflammatory cues, microglia are readily activated. Activated microglia are involved in regulating brain development and facilitate repair. However, in circumstances where primed microglia exist, cytokines entering the CNS may lead to overactivation of primed microglia. This may subsequently result in an exaggerated neuroinflammatory cascade, disrupting normal homeostasis and cell function and resulting in neuronal cell loss [28, 29]. Also, secretion of inflammatory mediators leads to changes in blood-brain barrier permeability and infiltration of peripheral immune cells into the CNS parenchyma. Overactive microglia induce detrimental neurotoxic effects by the excess secretion of a large variety of cytotoxic factors, such as superoxide, nitric oxide (NO), tumor necrosis factor-α (TNF-α) and glutamate [28, 30]. The finding that overactivation of primed microglia can lead to neurotoxicity corroborates with the fact that the elderly and patients with pre-existing cognitive failure, i.e., states associated with primed microglia, are most likely to suffer from long-term cognitive and functional decline after severe systemic inflammation.

Astrocytes also play a role in the neuroinflammatory response. Upon CNS injury, astrocytes become reactive and migrate to the damaged site to form a glial scar; this is called reactive astrogliosis. Astrocytes, as well as microglia, have two contrasting properties or phenotypes during inflammation. On the one hand, astrogliosis can have a neuroprotective role by preserving bioenergetics and trophic support, preventing excitotoxicity, and decreasing oxidative stress and apoptosis in neurons. Furthermore, astrocytes can downregulate microglial activation by secretion of anti-inflammatory substances, resembling a M2 phenotype. On the other hand, stimula-

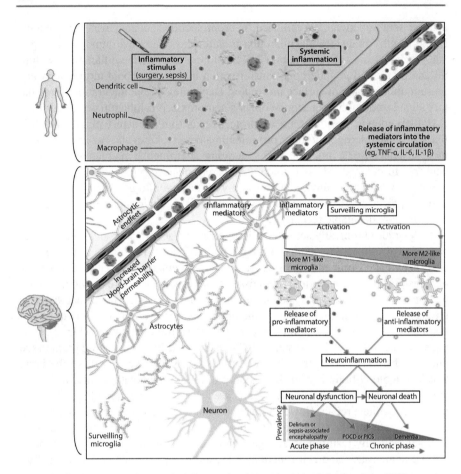

Fig. 2 Pathophysiology of systemic inflammation-induced cerebral dysfunction. *PICS*: post-intensive care syndrome; *POCD*: postoperative cognitive dysfunction; *TNF*: tumor necrosis factor; *IL*: interleukin

tion of astrocytes can enhance the production of reactive oxygen species (ROS), TNF-α, interleukin (IL)-1β, Il-6 and glutamate, thereby inducing neuronal loss [30]. Interestingly, activated astrocytes produce chemokines that are involved in the recruitment of microglia, monocytes, macrophages, T-cells and dendritic cells into the inflamed areas of the CNS. This results in a more complex and long-lasting immune response during neuroinflammation [31]. Finally, the presence of numerous astrocyte end-feet close to the blood-brain barrier allows for rapid regulation of blood-brain barrier permeability.

Although microglial and astrocyte activation is crucial for host defense and neuronal survival, the overactivation of microglia appears to account for detrimental and neurotoxic consequences. Understanding the pathophysiological role of neuroinflammation in the development of cerebral dysfunction after critical illness has become a recent focus of research in order to facilitate the discovery of novel therapeutic targets.

Measures of Neuroinflammation

Several methods to measure neuroinflammation are available. Unfortunately, the majority of the previous studies that have been performed were histological studies that require an invasive brain biopsy or a post-mortem specimen. Therefore most work has been done in rodents [24] and a few post-mortem human studies [26, 27] in which microglial activation in the brain following exposure to pathogens was assessed immunohistochemically, with flow-cytometry, quantitative polymerase chain reaction (qPCR) or Western blotting.

Until recently, due to the invasiveness of acquiring brain tissue, *in vivo* studies in humans were limited to the measurement of immune mediators in cerebrospinal fluid (CSF). Although CSF surrounds the brain and (waste)products of intracerebral biochemical pathways may end up in the CSF, analysis does not inform about the origin of these products. Recently, *in vivo* studies in humans have been extended with the use of cerebral microdialysis catheters, especially in patients with subarachnoid hemorrhage and TBI. These catheters are implanted in brain tissue and sample continuously free, unbound analyte concentrations in the extracellular fluid of the brain. Advantages of microdialysis are that sampling without fluid loss is possible due to the constant replacement of the sampling fluid, and the semipermeable membrane prevents cells, cellular debris and proteins from entering the dialysate. However, a limitation for immunological research is that implantation of the microdialysis catheter may alter tissue morphology (disruption of the blood-brain barrier) and may induce an inflammatory response [32]; therefore an optimal time window should be kept after probe insertion and before measurements.

Recently several nuclear imaging tracers have been developed that can quantitatively measure microglial and astrocytic activation *in vivo* and non-invasively, by targeting the mitochondrial 18 kDa translocator protein (TSPO). TSPO is localized primarily in the outer mitochondrial membrane of steroid-synthesizing tissue, including the brain. One of its main functions is the transport into mitochondria the substrate, cholesterol, which is required for steroid synthesis [33]. TSPO expression is minimal in healthy brain. Activation of microglia and astrocytes resulting in neuroinflammation is accompanied by markedly increased TSPO expression on these cells and, therefore, TSPO is currently under investigation as a biomarker of neuroinflammation. Many animal experiments have shown that different TSPO binding tracers can sensitively image microglial and astrocytic activation [33]. Interestingly, *in vitro* studies in mice showed that TSPO expression was selectively increased in microglia with the M1 phenotype, but not in microglia with the M2 phenotype. In agreement, TSPO transcript levels were not induced in an anti-inflammatory brain environment [34]. Nuclear imaging of neuroinflammation with a TSPO ligand therefore measures the deleterious pro-inflammatory activation of innate immune cells in the brain; however this should be confirmed in human *in vivo* studies.

The first study in humans using a TSPO tracer was published in 1995. Subsequently many studies in humans have been performed using TSPO tracers. The most commonly studied TSPO binding tracer is the first generation tracer, [^{11}C]-PK11195. Although [^{11}C]-PK11195 has been used in many human positron emission tomography (PET) studies as a marker of activated microglia for about two decades, it has high non-specific binding, high binding to plasma proteins and relatively poor blood-brain permeability. Furthermore the kinetic behavior of [^{11}C]-PK11195 limits the quantification of PET findings and hence the amount of microglial activation. Recently, several second generation tracers have been developed that overcome most of these drawbacks, have better pharmacokinetic and pharmacologic properties and have a much higher affinity to the TSPO receptor [33, 35]. As such, they have a superior ability to specifically image *in vivo* neuroinflammation. These tracers have been used in several human studies where they demonstrated increased microglial activation in several neurological diseases, such as stroke, TBI, Alzheimer's and Parkinson's disease and amyotrophic lateral sclerosis compared to healthy controls, which supports the role of neuroinflammation in the pathogenesis of these conditions.

Further microglial targets currently being explored for non-invasive imaging include the P2X7 receptor, the cannabinoid CB2 receptor, the cyclooxygenase-1 and -2 enzyme and matrix metalloproteinases [35].

Nuclear imaging of microglial activation is a safe and non-invasive method to assess the neuroinflammatory response in humans *in vivo*. It enables translational research, which will add to the understanding of the pathophysiology of neuroinflammation due to critical illnesses and its correlations with clinical outcomes in the next few years. Furthermore it may serve as a biomarker to evaluate therapy response in proof-of-principle phase II trials.

Neuroinflammation in Neurological Diseases

Although the brain was long regarded as an immune privileged organ, a strong association between the immune system and 'non-inflammatory' neurological diseases, such as stroke, TBI, Alzheimer's disease, Parkinson's disease, amyotrophic lateral sclerosis and Huntington's disease has been established over the last three decades [36].

Epidemiological studies have shown that infections, regardless of the severity, increase the risk of developing dementia in subsequent years by 2–3 fold [12–14, 37]. Alzheimer's disease is the most common cause of dementia in the elderly. Neuropathologically, it is characterized by the presence of senile plaques and neurofibrillary tangles, which are mainly composed of amyloid beta (Aβ) peptide and tau proteins, respectively. The current amyloid cascade-inflammatory hypothesis for the pathological mechanism of Alzheimer's disease proposes that Aβ induces an inflammatory response that is enhanced by the presence of tau. In Alzheimer's disease, microglia are not able to clear the excess of amyloid and since Aβ is a ligand for the Toll-like receptor (TLR)-4 receptor, a neuroinflammatory response is induced [38]. Indeed, nuclear imaging with TSPO tracers have shown that *in vivo* neuroinflammation correlates with cognitive decline in patients with neurodegenerative diseases [39].

Neuroinflammation in Sepsis

Sepsis models in rodents have shown that peripheral inflammatory stimuli cause microglial activation, concomitant with increases in inflammatory parameters in the brain. An increase in mRNA expression or protein levels of TLR-2 and TLR-4, TNF-α and IL-1β was associated with microglial activation [24]. Peripheral inflammatory stimuli resulted in deficits in cognitive performance on behavioral tests. Blood-brain barrier integrity was assessed using different approaches in several animal studies, however with conflicting results. Another sepsis model called cecal ligation and puncture (CLP), in which animals develop an abdominal sepsis due to fecal peritonitis, induces a neuroinflammatory response, also accompanied by cognitive impairment. This sepsis model has identified a role for the CD40-CD40 ligand pathway [40] and Nox-2 derived ROS [41] in the development of cognitive impairment after sepsis.

In humans, brain tissue of patients who died from sepsis showed a significant increase in activated microglia in the gray matter compared to non-septic controls [26]. Post-mortem brain tissue from patients with septic shock showed hemorrhages, hypercoagulability syndrome, micro-abscesses, multifocal necrotizing leukoencephalopathy and ischemia. Neuronal apoptosis was more pronounced in the autonomic nuclei of septic patients. In the five small brain areas studied, only occasional activated microglia and very few reactive astrocytes were revealed by immunostaining [27].

In healthy volunteers, endotoxemia significantly increased tracer binding to TSPO with 30–60% compared to baseline, 3 h after lipopolysaccharide (LPS) administration, demonstrating microglial activation throughout the brain. This was accompanied by an increase in serum levels of inflammatory cytokines, vital sign changes and sickness symptoms [25]. This is the first, and to date the only, *in vivo* evidence for robust increases in microglial activation after a systemic inflammatory stimulus. Despite this interesting finding, the human endotoxemia model is a simplified reproduction of a short-lived limited systemic inflammatory response compared to the complexity and duration of the inflammatory state during sepsis in the ICU population. Although the neuroinflammatory hypothesis is scientifically accepted, *in vivo* human data supporting the role of neuroinflammation in infected patients are still lacking.

Neuroinflammation in Postoperative Cognitive Dysfunction

Epidemiological studies have shown that POCD may occur following all types of surgery, but with higher incidences in cardiac surgery compared to non-cardiac surgery patients [15–17]. Rodent studies have shown that postoperative microglial activation and increases in systemic and hippocampal pro-inflammatory cytokines are associated with postoperative impairment of spatial and contextual learning and memory [42]. Inhibition of central pro-inflammatory cytokine signaling was shown to attenuate postoperative memory impairment in rodents [42]. The association between the peripheral inflammatory response to surgery and POCD was confirmed in patients [43].

In rats, POCD after cardiac surgery affects different cognitive domains compared to POCD after non-cardiac surgery and may therefore be more extensive rather than more severe [42]. Moreover, the effects of abdominal surgery seemed to be limited to hippocampal brain regions, whereas cardiac surgery was associated with more widespread alterations in the brain.

Interestingly, a recent study in patients undergoing prostatectomy was the first to explore, *in vivo,* the trajectory of microglial activation. Surprisingly, patients showed a global downregulation of TSPO tracer binding at 3 to 4 days postoperatively compared to baseline, which recovered or even increased relative to baseline after 3 months [44]. This unexpected result coincided with a transient reduction in immunoreactivity of peripheral blood cells, which is a well-known hallmark of an immunosuppressed state known as immunoparalysis [45]. Immunoparalysis has been described in patients with sepsis and trauma and likely contributes to the high mortality in critically ill patients. Indeed, critically ill patients who survive the initial cytokine response following sepsis, surgery or trauma often suffer from severe and sometimes lethal secondary infections due to this immunosuppressed state. This study [44] adds to the growing literature that links innate immune responses to neurological conditions and illustrates that immunoparalysis is not only a systemic phenomenon, but may also be present in the brain. This is still largely uncharted territory and needs confirmation in different patient groups. One may argue that the downregulated cerebral immune response may represent an endogenous protective mechanism to prevent immunopathology to the brain [46]. If so, reversing immunoparalysis by boosting the innate immune response in the acute phase of sepsis or post-surgery may be deleterious for the brain.

Future Perspectives

Although many studies on systemic inflammation-induced neuroinflammation have been performed, the majority of the evidence comes from animal studies. The trajectory of neuroinflammation after a systemic inflammatory stimulus in humans remains largely unclear. *In vivo* molecular imaging of microglial activity enables us to quantify the neuroinflammatory response non-invasively. However, the timing of PET data acquisition may be crucial especially when immunoparalysis indeed plays a role. Future translational studies should therefore focus on the trajectory of microglial activation after different peripheral inflammatory stimuli in humans *in vivo* to discover the correct timing of measurement and to elucidate the role of immunoparalysis in the neuroinflammatory response. Furthermore, the relationship of neuroinflammation and clinical outcomes, such as sepsis-associated encephalopathy, postoperative delirium, cognitive decline and deficits in other domains of the PICS, should be confirmed in patients who survived their critical illness. Although animal studies and studies in patients with neurodegenerative diseases suggest positive correlations with cerebral dysfunction and neuroinflammation, this has not yet been established in critically ill patients. Longitudinal prospective cohort studies with brain imaging data, neuropsychological examinations and monitoring of infectious events will add to the understanding of the cognitive effects and structural consequences to the brain during systemic inflammation. In order to discover novel therapeutic targets to prevent or treat cerebral dysfunction following systemic inflammation, it is essential that we improve our understanding of the biochemical pathways that are dysregulated during a neuroinflammatory response.

Promising Biochemical Compounds

Although the step from bench to bedside still has to be made for patients with states of systemic inflammation, several compounds are currently already under investigation, especially for other neurological conditions in which neuroinflammation may contribute to its pathogenesis. With the hypothesis that reducing neuroinflammation would improve patient outcomes, three approaches can be distinguished. First, reducing the (peripheral) systemic inflammatory stimulus could limit the detrimental neuroinflammatory response. The cerebral effects of registered drugs, such as steroids, non-steroid anti-inflammatory drugs (NSAIDs), TNF-α inhibitors (etanercept, infliximab) and IL-1 receptor antagonist (IL-1ra) are currently being investigated for this purpose [47]. However, in patients with critical illness, reducing the systemic inflammatory response, especially during the immunoparalytic period, could lead to severe secondary infections [45], hence this might not be the best approach in this population. Second, limiting the neuroinflammatory response itself by interfering in its pathways or capturing the neurotoxic end products of the response may benefit the inflamed brain. Examples of this treatment strategy currently under investigation are the following blood-brain barrier-crossing agents: anti-oxidants, erythropoietin, tetracyclines (minocycline, doxycycline), statins, cannabinoids and IL-1ra. The latter compound works on both treatment strategies mentioned above, because IL-1 is the cytokine that initiates macrophage activation [48]. As microglia are the tissue-resident macrophages of the brain, IL-1ra would antagonize both the peripheral immune response and the neuroinflammatory response. Third, indirect neuroprotection could be achieved through blood-brain barrier preservation by vascular endothelial growth factor (VEGF) inhibitors or neurokinin-1 (NK1) receptor blockade [47].

With respect to distinct microglial activity, promoting anti-inflammatory, while reducing pro-inflammatory microglial activity, may represent a viable and selective strategy to prevent neurotoxic effects during systemic inflammation. Targeting against the nuclear factor-κB (NF-κB) signaling pathway or enhancing the activation of cAMP-responsive element-binding protein (CREB) could selectively modulate microglia polarization to the M2 phenotype [49]. These potential therapeutic solutions are still far from clinical implementation. However, there are already some things clinicians can do or consider in the follow-up of ICU survivors. Physicians awareness of the physical, cognitive and mental impairments ICU survivors may face is important. Cognitive rehabilitation or treatment of psychiatric difficulties that could be driving the development of cognitive complaints could help to improve neuropsychological functioning [50]. Although appealing to consider, these approaches have not been properly studied in the context of cognitive impairment due to PICS.

Conclusion

Patients who survive severe systemic inflammatory states on the ICU are at risk of developing cerebral dysfunction. This includes acute cerebral dysfunction, such as sepsis-associated encephalopathy or postoperative delirium, but also long-term cognitive decline and an increased risk of dementia. Pathophysiologically, there is overwhelming evidence that systemic inflammation can induce an excessive neuroinflammatory response, which is characterized by the overactivation of M1-phenotypic or pro-inflammatory microglia and astrocytes. These innate immune cells of the brain secrete immune mediators and other compounds that can be neurotoxic to the brain and lead subsequently to cognitive impairment. This neuroinflammation has been associated with a variety of neurodegenerative diseases. Recently, novel nuclear imaging tracers have been developed that can quantitatively assess microglial activation in humans *in vivo*. However, data on the trajectory of the neuroinflammatory response after systemic inflammation in humans *in vivo* are currently lacking, as is the relationship with clinical outcomes, such as delirium and post-ICU cognitive impairment. Translational research to further unravel the pathophysiological mechanism of systemic inflammation-induced cerebral dysfunction is essential in order to facilitate the discovery and further development of novel therapeutic compounds. Clinically, physicians should be aware of the impairments ICU survivors may face following their critical illness and one may consider cognitive rehabilitation to improve neuropsychological functioning.

Acknowledgements

Dr. W. F. Abdo is supported by a research grant from the Netherlands Organization for Health Research and Development (ZonMw Clinical Fellowship Grant 90715610). This funding agency had no role in the concept, design and writing of this chapter, nor the collection or analysis of the literature presented.

References

1. Desai SV, Law TJ, Needham DM (2011) Long-term complications of critical care. Crit Care Med 39:371–379
2. Needham DM, Davidson J, Cohen H et al (2012) Improving long-term outcomes after discharge from intensive care unit: report from a stakeholders' conference. Crit Care Med 40:502–509
3. van den Boogaard M, Schoonhoven L, van der Hoeven JG, van Achterberg T, Pickkers P (2012) Incidence and short-term consequences of delirium in critically ill patients: a prospective observational cohort study. Int J Nurs Stud 49:775–783
4. Widmann CN, Heneka MT (2014) Long-term cerebral consequences of sepsis. Lancet Neurol 13:630–636
5. Wolters AE, Slooter AJ, van der Kooi AW, van Dijk D (2013) Cognitive impairment after intensive care unit admission: a systematic review. Intensive Care Med 39:376–386
6. Pandharipande PP, Girard TD, Jackson JC et al (2013) Long-term cognitive impairment after critical illness. N Engl J Med 369:1306–1316
7. Ehlenbach WJ, Hough CL, Crane PK et al (2010) Association between acute care and critical illness hospitalization and cognitive function in older adults. JAMA 303:763–770
8. Wilson RS, Hebert LE, Scherr PA, Dong X, Leurgens SE, Evans DA (2012) Cognitive decline after hospitalization in a community population of older persons. Neurology 78:950–956
9. Semmler A, Widmann CN, Okulla T et al (2013) Persistent cognitive impairment, hippocampal atrophy and EEG changes in sepsis survivors. J Neurol Neurosurg Psychiatry 84:62–69
10. Gunther ML, Morandi A, Krauskopf E et al (2012) The association between brain volumes, delirium duration, and cognitive outcomes in intensive care unit survivors: the VISIONS cohort magnetic resonance imaging study. Crit Care Med 40:2022–2032
11. Morandi A, Rogers BP, Gunther ML et al (2012) The relationship between delirium duration, white matter integrity, and cognitive impairment in intensive care unit survivors as determined by diffusion tensor imaging: the VISIONS prospective cohort magnetic resonance imaging study. Crit Care Med 40:2182–2189
12. Iwashyna TJ, Ely EW, Smith DM, Langa KM (2010) Long-term cognitive impairment and functional disability among survivors of severe sepsis. JAMA 304:1787–1794
13. Guerra C, Hua M, Wunsch H (2015) Risk of a diagnosis of dementia for elderly medicare beneficiaries after intensive care. Anesthesiology 123:1105–1112
14. Katan M, Moon YP, Paik MC, Sacco RL, Wright CB, Elkind MS (2013) Infectious burden and cognitive function: the Northern Manhattan Study. Neurology 80:1209–1215
15. Bruce K, Smith JA, Yelland G, Robinson S (2008) The impact of cardiac surgery on cognition. Stress Health 24:249–266
16. Monk TG, Weldon BC, Garvan CW et al (2008) Predictors of cognitive dysfunction after major noncardiac surgery. Anesthesiology 108:18–30
17. Moller JT, Cluitmans P, Rasmussen LS et al (1998) Long-term postoperative cognitive dysfunction in the elderly ISPOCD1 study. ISPOCD investigators. International Study of Post-Operative Cognitive Dysfunction. Lancet 351:857–861
18. Cao XZ, Ma H, Wang JK et al (2010) Postoperative cognitive deficits and neuroinflammation in the hippocampus triggered by surgical trauma are exacerbated in aged rats. Prog Neuropsychopharmacol Biol Psychiatry 34:1426–1432
19. Wan Y, Xu J, Ma D, Zeng Y, Cibelli M, Maze M (2007) Postoperative impairment of cognitive function in rats: a possible role for cytokine-mediated inflammation in the hippocampus. Anesthesiology 106:436–443
20. Sauer AM, Kalkman C, van Dijk D (2009) Postoperative cognitive decline. J Anesth 23:256–259
21. Mittelbronn M, Dietz K, Schluesener HK, Meyermann R (2001) Local distribution of microglia in the normal adult human central nervous system differs by up to one order of magnitude. Acta Neuropathol 101:249–255

22. Kettenmann H, Hanisch UK, Noda M, Verkhratsky A (2011) Physiology of microglia. Physiol Rev 91:461–553

23. Ransohoff RM (2016) A polarizing question: do M1 and M2 microglia exist? Nat Neurosci 19:987–991

24. Hoogland IC, Houbolt C, van Westerloo DJ, van Gool WA, van de Beek D (2015) Systemic inflammation and microglial activation: systematic review of animal experiments. J Neuroinflammation 12:114

25. Sandiego CM, Gallezot JD, Pittman B et al (2015) Imaging robust microglial activation after lipopolysaccharide administration in humans with PET. Proc Natl Acad Sci U S A 112:12468–12473

26. Lemstra AW, Groen in't Woud JC, Hoozemans JJ et al (2007) Microglia activation in sepsis: a case-control study. J Neuroinflammation 4:4

27. Sharshar T, Annane D, de la Grandmaison GL, Brouland JP, Hopkinson NS, Francoise G (2004) The neuropathology of septic shock. Brain Pathol 14:21–33

28. Bloc KML, Zecca L, Hong JS (2007) Microglia-mediated neurotoxicity: uncovering the molecular mechanisms. Nat Rev Neurosci 8:57–69

29. Godbout JP, Chen J, Abraham J et al (2005) Exaggerated neuroinflammation and sickness behavior in aged mice following activation of the peripheral innate immune system. Faseb J 19:1329–1331

30. Michels M, Steckert AV, Quevedo J, Barichello T, Dal-Pizzol F (2015) Mechanisms of long-term cognitive dysfunction of sepsis: from blood-borne leukocytes to glial cells. Intensive Care Med Exp 3:30

31. Gonzalez H, Elgueta D, Montoya A, Pacheco R (2014) Neuroimmune regulation of microglial activity involved in neuroinflammation and neurodegenerative diseases. J Neuroimmunol 274:1–13

32. Carson BP, McCormack WG, Conway C et al (2015) An in vivo microdialysis characterization of the transient changes in the interstitial dialysate concentration of metabolites and cytokines in human skeletal muscle in response to insertion of a microdialysis probe. Cytokine 71:327–333

33. Rupprecht R, Papadopoulos V, Rammes G et al (2010) Translocator protein (18 kDa) (TSPO) as a therapeutic target for neurological and psychiatric disorders. Nat Rev Drug Discov 9(12):971–988

34. Beckers L, Ory D, Geric I et al (2017) Increased expression of translocator protein (tspo) marks pro-inflammatory microglia but does not predict neurodegeneration. Mol Imaging Biol. https://doi.org/10.1007/s11307-017-1099-1 (Jul 10, Epub ahead of print)

35. Jacobs AH, Tavitian B (2012) Noninvasive molecular imaging of neuroinflammation. J Cereb Blood Flow Metab 32:1393–1415

36. Lehnardt S (2010) Innate immunity and neuroinflammation in the CNS: the role of microglia in Toll-like receptor-mediated neuronal injury. Glia 58:253–263

37. Tate JA, Snitz BE, Alvarez KA et al (2014) Infection hospitalization increases risk of dementia in the elderly. Crit Care Med 42:1037–1046

38. Bolos M, Perea JR, Avila J (2017) Alzheimer's disease as an inflammatory disease. Biomol Concepts 8:37–43

39. Stefaniak J, O'Brien J (2016) Imaging of neuroinflammation in dementia: a review. J Neurol Neurosurg Psychiatry 87:21–28

40. Michels M, Danielski LG, Vieira A et al (2015) CD40-CD40 ligand pathway is a major component of acute neuroinflammation and contributes to long-term cognitive dysfunction after sepsis. Mol Med 21:219–226

41. Hernandes MS, D'Avila JC, Trevelin SC et al (2014) The role of Nox2-derived ROS in the development of cognitive impairment after sepsis. J Neuroinflammation 11:36

42. Hovens IB, van Leeuwen BL, Mariani MA, Kraneveld AD, Schoemaker RG (2016) Postoperative cognitive dysfunction and neuroinflammation; Cardiac surgery and abdominal surgery are not the same. Brain Behav Immun 54:178–193

43. Peng L, Xu L, Ouyang W (2013) Role of peripheral inflammatory markers in postoperative cognitive dysfunction (POCD): a meta-analysis. PLoS One 8:e79624
44. Forsberg A, Cervenka S, Jonsson Fagerlund M et al (2017) The immune response of the human brain to abdominal surgery. Ann Neurol 81:572–582
45. Leentjens J, Kox M, van der Hoeven JG, Netea MG, Pickkers P (2013) Immunotherapy for the adjunctive treatment of sepsis: from immunosuppression to immunostimulation. Time for a paradigm change? Am J Respir Crit Care Med 187:1287–1293
46. Peters van Ton AM, Kox M, Pickkers P, Abdo WF (2017) Reduced glial activity after surgery: a sign of immunoparalysis of the brain? Ann Neurol 82:152
47. Hellewell S, Semple BD, Morganti-Kossmann MC (2016) Therapies negating neuroinflammation after brain trauma. Brain Res 1640(Pt A):36–56
48. Dinarello CA, Simon A, van der Meer JW (2012) Treating inflammation by blocking interleukin-1 in a broad spectrum of diseases. Nat Rev Drug Discov 11:633–652
49. Xia CY, Zhang S, Gao Y, Wang ZZ, Chen NH (2015) Selective modulation of microglia polarization to M2 phenotype for stroke treatment. Int Immunopharmacol 25:377–382
50. Jutte JE, Erb CT, Jackson JC (2015) Physical, cognitive, and psychological disability following critical illness: what is the risk? Semin Respir Crit Care Med 36:943–958

Opening a Window to the Injured Brain: Non-invasive Neuromonitoring with Quantitative Pupillometry

D. Solari, J.-P. Miroz, and M. Oddo

Introduction

Pupillary examination is an essential component of neurological follow-up in critically ill patients, which has crucial diagnostic and prognostic value [1]. The anatomical location of the oculomotor nuclei in the midbrain, closely related to the medial part of the temporal lobe, and the peripheral trajectory of the pupillomotor fibers along the third cranial nerve, make these structures extremely sensitive to compression [2]. Any form of severe brain injury (trauma, hypoxia/ischemia, hemorrhage) that causes brainstem compression may therefore lead to alterations in pupil size (anisocoria) and reactivity [3].

Despite its undisputable role, in clinical practice, pupillary examination has predominantly relied on pupil gauge penlights. The accuracy of these standard devices may be limited by several factors (e.g., influence of changing ambient lighting, examiner visual acuity and experience, the level of patient alertness and the method used to direct the light stimulus [intensity, duration, proximity, orientation]) that overall can reduce their reliability [4]. Most importantly, measurement of pupillary reactivity is qualitative (i.e., absent vs. present) and uses a non-standardized descriptive scale (i.e., brisk, sluggish). What if, instead, clinicians were offered a quantitative device for bedside neuromonitoring of pupillary size and reactivity?

Quantitative pupillometry has progressively evolved during recent years; however most clinical investigation has been in the field of anesthesia and analgesia [3]. Recently, there has been an increasing interest in the application of quantitative pupillometry in critical care, and emerging clinical data on its potential utility have become available.

The objective of this chapter is to provide a comprehensive summary of recent clinical investigation on automated infrared pupillometry in general critical care.

D. Solari · J.-P. Miroz · M. Oddo (✉)
Neuroscience Critical Care Research Group, Department of Intensive Care Medicine,
CHUV-Lausanne University Hospital
Lausanne, Switzerland
e-mail: mauro.oddo@chuv.ch

© Springer International Publishing AG 2018
J.-L. Vincent (ed.), *Annual Update in Intensive Care and Emergency Medicine 2018*,
Annual Update in Intensive Care and Emergency Medicine,
https://doi.org/10.1007/978-3-319-73670-9_38

We will first introduce device methodology and recent technological advancements, and discuss basic knowledge of pupil anatomy, function and pathophysiology. We will then illustrate the potential utility and clinical value of automated pupillometry as an additional complementary tool for bedside neuromonitoring of critically ill patients. We will particularly focus on the role of quantitative pupillary light reflex as a tool for: 1) detecting intracranial pressure(ICP)-related secondary insults; 2) predicting coma prognosis; and 3) potentially quantifying the extent of autonomic nervous dysfunction (a pathophysiologic determinant of intensive care unit (ICU)-acquired encephalopathy) in critically ill patients.

Anatomy and Pathophysiology of Pupillary Reactivity

Pupil size, accommodation, but also ocular blood flow and intraocular pressure, all are eye functions that undergo tightly controlled regulation by the autonomic nervous system [5]. The pupil size is regulated by the action of two antagonist smooth muscles: a) the sphincter pupillae, which is responsible for pupillary constriction and is activated by the parasympathetic nervous system; and b) the dilator pupillae (or radial muscle), which has lower strength than the sphincter pupillae and is involved in pupillary dilation and activated by the sympathetic nervous system. For the purpose of this review, we shall focus on the physiology of the pupillary light and dilation reflexes.

Pupillary Light Reflex

The anatomical pathway that controls the pupillary light reflex is illustrated in Fig. 1a. Briefly, the afferent light – sensed by intrinsic photosensitive cells in the retina (melanopsin-containing ganglions) – is conveyed via the optic nerve (2nd cranial nerve) to the pretectal nucleus. These neurons project axon fibers to midbrain pre-ganglionic cells of the Edinger-Westphal nucleus. Cells of the Edinger-Westphal nucleus have an intrinsic pacemaker activity that increases proportionally to the synaptic input [3]. They project through the oculomotor nerve (3rd cranial nerve), to post-ganglionic cells located in the ciliary ganglion (nicotinic synapse). A last short nerve leaves the ganglion up to the sphincter muscle (muscarinic synapse) that constricts the pupil. The parasympathetic nervous system is involved in this pathway and acetylcholine is the neurotransmitter in both synapses.

Although the pupillary light reflex is predominantly under the control of the parasympathetic nervous system, sympathetic nervous system inhibition (via the effect of the light stimulus on the sympathetic fibers) concurrently acts by reducing the tone of the radial muscle [6]. Pupil constriction is also in part influenced by the reticular activating system [7, 8].

a

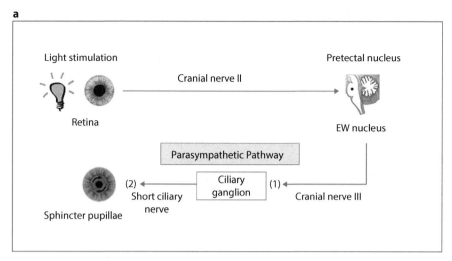

b

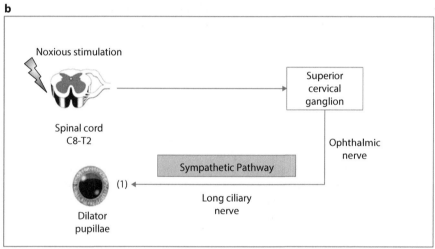

Fig. 1 Anatomy and physiology of pupillary light and dilation reflexes. **a** Pupillary light reflex. After receiving excitatory input from the retina, Edinger-Westphal (EW) neurons project to the sphincter pupillae inducing pupillary constriction. Along the efferent parasympathetic pathway (3rd cranial and short ciliary nerves) there are two cholinergic synapses: (1) a nicotinic synapse, mediating a fast transmission; (2) a muscarinic synapse, mediating a slow metabolic response. **b** Pupillary dilation reflex. After receiving excitatory input from the spinal cord, the superior cervical ganglion neurons project to the dilator pupillae inducing pupillary dilation. The efferent sympathetic pathway (ophthalmic and long ciliary nerves) acts through an $\alpha 1$-adrenergic synapse (1)

Pupillary Dilation Reflex

The pupillary dilation reflex is predominantly under the influence of the sympathetic nervous system (Fig. 1b). Sympathetic innervation of the radial muscle arises from pre-ganglionic neurons located in the C8-T2 segments of the spinal cord. An alerting stimulus (e.g., a painful maneuver) activates these groups of cells via a spinal reflex; their axons project to the sympathetic chain ganglia and travel in the sympathetic trunk to the superior cervical ganglion where they contact post-ganglionic neurons. From there, fibers leave the ganglion up to the radial muscle (alpha-1 adrenergic synapse) that dilates the pupil. Endogenous adrenergic agents are the neurotransmitters involved in the synapse. Importantly, it seems that, in addition to the spinal cord, the midbrain plays a key role in the regulation of the pupillary dilation reflex [9]. Indeed, in brain-dead patients where midbrain function is abolished, the pupillary dilation reflex cannot be elicited, thus confirming the hypothesis of a concomitant participation of supraspinal pathways in the control of the pupillary dilation reflex [10]. Furthermore, data from healthy volunteers undergoing desflurane anesthesia (an $\alpha 1$-adrenergic antagonist), suggest that in anesthetized persons, the pupillary dilation reflex may not be mediated by the sympathetic system [11].

Automated Infrared Pupillometry

Device Technology

The first application of infrared radiation (discovered by the German scientist Frederick William Herschel in 1800) to pupillary examination dates back to the 1950s, when Lowenstein and Loewenfeld first described the use of an infrared camera for pupillary imaging [9]. In those early years, pupillometers were heavy and not user-friendly, making them unsuitable for bedside utilization. Their use until the end of the 1990s was limited to anesthesiology research, to assess the effects of opiates and other psycho-pharmacological agents on pupillary reactivity [12–14].

More recently, automated infrared pupillometry has evolved towards non-invasive hand-held devices, easy to use, accurate, reproducible and readily available at the bedside for clinical purposes. Modern generation automated pupillometers are composed of an infrared light-emitting diode, a digital camera that senses the reflected infrared light from the iris, a data processor and a keyboard (Fig. 2). Several variables can be measured, including pupil size, maximum and minimum apertures,

Fig. 2 Schematic illustration of automated infrared pupillometry. The color liquid crystal screen displays a summary of measurements in response to a standardized light stimulation, including pupillary size (mm), constriction velocity (mm/s), latency (ms) and the percentage of pupillary response. The *green curve* illustrates the change in pupil size from the baseline (before the stimulus) to the minimum aperture (after the stimulus). The different variables that can be obtained after light and painful stimulation are also listed ▶

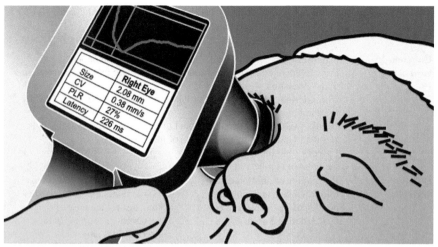

Size	Right Eye
CV	2.08 mm
PLR	0.38 mm/s
Latency	27%
	226 ms

Light stimulation

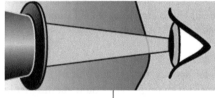

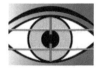

Variables

- Size (mm)
- Latency (ms)
- Constriction velocity (mm/s)
- Dilation velocity (mm/s)
- Percentage of constriction change (%)

Pupillary constriction

Painful stimulation

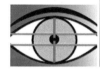

Variables

- Size (mm)
- Percentage of dilation change (%)

Pupillary dilation

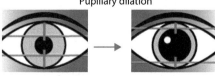

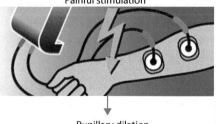

Table 1 Comparisons and technical differences between the NeuroLight Algiscan® (ID-Med, France) and the Npi-200® (Neuroptics, USA) pupillometer

	NeuroLight AlgiScan device	Npi-200 device
Common variables	**Size (mm)** mean pupil diameter during a latent period of 3–4″ **Percentage of constriction change (%)** difference in pupil diameter after light stimulation **Constriction velocity (mm/s)** the amount of the constriction divided by the duration of the constriction **Dilation velocity (mm/s)** the amount of pupil size recovery (after light stimulation) divided by the duration of the recovery **Latency (ms)** time interval between the application of light stimulus and the onset of pupillary constriction	
Different variables	**Percentage of dilation change (%)** difference in pupil diameter after a noxious stimulation (0 to 60 mA during 5 s max)	**NPi** algorithm that incorporates all above values and compares the reading against the mean distribution of scores obtained from healthy subjects. Values are standardized into *z scores* and combined to create an NPi score that ranges from 0 to 5
Differences in light stimulation	**Intensity of light stimulus:** 320 lx **Duration of light stimulus:** 1 s	**Intensity of light stimulus:** 1000 lx **Duration of light stimulus:** 0.7 s

and percentage of change, as well as the latency period and the constriction and dilation velocities. All these variables are shown on a color liquid crystal display in both graphical and numerical format.

Two models are currently available on the market (Table 1):

- The *NeurOptics NPi-200®* (Neuroptics, USA), which in addition to previous variables computes an additionally derived score, called Neurological Pupil index (NPi, from a minimum value of 0 to a maximum of 5);
- The *NeuroLight-Algiscan®* (ID-Med, France), which in addition to previous variables provides a quantitative pupillary dilation reflex measurement (upon a standardized painful stimulation of the cubital nerve). The pupillary dilation reflex may be of potential value in assessing the adequacy of analgesia [3], which will not be discussed in this review.

The two devices have similar accuracy (± 0.03 mm for the NeurOptics vs. ± 0.05 mm for the NeuroLight) and measurement range (1–9 mm vs. 0.5–10 mm, respectively).

Methodological Limitations

The pupillometer is monocular and therefore cannot measure consensual response. The measurement is best suited for comatose or sedated subjects, since uncontrolled movements, such as in non-cooperative, confused or agitated patients, will alter accuracy [15]. Trauma to the eye, periorbital or scleral edema, also may interfere with the measurement procedure. Finally, any pre-existing ophthalmic condition (e.g., cataract surgery) or disease that alters pupillary muscular dynamics (e.g., multiple sclerosis, sclerodermia, amyloidosis, multiple system atrophy) should be ruled out as these will intrinsically reduce reactivity of the pupil [16–18]

Pharmacological Effects

Several pharmacological agents may affect pupillary function and measurements [19], including analgesics and sedatives [20, 21]. In particular, opiates may significantly decrease pupil size and pupillary dilation reflex [22]. Opiates and benzodiazepines reduce constriction velocity, whereas neuromuscular blockers [20], calcium-channel blockers and oral psychotropic medications had no effects [21]. Induced burst-suppression with barbiturates may also considerably reduce constriction velocity [21]. In contrast, adrenergic drugs (except for high dose epinephrine) do not seem to alter pupillary dilation [3]. Finally, whereas mild hypothermia may not directly alter pupil dynamics, hyperthermia induces pupillary dilation and an increase in pupillary light reflex amplitude [3].

Normal Values in Healthy Subjects

Normal pupillometry values are derived from over 2400 paired measurements taken in 310 healthy volunteers, tested at variable conditions of ambient light [21]. Pupil diameter may vary from an average of 4.1 ($\pm$ 0.34) mm at rest to 2.7 ($\pm$ 0.21) mm after bright light stimulation. The average normal percentage pupillary light reflex is greater than 30%. Average constriction velocity is 1.48 ($\pm$ 0.33) mm/s, and latency varies between 120 and 360 ms.

Non-Invasive Monitoring of Brain Function in Critical Care: The Emerging Role of Bedside Automated Infrared Pupillometry

Detection of Anisocoria

Three independent single-center studies published in 2016 found relevant differences in pupillary examination between manual assessment and automated pupillometry measures. Olson et al. found marked inter-rater reliability among practitioners in pupillary assessments (size, shape and reactivity) between standard subjective measurement and automated pupillometer. Based on more than 2300 paired assessments, differences were more remarkable when pupils were abnormal [23]. After testing inter-rater variability, quantitative pupillometers appear very reliable [23]. Kerr et al. reported that critical care and neurosurgical nurses tended to underestimate pupil size using standard vs. quantitative assessments [24]. Differences between manual and automated examination were concerning in a French study by Couret et al. [25]. The authors reported that in neurocritical care patients, manual penlight failed to diagnose up to 50% of episodes with anisocoria that were actually detected by the pupillometer device. Discordances were also observed when assessing the pupillary light reflex, particularly in patients with small pupil size.

Whether a more accurate detection of anisocoria may prompt further investigation (e.g., computed tomography [CT] scan) and changes in patient management will need further study.

Detection of Refractory Elevated Intracranial Pressure

Alterations in pupil size (dilation and asymmetry) and reactivity (unresponsiveness) correlate with elevated ICP and brain herniation [26, 27], and are strong predictors of poor outcome [28–30]. Taylor et al. described the potential utility of quantitative pupillometry for detecting ICP elevations in a series of patients with severe traumatic brain injury (TBI). The authors found that patients who experienced sustained increases in ICP and had signs of brain herniation on the CT scan (> 3 mm midline shift) had significantly lower constriction velocity [21]. In the same work, it was found that pupillary asymmetry > 0.5 mm was always associated with ICP > 30 mmHg, whereas a pupillary light reflex < 10% correlated with ICP > 20 mmHg [21]. Because the ideal ICP threshold for injury and therapeutic intervention remains a debated subject [31, 32], quantitative pupillometry holds great promise. In this context, the use of the NPi score appears of particular interest. Chen et al. showed in a multicenter study (n = 134 patients) that patients with an NPi > 3 (normal pupillary reactivity) had an average ICP of 19.6 mmHg, whereas those with an NPi < 3 (reduced pupillary reactivity) had an average ICP of 30.5 mmHg. Importantly, the NPi abnormalities occurred on average 16 h before the actual ICP increase, highlighting the potential of quantitative pupillometry for timely prediction of severe intracranial hypertension [33].

Additional study is needed, but quantitative pupillometry appears promising for detecting elevated ICP non-invasively. Below we describe two clinical cases that illustrate the good relationship between quantitative pupillometry and parenchymal ICP.

Fig. 3 represents an abnormal brain CT scan showing temporal contusions and a left subdural hematoma from a 50-year old patient admitted after severe TBI (admission CT scan, upper panel). Also illustrated is the progressive increase in parenchymal ICP starting at day 3, with surges of refractory ICP > 25 mmHg. A second CT scan (lower panel) showed progression of left subdural hematoma with midline shift, which prompted emergent surgical evacuation. The evolution of quantitative pupillary light reflex is illustrated in parallel, showing the pathological decrease in pupillary light reflex (from 15% to < 5%) in the hours previous to refractory ICP. Successful treatment of high ICP was accompanied by a progressive post-surgery normalization of pupillary light reflex above normal ranges (> 30%).

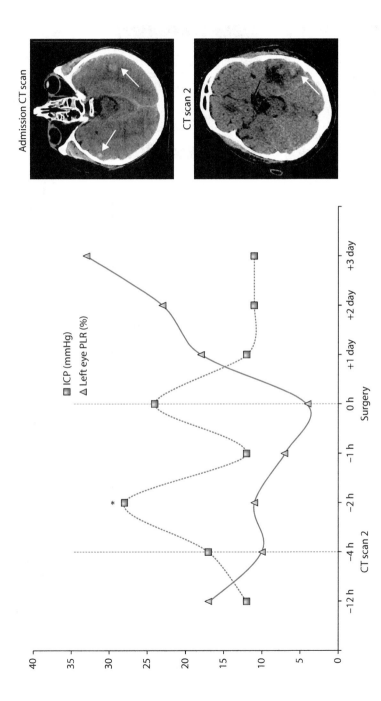

Fig. 3 Case 1, severe traumatic brain injury. Quantitative changes of left eye pupillary light reflex (PLR) and invasive intracranial pressure (ICP) over time in a 50-year old patient with severe traumatic brain injury. *Curves* show the progressive PLR reduction that parallels the ICP increase (*asterisk* = administration of osmotherapy). Progressive increase to normalization of PLR follows surgical evacuation of left subdural hematoma (time 0, *dashed gray line*)

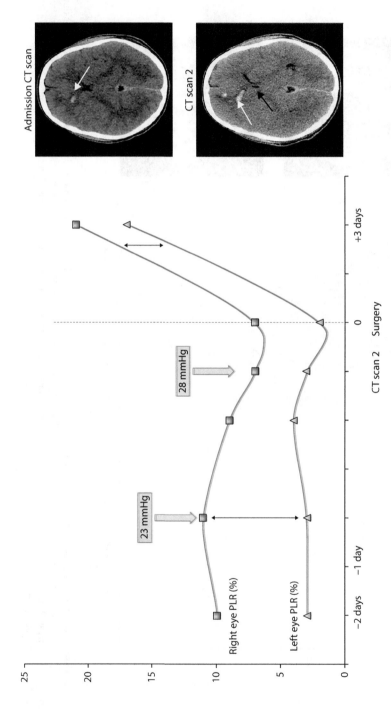

Fig. 4 Case 2, severe traumatic brain injury. Quantitative changes over time of pupillary light reflex (PLR) from both eyes in a 16-year old patient with severe traumatic brain injury. CT scans show frontal contusion. *Curves* show important pupillary asymmetry between the two eyes at times of elevated ICP, which progressively normalizes following ICP control post-decompressive craniectomy (time 0, *dashed gray line*). Timely evolution of PLR values (%) during ICP increase from 23 to 28 mmHg is also shown

Fig. 4 illustrates a case report of a 16-year old severe TBI patient with an abnormal brain CT scan showing multiple contusions (upper panel). ICP raised > 20 mmHg and became refractory to medical therapies (> 25 mmHg), prompting a 2nd CT scan, which diagnosed contusion progression with significant midline shift (lower panel), leading to emergent decompressive craniectomy. In the 48 h previous to decompressive craniectomy, pupillary light reflex was constantly $< 10\%$ and a marked pupillary light reflex asymmetry between the two eyes was observed. Pupillary light reflex asymmetry normalized following decompressive craniectomy.

Bedside continuous assessment of non-invasive pupillary light reflex, NPi, constriction velocities and asymmetry may become useful complements to invasive ICP monitoring for guiding timely interventions in patients with brain edema and midline shift.

Early Neuroprognostication

Abnormal pupillary reactivity is a strong predictor of poor outcome in critical care patients [1]. Quantitative pupillometry may thus be integrated in ICU multimodal prognostic assessment [34], e.g., in patients with coma after cardiac arrest, where absent pupillary response is strongly predictive of poor prognosis [35]. Indeed, using automated infrared pupillometry, it was recently shown that reduced quantitative pupillary light reflex is associated with unfavorable short-term [36, 37] and long-term [38] outcomes. Importantly, reduced pupillary light reflex (expressed as the percentage of pupillary response) was demonstrated to have excellent predictive value for poor outcome, as assessed by the Pittsburgh Cerebral Performance Categories [37, 38] (Table 2). Given the comparable prognostic performance of quantitative pupillometry compared to electro-physiologic exams [38], quantitative pupillometry may be integrated into multimodal assessment of prognosis, pending further confirmation by larger multicenter studies (e.g. ClinicalTrials.gov NCT02607878).

Table 2 Performance of early (48 h from ICU admission) quantitative pupillary reflex (PLR) to predict outcome of coma after cardiac arrest

First author [ref]	Number of patients	Threshold for quantitative PLR (%) at 48 h	Outcome	Specificity (95% CI)	Sensitivity (95% CI)
Heimburger [37]	82	$< 11\%$	3-month outcome (CPC 3–5)	83% (63–95)	70% (55–83)
Solari [38]	103	$< 13\%$	1-year mortality (CPC 5)	100% (93–100)	60.8% (48–75.2)

CPC: Cerebral Performance Categories

It is also conceivable to test the value of quantitative pupillometry for early outcome prognostication in other acute brain pathologies, such as head trauma or acute ischemic/hemorrhagic stroke. Additional indications may be in conditions where hypoxic-ischemic neurological complications and the rate of poor outcome are frequent, such as following emergent arteriovenous extracorporeal membrane oxygenation (ECMO) for refractory cardiac arrest [39]. In this particular setting, the decisional criteria to insert ECMO are primarily based on no-flow and low-flow times, which represent approximate estimates of the duration of circulatory arrest. With the advent of automated infrared pupillometry, it is now possible to quantify pupillary light response during cardiopulmonary resuscitation (CPR) or immediately after the return of spontaneous circulation. Indeed, preliminary clinical data in patients undergoing CPR demonstrated that the recovery of a quantitative pupillary light reflex was associated with early survival and favorable neurological outcome, while a persistently absent pupillary light reflex correlated with early mortality [40]. Whether the use of quantitative pupillometry may help with decision-making in this setting needs further exploration.

Early Detection of ICU-related Encephalopathy

Critical illness-related encephalopathy is frequently observed in sedated mechanically ventilated patients [41, 42] and is associated with worse morbidity [43] and neurological prognosis [44]. Although a comprehensive description of the pathophysiology of ICU-related encephalopathy is beyond the scope of this review, autonomic nervous system dysfunction is likely an important pathogenic determinant [45]. Findings of experimental studies demonstrated that cholinergic activity attenuated inflammation while, in contrast, stimulation of the adrenergic pathways led to amplification of the inflammatory response [46, 47]. Microglia cells are usually kept in a quiescent state by a cholinergic inhibitory control. Several factors (e.g., the administration of anticholinergic drugs, systemic infection, incipient neurodegenerative diseases) contribute to the development of a neurotransmitter imbalance, that is, an increase in mono-aminergic activity and a parallel deficit in cholinergic activity. Microglia escape from cholinergic control, promoting macrophage proliferation and the secretion of several inflammatory mediators, thus leading to neuroinflammation, blood-brain barrier disruption and, in the long-term, neuro-degeneration (Fig. 5).

Given that pupillary light reflex is regulated by the cholinergic system (see earlier), then a deficit in cholinergic activity should lead to a decrease in pupillary light reflex, which could serve as a potential marker of ICU-related encephalopathy. This provides the rationale for testing quantitative pupillometry as a bedside monitoring tool to detect patients at higher risk for ICU-acquired acute brain dysfunction who may subsequently develop delirium. Confirmation of the utility of such an approach may have relevant clinical implications since, despite major advances in the comprehension of ICU-related encephalopathy, its diagnosis is currently solely based on predictive scores [48] based on *a posteriori* assessment.

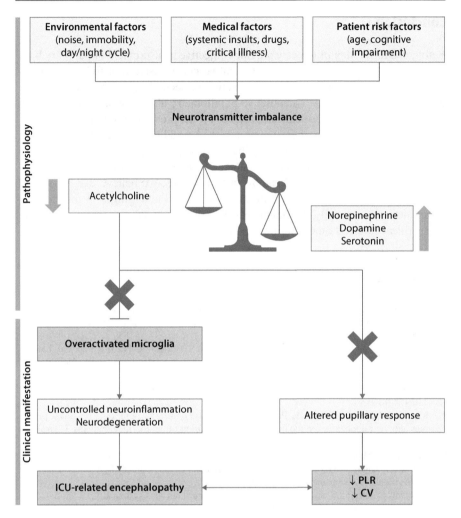

Fig. 5 Potential mechanisms by which reduced pupillary light reflex (PLR) and constriction velocity (CV) measured by quantitative pupillometry may be a clinical marker of intensive care unit (ICU)-related encephalopathy. Different intrinsic and external factors contribute to ICU-related acute brain dysfunction. The most acclaimed hypothesis focuses on neurotransmitter imbalance. The cholinergic pathway attenuates the immune response and is considered anti-inflammatory: a reduction in cholinergic activity leads to uncontrolled inflammation, which weakens astrocytic tight junctions affecting neuronal functioning, thus causing delirium. Given acetylcholine is the main mediator of pupillary light reflex, reduced PLR may be a marker of acute brain dysfunction and could be of value in predicting ICU-related encephalopathy

Conclusion

Automated infrared pupillometry provides objective measurement of pupillary light reflex at the bedside and offers a quantitative non-invasive tool for the monitoring of brain injured patients and the detection of secondary cerebral insults, such as refractory elevated ICP. Quantitative pupillometry also may be useful for early neuroprognostication in critical care, such as for the prediction of functional neurological recovery in coma after cardiac arrest. An additional area of investigation where quantitative pupillometry may be promising is for the detection of ICU-related encephalopathy. Multicenter validation assessment of quantitative pupillometry is currently ongoing. Pending further studies, we believe that automated infrared pupillometry holds great promise as a novel emerging tool for the neuromonitoring of critically ill patients and may have clinical relevance for guiding neurocritical care and timely surgical interventions.

References

1. Sharshar T, Citerio G, Andrews PJ et al (2014) Neurological examination of critically ill patients: a pragmatic approach. Report of an ESICM expert panel. Intensive Care Med 40:484–495
2. Chen JW, Gombart ZJ, Rogers S, Gardiner SK, Cecil S, Bullock RM (2011) Pupillary reactivity as an early indicator of increased intracranial pressure: the introduction of the Neurological Pupil index. Surg Neurol Int 2:82
3. Larson MD, Behrends M (2015) Portable infrared pupillometry: a review. Anesth Analg 120:1242–1253
4. Martinez-Ricarte F, Castro A, Poca MA et al (2013) Infrared pupillometry. Basic principles and their application in the non-invasive monitoring of neurocritical patients. Neurologia 28:41–51
5. McDougal DH, Gamlin PD (2015) Autonomic control of the eye. Compr Physiol 5:439–473
6. Clarke RJ, Zhang H, Gamlin PD (2003) Characteristics of the pupillary light reflex in the alert rhesus monkey. J Neurophysiol 89:3179–3189
7. Koss MC (1986) Pupillary dilation as an index of central nervous system alpha 2-adrenoceptor activation. J Pharmacol Methods 15:1–19
8. Gu Q (2002) Neuromodulatory transmitter systems in the cortex and their role in cortical plasticity. Neuroscience 111:815–835
9. Loewenfeld IE (1958) Mechanisms of reflex dilatation of the pupil; historical review and experimental analysis. Doc Ophthalmol 12:185–448
10. Yang LL, Niemann CU, Larson MD (2003) Mechanism of pupillary reflex dilation in awake volunteers and in organ donors. Anesthesiology 99:1281–1286
11. Larson MD, Tayefeh F, Sessler DI, Daniel M, Noorani M (1996) Sympathetic nervous system does not mediate reflex pupillary dilation during desflurane anesthesia. Anesthesiology 85:748–754
12. Grunberger J, Linzmayer L, Cepko H, Saletu B (1986) Pupillometry in psychopharmacologic experiments. Arzneimittelforschung 36:141–146
13. Grunberger J, Linzmayer L, Gathmann P, Saletu B (1985) Computer-assisted static and light-evoked dynamic pupillometry in psychosomatic patients. Wien Klin Wochenschr 97:775–781
14. Pickworth WB, Welch P, Henningfield JE, Cone EJ (1989) Opiate-induced pupillary effects in humans. Methods Find Exp Clin Pharmacol 11:759–763

15. Meeker M, Du R, Bacchetti P et al (2005) Pupil examination: validity and clinical utility of an automated pupillometer. J Neurosci Nurs 37:34–40

16. de Seze J, Stojkovic T, Gauvrit JY et al (2001) Autonomic dysfunction in multiple sclerosis: cervical spinal cord atrophy correlates. J Neurol 248:297–303

17. Davies DR, Smith SE (1999) Pupil abnormality in amyloidosis with autonomic neuropathy. J Neurol Neurosurg Psychiatry 67:819–822

18. Dutsch M, Hilz MJ, Rauhut U, Solomon J, Neundorfer B, Axelrod FB (2002) Sympathetic and parasympathetic pupillary dysfunction in familial dysautonomia. J Neurol Sci 195:77–83

19. Fountas KN, Kapsalaki EZ, Machinis TG, Boev AN, Robinson JS, Troup EC (2006) Clinical implications of quantitative infrared pupillometry in neurosurgical patients. Neurocrit Care 5:55–60

20. Gray AT, Krejci ST, Larson MD (1997) Neuromuscular blocking drugs do not alter the pupillary light reflex of anesthetized humans. Arch Neurol 54:579–584

21. Taylor WR, Chen JW, Meltzer H et al (2003) Quantitative pupillometry, a new technology: normative data and preliminary observations in patients with acute head injury. Technical note. J Neurosurg 98:205–213

22. Larson MD, Berry PD (2000) Supraspinal pupillary effects of intravenous and epidural fentanyl during isoflurane anesthesia. Reg Anesth Pain Med 25:60–66

23. Olson DM, Stutzman S, Saju C, Wilson M, Zhao W, Aiyagari V (2016) Interrater reliability of pupillary assessments. Neurocrit Care 24:251–257

24. Kerr RG, Bacon AM, Baker LL et al (2016) Underestimation of pupil size by critical care and neurosurgical nurses. Am J Crit Care 25:213–219

25. Couret D, Boumaza D, Grisotto C et al (2016) Reliability of standard pupillometry practice in neurocritical care: an observational, double-blinded study. Crit Care 20:99

26. Fisher CM (1980) Oval pupils. Arch Neurol 37:502–503

27. Marshall LF, Barba D, Toole BM, Bowers SA (1983) The oval pupil: clinical significance and relationship to intracranial hypertension. J Neurosurg 58:566–568

28. Choi SC, Narayan RK, Anderson RL, Ward JD (1988) Enhanced specificity of prognosis in severe head injury. J Neurosurg 69:381–385

29. Tien HC, Cunha JR, Wu SN et al (2006) Do trauma patients with a Glasgow Coma Scale score of 3 and bilateral fixed and dilated pupils have any chance of survival? J Trauma 60:274–278

30. Jennett B, Teasdale G, Fry J et al (1980) Treatment for severe head injury. J Neurol Neurosurg Psychiatry 43:289–295

31. Guiza F, Depreitere B, Piper I et al (2015) Visualizing the pressure and time burden of intracranial hypertension in adult and paediatric traumatic brain injury. Intensive Care Med 41:1067–1076

32. Carney N, Totten AM, O'Reilly C et al (2017) Guidelines for the management of severe traumatic brain injury, fourth edition. Neurosurgery 80:6–15

33. Chen JW, Vakil-Gilani K, Williamson KL, Cecil S (2014) Infrared pupillometry, the Neurological Pupil index and unilateral pupillary dilation after traumatic brain injury: implications for treatment paradigms. Springerplus 3:548

34. Rossetti AO, Rabinstein AA, Oddo M (2016) Neurological prognostication of outcome in patients in coma after cardiac arrest. Lancet Neurol 15:597–609

35. Kamps MJ, Horn J, Oddo M et al (2013) Prognostication of neurologic outcome in cardiac arrest patients after mild therapeutic hypothermia: a meta-analysis of the current literature. Intensive Care Med 39:1671–1682

36. Suys T, Bouzat P, Marques-Vidal P et al (2014) Automated quantitative pupillometry for the prognostication of coma after cardiac arrest. Neurocrit Care 21(2):300–308

37. Heimburger D, Durand M, Gaide-Chevronnay L et al (2016) Quantitative pupillometry and transcranial Doppler measurements in patients treated with hypothermia after cardiac arrest. Resuscitation 103:88–93

38. Solari D, Rossetti AO, Carteron L et al (2017) Early prediction of coma recovery after cardiac arrest with blinded pupillometry. Ann Neurol 81:804–810

39. Abrams D, Brodie D (2017) Extracorporeal membrane oxygenation for adult respiratory failure: 2017 update. Chest 152:639–649
40. Behrends M, Niemann CU, Larson MD (2012) Infrared pupillometry to detect the light reflex during cardiopulmonary resuscitation: a case series. Resuscitation 83:1223–1228
41. Tasker RC, Menon DK (2016) Critical care and the brain. JAMA 315:749–750
42. Smith M, Meyfroidt G (2017) Critical illness: the brain is always in the line of fire. Intensive Care Med 43:870–873
43. Mehta S, Cook D, Devlin JW et al (2015) Prevalence, risk factors, and outcomes of delirium in mechanically ventilated adults. Crit Care Med 43:557–566
44. Pandharipande PP, Girard TD, Jackson JC et al (2013) Long-term cognitive impairment after critical illness. N Engl J Med 369:1306–1316
45. van Gool WA, van de Beek D, Eikelenboom P (2010) Systemic infection and delirium: when cytokines and acetylcholine collide. Lancet 375:773–775
46. Willard LB, Hauss-Wegrzyniak B, Wenk GL (1999) Pathological and biochemical consequences of acute and chronic neuroinflammation within the basal forebrain cholinergic system of rats. Neuroscience 88:193–200
47. Tracey KJ (2002) The inflammatory reflex. Nature 420:853–859
48. van den Boogaard M, Pickkers P, Slooter AJ et al (2012) Development and validation of PRE-DELIRIC (PREdiction of DELIRium in ICu patients) delirium prediction model for intensive care patients: observational multicentre study. BMJ 344:e420

Brain Ultrasound: How, Why, When and Where?

C. Robba and G. Citerio

Introduction

Brain ultrasound is a safe, quick, bedside technique, which enables identification of several structures within the brain parenchyma and monitoring of various aspects of cerebrovascular pathophysiology [1, 2]. The non-invasiveness of this technique, together with its safety and relatively low cost as a neuromonitoring system, determine its applicability in multiple settings, including neuro- and general intensive care, as well as in the operating room and the emergency department. At present, brain ultrasound is still a poorly developed technique and is not routinely performed in critical care. The main obstacle to ultrasound penetration of the skull is bone. Therefore, the basic technique for brain ultrasound examination consists of insonating the brain structure through different 'windows', through which sound waves will be transmitted, found at various locations in the skull.

The aim of this chapter is to provide an overview of basic and advanced principles, methodology and clinical applications of brain ultrasound in the monitoring and treatment of critical care patients, including those with intracranial hemorrhage, intracranial space occupying lesions, hydrocephalus, and midline shift in both acute and chronic clinical settings.

C. Robba
Neurocritical Care Unit, Addenbrooke's Hospital
Cambridge, UK

G. Citerio (✉)
School of Medicine and Surgery, University of Milan-Bicocca
Milan, Italy
Neurointensive Care, San Gerardo Hospital, ASST-Monza
Monza, Italy
e-mail: giuseppe.citerio@unimib.it

© Springer International Publishing AG 2018   519
J.-L. Vincent (ed.), *Annual Update in Intensive Care and Emergency Medicine 2018*,
Annual Update in Intensive Care and Emergency Medicine,
https://doi.org/10.1007/978-3-319-73670-9_39

How and Why?

Ultrasound examination should be performed with the patient in a supine position using a low-frequency 2.0–2.5 MHz probe. The acoustic window is generally located in the anterior part of the temporal bone, close to the vertical portion of the zygomatic bone. If the patient has previously had decompressive craniectomy, a standard abdominal convex phased array probe with a mean central frequency of 4 MHz and an abdominal setting should be used. Initially, the operator needs to make sure that he/she is in the correct acoustic window, by identifying the contralateral bone and the main brain structures (Figs. 1 and 2). The mesencephalic

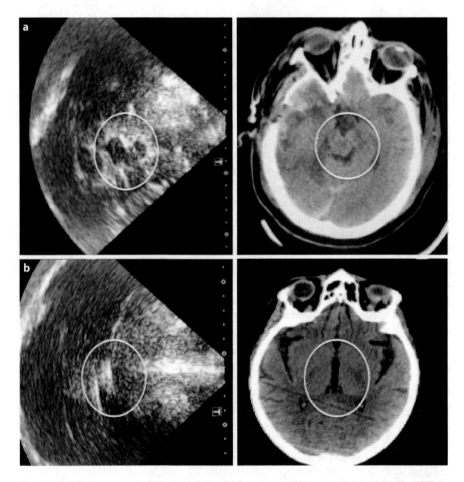

Fig. 1 a Midbrain transverse ultrasound scan and corresponding computed tomography (CT) in the same plane. The butterfly-shaped mesencephalic brainstem surrounded by the echogenic basal cisterns is shown in the *circle*. **b** Diencephalic transverse scan and corresponding CT image. The third ventricle is shown in the *circle*

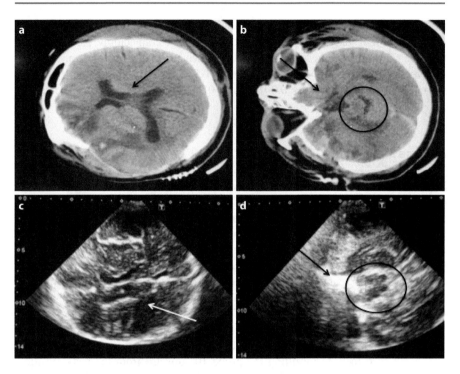

Fig. 2 Brain US images in a decompressed patient (**c, d**) and corresponding CT head in the same plane (**a, b**). **a–c**: The *arrows* show the lateral ventricles, slightly dilated. **b–d**: The mesencephalon is shown in the *circle* and the basal cisterns are indicated by the *arrow*

brainstem can be observed in most patients and represents the main landmark for the ultrasound examination (mesencephalic plane). It is generally observed in the axial plane parallel to the 'orbitomeatal line' (Fig. 1) as a butterfly-shaped structure surrounded by the echogenic basal cisterns. The third ventricle can be visualized by tilting the probe about 10° upwards and it looks like a highly echogenic double line image, because of the hyperechogenic ependyma walls (Fig. 1), and is surrounded by the hypoechogenic/isoechogenic thalami (diencephalic plane). Moving the probe slightly anteriorly, it is possible to visualize the frontal horn of the contralateral lateral ventricle, which is recognized as a hypoechogenic structure, between two hyperechogenic parallel lines.

Hydrocephalus

Visualization of the third ventricle on the diencephalic plane enables measurement of the diameter of the ventricles for the diagnosis of hydrocephalus. Several studies have compared ventricular diameter measurements using ultrasound and computed tomography (CT), and found good correlation, in particular for the measurement of the third ventricle, because direct measurement of lateral ventricles is more difficult [3, 4]. In a recent study, in patients after decompressive craniectomy, the correlation between CT versus sonographic technique in measuring the diameters of all cerebral ventricles was found to be excellent (r = 0.978 for the right lateral, p < 0.001; r = 0.975 for the left lateral, p < 0.001; and r = 0.987, p < 0.001 for the third ventricle) [1].

Midline Shift

Rapid progression of midline shift from edema or hemorrhage is a life-threatening condition that requires urgent diagnosis and treatment. A midline shift ≥ 1 cm is associated with increased mortality, and a midline shift ≥ 0.5 cm on the initial brain CT scan has been shown to be a predictor of poor neurological outcome [4]. Therefore, early detection of midline shift in neurosurgical ICU patients is crucial as it allows an aggressive treatment plan of surgical evacuation of the hematomas and masses. Head CT scan is considered to be the gold standard to diagnose midline shift. However, CT is not always immediately available. Therefore, several authors studied use of ultrasound for detection of midline shift [5, 6].

The third ventricle should be considered as a marker of the midline. As previously described, it can be visualized through the temporal acoustic bone window at a depth of 6 to 8 cm by tilting the probe 10° upward from the basal position and the middle cerebral artery. The midline shift is calculated according to the formula $(A - B)/2$, where A is the distance between the probe and the center of the

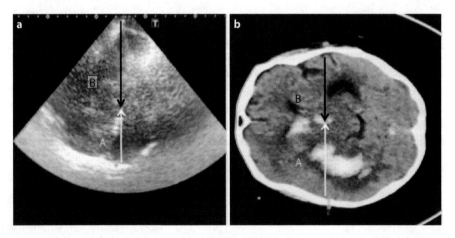

Fig. 3 Measurement of the midline shift on ultrasound (**a**) and computed tomography (CT) (**b**). The third ventricle should be considered as a marker of the midline. The distance between the third ventricle and the external side of the temporal bone (*A*) has to be measured. The same calculation can be repeated for the contralateral side (*B*). A midline shift is then estimated according to the formula midline shift $= (A - B)/2$

third ventricle in a perpendicular line to its margins, and B is the contralateral distance between the third ventricle and the temporal bone (Fig. 3). Motuel et al. [7], in a prospective study comparing transcranial sonographic measurement of midline shift with CT in 52 neurosurgical patients reported a correlation coefficient between ultrasound and CT scan of 0.65 ($p < 0.001$), with a sensitivity of 84.2% and specificity of 84.8% using a cut-off of 0.35 cm. In patients who have had decompressive craniectomy, the accuracy of ultrasound to assess the midline shift has been demonstrated to be even better, with the mean difference between CT and ultrasound of 0.3 ± 1.6 mm [1], suggesting that echography may be a valid alternative to CT in patients who have had decompressive craniectomy [7, 8].

Intracranial Hemorrhage

Brain ultrasound can have a role even in the monitoring of the volume of intracranial hemorrhage. Intracranial blood is visualized as a hyperechoic sharply demarcated mass within the brain parenchyma. Caricato et al. [1] found an excellent correlation between CT and transcranial sonography in assessing volumes of hyperdense lesions (intraclass correlation coefficient 0.993; $p < 0.001$) in a cohort of decompressed patients. In non-decompressed patients, the accuracy is limited, as the temporal window does not enable visualization of the whole brain. Mäurer et al. [9] in a large study including 151 stroke patients, found that 12% had an insufficient temporal bone window for transcranial insonation; however, brain sonography was able to correctly differentiate between ischemia and hemorrhage in most cases.

Ultrasonography of the Eye: Optic Nerve Sheath Diameter

The optic nerve sheath is in direct continuity with the dura mater and the subarachnoid space of the brain and contains cerebrospinal fluid (CSF) [10]. Because the optic nerve sheath is distensible, CSF pressure increases the optic nerve sheath diameter, particularly in the anterior, retro-bulbar compartment, about 3 mm behind the globe (Fig. 4). Therefore, when intracranial pressure (ICP) increases, the pressure is transmitted to the subarachnoid compartment of the nerve, resulting in an enlargement of the optic nerve sheath diameter [11]. Several authors have studied the relationship between ICP and the optic nerve sheath diameter, and reported a linear relationship between the perioptic CSF pressure and ICP during infusion tests [12–14], during administration of osmotic therapy or following CO_2 variation [15]. Measurement of optic nerve sheath diameter using ultrasound with a 7.5 MHz linear probe has the advantage of being non-invasive, safe and repeatable. Several studies have directly correlated optic nerve sheath diameter measurements on ultrasound with invasively measured ICP, in adult and pediatric populations [12–14]. In most of the studies, the authors found good correlation coefficients and good specificity and sensitivity, demonstrating high accuracy for this method; the cut-off value for normal ICP (ICP ≤ 20 mmHg) assessed with optic nerve sheath diameter

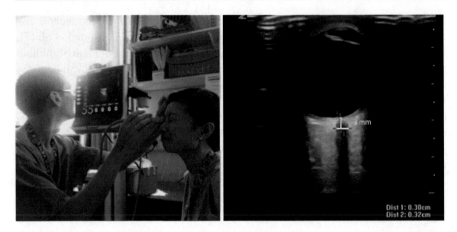

Fig. 4 Insonation of the optic nerve sheath diameter. There should not be any direct contact of the probe with the eyelid nor should pressure be exerted on the globe. Subtle movements scan from side to side (i.e., temporal to nasal), slowly angling the probe superiorly or inferiorly to bring the optic nerve into view. The goal is to center the image on the monitor. Once the image is obtained, first locate a point 3 mm posterior to the optic disk, and place the calipers at 90 degrees to the axis of the optic nerve to measure the diameter of the optic nerve and the optic nerve sheath

ranged from 4.8 to 6 mm in adults and the upper limit of normality for children was 4.0 mm in infants aged less than 1 year, and 4.5 mm in elder children [14, 15]. Also, compared to other non-invasive ultrasound based methods, such as methods derived from transcranial Doppler (TCD) [16], optic nerve sheath diameter has shown the best accuracy in the detection of ICP. However, this technique has several limitations, including its operator-dependency [17] and, therefore, does not seem to be accurate enough to be used as a replacement for invasive ICP measurement.

Transcranial Doppler–Echo Duplex: Arterial and Venous

TCD ultrasonography is a readily available, accessible tool able to evaluate cerebral blood flow (CBF) velocity in the basal cerebral arteries [18]. TCD is based on the Doppler effect, according to which when a sound wave emitted with a certain frequency strikes a moving object, such as red blood cells moving inside an insonated blood vessel, the wave is then reflected with a different frequency (the Doppler shift), directly proportional to the velocity of the object.

TCD is a well-known technique and has been applied in various critical care conditions (Box 1) [18, 19]. The two main assumptions and limitations that govern the use of TCD are a constant vessel diameter and an unchanged angle of insonation. The basic technique for TCD examination consists of insonating the basal portions of the major cerebral arteries of the circle of Willis through different acoustic windows at various locations in the skull (Table 1). Low frequencies, 1–2 MHz, reduce the attenuation of the ultrasound wave caused by bone (Fig. 5).

Box 1 Clinical applications of transcranial Doppler

Clinical Applications of Transcranial Doppler
Detection and follow-up of stenosis or occlusion in a major intracranial artery in the circle of Willis and vertebrobasilar system, including monitoring of thrombolytic therapy for acute stroke patients
Detection of cerebral vasculopathy
Detection and monitoring of vasospasm in patients with spontaneous or traumatic subarachnoid hemorrhage
Assessment of intracranial pressure and hydrocephalus
Evaluation of collateral pathways of intracranial blood flow, including after surgery monitoring
Detection of circulating cerebral microemboli
Detection of right-to-left cardiac shunts (e.g., patent foramen ovale)
Assessment of cerebrovascular autoregulation and vasomotor reactivity
Adjunct in the confirmation of the clinical diagnosis of brain death
Intraoperative and periprocedural monitoring to detect cerebral embolization, thrombosis, hypoperfusion and hyperperfusion
Evaluation of sickle cell disease to determine stroke risk
Assessment of arteriovenous malformations
Detection and follow-up of intracranial aneurysms
Evaluation of positional vertigo or syncope
Assessment of dural venous sinus patency

Table 1 Criteria for the identification of the main cerebral vessels

Artery	Window	Depth (mm)	Direction of flow (relative to transducer)	Velocity (cm/s)
MCA	Transtemporal	45–65	Toward	46–86
MCA/ACA bifurcation	Transtemporal	60–65	Bidirectional	–
ACA	Transtemporal	60–75	Away	41–76
PCA (P1)	Transtemporal	60–75	Toward	33–64
PCA (P2)	Transtemporal	60–75	Away	33–64
Ophthalmic artery	Transocular	45–60	Toward	21–49
Vertebral artery	Transoccipital	65–85	Away	27–55
Basilar artery	Transoccipital	90–120	Away	30–57

MCA: middle cerebral artery; *ACA*: anterior cerebral artery; *PCA*: posterior cerebral artery

Transcranial color duplex is a well-established diagnostic method, allowing direct non-invasive imaging of intracranial vascular structures (Figs. 5 and 6). This visual approach allows more rapid and reliable vessel identification, shortening the examination time and permitting exact localization of the vessel. The hypoechoic butterfly-shaped mesencephalon and echogenic basilar cisterns are the reference landmarks for the circle of Willis (Fig. 5). The posterior cerebral artery (PCA) is seen coursing around the cerebral peduncles. The middle cerebral artery (MCA) has a flow directed towards the transducer and is normally insonated at 2 to 5 mm

Fig. 5 Transcolor duplex
Doppler. Insonation of
the middle cerebral artery
(MCA). a Identification of
the butterfly-shaped mesencephalic (M); b Using the
power color Doppler, the
main vessels of the Wills
circle are identified and
visualized; c MCA TCD
waveform with color Doppler

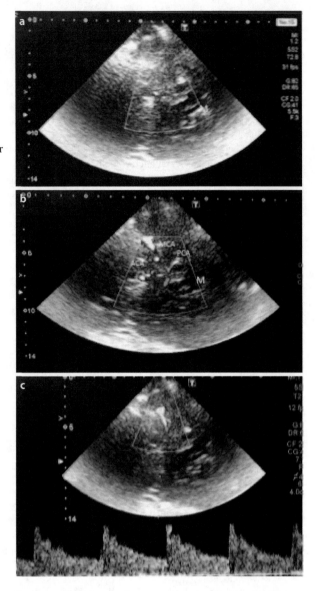

Fig. 5 Transcolor duplex Doppler. Insonation of the middle cerebral artery (MCA). a Identification of the butterfly-shaped mesencephalic (M); b Using the power color Doppler, the main vessels of the Wills circle are identified and visualized; c MCA TCD waveform with color Doppler

intervals from its most superficial point below the calvarium to the bifurcation of the anterior cerebral artery (ACA) and the MCA.

The spectral waveform derived from TCD is made of three components: peak systolic velocity, mean flow velocity and end-diastolic velocity values; simultaneous monitoring of these signals as well as ICP and arterial blood pressure, can give valuable information regarding the state of cerebral hemodynamics [20, 21]. Based on the pulse waveforms derived from CBF velocity signals, several basic

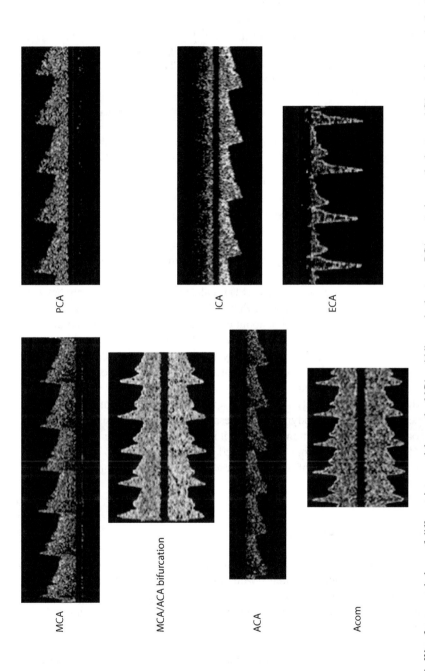

Fig. 6 Waveform morphology of different intracranial vessels. *MCA*: middle cerebral artery; *PCA*: posterior cerebral artery; *ACA*: anterior cerebral artery; *ICA*: internal carotid artery; *Acom*: anterior communicating artery; *ECA*: external carotid artery. Images provided by Dr. Rigamonti

Box 2 Basic and advanced methods derived from transcranial Doppler waveform analysis used in the diagnosis and monitoring of cerebrovascular diseases

Basic methods	Flow velocity (FV)
	Pulsatility index (PI)
Advanced methods	Critical closing pressure (CrCp); the lower threshold of arterial blood pressure, below which small brain vessels collapse and cerebral blood flow ceases
	Autoregulation (Mx index)
	Cerebral compliance (Ca); the ability of the brain to adapt to changes in volume in response to a change in pressure
	Cerebrovascular time constant (Tau); a non-invasive TCD-based index theoretically indicating the time to establish a change in cerebral blood volume after a sudden change in arterial blood pressure during one cardiac cycle
	Non-invasive cerebral perfusion pressure (nCPP)
	Non-invasive intracranial pressure (nICP)

and advanced model-based analyses of cerebral hemodynamics have been introduced, which enable assessment of different aspects of cerebral pathophysiology [20–22] (Box 2). The pulsatility index (PI) is calculated as the relationship between the difference in systolic and diastolic flow velocities divided by the mean flow velocity and can provide information about cerebral vascular resistance and describe changes in the morphology of the TCD waveform resulting from cerebral perfusion pressure changes [22]. The pulsatility index has been traditionally used for assessment of distal cerebrovascular resistance and for the assessment of ICP. Some authors demonstrated a strong correlation coefficient with ICP ($R = 0.94$ $p < 0.05$) [22]. However, the pulsatility index is not specific for the assessment of ICP, and is influenced by many hemodynamic and respiratory parameters (such as CO_2) and many other authors have demonstrated that it is not a good index for ICP assessment [23, 24]. Similarly, many other TCD-derived parameters have been assessed for the non-invasive measurement of ICP, but their accuracy and clinical application is not clear [25, 26].

Venous Transcranial Doppler

Venous TCD is a poorly developed technique. It has been traditionally used for diagnosis and follow-up of patients with stroke, cerebral venous thrombosis and head trauma. However, in the neurointensive care setting, growing evidence suggests a relationship between venous blood flow and ICP [27]. Increasing ICP can influence venous hemodynamics, because the venous system and, in particular, the subarachnoid bridging veins are sensitive and affected by elevated ICP. Cerebral compliance and ICP strongly depend on the compressibility of the low-pressure venous compartment, as stasis in the pial veins is an early compensatory mechanism in case of increased ICP. Therefore, venous blood may be pushed toward larger venous vessels (straight sinus and Rosenthal vein) determining an increase in venous CBF velocity. Schoser et al. found a linear relationship between mean ICP and maximal venous flow velocity in the basal vein of Rosenthal ($r = 0.645$; $p = 0.002$) and in the straight sinus ($r = 0.928$; $p < 0.001$) [27]. However, insonation of the straight sinus is only possible in 72% of patients, reflecting anatomic variations in cerebral venous anatomy.

Brain Perfusion

Brain contrast-enhanced ultrasonography is a non-invasive imaging technique that is able to provide real-time information on changes in cerebral perfusion [29]. Contrast-enhanced ultrasonography is performed by the injection in a peripheral vein of a dedicated contrast agent (air microbubbles). Brain imaging is obtained using an ultrasound machine with a low mechanical index and 2–4 MHz multifrequency probe transducer with second harmonic contrast-imaging mode; images are obtained 1 min after infusion. Using a low frame rate (20FR), video cine loops of 20 s sequences, starting immediately before contrast injection and continuing up to complete contrast wash-out, are then recorded and images are analyzed off-line. Time-intensity curves are reconstructed and time to peak, defined as the time needed from the beginning of contrast injection to reach maximum enhancement, and peak intensity, the value of the maximum intensity in the brain, are used to evaluate changes in perfusion of microcirculation. Bilotta et al. [29] performed contrast-enhanced ultrasonography in 12 patients treated with decompressive craniotomy after acute ischemic stroke at baseline conditions and after the administration of vasoconstrictor and vasodilator drugs and mild hyperventilation. The authors found that contrast-enhanced ultrasonography was able to detect a significant difference in the response to vascular changes between the two hemispheres, related to the loss of autoregulation in the damaged zone of the brain; they concluded that contrast-enhanced ultrasonography is a safe, fast, bedside, dynamic, feasible and repeatable technique to assess cerebral perfusion. However, contrast-enhanced ultrasonography requires use of specific echographic equipment, including dedicated software that can analyze time intensity/curves; moreover, accurate assessment of global cerebral perfusion is feasible only in patients who have undergone decompressive craniectomy.

When and Where: Clinical Applications

Neurocritical Care

The clinical applications of brain ultrasound traditionally and primarily relate to neurocritical care settings (Box 1).

Vasospasm

TCD is considered an established technique for the detection and monitoring of angiographic vasospasm after spontaneous aneurysmal subarachnoid hemorrhage. Vasospasm after subarachnoid hemorrhage causes increased flow velocity inside intracranial vessels, that can be detected by TCD imaging, and mean flow velocity is directly proportional to flow and inversely proportional to the section of the vessels [30]. Threshold velocities above which vasospasm comes into place are well defined for MCA. A mean flow velocity between 100 and 120 cm/s indicates the presence of a slight reduction in the vessel lumen, which cannot be detected with digital subtraction angiography (DSA); velocities between 120 and 200 cm/s indicate moderate vasospasm, which leads to a reduction in the lumen of between 25 and 50%; mean velocities > 200 cm/s indicate severe vasospasm with a reduction of the lumen exceeding 50% [31].

Nevertheless, an increase in velocity alone is not often sufficient to confirm a diagnosis of vasospasm: in fact, hyperemia also presents with an increased flow velocity pattern, which is not obviously due to reduction in the vessel lumen. To differentiate between vasospasm and hyperemia, the Lindegaard Index has therefore been introduced. This index is calculated as the ratio between the mean flow velocity in the MCA and the mean flow velocity in the internal carotid artery (ICA). Thus, a Lindegaard Index < 3 indicates hyperemia, between 3 and 6 moderate vasospasm and > 6 serious vasospasm.

Autoregulation

Evaluation of cerebrovascular autoregulation can give useful prognostic information in several neurocritical care conditions [32]. When autoregulation is compromised, patients are at risk of developing ischemia and cerebral edema [33].

Changes in flow velocity in response to fluctuations in arterial blood pressure have been used as markers of cerebrovascular regulation. Thus, autoregulation of the cerebral circulation can be assessed by examining the changes in flow velocity in response to changes in mean arterial pressure (MAP). TCD enables assessment of both static (observing changes in flow velocity caused by pharmacologically/mechanically induced episodes of hypertension and hypotension) and dynamic autoregulation [34]. The dynamic component of autoregulation can be measured using the mean flow velocity index (Mx index), which expresses the correlation (coefficient) between cerebral perfusion pressure (CPP) and TCD-detected mean flow velocity in the MCA. A positive correlation means that blood flow is pressure-dependent and there is no autoregulation, a negative correlation is found when autoregulatory function is preserved [32–34]. Mx has been used in subjects affected by ICA stenosis; derangement of autoregulatory function can represent a marker of high risk of stroke, so it can be used to guide treatment toward revascularization.

Non-invasive ICP Measurement

Another important application of brain ultrasound techniques is the non-invasive assessment of ICP. TCD waveform analysis has been investigated as a technique for non-invasive ICP estimation; increased ICP could affect the waveform of blood flow velocity in major cerebral vessels, which have compliant walls. Different methods have been studied to non-invasively assess ICP [16], with contrasting results. However, both the optic nerve sheath diameter and the venous velocity in the straight sinus seem to be correlated with ICP [16]. In a recent prospective study in 64 brain injury patients [16], different ultrasound-based methods to assess ICP were compared, including insonation of the straight sinus, the optic nerve sheath diameter and arterial TCD-derived indices. The authors found that the systolic flow velocity on the straight sinus (FVsv) had a good correlation with ICP ($r = 0.72$). Non-invasive ICP was calculated as $0.38 \times FVsv + 0.0005$ (mmHg) with an area under the curve of 0.81 for a threshold of 20 mmHg of ICP. Moreover, the combination of FVsv and the optic nerve sheath diameter resulted in an even higher accuracy to assess ICP ($r = 0.81$):

$$\text{non-invasive ICP (mmHg)} = 4.23 \times \text{optic nerve sheath diameter (mm)} \\ + 0.14 \times FVsv - 14.51$$

The combination of these two methods represents, so far, one of the most accurate methods to non-invasively assess ICP.

Non-neurocritical Care Settings

Emergency Department and Prehospital

A recent case report and literature review suggested that prehospital CT studies (performed in an ambulance equipped with a CT scan) or in general, prehospital brain imaging, can be useful in the management of patients with neurologic disorders [35]. Similarly, optic nerve sheath diameter on CT has been shown to have a potential role as an initial triage tool in the emergency department as well as a method of determining the need for sequential CT in patients with mild traumatic brain injury (TBI), and is useful to improve the prognostic value of gray-to-white matter for predicting poor neurologic outcomes in post-cardiac arrest.

Compared to CT, ultrasound is quick, safe, easy, available and repeatable; therefore its potential use in the emergency department and prehospital setting has been proposed [35]. Bouzat et al. demonstrated that the early use of TCD in patients with mild to moderate TBI was able to predict neurologic worsening and suggested its use for in-hospital triage [36].

Operating Room

Intraoperatively, the optic nerve sheath diameter and TCD have been applied in patients undergoing different procedures at risk of increased ICP, including laparoscopic procedures with pneumoperitoneum and Trendelenburg position, and in patients in prone position at different levels of positive end-expiratory pressure (PEEP) [37]. A prospective observational study showed that non-invasive ICP measured using the optic nerve sheath diameter and TCD-derived methods was able to detect changes in ICP during laparoscopic procedures. Therefore, these data suggest, that especially in patients at risk of increased ICP (such as with brain injury or intracerebral masses), intraoperative use of brain ultrasound should be recommended.

General and Cardiac ICU

Brain ultrasound can have several applications in general and cardiac ICUs. Brain injury is frequently observed after non-primary neurological diseases, including sepsis, metabolic coma, liver failure and acute respiratory distress syndrome (ARDS), through direct effects of the systemic insult on the brain (brain edema, ischemia, seizures) or by indirect injuries (e.g., hypotension, hypoxemia, hypocapnia, hyperglycemia).

Hepatic encephalopathy is associated with cerebral edema, increased ICP and subsequent neurologic complications. Patients with liver failure would benefit from non-invasive neuromonitoring, as liver failure determines severe coagulopathy and risk of bleeding. TCD has also been used in the general ICU to monitor patients with meningitis at risk of neurological complications [38]. In the cardiac ICU, brain ultrasound can have a role in the assessment of neurological complications after cardiac or carotid surgery or during cardiopulmonary bypass (CPB).

TCD has also been shown be useful in the prediction of development of ischemic events in patients suffering from spontaneous carotid arterial dissection without stroke [39]. Cerebrovascular complications are very high even in patients treated with extracorporeal membrane oxygenation (ECMO) related to ischemic stroke as well as intracranial hemorrhage. As the use of ECMO is increasing even in patients with TBI [40], brain ultrasound could potentially became an invaluable tool in the assessment of cerebral complications.

Conclusion

The non-invasiveness, repeatability, and portability of ultrasound make this technique an excellent tool for bedside assessment of brain pathology. These characteristics determine its wide applicability in the monitoring of multiple emergency settings including ICUs, operating rooms and emergency departments. Operator dependence and the need for an adequate temporal acoustic window (lacking in 5–18% of patients) are the main limitations of brain ultrasound. However, its use should be developed further and, especially in patients who undergo decompressive craniectomy, should become a standard of care.

References

1. Caricato A, Mignani V, Bocci MG et al (2012) Usefulness of transcranial echography in patients with decompressive craniectomy. Crit Care Med 40:1745–1752
2. Naqvi J, Yap KH, Ahmad G, Ghosh J (2013) Transcranial Doppler ultrasound: a review of the physical principles and major applications in critical care. Int J Vasc Med 2013:629378
3. Kiphuth IC, Huttner HB, Struffert T, Schwab S, Köhrmann M (2011) Sonographic monitoring of ventricle enlargement in posthemorrhagic hydrocephalus. Neurology 76:858–862
4. Gerriets T, Stolz E, König S et al (2001) Sonographic monitoring of midline shift in space-occupying stroke. An early otcome predictor. Stroke 32:442–447
5. Kazdal H, Kanat A, Findik H et al (2016) Transorbital ultrasonographic measurement of optic nerve sheath diameter for intracranial midline shift in patients with head trauma. World Neurosurg 85:292–297
6. Seidel G, Kaps M, Gerriets T, Hutzelmann A (1995) Evaluation of the ventricular system in adults by transcranial duplex sonography. J Neuroimaging 5:105–108
7. Motuel J, Biette I, Srairi M et al (2014) Assessment of brain midline shift using sonography in neurosurgical ICU patients. Crit Care 18:676
8. Bendella H, Maegele M, Hartmann A et al (2017) Cerebral ventricular dimensions after decompressive craniectomy: a comparison between bedside sonographic duplex technique and cranial computed tomography. Neurocrit Care 26:321–329
9. Mäurer M, Shambal S, Berg D et al (1998) Differentiation between intracerebral hemorrhage and ischemic stroke by transcranial color-coded duplex-sonography. Stroke 29:2563–2567
10. Puntis M, Reddy U, Hirsch N (2016) Cerebrospinal fluid and its physiology. Anaesth Intensive Care Med 17:611–612
11. Helmke K, Hansen HC (1996) Fundamentals of transorbital sonographic evaluation of optic nerve sheath expansion under intracranial hypertension. I. Experimental study. Pediatr Radiol 26:701–705
12. Hansen H-C, Helmke K (1997) Validation of the optic nerve sheath response to changing cerebrospinal fluid pressure: ultrasound findings during intrathecal infusion tests. J Neurosurg 87:34–40
13. Launey Y, Nesseler N, Le Maguet P, Malledant Y, Seguin P (2014) Effect of osmotherapy on optic nerve sheath diameter in patients with increased intracranial pressure. J Neurotrauma 31:984–988
14. Ballantyne J, Hollman AS, Hamilton R et al (1999) Transorbital optic nerve sheath ultrasonography in normal children. Clin Radiol 54:740–742
15. Newman WD (2002) Measurement of optic nerve sheath diameter by ultrasound: a means of detecting acute raised intracranial pressure in hydrocephalus. Br J Ophthalmol 86:1109–1113
16. Robba C, Cardim D, Tajsic T et al (2017) Ultrasound non-invasive measurement of intracranial pressure in neurointensive care: a prospective observational study. PloS Med 14:e1002356
17. Ballantyne SA, O'Neill G, Hamilton R, Hollman AS (2002) Observer variation in the sonographic measurement of optic nerve sheath diameter in normal adults. Eur J Ultrasound 15:145–149
18. Moppett IK, Mahajan RP (2004) Transcranial Doppler ultrasonography in anaesthesia and intensive care. Br J Anaesth 93:710–724
19. Bhatia A, Gupta AK (2007) Neuromonitoring in the intensive care unit. I. Intracranial pressure and cerebral blood flow monitoring. Intensive Care Med 33:1263–1271
20. Hoffmann O, Zierski JT (1982) Analysis of the ICP pulse-pressure relationship as a function of arterial blood pressure: clinical validation of a mathematical model. Acta Neurochir (Wien) 66:1–21
21. Bekker A, Wolk S, Turndorf H, Kristol D, Ritter A (1996) Computer simulation of cerebrovascular circulation: assessment of intrac rani al hemodynamics during induction of anesthesia. J Clin Monit 12:433–444

22. Bellner J, Romner B, Reinstrup P, Kristiansson KA, Ryding E, Brandt L (2004) Transcranial Doppler sonography pulsatility index (PI) reflects intracranial pressure (ICP). Surg Neurol 62:45–51

23. Cardim D, Robba C, Bohdanowicz M et al (2016) Non-invasive monitoring of intracranial pressure using transcranial doppler ultrasonography: is it possible? Neurocrit Care 25:473–491

24. De Riva N, Budohoski KP, Smielewski P et al (2012) Transcranial doppler pulsatility index: what it is and what it isn't. Neurocrit Care 17:58–66

25. Rasulo FA, Bertuetti R, Robba C et al (2017) The accuracy of transcranial Doppler in excluding intracranial hypertension following acute brain injury: a multicenter prospective pilot study. Crit Care 21:44

26. Cardim D, Robba C, Donnelly J et al (2015) Prospective study on non-invasive assessment of ICP in head injured patients: comparison of four methods. J Neurotrauma 33:792–802

27. Schoser BG, Riemenschneider N, Hansen HC (1999) The impact of raised intracranial pressure on cerebral venous hemodynamics: a prospective venous transcranial Doppler ultrasonography study. J Neurosurg 91:744–749

28. Rim SJ, Leong-Poi H, Lindner JR et al (2001) Quantification of cerebral perfusion with "Real-Time" contrast-enhanced ultrasound. Circulation 104:2582–2587

29. Bilotta F, Robba C, Santoro A, Delfini R, Rosa G, Agati L (2016) Contrast-enhanced ultrasound imaging in detection of changes in cerebral perfusion. Ultrasound Med Biol 42:2708–2716

30. Sloan MA, Alexandrov AV, Tegeler CH et al (2004) Assessment: transcranial Doppler ultrasonography: report of the therapeutics and technology assessment subcommittee of the American Academy of Neurology. Neurology 62:1468–1481

31. Lysakowski C, Walder B, Costanza MC, Tramèr MR (2001) Transcranial Doppler versus angiography in patients with vasospasm due to a ruptured cerebral aneurysm. Stroke 32:2292–2298

32. Donnelly J, Aries MJ, Czosnyka M (2015) Further understanding of cerebral autoregulation at the bedside: possible implications for future therapy. Expert Rev Neurother 15:169–185

33. Jaeger M, Schuhmann MU, Soehle M, Nagel C, Meixensberger J (2007) Continuous monitoring of cerebrovascular autoregulation after subarachnoid hemorrhage by brain tissue oxygen pressure reactivity and its relation to delayed cerebral infarction. Stroke 38:981–986

34. Panerai RB (1998) Assessment of cerebral pressure autoregulation in humans – a review of measurement methods. Physiol Meas 19:305

35. Schwindling L, Ragoschke-Schumm A, Kettner M et al (2016) Prehospital imaging-based triage of head trauma with a mobile stroke unit: first evidence and literature review. J Neuroimaging 26:489–493

36. Bouzat P, Francony G, Declety P et al (2011) Transcranial Doppler to screen on admission patients with mild to moderate traumatic brain injury. Neurosurgery 68:1603–1609

37. Robba C, Cardim D, Donnelly J et al (2016) Effects of pneumoperitoneum and Trendelenburg position on intracranial pressure assessed using different non-invasive methods. Br J Anaesth 117:783–791

38. Kiliç T, Elmaci I, Özek MM, Pamir MN (2002) Utility of transcranial Doppler ultrasonography in the diagnosis and follow-up of tuberculous meningitis-related vasculopathy. Childs Nerv Syst 18:142–146

39. Brunser AM, Lavados PM, Hoppe A et al (2017) Transcranial Doppler as a predictor of ischemic events in carotid artery dissection. J Neuroimaging 27:232–236

40. Robba C, Ortu A, Bilotta F et al (2017) Extracorporeal membrane oxygenation for adult respiratory distress syndrome in trauma patients. J Trauma Acute Care Surg 82:165–173

Continuous Electroencephalography Monitoring in Adults in the Intensive Care Unit

A. Caricato, I. Melchionda, and M. Antonelli

Introduction

Neurologic monitoring in the intensive care unit (ICU) is based on the acquisition of several parameters from multiple brain devices. Electroencephalography (EEG) is one of the simplest ways to investigate cerebral activity, easily recorded at the bedside and sensitive to changes in both brain structure and function [1]. Due to these features and its simple utilization, use of continuous EEG (cEEG) recording in critically ill patients has increased over the past decade [2, 3]. Recently, it was recommended by international guidelines with well-defined indications [4–6]. Nonetheless, few academic centers use it, and the expertise of neurointensivists for continuous real-time interpretation of EEG patterns is uncommon [7].

This chapter summarizes recent results on this topic, focusing on indications, duration of monitoring and technical issues.

Indications

Non-convulsive Seizures and Non-convulsive Status Epilepticus

Recent classifications define convulsive status epilepticus as a condition of abnormally prolonged seizures lasting more than 5 min. Non-convulsive status epilepticus (NCSE) is defined as abnormally prolonged seizures without prominent motor symptoms. The limit for 'prolonged' remains to be determined: in selected cases of NCSE, for example, focal status epilecticus with impaired consciousness, it was defined as 10 min by a Task Force from the International League against Epilepsy [8].

A. Caricato (✉) · I. Melchionda · M. Antonelli
Dept. of Anesthesiology and Intensive Care Medicine, Fondazione Policlinico Universitario A. Gemelli, Università Cattolica del Sacro Cuore
Rome, Italy
e-mail: anselmo.caricato@unicatt.it

© Springer International Publishing AG 2018
J.-L. Vincent (ed.), *Annual Update in Intensive Care and Emergency Medicine 2018*,
Annual Update in Intensive Care and Emergency Medicine,
https://doi.org/10.1007/978-3-319-73670-9_40

Several authors have reported that NCSE is a common finding in critically ill patients, associated with increased mortality and increased risk of poor neurological outcome [9–11].

To exclude this condition, a consensus statement of the American Clinical Neurophysiology Society recommend use of cEEG [4]:

1. after seizures, if impaired consciousness persists after initial treatment
   Evidence is strong for this recommendation. In ICU patients admitted for seizures, DeLorenzo et al. reported that non-convulsive seizures were observed on cEEG in 48% of cases, and NCSE in 14% of cases [12]. Claassen et al. identified non-convulsive seizures on cEEG monitoring in 25% of 570 critical care patients; in a subgroup of 110 patients who had seizures before monitoring, non-convulsive seizures were observed on cEEG in 43% of the cases [13]. Several authors have confirmed these results, providing solid arguments for extended EEG monitoring in this condition [4].
2. in cases of unexplained alteration of mental status without known acute brain injury
   In one prospective study, 75% of diagnoses of NCSE or non-convulsive seizures on cEEG were not preceded by clinical seizures. In these cases, symptoms may be minor or absent, or include aphasia, confusion, agitation or behavioral abnormalities [13]. Neurological fluctuation is a typical finding, and may help in diagnosis. When coma is present, NCSE is observed in 0–14% of the cases [14, 15]
3. When specific EEG patterns are recognized on routine recording: generalized periodic discharges (GPDs), lateralized periodic discharges (LPDs), or BIPDs (bilateral independent periodic discharges) (Fig. 1)
   In a large retrospective multicenter study in 4722 critically ill patients, based on the Critical Care EEG Monitoring Research Consortium multicenter database, there was significant relationship of seizures with some periodic and rhythmic patterns: GPDs, LPDs and lateralized rhythmic delta activity (LRDA) [16]. In these cases, the incidence of seizures ranged from 50% and 88% on routine EEG [4]. In particular, data showed that most of the seizures were non-convulsive. A detailed EEG description using standardized nomenclature is of paramount importance for a correct interpretation of EEG tracings, and for seizure risk stratification. These results strongly support the use cEEG to detect seizure occurrence when these pattern are found.
4. In comatose patients after acute brain injury
   Several conditions have been reported to be correlated with NCSE, with incidences of up to 30% in subarachnoid hemorrhage, head injury, intracerebral hemorrhage, central nervous system infections [3]. The incidence may be even higher in post-anoxic encephalopathy, ranging from 10 to 60%.
5. When neuromuscular blocking drugs (NMBD) are used in high risk patients

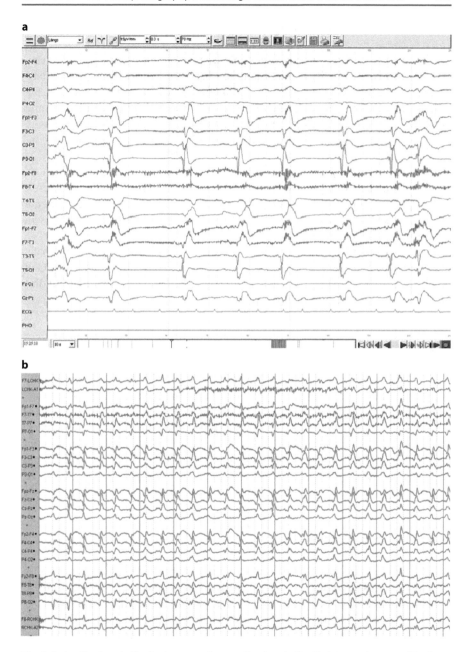

Fig. 1 Lateralized periodic discharges and generalized periodic discharges. An example of two periodic patterns: **a** temporo-parietal lateralized periodic discharges and **b** generalized periodic discharges. Continuous EEG recording is recommended in these cases

Duration of cEEG Monitoring

cEEG should be initiated as soon as possible when non-convulsive seizures are suspected, as higher morbidity and mortality has been observed, and early treatments are likely to be more effective [17]. Recording for at least 24 h is recommended, but in some cases shorter or longer periods may be necessary. Traditional 30–60 min EEG recordings identify non-convulsive seizures in only 45–58% of patients in whom seizures are eventually recorded. About 80–95% of patients with non-convulsive seizures can be identified within 24–48 h [18, 19].

In 625 critically ill patients, the probability of seizures was strongly influenced by findings detected very early in the course of monitoring. In case of absence of epileptiform abnormalities during the first 15 min recording, the 72-h seizure probability was less than 10%, and less than 5% if no abnormality was present during the first 2 h recording [20].

In selected populations, the duration of monitoring is still a matter of debate. Thirty-minute serial EEGs have been demonstrated to have similar yield to cEEG in adult post-cardiac arrest patients undergoing hypothermia [21]. Additional studies need to draw definitive data on this topic.

Diagnosis of Ischemia

EEG is very sensitive in detecting changes in cerebral blood flow (CBF), generally showing regional attenuation of faster frequencies and increases in slow activity; based on these observations, many authors have suggested cEEG for ischemia identification during surgical or neuroradiological procedures, during intracranial hypertension and for the diagnosis of delayed cerebral ischemia (DCI) after subarachnoid hemorrhage [22–24]. Although many studies have tried to show a specific ischemic pattern in various conditions, current recommendations suggest cEEG to detect ischemia only for the diagnosis of DCI after subarachnoid hemorrhage [5].

Delayed Cerebral Ischemia

DCI is a severe complication that occurs after subarachnoid hemorrhage in 20–30% of cases. Diagnosis is based on clinical symptoms and is characterized by a decrease in consciousness, new focal deficit, or both. No radiological examination can confirm or exclude DCI at the time of clinical deterioration; theoretically EEG is able to detect electrical changes before structural damage occurs, providing a window of opportunity for therapeutic interventions [25].

Several authors have investigated this hypothesis in small prospective studies using cEEG, and many quantitative EEG parameters have been evaluated. According to Claassen et al., a 10% reduction in the alpha-delta power ratio had a sensitivity of 100% for DCI, with a specificity of 76% [26]. Rots et al. confirmed these results in 20 patients with subarachnoid hemorrhage, reporting that a reduction in the alpha-delta ratio over time in any channel was the single most accurate prognostic indicator; patients in the DCI group showed a median decrease of 62% in the ratio, compared with a median increase of 27% in the control group [27]. Changes in alpha variability were also associated with DCI in these patients.

According to Rots et al. [27] and Gollwitzer et al. [28], EEG changes appearing before ischemia were identified in around 70% of cases; the median time between quantitative EEG (qEEG) changes and the clinical diagnosis of DCI ranged from 5 to 60 h. At the Massachusetts General Hospital, an institutional protocol for patients with subarachnoid hemorrhage included cEEG recording, and prediction of DCI was suggested if there was an alpha-delta ratio decrease of 10% lasting 6 h (100% sensitivity and 76% specificity) or when at least 50% decrements in the alpha-delta ratio were observed for 2 h or more (89% sensitivity and 84% specificity) [29].

Recent international recommendations suggest use of cEEG to detect DCI in conjunction with other conventional examinations in comatose patients, in whom neurological examination is unreliable, and suggest that it may predict DCI 24–48 h prior to other diagnostic tools [5].

Prognostication

Some of the data obtained from EEG, such as sleep architecture, the presence of a sleep/awake cycle, reactivity to external stimuli, and detection of epileptiform changes can be used for prognostic evaluation in comatose patients [30]. In this setting, postanoxic encephalopathy has been extensively studied, and selected EEG patterns were found to be associated with a poor neurological outcome. A statement from the European Society of Intensive Care Medicine and the European Resuscitation Council suggests that the absence of EEG reactivity to external stimuli and the presence of burst-suppression or status epilepticus at 72 h after cardiac arrest significantly predict poor outcome, defined as severe neurological disability, persistent vegetative state or death, with a false positive ratio ranging from 0 to 6% [31].

Recently, Westhall et al. reported that the presence of a highly malignant EEG pattern, defined according to the EEG terminology standardized by the American Clinical Neurophysiology Society as suppressed background without discharges, suppressed background with continuous periodic discharges, or burst-suppression background with or without discharges, predicted poor outcome in comatose patients after cardiac arrest without false-positives [32].

Several studies have investigated the prognostic significance of EEG recordings in patients with subarachnoid hemorrhage [9, 10, 26–28]. Claassen et al. reported that outcome was poor (modified Rankin Scale 4 to 6) in all patients with absent EEG reactivity, GPDs, or BIPDs, and in 92% of patients with NCSE [33]. DeMarchis et al. confirmed these results, observing that patients with subarachnoid hemorrhage with seizures had more than 3-times higher odds of disability or death [10]. Whether cEEG adds information to serial EEG on this topic is not known. Duration of monitoring has not been investigated, and no definitive data can be drawn.

Methods

Based on the clinical scenario and available resources, different types of EEG monitoring can be chosen for recording in the ICU. It can be performed with portable EEG, mobile desktop EEG, and EEG workstations; in its most complete configuration, it is associated to a video-camera for a synchronous recording of video and EEG trace in order to minimize artifacts and recognize clinical correspondence with the EEG signal. Telemedicine programs may create connections between workstations remotely located in different places within or outside the hospital. This is of paramount importance, in particular when resources are lacking and neurologists and/or neurophysiologists are not always available.

Electrode Positioning

Most EEG recordings follow the American Clinical Neurophysiology Society International 10–20 system guidelines for head measurements and electrode applications [34]. The positions are determined as follows: reference points are the *nasion*, which is the depression at the top of the nose, at the eye level; and the *inion*, which is the bony lump at the base of the skull on the midline at the back of the head. From these points, the skull perimeters are measured in the transverse and median planes. The 10 and 20 refers to the electrode location, which is determined by dividing these perimeters into 10% and 20% intervals.

Different types of electrodes are available [35]. Disk or cup electrodes are classically used, and those with a central hole are best to permit periodic refilling with electrode conductive gel. When possible, computed tomography (CT) or magnetic resonance imaging (MRI) compatible electrodes should be used; they can remain in place during imaging, reducing time spent removing and reapplying, and may also reduce skin breakdown caused by frequent electrode removal and reapplication. Subdermal needle electrodes can be applied rapidly and do not require scalp abrasion. Needles are inserted just beneath the skin, parallel to the surface of the scalp and should be secured with adhesive paste. They are not recommended for awake patients or prolonged recording, but are very useful because of their rapid positioning and for brief recording in some comatose patients.

Subdermal wire electrodes are thin wires with a silver chloride tip, and are placed in a similar manner to that of the standard subdermal needle electrode. They are hooked into the lumen of a 25G or 27G needle; after positioning the needle is removed and the wire remains in the subdermal tissue. On the skin, some fixation with patches or glue may be useful. They may reduce skin breakdown and provide better recording performance compared to disc electrodes during prolonged cEEG monitoring [36]. An electrode cap and template system may be used when rapid initiation of EEG recording is essential. Their use may be limited by the presence of scalp wounds, dressings or intracranial devices (Fig. 2).

The number of electrodes used in cEEG studies varies considerably. Usually the 10–20 system places 21 electrodes. Alternatives to this full montage have been

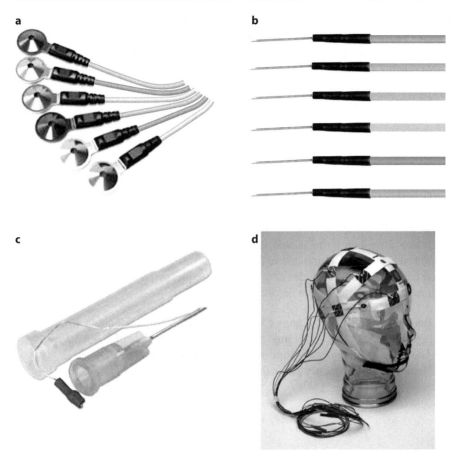

Fig. 2 Type of EEG electrodes. Examples of classic cup electrodes (**a**), subdermal needle electrodes (**b**), subdermal wire electrodes (**c**) and an EEG template system (**d**)

described. One of these is a sub-hairline recording, which uses four bipolar derivations: left temporal (left anterior temporal electrode to left mastoid electrode), left frontal (left frontal electrode to left anterior temporal electrode), right frontal (right frontal electrode to right anterior temporal electrode) and right temporal (right frontal anterior temporal electrode to right mastoid electrode) [37]. A montage with eight recording electrodes uses four couples of electrodes: forehead FP1, FP2; central C3, C4; temporal T3, T4; and occipital O1, O2. The reference electrodes should be at the bilateral earlobe or mastoid levels. The grounding electrode should be placed at the midpoint of the frontal pole (FPz), and the common reference electrode should be placed at the median central point (Cz) [37].

A full electrode configuration improves the ability to distinguish brain signals from artifact, aids in spatial localization of pathological activity, and provides redundancy, enabling continued interpretation in case one or more leads fail. However, in several cases, EEG recording is performed with a reduced number of electrodes, or in altered positions, in particular when surgical wounds, ventricular drains, or neuromonitoring devices limit the available surface of the skull. Under these conditions, electrode positioning is faster and easier to maintain. However, it is critical to maintain the symmetry of the left and right side electrodes.

For the application of long-term EEG monitoring, a 12–24 h suspension may be needed after 24–48 h of continuous monitoring. Sometimes, it is necessary to clean the skin or change the location of some electrodes to avoid scalp ulceration or infection.

EEG Analysis

EEGs may be categorized based on amplitude, frequency, symmetry and patterns. Although amplitude is measured quantitatively in microvolts, it is generally reported as low or high compared to a previously measured baseline. Amplitude has been somewhat arbitrarily divided into four frequency ranges (Fig. 3). From the highest to the lowest frequencies these waves are:

- Beta waves – frequency range 15–30 Hz and an amplitude of about 30 μv
- Alpha waves – frequency range 8–14 Hz and an amplitude of about 30–50 μv
- Theta waves – frequency range 3–8 HZ and an amplitude of about 50–100 μv
- Delta waves – frequency range 0.5–4 Hz and an amplitude of about 100–200 μv.

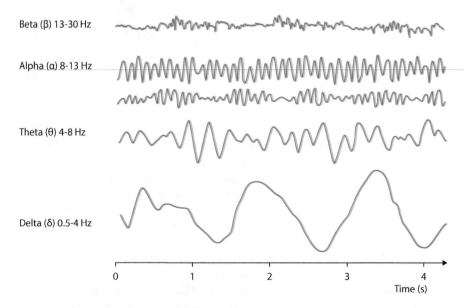

Fig. 3 EEG waveform frequency. Examples of traditional classification of alpha, beta, theta, delta EEG frequencies

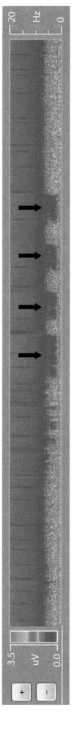

Fig. 4 Color density spectral array. In this frequency(*y*) *vs* time(*x*) graph, each pixel shows the amplitude of EEG recording, according to its color (*purple* low, *red* high). The color range for the amplitude scale is shown on the *left*. Waveform frequency is displayed on the *right*. Phases of sudden reduction of faster frequencies during sedation can be easily recognized (*arrows*)

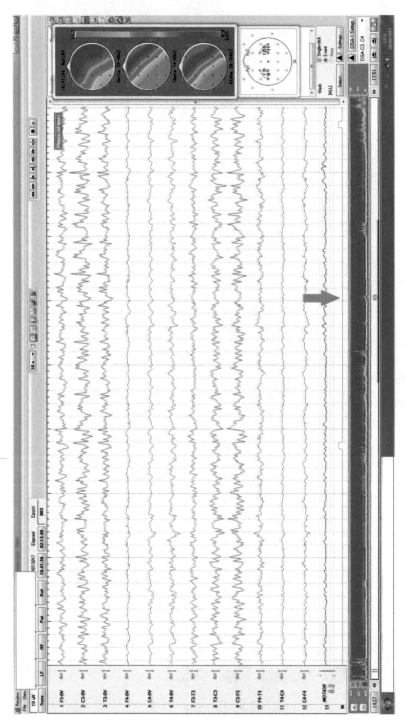

Fig. 5 Focal increase in EEG fast frequencies. In this raw EEG, fast frequencies in the left temporal region are shown. By DSA compression, these are easily observed as a sudden modification in the EEG recording (*arrow*). Topographic maps of spectral power are displayed on the *right*; they are spatial representations of the amplitude of traditional waveform frequencies (delta, theta, alpha), referred to the raw EEG displayed on the screen. Focal asymmetries can be easily identified. The color range of the amplitude scale is shown on the *right*

Monitoring an ICU patient for several days generates gigabytes of data that, in their raw form, are nearly impossible for a neurophysiologist to review and to analyze at the bedside. Thus, several qEEG analyses have been implemented for use in cEEG monitoring. This involves fast Fourier transformation of raw EEG data performed in near real-time and subsequently displayed in compressed form. In this way, several hours of raw EEG recordings can be reduced to a single screen of time-frequency values.

Color density spectral array (DSA) is a graphical picture of the EEG that compresses hours of activity into time, distribution of frequency, and power measurements. It is an X-Y graph, (frequency vs time), on which each pixel is colored according to the amplitude of the EEG recording. We can, therefore, easily observe amplitude in a particular range of frequency. Color DSA is very useful for rapid screening of EEG recordings, so as to identify significant abnormalities, such as seizures, effects of sedation, sleep-wake cycle muscle artifacts (Fig. 4). In addition, it enables identification of gradual changes in the EEG trace, which are difficult to detect when reading EEG at a conventional review speed of 10 s per page.

Topographic maps of spectral power are graphical spatial representations, one for each classic frequency range (alpha, theta and delta), where each pixel is colored according to the amplitude of the signal, as with DSA. The maps enable rapid identification of asymmetries (Fig. 5).

Other graphical displays include ratios of power in certain bands over a broader spectrum of EEG power, envelope trends, amplitude-integrated EEG, and spectral edge displays. qEEG trends can be generated for individual EEG channels or combinations of channels to provide overviews of homologous left and right brain regions [38].

Conclusion

Use of cEEG has become more frequent over the last decade, and cEEG is considered one of the most important tools in multiparametric monitoring of neurocritical care patients. Since its introduction into clinical practice, several challenges have been solved, and international recommendations now use standardized terminology and indications and refer to the same technical issues. Nevertheless, clinical indications for cEEG are often not followed, and it still represents an underused tool.

One of the most important issues for its widespread diffusion is the 24/7 need for a technician to position and verify the electrodes, and a neurophysiologist to read the EEG. Several articles have shown that, after a relatively short period of training, ICU physicians and nurses can achieve an acceptable level in solving technical problems and identifying the main EEG patterns [39, 40]. This is an interesting challenge for neurointensivists. Further, at this time evidence that cEEG may improve patient outcome is still lacking. Nevertheless, its limited invasiveness, bedside availability and relatively low costs make cEEG an attractive tool with many potential areas of interest in the multiparametric monitoring of neurocritical care patients.

References

1. Nuwer MR (1994) EEG and evoked potentials: monitoring cerebral function in the neurosurgical ICU. In: Martin NA (ed) Neurosurgical Intensive Care. W.B. Saunders, Philadelphia, pp 647–659
2. Ney JP, van der Goes DN, Nuwer MR, Nelson L, Eccher MA (2013) Continuous and routine EEG in intensive care: utilization and outcomes, United States 2005–2009. Neurology 81:2002–2008
3. Kinney MO, Kaplan PW (2017) An update on the recognition and treatment of non-convulsive status epilepticus in the intensive care unit. Exp Rev Neurother 17:987–1002
4. Herman ST, Abend N, Bleck TP (2015) Consensus statement on continuous eeg in critically ill adults and children, Part I: Indications. J Clin Neurophysiol 32:87–95
5. Claassen J, Taccone FS, Horn P, Holtkamp M, Stocchetti N, Oddo M (2013) Recommendations on the use of EEG monitoring in critically ill patients: consensus statement from the neurointensive care section of the ESICM. Intensive Care Med 39:1337–1351
6. André-Obadia N, Parain D, Szurhaj W (2015) Continuous EEG monitoring in adults in the intensive care unit. Neurophysiol Clin 45:39–46
7. Gavvala J, Abend N, LaRoche S et al (2014) Continuous EEG monitoring: a survey of neurophysiologists and neurointensivists. Epilepsia 55:1864–1871
8. Trinka E, Cock H, Hesdorffer D et al (2015) A definition and classification of status epilepticus – report of the ILAE task force on classification of status epilepticus. Epilepsia 56:1515–1523
9. Claassen J, Albers D, Schmidt JM et al (2014) Non convulsive seizures in subarachnoid hemorrhage link inflammation and outcome. Ann Neurol 75:771–781
10. De Marchis GM, Pugin D, Meyers E et al (2016) Seizure burden in subarachnoid hemorrhage associated with functional and cognitive outcome. Neurology 86:253–260
11. Payne ET, Zhao XY, Frndova H et al (2014) Seizure burden is independently associated with short term outcome in critically ill children. Brain 137:1429–1438
12. DeLorenzo RJ, Waterhouse EJ, Towne AR et al (1998) Persistent nonconvulsive status epilepticus after the control of convulsive status epilepticus. Epilepsia 39:833–840
13. Laccheo I, Sonmezturk H, Bhatt AB et al (2015) Non-convulsive status epilepticus and nonconvulsive seizures in neurological ICU patients. Neurocrit Care 22:202–211
14. Towne AR, Waterhouse EJ, Boggs JG et al (2000) Prevalence of nonconvulsive status epilepticus in comatose patients. Neurology 54:340–345
15. Oddo M, Carrera E, Claassen J, Mayer SA, Hirsch LJ (2009) Continuous electroencephalography in the medical intensive care unit. Crit Care Med 37:2051–2056
16. Rodriguez Ruiz A, Vlachy J, Lee JW et al (2017) Association of periodic and rhythmic electroencephalographic patterns with seizures in critically ill patients. JAMA Neurol 74:181–188
17. Vespa PM, McArthur DL, Xu Y et al (2010) Nonconvulsive seizures after traumatic brain injury are associated with hippocampal atrophy. Neurology 75:792–798
18. Claassen J, Mayer SA, Kowalski RG, Emerson RG, Hirsch LJ (2004) Detection of electrographic seizures with continuous EEG monitoring in critically ill patients. Neurology 62:1743–1748
19. Fogang Y, Legros B, Depondt C et al (2017) Yield of repeated intermittent EEG for seizure detection in critically ill adults. Clin Neurophysiol 47:5–12
20. Westover MB, Shafi MM, Bianchi MT et al (2015) The probability of seizures during EEG monitoring in critically ill adults. Clin Neurophysiol 126:463–471
21. Alvarez V, Sierra-Marcos A, Oddo M, Rossetti AO (2013) Yield of intermittent versus continuous EEG in comatose survivors of cardiac arrest treated with hypothermia. Crit Care 17:R190
22. Diedler J, Sykora M, Bast T et al (2009) Quantitative EEG correlates of low cerebral perfusion in severe stroke. Neurocrit Care 11:210–216
23. Skordilis M, Rich N, Viloria A et al (2011) Processed electroencephalogram response of patients undergoing carotid endarterectomy: a pilot study. Ann Vasc Surg 25:909–912

24. Mishra M, Banday M, Derakhshani R, Croom J, Camarata PJ (2011) A quantitative EEG method for detecting post clamp changes during carotid endarterectomy. J Clin Monit Comput 25:295–308

25. Gaspard N (2016) Current clinical evidence supporting the use of continuous eeg monitoring for delayed cerebral ischemia detection. J Clin Neurophysiol 33:211–216

26. Claassen J, Hirsch LJ, Kreiter KT et al (2004) Quantitative continuous EEG for detecting delayed cerebral ischemia in patients with poor-grade subarachnoid hemorrhage. Clin Neurophysiol 115:2699–2710

27. Rots ML, van Putten MJAM, Hoedemaekers CWE, Horn J (2016) Continuous EEG monitoring for early detection of delayed cerebral ischemia in subarachnoid hemorrhage: a pilot study. Neurocrit Care 24:207–216

28. Gollwitzer S, Groemer T, Rampp S et al (2015) Early prediction of delayed cerebral ischemia in subarachnoid hemorrhage based on quantitative EEG: a prospective study in adults. Clin Neurophysiol 126:1514–1523

29. Muniz CF, Shenoy AV, O'Connor KL et al (2016) Clinical development and implementation of an institutional guideline for prospective EEG monitoring and reporting of delayed cerebral ischemia. J Clin Neurophysiol 33:217–226

30. Velly L, Pellegrini L, Bruder N (2012) EEG en reanimation: quelles indications, quel materiel? Ann Franc Anesth Reanim 31:e145–e153

31. Sandroni C, Cariou A, Cavallaro F et al (2014) Prognostication in comatose survivors of cardiac arrest: an advisory statement from the European Resuscitation Council and the European Society of Intensive Care Medicine. Intensive Care Med 40:1816–1831

32. Westhall E, Rossetti AO, Van Rootselaar AF (2016) Standardized EEG interpretation accurately predicts prognosis after cardiac arrest. Neurology 86:1482–1490

33. Claassen J, Hirsch LJ, Frontera JA et al (2006) Prognostic significance of continuous EEG monitoring in patients with poor-grade subarachnoid hemorrhage. Neurocrit Care 4:103–112

34. American Clinical Neurophysiology Society (2006) Guideline 1: Minimum technical requirements for performing clinical electroencephalography. J Clin Neurophysiol 23:86–91

35. Vulliemoz S, Perrig S, Pellise D et al (2009) Imaging compatible electrodes for continuous electroencephalogram monitoring in the intensive care unit. J Clin Neurophysiol 26:236–243

36. Young GB, Ives JR, Chapman MG, Mirsattari SM (2006) A comparison of subdermal wire electrodes with collodion-applied disk electrodes in long-term EEG recordings in ICU. Clin Neurophysiol 117:1376–1379

37. Tanner AE, Sarkela MO, Virtanen J et al (2014) Application of subhairline EEG montage in intensive care unit: comparison with full montage. J Clin Neurophysiol 31:181–186

38. Scheuer ML, Wilson SB (2004) Data analysis for continuous EEG monitoring in the ICU: seeing the forest and the trees. J Clin Neurophysiol 21:353–378

39. Dericioglu N, Yetim E, Bas DF et al (2015) Nonexpert use of quantitative EEG displays for seizure identification in the adult neuro-intensive care unit. Epilepsy Res 109:48–56

40. Citerio G, Patruno A, Beretta S et al (2017) Implementation of continuous qEEG in two neurointensive care units by intensivists: a feasibility study. Intensive Care Med 43:1067–1068

Respiratory Management in Patients with Severe Brain Injury

K. Asehnoune, A. Roquilly, and R. Cinotti

Introduction

Severe brain injuries, such as traumatic brain injury (TBI), intracranial hemorrhage or stroke are a common cause of intensive care unit (ICU) admission and mechanical ventilation initiation [1]. Mechanical ventilation is frequently applied to protect the airway from the risk of aspiration and to prevent both hypoxemia and hypercapnia, which are two major systemic factors of secondary brain insult. Recent guidelines [2] recommend that prolonged prophylactic hyperventilation with $PCO_2 \leq 25$ mmHg should be avoided, but the ventilator settings, including those to set tidal volume or positive end-expiratory pressure (PEEP), remain undetailed. Observational data suggest that brain injury patients are delivered higher tidal volume and lower PEEP levels than non-neurological patients [3] but they have longer mechanical ventilation duration, and higher rates of hospital-acquired pneumonia [4, 5], tracheostomy and mortality than non-neurologic patients [3]. The respiratory management is further complex because weaning these patients from mechanical ventilation and the decision to extubate remain two challenging issues [6]. Indeed, guidelines for the weaning of mechanical ventilation in ICU patients were developed 10 years ago [7], but owing to the lack of robust evidence in the literature, no clear recommendations are currently available in the neuro-ICU setting.

K. Asehnoune (✉) · A. Roquilly
Intensive Care Unit, Anesthesia and Critical Care Department, Hôtel Dieu, University Hospital of Nantes
Nantes, France
Laboratoire UPRES EA 3826 "Thérapeutiques cliniques et expérimentales des infections",
University Hospital of Nantes
Nantes, France
e-mail: karim.asehnoune@chu-nantes.fr

R. Cinotti
Intensive Care Unit, Anesthesia and Critical Care Department, Hôtel Dieu, University Hospital of Nantes
Nantes, France

© Springer International Publishing AG 2018   549
J.-L. Vincent (ed.), *Annual Update in Intensive Care and Emergency Medicine 2018*,
Annual Update in Intensive Care and Emergency Medicine,
https://doi.org/10.1007/978-3-319-73670-9_41

Interest in the respiratory management of brain injury patients has increased recently. In particular, the use of protective ventilation in the early phase of brain injury [8, 9] has been evaluated, and new data regarding the criteria compatible with successful extubation [10–12] have been gathered.

In this chapter, we will focus on the most recent data available in the neuro-ICU field regarding respiratory management, from the early phase of mechanical ventilation initiation to liberation from mechanical ventilation and extubation.

Historical Practices in Mechanical Ventilation

Tidal Volume

After brain injury, impaired consciousness and brain-stem reflexes induce hypoventilation and lead to aspiration. The first aim of mechanical ventilation is to protect the airway through tracheal intubation. Current guidelines recommend that endotracheal intubation should be performed systematically when the Glasgow Coma Score (GCS) is ≤ 8 [2]. In the first days after brain injury, hypoxemia and hyper/hypocapnia lead to secondary brain insults, which alter the outcome [13]. Treatment of hypoxemia consists of increasing the inspired oxygen fraction (FiO_2) delivery with a target of $PaO_2 > 60$ mmHg [2], which can be modified if brain ischemia is diagnosed by multimodal monitoring (low tissue oxygen tension [$PtiO_2$] and low jugular venous oxygen saturation [$SvjO_2$]) [14]. $PaCO_2$ is a powerful determinant of cerebral blood flow (CBF), which impacts intracranial pressure (ICP) [2]. An adequate control of $PaCO_2$ within a 32–45 mmHg range, even at the very early phase, was associated with a better outcome [15]. The maintenance of normal levels of $PaCO_2$ is thus recommended throughout the TBI course [2]. Nonetheless, no consensus is available to set the respiratory rate and the tidal volume in order to reach the $PaCO_2$ target, and in daily practice, practitioners usually increase tidal volume, in order to provide better $PaCO_2$ control (Table 1).

In a multicenter nationwide observational study, patients with brain injury had a comparable mean tidal volume compared to non-neurologic patients, with a median of 9 ml/kg of ideal predicted body weight [3]. However, a significantly lower proportion of patients with intracranial hemorrhage (15%) received protective ventilation on day 1 of mechanical ventilation, probably because of the fear of hypercapnia [3]. Because lung injuries were observed in animal models of brain injury and associated with the release of danger-associated molecular patterns (DAMPs) and with lung injury [16], it is reasonable to propose that brain injury is a risk factor for ventilator-induced lung injury (VILI) and that low tidal volume could be of interest in these patients. Indeed, it is now well established that high tidal volume ventilation leads to VILI [17] and, in neurologic ICU studies, the use of high tidal volume is associated with an increased rate of acute respiratory distress syndrome (ARDS), worsening outcomes [18].

Table 1 Evolution of respiratory care bundle in patients with brain injury [8–12]

	Current practice	Evolution of practice
Tidal volume	> 8 ml/kg IBW	6–7 ml/kg IBW
PEEP	0–3 cmH$_2$O	≥ 5 cmH$_2$O
Extubation management	Awaiting recovery or awareness	Negative fluid balance Cough Gag reflex VISAGE score: – Age < 40 – GGS > 10 – Visual pursuit – Swallowing
Tracheostomy management	?	?

PEEP: positive end-expiratory pressure; *GCS*: Glasgow Coma Score; *IBW*: ideal body weight

Low Positive End-expiratory Pressure

PEEP increases the intrathoracic pressure and consequently may impair the central venous return leading to increased ICP. In a study performed in nine patients with brain injury [19], the authors showed a positive correlation between PEEP and ICP during recruitment maneuvers. However, in an experimental study in healthy pigs, PEEP increase did not affect ICP [20]. In patients with subarachnoid hemorrhage [20], PEEP impaired CBF by a decrease in mean arterial pressure (MAP) although ICP was not altered. It has therefore been advocated to use low or null PEEP in mechanically ventilated patients with brain injury, and 80% of patients with brain injury receiving mechanical ventilation, are delivered a PEEP ≤ 5 cmH$_2$O [3].

Weaning from Invasive Mechanical Ventilation and Extubation

The population of severe brain injury patients is at high risk of extubation failure with rates up to 38% [21]. Currently, no strategy has been described regarding weaning or extubation and brain injury patients were hardly described in the latest guidelines [7]. The clinical features and level of arousal compatible with successful extubation are still debated in brain injury patients and, therefore, the rates of extubation failure and delayed extubation remain high in this population. Extubation failure is associated with significant morbidity: nosocomial pneumonia, longer mechanical ventilation duration, increased ICU length of stay and higher mortality [6, 10, 11], but the cause of extubation failure is probably more deleterious than the failure itself [6]. The fear of extubation failure explains the high rate of delayed extubation in neuro-ICU patients (extubation is considered as delayed when patients are not extubated within 48 h of meeting defined readiness criteria [6]), even though delaying extubation is not a guarantee of success [6]. Delaying extubation leads to an increased rate of pneumonia altering the neurological outcome; the high rate of delayed extubation also increases healthcare costs [6].

New Perspectives: How to Set Mechanical Ventilation in Clinical Practice

There was a recent reappraisal about the effects of PEEP on cerebral perfusion pressure (CPP). In a retrospective study in 341 patients [22], the authors noted a statistically significant decrease in CPP with increase in PEEP, but CPP remained within the therapeutic target. Moreover, no data were provided about the patients' volemic status; this is important because PEEP may alter CPP in hypovolemic conditions. In a pilot prospective study performed in 20 patients with TBI and ARDS [23], the authors increased PEEP up to 15 cmH$_2$O. There was no significant change in ICP or CPP and, importantly, the authors reported a significant improvement in brain tissue oxygenation with higher levels of PEEP. In conclusion, it seems that an increase in PEEP can be safely applied in ARDS patients with brain injury, provided that they are normovolemic, and may even have beneficial cerebral effects. Our group recently confirmed the safety of PEEP by showing that PEEP > 5 cmH$_2$O did not alter the ICP in patients with severe brain injury [9].

The use of low tidal volume within a protective ventilation strategy in the general ICU population with ARDS [24] or in the perioperative setting [25], is strongly associated with improved outcomes. Our group recently evaluated, in two before-after studies, the efficacy of a protective ventilation strategy in patients with brain injury:

1) A study [8] in two ICUs including 499 patients evaluated a bundle of care with a protective ventilation strategy (tidal volume between 6–8 ml/kg of ideal predicted bodyweight and PEEP > 3 cmH$_2$O) and early extubation (when GCS ≥ 10 and cough was obtained). An improvement in the number of ventilatory-free days was observed during the intervention period.

2) A multicenter nationwide before-after study in 749 brain injury patients was conducted to evaluate the effects of protective ventilation (≤ 7 ml/kg of ideal predicted body weight and a PEEP between 6–8 cmH$_2$O) associated with early extubation [9]. There was no difference in the number of ventilatory-free days at day 90 between the two periods. However, in the subgroup of patients in which all the recommendations were applied (protective ventilation and early extubation), there was a significant improvement in the number of ventilator free days at day 90 and in the mortality rate.

In both these studies [8, 9], the use of protective ventilation did not alter outcomes or impair ICP provided that the level of PaCO$_2$ was monitored and maintained within normal ranges. These results also provide important, simple and applicable data to attending physician on how to reach the goals of PaCO$_2$ suggested by international guidelines [2] with a strategy of modifying respiratory rate rather than tidal volume.

When Should we Perform Extubation After Brain Injury?

The level of arousal is a major issue in deciding when to safely perform extubation, but multiple pitfalls persist in its bedside evaluation. Coplin et al. pointed out that delaying extubation, in order to wait for sufficient neurological recovery, did not guarantee successful extubation and was associated with increased nosocomial pneumonia, ICU and hospital lengths of stay and costs [6]. Navalesi et al. proposed algorithm-based extubation when patients displayed a GCS $\geq$ 8 with audible cough during suctioning, and showed a significant improvement in extubation success [26]. Namen et al. showed that a GCS of 8 had the highest area under the receiver operating curve for predicting successful extubation [21].

Surprisingly, in a multicenter study including 192 patients, and in a monocenter cohort of 140 patients [11], higher GCS was not associated with extubation success [12]. A major limitation potentially explaining the discrepancies between these studies is that the GCS has never been validated in intubated patients, and it should be remembered that quantification of the verbal component is impossible in intubated patients, especially after brain injury. Some authors have arbitrarily decided to score the verbal component as 1 in all intubated patients [6], whereas others chose to score the verbal component as 1 in non-communicating patients and as 4 in patients who tried to speak with the endotracheal tube [10]. In other studies [21, 26], the evaluation of the verbal component is not available. This observation may explain why the GCS has been inconsistently reported as a factor associated with extubation success, and other tools of arousal evaluation are mandatory.

Further specific neurologic features compatible with safe extubation have been identified. In a multicenter study performed in 437 patients, our group aimed to develop a standardized specific physical examination on the day of extubation that could predict extubation success [10]. Age < 40 years old, visual pursuit, attempts to swallow and a GCS > 10 on the day of extubation were independent markers of successful extubation. Based on these four items, the predictive VISAGE score was built, which predicted at least 90% of episodes of extubation success when three items were present. In another monocenter study in 140 patients [11], visual pursuit and preserved upper airway reflexes were predictive factors of extubation success. In 192 patients [12], in another monocenter study, younger age, negative fluid balance and the presence of cough were predictive factors. Cough was also identified as predictive in a monocenter study in 311 patients with TBI [27]. We summarize the clinical features that may predict successful extubation after brain injury in Table 1. Large multicenter studies need to be performed to better delineate the impact of predictive factors of extubation success in order to enhance the benefit/risk balance in the decision to extubate and improve outcomes of brain injury patients (Table 2).

Table 2 Description of extubation failure rates and in-intensive care unit (ICU) mortality in brain-injured patients

First author [ref]	Number of patients with brain injury	Baseline GCS	GCS at extubation	Extubation failure rate (%)	In-ICU mortality rate (%)
Navalesi [26] (intervention/control groups)	165/153	9.4 ± 1.9/ 9.3 ± 1.9	10.6 ± 0.7/ 10.5 ± 0.9	5/12	1/4
Qureshi [32]	69	Unknown	Unknown	67	39
Reis [35] (success/failure groups)	311	9.7 ± 4.4	Unknown	13.8	3/14
Coplin [6]	136	Unknown	Unknown	17.4	16.1
Namen [21] (intervention/control groups)	100	Unknown	8.3 ± 2.6	38	41/31
Karanjia [36]	1,265	Unknown	11 ± 3	6.1	Unknown
Wendell [37] (success/failure groups)	37	11 (8–14)/11.5 (7–14)	13 (9–14)/10.5 (8–14)	21	8/20
Godet [11] (success/failure groups)	140	8 (5–11)/6 (4–9)	9 (8–10)/9 (7–10)	31	1/19
McCredie [12] (success/failure groups)	192	7 (4–9)/7(6–9)	9(8–10)/9(8–10)	21	1/13
Asehnoune [10] (success/failure groups)	437	7(5–10)/7(3–10)	11 (10–14)/11 (9–13)	22.6	1.2/11.1

GCS: Glasgow Coma Scale expressed as mean (±standard deviation) or median (interquartile) accordingly. In-ICU mortality is displayed for the entire cohort or according to the extubation success/failure group and the intervention/control group whenever appropriate

When Should we Perform Tracheostomy After Brain Injury?

Owing to the complicated extubation process in patients with brain injury, tracheostomy appears an interesting approach. Debate remains over the benefit of early versus late tracheostomy [28] because early tracheostomy may be associated with an increase in the number of ventilator-free days. Data on the subject are scarce in the neuro-ICU literature (Table 3). Two recent studies have used large databases to assess the potential effects of early versus late tracheostomy. In the first monocenter retrospective study performed in a trauma population [29], a propensity analysis matched for head and chest injury favored early tracheostomy with less pneumonia, lower mechanical ventilation duration and ICU length of stay. The second retrospective multicenter study in 1811 TBI patients [30] also supported an early tracheostomy policy. The mortality rate was similar between patients with early and late tracheostomy in both studies. The main issue is that these analyses are

Table 3 Description of tracheostomy and mortality rates in patients with severe brain injury

First author [ref]	Number of patients	Tracheostomy, n (%)	General in-ICU mortality, n (%)	In-ICU mortality in patients with tracheostomy, n (%)
Navalesi [26]	318	16 (5)	8 (2)	Unknown
Qureshi [32]	69	23 (33)	27 (39)	Unknown
Reis [35]	311	29 (9)	21 (6)	Unknown
Coplin [6]	136	4 (3)	22 (16.1)	Unknown
Namen [21]	100	29 (29)	36 (36)	Unknown
Karanjia [36]	1,265	181 (14)	Unknown	Unknown
Wendell [37]	37	3 (8)	5 (13.5)	Unknown
Godet [11]	140	9 (6.4)	9 (6.4)	Unknown
Asehnoune [10]	437	40 (9.1)	15 (3.4)	2 (0.4)

ICU: intensive care unit

extracted from databases in which the reason why tracheostomy was performed is unknown. These results were challenged in a randomized parallel-group, controlled, open study in stroke patients [31] in which early tracheostomy did not result in a reduction in the ICU length of stay, which was the primary outcome, but resulted in lower mortality. This result should be cautiously interpreted because only 60 patients were included and mortality was a secondary outcome.

In clinical practice, early tracheostomy is not recommended but could be considered in situations with high risk of extubation failure like infra-tentorial lesions [32], protracted mechanical ventilation or in patients with poor neurological recovery and/or after extubation failure.

Extubation, Tracheostomy and Withdrawal of Life-sustaining Therapies After Brain Injury

A major clinical issue regarding extubation and tracheostomy in the neuro-ICU setting, is that physicians fear that tracheostomy may facilitate weaning the patient from mechanical ventilation but sometimes with unacceptable neurologic damage. Extubation may be the last step of withdrawal of life-sustaining therapies. This practical aspect of end-of-life care has not been adequately addressed in neuro-ICU patients. A descriptive monocenter study confirmed that mechanical ventilation discontinuation accounted for 50% of deaths in a population of neurovascular patients (stroke, intracerebral hemorrhage or subarachnoid hemorrhage) [33]. In most studies regarding extubation in brain injury patients, patients undergoing withdrawal of life-sustaining therapies are not included [10, 11], but the timing, modalities and consequences of extubation in this context are not addressed in the neuro-ICU literature.

Withdrawal of life-sustaining therapies is a complex process and its modalities after brain injury cannot be reduced only to extubation, which could remain successful even in comatose patients [6, 10–12].

Conclusion

Revisiting current strategies for respiratory management in patients with acute brain injury is important because no clear recommendations are currently available and respiratory management in general may impact neurological outcomes. It is now clear that PEEP has minor effects on CPP in euvolemic patients and could even have positive consequences on brain tissue oxygenation. Protective ventilation, with low tidal volumes (6–8 ml/kg of ideal body weight), can be safely performed after brain injury, but its positive effects on outcome have to be better delineated. Extubation remains challenging in the neuro-ICU setting. Waiting for a patient's full neurological recovery is not mandatory and some specific features, such as visual pursuit, cough, and deglutition, may help the attending physician to perform extubation. Tracheostomy can be considered, but the best timing and the selection of patients who might benefit from this strategy remain unknown. Finally, the development of quality improvement projects is a crucial step in improving outcomes of patients with acute brain injury [34].

References

1. Esteban A, Anzueto A, Frutos F et al (2002) Characteristics and outcomes in adult patients receiving mechanical ventilation: a 28-day international study. JAMA 287:345–355
2. Carney N, Totten AM, O'Reilly C et al (2017) Guidelines for the management of severe traumatic brain injury, fourth edition. Neurosurgery 80:6–15
3. Pelosi P, Ferguson ND, Frutos-Vivar F et al (2011) Management and outcome of mechanically ventilated neurologic patients. Crit Care Med 39:1482–1492
4. Lepelletier D, Roquilly A, Demeure dit latte D et al (2010) Retrospective analysis of the risk factors and pathogens associated with early-onset ventilator-associated pneumonia in surgical-ICU head-trauma patients. J Neurosurg Anesthesiol 22:32–37
5. Cinotti R, Dordonnat-Moynard A, Feuillet F et al (2014) Risk factors and pathogens involved in early ventilator-acquired pneumonia in patients with severe subarachnoid hemorrhage. Eur J Clin Microbiol Infect Dis 33:823–830
6. Coplin WM, Pierson DJ, Cooley KD et al (2000) Implications of extubation delay in brain-injured patients meeting standard weaning criteria. Am J Respir Crit Care Med 161:1530–1536
7. Boles J-M, Bion J, Connors A et al (2007) Weaning from mechanical ventilation. Eur Respir J 29:1033–1056
8. Roquilly A, Cinotti R, Jaber S et al (2013) Implementation of an evidence-based extubation readiness bundle in 499 brain-injured patients. a before–after evaluation of a quality improvement project. Am J Respir Crit Care Med 188:958–966
9. The BI-VILI study group, Asehnoune K, Mrozek S et al (2017) A multi-faceted strategy to reduce ventilation-associated mortality in brain-injured patients. The BI-VILI project: a nationwide quality improvement project. Intensive Care Med 287:345–314
10. Asehnoune K, Seguin P, Lasocki S et al (2017) Extubation success prediction in a multicentric cohort of patients with severe brain injury. Anesthesiology 127:338–346
11. Godet T, Chabanne R, Marin J et al (2017) Extubation failure in brain-injured patients: risk factors and development of a prediction score in a preliminary prospective cohort study. Anesthesiology 126:104–114

12. McCredie VA, Ferguson ND, Pinto RL et al (2017) Airway management strategies for brain-injured patients meeting standard criteria to consider extubation. a prospective cohort study. Ann Am Thorac Soc 14:85–93
13. Rosenfeld JV, Maas AI, Bragge P et al (2012) Early management of severe traumatic brain injury. Lancet 380:1088–1098
14. Longhi L, Pagan F, Valeriani V et al (2007) Monitoring brain tissue oxygen tension in brain-injured patients reveals hypoxic episodes in normal-appearing and in peri-focal tissue. Intensive Care Med 33:2136–2142
15. Davis DP, Idris AH, Sise MJ et al (2006) Early ventilation and outcome in patients with moderate to severe traumatic brain injury. Crit Care Med 34:1202–1208
16. López-Aguilar J, Villagrá A, Bernabé F et al (2005) Massive brain injury enhances lung damage in an isolated lung model of ventilator-induced lung injury. Crit Care Med 33:1077–1083
17. Gattinoni L, Protti A, Caironi P, Carlesso E (2010) Ventilator-induced lung injury: The anatomical and physiological framework. Crit Care Med 38:S539–S548
18. Mascia L, Zavala E, Bosma K et al (2007) High tidal volume is associated with the development of acute lung injury after severe brain injury: an international observational study. Crit Care Med 35:1815–1820
19. Zhang XY, Yang ZJ, Wang QX, Fan HR (2011) Impact of positive end-expiratory pressure on cerebral injury patients with hypoxemia. Am J Emerg Med 29:699–703
20. Muench E, Bauhuf C, Roth H et al (2005) Effects of positive end-expiratory pressure on regional cerebral blood flow, intracranial pressure, and brain tissue oxygenation. Crit Care Med 33:2367–2372
21. Namen AM, Ely EW, Tatter SB et al (2001) Predictors of successful extubation in neurosurgical patients. Am J Respir Crit Care Med 163:658–664
22. Boone MD, Jinadasa SP, Mueller A et al (2016) The effect of positive end-expiratory pressure on intracranial pressure and cerebral hemodynamics. Neurocrit Care 26:174–181
23. Nemer SN, Caldeira JB, Santos RG et al (2015) Effects of positive end-expiratory pressure on brain tissue oxygen pressure of severe traumatic brain injury patients with acute respiratory distress syndrome: a pilot study. J Crit Care 30:1263–1266
24. Bellani G, Laffey JG, Pham T et al (2016) Epidemiology, patterns of care, and mortality for patients with acute respiratory distress syndrome in intensive care units in 50 countries. JAMA 315:788
25. Futier E, Constantin J-M, Paugam-Burtz C et al (2013) A trial of intraoperative low-tidal-volume ventilation in abdominal surgery. N Engl J Med 369:428–437
26. Navalesi P, Frigerio P, Moretti MP et al (2008) Rate of reintubation in mechanically ventilated neurosurgical and neurologic patients: evaluation of a systematic approach to weaning and extubation. Crit Care Med 36:2986–2992
27. Reis dos HFC, Gomes-Neto M, Almeida MLO et al (2017) Development of a risk score to predict extubation failure in patients with traumatic brain injury. J Crit Care 42:218–222
28. Young D, Harrison DA, Cuthbertson BH et al (2013) Effect of early vs late tracheostomy placement on survival in patients receiving mechanical ventilation: the TracMan randomized trial. JAMA 309:2121–2129
29. Hyde GA, Savage SA, Zarzaur BL et al (2015) Early tracheostomy in trauma patients saves time and money. Injury 46:110–114
30. Alali AS, Scales DC, Fowler RA et al (2014) Tracheostomy timing in traumatic brain injury. J Trauma Acute Care Surg 76:70–78
31. Bosel J, Schiller P, Hook Y et al (2012) Stroke-related early tracheostomy versus prolonged orotracheal intubation in neurocritical care trial (SETPOINT): a randomized pilot trial. Stroke 44:21–28
32. Qureshi AI, Suarez JI, Parekh PD, Bhardwaj A (2000) Prediction and timing of tracheostomy in patients with infratentorial lesions requiring mechanical ventilatory support. Crit Care Med 28:1383–1387

33. Holloway RG, Ladwig S, Robb J et al (2010) Palliative care consultations in hospitalized stroke patients. J Palliat Med 13:407–412
34. Middleton S, McElduff P, Ward J et al (2011) Implementation of evidence-based treatment protocols to manage fever, hyperglycaemia, and swallowing dysfunction in acute stroke (QASC): a cluster randomised controlled trial. Lancet 378:1699–1706
35. Reis HF, Almeida MLO, Silva MFD, de Rocha MS (2013) Extubation failure influences clinical and functional outcomes in patients with traumatic brain injury. J Bras Pneumol 39:330–338
36. Karanjia N, Nordquist D, Stevens R, Nyquist P (2011) A clinical description of extubation failure in patients with primary brain injury. Neurocrit Care 15:4–12
37. Wendell LC, Raser J, Kasner S, Park S (2011) Predictors of extubation success in patients with middle cerebral artery acute ischemic stroke. Stroke Res Treat 2011:1–5

Part XII
Therapeutic Issues

Central α2-adrenoreceptor Agonists in Intensive Care

D. Liu and M. C. Reade

Introduction

α_2-adrenoceptor agonists are well-established as veterinary anesthetics but have only slowly entered human intensive care unit (ICU) and perioperative practice over the last 17 years. With many attractive properties in addition to sedation, including preservation of rousability, respiratory drive and airway reflexes at useful hypnotic doses, analgesia, anti-inflammatory effects and potentially neuroprotective and anti-delirium actions, they also avoid many of the adverse consequences of gamma-aminobutyric acid (GABA)-agonists, such as benzodiazepines and propofol. In this chapter, we will examine existing clinical evidence for use of α_2-adrenoceptor agonists for various indications, along with highlighting important studies currently underway. Suggestions for current clinical practice and for future research are made.

Medications

Clonidine (trade names include Catapres and Kapvay) is the prototypical α_2-adrenoreceptor agonist, first synthesized in the 1960s as a nasal decongestant before being approved in the USA in 1974 for the treatment of hypertension [1].

D. Liu
Faculty of Medicine, The University of Queensland
Herston, Queensland, Australia

M. C. Reade (✉)
Faculty of Medicine & Burns, Trauma and Critical Care Research Centre, The University of Queensland
Brisbane, Queensland, Australia
Australian Defence Force Joint Health Command
Canberra, Australian Capital Territory, Australia
Department of Intensive Care, Royal Brisbane and Women's Hospital
Brisbane, Queensland, Australia
e-mail: m.reade@uq.edu.au

© Springer International Publishing AG 2018
J.-L. Vincent (ed.), *Annual Update in Intensive Care and Emergency Medicine 2018*,
Annual Update in Intensive Care and Emergency Medicine,
https://doi.org/10.1007/978-3-319-73670-9_42

It is marketed in enteral, intravenous and transdermal (depending upon market) formulations.

Dexmedetomidine (trade names include Dexdor® and Precedex®) is the dextro-enantiomer of medetomidine, a sedative and analgesic used in veterinary medicine. It was originally approved in the USA in 1999 for intravenous sedation of mechanically ventilated ICU patients for up to 24 h, with an additional indication granted in 2008 for sedation of non-intubated patients prior to and/or during surgical procedures [2]. European approval was granted in 2011 for sedation, while remaining rousable in response to verbal stimulation, of adult patients in the ICU [3].

Clonidine and dexmedetomidine are the main α_2-adrenoreceptor agonists of relevance to intensive care medicine. Other α_2-adrenoreceptor agonists exist – e.g., guanfacine, guanabenz, lofexidine, tizanidine, and xylazine (veterinary use) – but there is no information on their use in critically ill patients. Guanfacine (trade names include Tenex® and Intuniv®) is currently available in an extended release enteral formulation for the treatment of attention-deficit/hyperactivity disorder (ADHD) in the USA, Europe and Australia. Lofexidine (trade names BritLofex® and Dimatex®) is approved in the UK and Italy for rapid opioid detoxification.

Atipamezole is a selective α_2-adrenoreceptor antagonist that can reverse the effects of agonists such as dexmedetomidine, but is currently only approved for veterinary use [2].

Pharmacology, Pharmacokinetics and Pharmacodynamics

As α_2-adrenoreceptor agonists, clonidine and dexmedetomidine both act to reduce norepinephrine release from sympathetic nerve terminals [1, 2]. This reduces neuronal signaling in the central nervous system (CNS), prominently in the locus ceruleus, causing both sedation and anxiolysis. Both central and spinal inhibition of noradrenergic transmission also reduces conduction and perception of pain impulses. Stimulation of α_2-receptors also reduces cardiovascular sympathetic tone, causing bradycardia and hypotension. The 2A subtype of the α_2-receptor is the major mediator of sedation and analgesia. Dexmedetomidine has a higher affinity than clonidine for this receptor subtype, explaining its lesser cardiovascular effects for equal levels of sedation. Combining analgesic, hypnotic and (possibly, as discussed below) direct anti-delirium affects, α_2-adrenoreceptor agonists are the only agents to address simultaneously each of the three components of the "ICU cognitive triad" (Fig. 1).

At clinical intravenous doses, the distribution half-lives in adults of dexmedetomidine and clonidine are 6 min and 20 min, respectively. The elimination half-life of dexmedetomidine in adults is approximately two hours, with hepatic metabolism by glucuronidation and cytochrome P450 hydroxylation followed by almost exclusively renal elimination of metabolites that are not known to have any biological activity. The elimination half-life of clonidine in adults is much longer, 12–16 h, with 50% renally excreted unchanged and 50% undergoing hepatic metabolism. Intravenous clonidine is therefore more suitable than dexmedetomidine for bolus

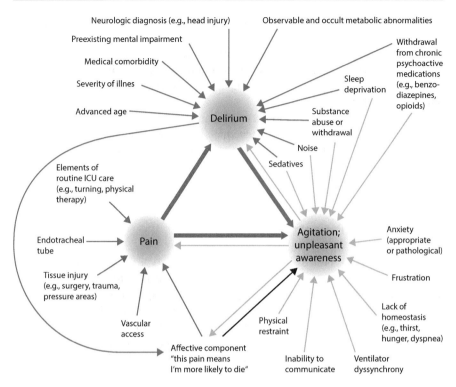

Fig. 1 Causes and interactions of pain, agitation and delirium. Drugs and other treatments for pain, agitation and delirium form a "triad of ICU" cognitive management analogous to the "triad of anesthesia," which highlights interactions among hypnotics, analgesics and muscle relaxants to encourage balanced anesthesia. The "triad of ICU" concept highlights that treating one element is unlikely to be as effective as a coordinated approach. Unique amongst medications used in the ICU, α_2-adrenoreceptor agonists affect each component of the triad. From [51] with permission

intravenous dosing, and when given by infusion has a greater potential to accumulate, particularly in renal impairment. Clonidine is 70–80% orally bioavailable, with peak plasma concentrations attained after 1–3 h. In contrast, dexmedetomidine is only 15% bioavailable via the oral route, but well-absorbed and tolerated buccally or intranasally (82% in both cases).

Indications

The approved indications for dexmedetomidine in critical care are for sedation in the ICU and perioperative period, and for procedural sedation [2], but off-label applications reported in the literature include treating pain, withdrawal syndromes, and more recently, treatment of delirium and improvement of sleep quality. In Europe, dexmedetomidine is most commonly used for sedation in the ICU (79%), perioperatively (16%), and for procedural sedation (5%), with other applications accounting for < 1% [3].

Clonidine is approved for use as an anti-hypertensive agent. However, in some parts of the world – notably the UK – it is commonly used for its sedative effects, particularly in agitated patients with sympathetic hyperactivity due to CNS-depressant withdrawal states.

Recent research on α_2-adrenoreceptor agonists in critical care has focused primarily on dexmedetomidine, although there is renewed interest in repurposing clonidine – especially in its enteral formulation, which has a lower risk of hemodynamic side effects, minimizes cost, and can be administered safely outside the ICU [1].

Sedation of ICU Patients

Dexmedetomidine produces a qualitatively different type of sedation to that of GABA-agonists, characterized by minimal respiratory depression, greater rousability at similar levels of unstimulated hypnosis, and analgesia. Compared to benzodiazepine-based strategies, several studies have found dexmedetomidine to be associated with reduced duration of mechanical ventilation, shorter ICU length of stay and reduced incidence of delirium [4–6]. The recent European DexDUS audit reported that dexmedetomidine-based sedation was highly effective, achieving its intended effect in 85% of adults and 91% of pediatric patients [3]. However, dexmedetomidine was discontinued or replaced with another sedative due to lack of efficacy in 10% and 6% of administrations in adults and pediatrics, respectively [3].

Long-term (> 24 h) sedation using dexmedetomidine is an off-label use. Recent systematic reviews and meta-analyses [4, 7] have reported that in long-term mechanically ventilated adult ICU patients, dexmedetomidine reduces the duration of mechanical ventilation by 22% (95% CI 10–33%) and ICU length of stay by 14% (95% CI 1–24%). There is no evidence of reduced risk of delirium (RR 0.85, 95% CI 0.63–1.14) or mortality (RR 0.99; 95% CI 0.79–1.24), but dexmedetomidine was associated with a substantially greater incidence of bradycardia (RR 2.11; 95% CI 1.39–3.20). The overall quality of evidence for long-term sedation with dexmedetomidine was low.

In mechanically ventilated neurocritical care patients, sedation with α_2-adrenoreceptor agonists is generally successful and appears to also reduce requirements for adjunctive sedative and analgesic agents, although the supporting data are limited [8]. Dexmedetomidine does not appear to cause severe, uncompensated hemodynamic changes (cerebrally or systemically), but reporting of pharmacological compensation required from vasopressors in trials has been limited. Of note, in a randomized, double-blinded cross-over study of 30 intubated patients, dexmedetomidine-based sedation improved Adaptive Cognitive Exam (ACE) scores by a mean of 6.8 (95% CI 1.2–12.4) measured at 30 min after attaining sedation targets following commencement of infusion, compared to baseline scores with only as-required fentanyl analgesia. In contrast, propofol-based sedation reduced scores by −12.4 (95% CI −8.3 to −16.5) compared to baseline [9]. Comparative cognitive assessments with long-term sedation using dexmedetomidine have not been reported.

Dexmedetomidine dosing for sedation is an intravenous infusion initially at 0.7 mcg/kg/h, titrated to effect to between 0.2–1.4 mcg/kg/h (the labeled usage for Dexdor® [2]) or up to 0.7 mcg/kg/h (ICU sedation in the USA) or 1.0 mcg/kg/h (procedural sedation in the USA; all use in Australia) (Table 1). Although the Precedex® labeled dosage in the USA incorporates a loading dose of 1.0 mcg/kg, most European administrations of dexmedetomidine (>98%) do not use a loading dose [3] due to concerns over bradycardia and hypotension.

Evidence supporting use of clonidine for sedation of critically ill patients is limited [10]. Intravenous and enteral clonidine have been used successfully for sedation in small clinical trials [1, 10], but the benefits associated with dexmedetomidine – such as shorter duration of mechanical ventilation and reduction of ICU length of stay – have not been reported with clonidine-based sedation [10]. As with dexmedetomidine, no ICU mortality differences have been reported with clonidine. Clonidine use, however, is associated with an increased incidence of clinically significant hypotension (RR 3.11, 95% CI 1.64–5.87).

Only one trial has directly compared sedation using dexmedetomidine versus clonidine [11]. In this 120-patient intraoperative trial of patients undergoing abdominal surgery with spinal anesthesia, those sedated with dexmedetomidine (1 mcg/kg loading dose followed by 0.5 mcg/kg/h infusion) were aroused from sedation more quickly (37.23 ± 2.42 min vs. 57.26 ± 4.11 min), and had prolonged postoperative analgesic effects (198.23 ± 33.15 min vs. 150.65 ± 28.55 min), compared to intravenous clonidine (1 mcg/kg loading dose followed by 1 mcg/kg/h infusion) sedation. These findings are consistent with the longer elimination half-life of clonidine, and greater affinity for α_{2A}-adrenoreceptors by dexmedetomidine [11].

A major advantage of clonidine over dexmedetomidine is the availability of an enteral formulation, which can be used to provide sedation while transitioning from intravenous infusions (discussed in further detail, below). Recommended intravenous clonidine dosing for sedation is 0.5–2.0 mcg/kg/h, i.e., 0.96–3.8 mg/day for an 80 kg patient ([12]; Table 1). Recommended enteral dosing is 0.1–0.3 mg every 6–8 h initially, titrated up to 0.4 mg every 6 h based on clinical response [1].

Disadvantages of clonidine for sedation compared to dexmedetomidine include its substantially longer half-life, making it more difficult to titrate to clinical effect, and the risk of patients developing clonidine withdrawal syndrome (hypertension and symptoms mimicking sympathetic hyperactivity) [1]. Well-designed trials are needed to properly assess the efficacy of clonidine as a sedative in the ICU, and to identify subgroups that would more likely benefit from the use of dexmedetomidine [4]. A large randomized 3-arm effectiveness trial comparing clonidine, dexmedetomidine and standard care (the A to B trial) is planned for the UK, beginning in 2018.

Table 1 Dosing of α_2-adrenoreceptor agonists, dexmedetomidine and clonidine, in intensive care

Indication	Dosage	
	Dexmedetomidine	Clonidine
ICU sedation	*Intravenous infusion:* 0.7 mcg/kg/h, titrated to effect between: – 0.2–1.4 mcg/kg/h (Dexdor®), or – up to 0.7 mcg/kg/h (ICU sedation in the USA), or – 1.0 mcg/kg/h (procedural sedation in the USA; all use in Australia)	*Intravenous infusion:* 0.5–2.0 mcg/kg/h [12] *Enteral:* 0.1–0.3 mg every 6–8 h initially, titrated up to 0.4 mg every 6 h [1]
Procedural sedation	*Intravenous infusion:* 1.0 mcg/kg over 10 min, maintenance infusion at 0.6 mcg/kg/h titrated to clinical effect between 0.2–1.0 mcg/kg/h Loading doses $\geq$ 1.0 mcg/kg may be associated with bradycardia [15]	*Intravenous bolus:* 1.0 mcg/kg (up to 6.0 mcg/kg) for laryngoscopy *Intravenous infusion:* 0.3 mcg/kg/h infusion perioperatively [22] *Intrathecal bolus:* 1.0 mcg/kg (maximum 150 mcg) [22] *Intrathecal infusion:* 30 mcg/h added to the usual local anesthetic agent [22]
Delirium and sleep	**Prophylaxis** *Intravenous:* 0.1 mcg/kg/h untitrated to prevent postoperative delirium and improve sleep quality [30, 36] **Treatment of delirium** *Intravenous:* 0.5 mcg/kg/h titrated between 0.0–1.5 mcg/kg/h to effect [33, 34]	No evidence supporting use
Transitioning from dexmedetomidine	N/A	*Enteral:* initially 0.2–0.5 mg clonidine every 6 h titrated to effect, reducing dexmedetomidine rate by 25% of baseline every 6 h if tolerated. Taper clonidine dose by extending dosing interval (q6h → q8h → q12h → q24h) every 1–2 days (to avoid withdrawal syndrome). Resume previous dose if agitation, pain, delirium or withdrawal occurs, then re-taper
Pediatric [23]	**Premedication for anxiolysis** *Buccal:* 1 mcg/kg *Intranasal:* 0.5–2.0 mcg/kg **Intraoperative** *Intravenous:* 0.5–2.0 mcg/kg over 10 min prior to airway procedures, followed by a maintenance infusion of 0.5–3.0 mcg/kg/h intraoperatively **Emergence and recovery** *Intravenous:* 0.2–1.0 mcg/kg for emergence agitation, or 0.5 mcg/kg for postoperative shivering	**Analgesia and sedation** [24] *Intravenous:* 0.1–2.0 mcg/kg/h *Nasogastric:* 1.0–5.0 mcg/kg every 8 h

Perioperative Adjunct and Procedural Sedation

The sympatholytic properties of α_2-adrenoreceptor agonists, along with rousability and minimal risk of respiratory depression, makes them attractive for perioperative and procedural sedation [2, 13]. When used as premedication, they can attenuate the sympathetic response to noxious stimuli, such as from laryngoscopy, intubation and skin incision [14]. Multiple studies have reported that α_2-adrenoreceptor agonists are more effective than fentanyl or placebo at blunting the intubation response [15]. Both clonidine and dexmedetomidine have been found to be effective at reducing the incidence of postoperative shivering compared to placebo [16]. However, inadvertent sedation in the post-anesthesia care unit appears to be more common with dexmedetomidine: all seven dexmedetomidine studies found statistically significant increases in sedation scores compared to controls, but this was not reported in either of the two clonidine studies [16].

Dexmedetomidine is often used in combination with another drug, such as propofol or ketamine, to provide optimum sedation conditions rapidly with less bradycardia and hypotension than when a loading dose of dexmedetomidine is used to achieve a similar speed of onset. Amnesic effects may be desirable in some situations and can be provided with low-dose benzodiazepine [13]. For example, dexmedetomidine has been demonstrated to be both effective and safe when used in combination with propofol [14] or midazolam [17]. There are well-documented postoperative analgesia sparing effects in adult [18] and pediatric [2] patients and when used as an epidural adjunct [19]. There are also reports of reduced postoperative nausea and vomiting [20] and shivering [16] with dexmedetomidine. Precedex® labeled dosing for procedural sedation is 1.0 mcg/kg over 10 min, followed by maintenance infusion at 0.6 mcg/kg/h titrated to clinical effect between 0.2–1.0 mcg/kg/h (Table 1). Loading doses $\geq$ 1.0 mcg/kg may be associated with bradycardia [15].

Clonidine has similar sedative and analgesia-sparing effects to dexmedetomidine when used as a perioperative adjunct and during procedural sedation [21]. Trials of enteral clonidine have also reported reduced benzodiazepine use in general ICU patients [1]. Dosing intravenously for adult procedural sedation ranges from 1.0–6.0 mcg/kg, although 1.0 mcg/kg has been shown to be effective at attenuating the intubation response (Table 1) [15]. Perioperatively in adults, an intravenous infusion of 0.3 mcg/kg/h can be used. Alternatively, epidural/intrathecal bolus doses of 1.0 mcg/kg (maximum 150 mcg) or infusion of 30 mcg/h can be used, either option added to the usual local anesthetic agent [22].

In a trial comparing 1.0 mcg/kg clonidine versus dexmedetomidine at 0.5 mcg/kg and 1.0 mcg/kg in ASA I and II patients undergoing surgery, all three treatments were equally effective at attenuating laryngoscopy and intubation responses [15]. However, there were fewer incidences of bradycardia and hypotension requiring treatment in the clonidine group versus both dexmedetomidine groups. For epidural analgesia, dexmedetomidine has been reported in multiple studies to have faster onset of sensory block than clonidine [19].

Pediatrics

Dexmedetomidine is not labeled for use in children, but there is increasing literature demonstrating its effectiveness [2, 23] with indications and benefits similar to those found in adults. In the DexDUS audit, pediatric patients accounted for 6% of all administrations of dexmedetomidine [3].

Buccal (1 mcg/kg) and intranasal (0.5–2.0 mcg/kg) routes of administration of dexmedetomidine are effective for preoperative anxiolysis [23]. A trial of preoperative intranasal dexmedetomidine vs. intraoperative intravenous dexmedetomidine vs. placebo, assessing postoperative behavior up to 28 days, is currently underway (ACTRN12616000096459). Intraoperatively, dexmedetomidine can be administered before pediatric airway procedures as a loading dose of 0.5–2.0 mcg/kg over 10 min, followed by a maintenance infusion of 0.5–3.0 mcg/kg/h ([23]; Table 1). As an intraoperative adjunct, it is commonly administered at rates of 0.1–0.5 mcg/kg/h [23]. During the recovery period, 0.2–1.0 mcg/kg is used to treat postoperative emergence of agitation, and 0.5 mcg/kg for postoperative shivering [23].

Clonidine is commonly used in pediatric anesthesia and intensive care medicine across Europe, but evidence supporting this practice is limited. Consensus guidelines recommend intravenous dosing at 0.1–2.0 mcg/kg/h, or nasogastric dosing at 1.0–5.0 mcg/kg every 8 h ([24]; Table 1). Other non-parenteral routes of administration are available [25]. Larger, high quality studies such as the CLOSED trial (NCT02509273) are in progress.

Delirium Prophylaxis and Treatment

Several trials of dexmedetomidine as an ICU sedative have reported lower rates of delirium with its use compared to benzodiazepine-based sedation [5, 6, 26]. Based on animal models, it was thought the neuroprotective properties of dexmedetomidine result from reduced cerebral catecholamine and glutamate release, modulation of apoptosis-regulating proteins [2], and potentially reduced neuroinflammation [27].

The prophylactic effect of dexmedetomidine on delirium in surgical patients is less clear [28]. In a single-blinded randomized controlled trial (RCT) involving elderly postoperative cardiac surgery patients followed for five days, dexmedetomidine sedation (0.4 mcg/kg loading dose followed by 0.2–0.7 mcg/kg/h infusion) resulted in substantially less delirium (OR 0.46, 95% CI 0.23–0.92, p = 0.028) compared to propofol (25–50 mcg/kg/min) [29]. In a doubled-blind RCT with 700 postoperative non-cardiac surgical ICU patients, dexmedetomidine administered at a low dose (0.1 mcg/kg/h, no loading dose and un-titrated) – considered subtherapeutic as a sedative – only on the evening after surgery resulted in a substantial reduction in the incidence of delirium over the following seven days compared to placebo (OR 0.35, 95% CI 0.22–0.54, p < 0.0001) [30]. However, in another trial where dexmedetomidine (0.5 mcg/kg/h) was instead administered only intraoperatively and for two hours postoperatively, there was no difference in postoperative delirium over five days of follow up (12.2% vs 11.4%, p = 0.94) [31].

Dexmedetomidine is one of only two drugs (the other being quetiapine [32]) to have shown superiority over placebo in treating established ICU delirium. In a double-blinded RCT involving mechanically ventilated ICU patients with severe agitated delirium who were otherwise ready to be extubated, dexmedetomidine (0.5 mcg/kg/h titrated between 0.0–1.5 mcg/kg/h to physician-prescribed sedation goals for up to seven days) was compared to placebo [33]. Patients in the dexmedetomidine group had more ventilator-free hours at seven days (median difference, 17.0 h, 95% CI 4.0–33.2 h, p = 0.01), reduced time to extubation (median difference, –19.5 h, 95% CI –5.3 to –31.1 h, p < 0.001), and accelerated resolution of delirium (median difference, –16.0 h, 95% CI –3.0 to –28.0 h, p = 0.01).

Dexmedetomidine also appears effective in treating agitated delirium in nonintubated ICU patients [34]. In a novel non-randomized trial design, 132 patients with agitated delirium were initially treated with haloperidol. Those who responded continued with haloperidol bolus ± infusion as required; those who did not respond received dexmedetomidine up to 0.7 mcg/kg/h. The dexmedetomidine patients (presumably with the greater severity of agitation at trial entry) spent significantly more time without delirium, and significantly more time satisfactorily sedated. Adverse events, primarily oversedation, were greater in the haloperidol group.

In contrast to the above ICU studies, dexmedetomidine appears unsuitable to control agitation in the emergency department. In a small case series of patients who had failed behavioral control with other drugs, only two of five had effective sedation after a loading dose alone. Of eight who had an infusion continued, only two had effective sedation with no adverse effects; in others dexmedetomidine was either ineffective or caused problematic bradycardia and hypotension [35].

There are no data on whether clonidine can also prevent or treat delirium in the ICU, but trials are currently in progress with geriatric and pediatric patients in the LUCID (NCT01956604) and CLOSED (NCT02509273) trials, respectively.

Improving Sleep

Sedation with α_2-adrenoreceptor agonists is often cited as influencing endogenous sleep-promoting pathways, improving sleep architecture by creating a state resembling natural sleep that mimics the deep recovery sleep seen after sleep deprivation [2]. The physiological sleep-wake cycles that patients receiving α_2-adrenoreceptor agonists such as dexmedetomidine experience are thought to contribute to reduced risk of delirium [2].

Dexmedetomidine has been shown in recent trials to improve the quality and quantity of sleep in the ICU. A trial of 76 elderly, non-ventilated patients admitted to the ICU after non-cardiac surgery compared low-dose dexmedetomidine infusion (0.1 mcg/kg/h, i.e., the same dose used to prevent delirium in another trial [30]) to placebo for 15 h, measuring sleep quality and duration with polysomnography [36]. Dexmedetomidine resulted in improved sleep architecture with 14.7% greater median time spent in N2 sleep stage (95% CI 0.0–31.9%, p = 0.048). Dexmedetomidine also increased the total sleep time (median difference 69 min, 7–132 min, p = 0.028) and subjective sleep quality on the first morning after surgery.

There are no data on whether clonidine administration would also improve the quality and duration of patients' sleep in the ICU.

Substance Withdrawal Syndromes

Withdrawal syndromes from opiates, alcohol and nicotine involve excessive and elevated sympathetic activity, so α_2-adrenoreceptor agonists may have a role in the treatment of severe withdrawal syndromes due to their sympatholytic effects [37, 38]. The body of evidence supporting this, however, is limited and current data do not support routine use of α_2-adrenoreceptor agonists as the primary or sole agents for the treatment of withdrawal syndromes [37].

For the treatment of iatrogenic opioid abstinence syndrome, case series and retrospective studies of dexmedetomidine show promise but there have been no prospective studies [37]. Small studies suggest that clonidine (primarily in a transdermal formulation) may be useful in heroin detoxification, but a recent trial comparing clonidine to placebo for opiate and benzodiazepine withdrawal in a pediatric ICU found no differences in outcomes [39]. Although lofexidine is approved in the UK and Italy for opiate withdrawal and is more effective than placebo, data supporting its role as a primary agent in the ICU are limited [39].

For the treatment of severe alcohol withdrawal syndromes, limited data suggest that clonidine and dexmedetomidine may both be useful as adjuncts in combination with benzodiazepines [37]. Benzodiazepines are recognized to be deliriogenic, but the risk of seizures in alcohol withdrawal is thought to warrant their use. Whether the sedation caused by α_2-adrenoreceptor agonists alone would be sufficient is not known. Prospective well-controlled trials are required to define the clinical role of either agent in treatment of alcohol withdrawal.

Smokers in the ICU have a higher incidence of agitation, and often require more interventions, such as sedatives, analgesics, neuroleptic agents and physical restraints than non-smokers [37]. Transdermal clonidine patches effectively promote smoking cessation compared to placebo, but are only recommended as second-line therapy due to dose-dependent unwanted sedation and postural hypotension [37]. Furthermore, there are few data comparing α_2-adrenoreceptor agonists to nicotine replacement therapy, and clinical studies demonstrating their effectiveness are lacking [38].

Future Applications

Dexmedetomidine as Part of an 'Early, Goal-directed' Light Sedation Protocol

To date, trials of dexmedetomidine as a sedative have mostly enrolled patients up to 48 h (and some after 96 h) after ICU admission. However, deep sedation in the first 48 h of an ICU admission is an independent predictor of hospital and 180-day mortality [40], suggesting a protocol that prioritizes light sedation during this time might improve mortality. Dexmedetomidine's ability to induce a rousable state of calmness makes it an attractive drug with which to target this goal. The SPICE trial (NCT01728558) is randomizing 4,000 patients to dexmedetomidine-based early light sedation or standard care, powered to detect a mortality difference at 180 days. SPICE should be completed by the end of 2018.

Patient-Controlled Sedation and Analgesia Using Dexmedetomidine

As a combined analgesic and sedative, dexmedetomidine is potentially attractive as a patient-controlled drug to treat both pain and anxiety, either as a single agent or an adjuvant to conventional patient-controlled opioids. A study of 100 patients undergoing hysterectomy randomized to postoperative morphine or morphine + dexmedetomidine reported that the addition of dexmedetomidine enhanced analgesia and reduced both morphine consumption and nausea [41]. The feasibility of using dexmedetomidine as a single patient-controlled drug for burns dressings is currently under investigation (NCT02409810).

Burns and Sepsis

α_2-adrenoreceptor agonists have been theorized to be useful in the treatment of burns and sepsis in critically ill patients, by mitigating sympathetic outflow and preventing unregulated sympathetic tone from becoming detrimental to the patient [42]. This is supported by animal models showing that dexmedetomidine and clonidine can reduce norepinephrine requirements, and clonidine can reduce angiotensin II requirements, but the clinical evidence is limited [43].

A recent open-label RCT comparing sedation with and without dexmedetomidine in 201 mechanically-ventilated septic patients found no statistically significant differences in either mortality at 28 days (HR 0.69, 95% CI 0.38–1.22, p = 0.20) or ventilator-free days at 28 days [44]. Well-controlled sedation was, however, significantly higher in the dexmedetomidine group. This was a disappointing result given theorized positive effects of α_2-adrenoreceptor agonists on inflammation in sepsis. However, the study was underpowered to detect differences in mortality, having based its power calculation on sepsis mortality data from 10 years earlier (when case fatality rates were significantly higher). Furthermore, only 78% of patients received dexmedetomidine as prescribed on day one, and the maximum dose was only 0.7 mcg/kg/h, lower than that used in most trials. This trial is important, however, as it showed a beneficial mortality effect in the subsets of patients with APACHE II scores $\geq$ 23, and those with shock – dispelling the concern that possible cardiovascular effects of dexmedetomidine contraindicate its use in the most unwell septic patients. Of note, a 530-patient trial in 10 US ICUs comparing propofol with dexmedetomidine in patients with known or suspected infection (MENDS 2; NCT01739933) is due to complete enrolment in December 2018.

Prevention of Acute Kidney Injury

Recent trials of dexmedetomidine in cardiac surgery have reported reno-protective effects. For example, in an RCT of 200 patients undergoing valvular heart surgery, the incidence of acute kidney injury (AKI) during the postoperative 48-hours was significantly reduced with dexmedetomidine use versus placebo (OR 0.33, 95% CI 0.16–0.67, p = 0.002) [45]. This benefit was attributed to the sympatholytic effect of pre-emptive dexmedetomidine infusion.

No studies have investigated the reno-protective potential of clonidine. Further data are required before clinical recommendations regarding the role of α_2-adrenoreceptor agonists in AKI prophylaxis can be made.

Fever

Animal studies have demonstrated that α_2-adrenoreceptor agonists, both dexmedetomidine and clonidine, have inhibitory effects on fever [46]. A *post hoc* analysis of an RCT compared enteral clonidine (0.1 mg every 8 h, increased to 0.2 mg if hemodynamically stable) to placebo in 40 ICU patients. The placebo group were more likely to develop fever $\geq$ 38.3 °C (OR 3.96, p = 0.049), and had a higher mean body temperature (0.52 °C, p = 0.006) compared to the clonidine group [46]. Prospective trials are required to define the role of α_2-adrenoreceptor agonists in the prevention and management of fever in critically ill patients.

Transitioning from Dexmedetomidine to Clonidine

While dexmedetomidine has been shown to be effective in the ICU, there may be advantages of transitioning stable patients to an enteral or transdermal formulation of an α_2-agonist in order to save drug costs, nursing time, facilitate earlier ICU discharge, and avoid the risks of intravenous medication administration [12]. At present, only clonidine is available in these forms. Indications for transition to enteral clonidine include the absence of excessive agitation or over-sedation, ability to obey simple commands, and favorable response to dexmedetomidine for at least 12–24 h. Contraindications include hemodynamic instability, atrioventricular conduction defects greater than 1st degree block, or patients' inability to consume enteral/sublinguinal clonidine.

During weaning, initial doses of enteral clonidine range from 0.2–0.5 mg every 6 h (depending upon current dexmedetomidine dose, body mass and age), titrated to clinical effect [12]. The dexmedetomidine infusion rate is reduced by 25% of baseline every 6 h if no agitation requiring rescue medications occurs. The clonidine dose is tapered down until the patient is no longer agitated or requiring sedation, by slowly increasing the dosing interval every 24–48 h (to avoid withdrawal syndrome). For example, oral clonidine 0.3 mg every 6 h can be titrated down to 0.3 mg every 8 h for 1–2 days, then 0.3 mg every 12 h for 1–2 days, then 0.3 mg every 24 h for 1–2 days, then finally stopping altogether. If agitation, pain, delirium or withdrawal syndromes occur, the previous dose can be resumed before re-tapering.

Although small cohort studies have demonstrated that this approach is feasible, there have been no large prospective RCTs investing the effectiveness of weaning using clonidine, therefore it cannot be recommended as routine clinical practice [1].

Economic Analyses

Dexmedetomidine is still covered by patent and so is expensive. For example, in 2017 in Australia, dexmedetomidine costs A$52 for a 200 mcg ampoule. For a 70 kg patient requiring 1.0 mcg/kg/h, dexmedetomidine costs would therefore amount to A$468/day. Similar costs were reported in Canada in 2014, with full sedation with dexmedetomidine costing C$452/day (compared to C$126/day for midazolam and $230/day for propofol) [47]. By comparison, clonidine is inexpensive: A$5.70 for 150 mcg intravenous preparation and A$0.39 for 150 mcg oral preparation. Using a sedative dose of 1.0 mcg/kg/h for 24 hrs would cost A$64.

The cost of dexmedetomidine might be offset in healthcare systems that reimburse hospitals according to patient activity if duration of mechanical ventilation or ICU stay is shortened [48]. These cost-minimization approaches of economic analysis are controversial, however, because they focus primarily on drug costs and top-down approaches to costing resource utilization [49]. They may substantially overestimate potential cost savings [50] by not taking into account factors such as ICU admissions and mechanical ventilation incurring most of its cost on the first rather than the last day. Cost-effectiveness of ICU interventions remains an ongoing area of research.

Conclusion

Both dexmedetomidine and clonidine show promise as sedatives, analgesics and anti-delirium agents in critically ill and surgical patients. In part, their superiority may rest on avoidance of the adverse neurocognitive effects of the commonly-used alternatives, propofol and benzodiazepines. However, *in vitro* evidence and an anti-delirium effect in comparison to placebo suggest there may also be an element of neuroprotection. Certain types of patient may derive particular benefit, such as those with sepsis, burns, and acute substance withdrawal states, but specific trial evidence in these populations is still lacking. Concerns over adverse hemodynamic effects appear overstated, especially when (as with all ICU infusions) doses are carefully titrated. Clonidine may be as effective as dexmedetomidine, particularly in patients with heightened sympathetic activity, but head-to-head trials testing this are only just about to begin. For now, the strongest advice is:

- Dexmedetomidine is superior to benzodiazepines as an ICU sedative. Severity of illness is not a contraindication as long as the infusion rate is carefully titrated.
- Dexmedetomidine is an effective treatment for refractory ICU agitated delirium.
- Dexmedetomidine at low (0.1 mcg/kg/h) non-titrated doses effectively promotes sleep and reduces delirium in the immediate postoperative period.
- There is little comparative evidence suggesting clonidine can achieve the same sedative and anti-delirium effects as dexmedetomidine, but given extensive experience with clonidine in some countries this appears to be a reasonable alternative, pending trial results, as long as the infusion rate is carefully titrated.
- Both dexmedetomidine and clonidine are effective adjuvants to other analgesics.
- The cost-effectiveness of dexmedetomidine and clonidine must be assessed in individual healthcare systems, as this will depend on ICU admission policies and re-imbursement methods.

References

1. Gagnon DJ, Fontaine GV, Riker RR, Fraser GL (2017) Repurposing valproate, enteral clonidine, and phenobarbital for comfort in adult ICU patients: a literature review with practical considerations. Pharmacotherapy 37:1309–1321
2. Weerink MAS, Struys M, Hannivoort LN, Barends CRM, Absalom AR, Colin P (2017) Clinical pharmacokinetics and pharmacodynamics of dexmedetomidine. Clin Pharmacokinet 56:893–913
3. Weatherall M, Aantaa R, Conti G et al (2017) A multinational, drug utilization study to investigate the use of dexmedetomidine (Dexdor®) in clinical practice in the EU. Br J Clin Pharmacol 83:2066–2076
4. Cruickshank M, Henderson L, MacLennan G et al (2016) Alpha-2 agonists for sedation of mechanically ventilated adults in intensive care units: a systematic review. Health Technol Assess 20:v–xx (S 1–117)
5. Pandharipande PP, Pun BT, Herr DL et al (2007) Effect of sedation with dexmedetomidine vs lorazepam on acute brain dysfunction in mechanically ventilated patients: the MENDS randomized controlled trial. JAMA 298:2644–2653
6. Riker RR, Shehabi Y, Bokesch PM et al (2009) Dexmedetomidine vs midazolam for sedation of critically ill patients: a randomized trial. JAMA 301:489–499
7. Chen K, Lu Z, Xin YC, Cai Y, Chen Y, Pan SM (2015) Alpha-2 agonists for long-term sedation during mechanical ventilation in critically ill patients. Cochrane Database Syst Rev CD010269
8. Tran A, Blinder H, Hutton B, English SW (2017) A systematic review of alpha-2 agonists for sedation in mechanically ventilated neurocritical care patients. Neurocrit Care. https://doi.org/10.1007/s12028-017-0388-5 (May 25, Epub ahead of print)

9. Mirski MA, Lewin JJ 3rd, Ledroux S et al (2010) Cognitive improvement during continuous sedation in critically ill, awake and responsive patients: the Acute Neurological ICU Sedation Trial (ANIST). Intensive Care Med 36:1505–1513

10. Wang JG, Belley-Cote E, Burry L et al (2017) Clonidine for sedation in the critically ill: a systematic review and meta-analysis. Crit Care 21:75–85

11. Kaur S, Gupta KK, Singh A, Sunita, Baghla N (2016) Arousal from sedation in lower abdominal surgeries under spinal anesthesia: comparison between dexmedetomidine and clonidine. Anesth Essays Res 10:98–103

12. Gagnon DJ, Riker RR, Glisic EK, Kelner A, Perrey HM, Fraser GL (2015) Transition from dexmedetomidine to enteral clonidine for ICU sedation: an observational pilot study. Pharmacotherapy 35:251–259

13. Chawla N, Boateng A, Deshpande R (2017) Procedural sedation in the ICU and emergency department. Curr Opin Anaesthesiol 30:507–512

14. Kim KN, Lee HJ, Kim SY, Kim JY (2017) Combined use of dexmedetomidine and propofol in monitored anesthesia care: a randomized controlled study. BMC Anesth 17:34–40

15. Kakkar A, Tyagi A, Nabi N, Sethi AK, Verma UC (2016) Comparision of clonidine and dexmedetomidine for attenuation of laryngoscopy and intubation response – a randomized controlled trial. J Clin Anesth 33:283–288

16. Lewis SR, Nicholson A, Smith AF, Alderson P (2015) Alpha-2 adrenergic agonists for the prevention of shivering following general anaesthesia. Cochrane Database Syst Rev CD011107

17. Barends CR, Absalom A, van Minnen B, Vissink A, Visser A (2017) Dexmedetomidine versus midazolam in procedural sedation. a systematic review of efficacy and safety. PLoS One 12:e169525

18. Bellon M, Le Bot A, Michelet D et al (2016) Efficacy of intraoperative dexmedetomidine compared with placebo for postoperative pain management: a meta-analysis of published studies. Pain Ther 5:63–80

19. Zhang X, Wang D, Shi M, Luo Y (2017) Efficacy and safety of dexmedetomidine as an adjuvant in epidural analgesia and anesthesia: a systematic review and meta-analysis of randomized controlled trials. Clin Drug Investig 37:343–354

20. Jin S, Liang DD, Chen C, Zhang M, Wang J (2017) Dexmedetomidine prevent postoperative nausea and vomiting on patients during general anesthesia: A PRISMA-compliant meta analysis of randomized controlled trials. Medicine (Baltimore) 96:e5770

21. Patel J, Thosani R, Kothari J, Garg P, Pandya H (2016) Clonidine and ketamine for stable hemodynamics in off-pump coronary artery bypass. Asian Cardiovasc Thorac Ann 24:638–646

22. Australian Medicines Handbook Pty (2017) Clonidine (anaesthesia). In: Australian Medicines Handbook. Australian Medicines Handbook Pty, Adelaide

23. Mahmoud M, Mason KP (2015) Dexmedetomidine: review, update, and future considerations of paediatric perioperative and periprocedural applications and limitations. Br J Anaesth 115:171–182

24. Playfor S, Jenkins I, Boyles C et al (2006) Consensus guidelines on sedation and analgesia in critically ill children. Intensive Care Med 32:1125–1136

25. Hanning SM, Orlu Gul M, Toni I, Neubert A, Tuleu C (2017) A mini-review of non-parenteral clonidine preparations for paediatric sedation. J Pharm Pharmacol 69:398–405

26. Mo Y, Zimmermann AE (2013) Role of dexmedetomidine for the prevention and treatment of delirium in intensive care unit patients. Ann Pharmacother 47:869–876

27. Li B, Li Y, Tian S et al (2015) Anti-inflammatory effects of perioperative dexmedetomidine administered as an adjunct to general anesthesia: a meta-analysis. Nat Sci Reports 5:12342

28. Berian JR, Rosenthal RA, Robinson TN (2017) Confusion regarding surgical delirium-is dexmedetomidine the answer? JAMA Surg 152:e171511

29. Djaiani G, Silverton N, Fedorko L et al (2016) dexmedetomidine versus propofol sedation reduces delirium after cardiac surgery: a randomized controlled trial. Anesthesiology 124:362–368

30. Su X, Meng ZT, Wu XH et al (2016) Dexmedetomidine for prevention of delirium in elderly patients after non-cardiac surgery: a randomised, double-blind, placebo-controlled trial. Lancet 388:1893–1902

31. Deiner S, Luo X, Lin HM et al (2017) Intraoperative infusion of dexmedetomidine for prevention of postoperative delirium and cognitive dysfunction in elderly patients undergoing major elective noncardiac surgery: a randomized clinical trial. JAMA Surg 152:e171505

32. Devlin JW, Roberts RJ, Fong JJ et al (2010) Efficacy and safety of quetiapine in critically ill patients with delirium: a prospective, multicenter, randomized, double-blind, placebo-controlled pilot study. Crit Care Med 38:419–427

33. Reade MC, Eastwood GM, Bellomo R et al (2016) Effect of dexmedetomidine added to standard care on ventilator-free time in patients with agitated delirium: a randomized clinical trial. JAMA 315:1460–1468

34. Carrasco G, Baeza N, Cabre L et al (2016) Dexmedetomidine for the treatment of hyperactive delirium refractory to haloperidol in nonintubated ICU Patients: a nonrandomized controlled trial. Crit Care Med 44:1295–1306

35. Calver L, Isbister GK (2012) Dexmedetomidine in the emergency department: assessing safety and effectiveness in difficult-to-sedate acute behavioural disturbance. Emerg Med J 29:915–918

36. Wu XH, Cui F, Zhang C et al (2016) Low-dose dexmedetomidine improves sleep quality pattern in elderly patients after noncardiac surgery in the intensive care unit: a pilot randomized controlled trial. Anesthesiology 125:979–991

37. Albertson TE, Chenoweth J, Ford J, Owen K, Sutter ME (2014) Is it prime time for alpha2-adrenocepter agonists in the treatment of withdrawal syndromes? J Med Toxicol 10:369–381

38. Awissi DK, Lebrun G, Fagnan M, Skrobik Y (2013) Alcohol, nicotine, and iatrogenic withdrawals in the ICU. Crit Care Med 41:S57–S68

39. Chiu AW, Contreras S, Mehta S et al (2017) Iatrogenic opioid withdrawal in critically ill patients: a review of assessment tools and management. Ann Pharmacother 51:1099–1111

40. Shehabi Y, Bellomo R, Reade MC et al (2012) Early intensive care sedation predicts long-term mortality in ventilated critically ill patients. Am J Respir Crit Care Med 186:724–731

41. Lin TF, Yeh YC, Lin FS et al (2009) Effect of combining dexmedetomidine and morphine for intravenous patient-controlled analgesia. Br J Anaesth 102:117–122

42. Ferreira J (2017) The theory is out there: the use of alpha-2 agonists in treatment of septic shock. Shock. https://doi.org/10.1097/SHK0000000000000979 (Aug 29, Epub ahead of print)

43. Scibelli G, Maio L, Sasso M, Lanza A, Savoia G (2017) Dexmedetomidine: current role in burn ICU. Transl Med UniSa 16:1–10

44. Kawazoe Y, Miyamoto K, Morimoto T et al (2017) Effect of dexmedetomidine on mortality and ventilator-free days in patients requiring mechanical ventilation with sepsis: a randomized clinical trial. JAMA 317:1321–1328

45. Meersch M, Schmidt C, Zarbock A (2017) Perioperative acute kidney injury: an under-recognized problem. Anesth Analg 125:1223–1232

46. Mokhtari M, Sistanizad M, Farasatinasab M (2017) Antipyretic effect of clonidine in intensive care unit patients: a nested observational study. J Clin Pharmacol 57:48–51

47. Canadian Agency for Drugs and Technologies in Health (2014) Dexmedetomidine for sedation in the ICU or PICU: a review of cost-effectiveness and guidelines. Canadian Agency for Drugs and Technologies in Health, Ottawa

48. Turunen H, Jakob SM, Ruokonen E et al (2015) Dexmedetomidine versus standard care sedation with propofol or midazolam in intensive care: an economic evaluation. Crit Care 19:67–76

49. Wilcox ME, Rubenfeld GD (2015) Is critical care ready for an economic surrogate endpoint? Crit Care 19:248–250

50. Ming LC, Yeoh SF, Patel RP, Zaidi ST (2017) Revisiting the clinical evidence and economics of dexmedetomidine use. J Med Mark 15:90–92
51. Reade MC, Finfer S (2014) Sedation and delirium in the intensive care unit. N Engl J Med 370:442–452

Rituximab-related Severe Toxicity

E. Ghrenassia, E. Mariotte, and E. Azoulay

Introduction

Rituximab is an immunoglobulin G (IgG)1κ monoclonal chimeric human/murine antibody targeting CD20 antigen [1]. CD20 is a surface antigen specific to mature B lymphocytes, from pre-B cells to memory B cells [2]. Rituximab induces early (24–48 h) and prolonged (2–6 month) B cell depletion via different mechanisms: antibody-dependent cellular cytotoxicity, direct cross-linking of CD20, complement dependent cytotoxicity, and opsonization-induced phagocytosis ([3]; Fig. 1).

Rituximab is increasingly used in various types of patients with hematology, internal medicine, rheumatology or orphan diseases (Table 1). Rituximab was conceptually designed for the treatment of non-Hodgkin lymphomas of B cell lineage and remains a major drug in this indication [4]. Indeed rituximab, in association with polychemotherapy, provides benefit for the treatment induction of various non-Hodgkin lymphomas, such as diffuse large B cell lymphoma [5, 6], chronic lymphocytic leukemia (CLL) [7], or for maintenance therapy of non-Hodgkin lymphomas, such as follicular lymphoma [8]. Moreover, rituximab is now recognized to be effective and is widely used in many autoimmune diseases such as rheumatoid arthritis [9] or anti-neutrophil cytoplasmic antibody (ANCA)-associated vasculitis [10, 11].

Critical care physicians may be using rituximab in severe forms of autoimmune diseases requiring emergency treatment along with the management of acute respiratory failure, acute kidney injury (AKI) and neurologic or cardiac involvement. In a recent series of 381 patients with systemic autoimmune disease (connective tissue

E. Ghrenassia · E. Azoulay (✉)
Intensive Care Unit, APHP, Hôpital Saint-Louis
Paris, France
Paris Diderot University
Paris, France
e-mail: elie.azoulay@sls.aphp.fr

E. Mariotte
Intensive Care Unit, APHP, Hôpital Saint-Louis
Paris, France

© Springer International Publishing AG 2018
J.-L. Vincent (ed.), *Annual Update in Intensive Care and Emergency Medicine 2018*,
Annual Update in Intensive Care and Emergency Medicine,
https://doi.org/10.1007/978-3-319-73670-9_43

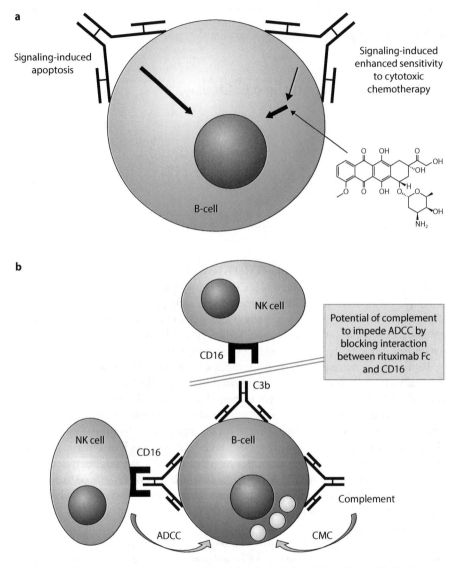

Fig. 1 a Mechanisms of action related to direct rituximab-induced signaling. **b** Mechanisms of action related to rituximab-induced CMC and ADCC with potential that these two mechanisms can be antagonistic. *CMC*: complement dependent cytotoxicity; *ADCC*: antibody-dependent cellular cytotoxicity. From [83] with permission

disease or multisystemic vasculitis) requiring admission to the intensive care unit (ICU), 3.9% received rituximab in the ICU [12]. In the ICU setting, anti-CD20 antibodies are also administered in patients with aggressive lymphomas receiv-

Table 1 Cinical conditions for which rituximab has been approved

Approved therapeutic indications for rituximab (EMA, FDA)	
HEMATOLOGY	**IMMUNOLOGY**
Follicular lymphoma	Rheumatoid arthritis
Diffuse large B-cell lymphoma	Granulomatosis with polyangiitis
Chronic lymphocytic leukemia	Microscopic polyangiitis
Other potential indications for rituximab (off-label)	
Burkitt lymphoma	Cardiac and renal transplantation
MALT lymphoma	Autoimmune hemolytic anemia
Central nervous system lymphoma	Immune thrombocytopenia
Hodgkin lymphoma	Thrombotic thrombocytopenic purpura
Post-transplant lymphoproliferative disorder	Lupus nephritis
Graft versus host disease	Membranous nephropathy

FDA: US Food and Drug Administration; *EMA*: European Medicines Agency

ing chemotherapy in the ICU or patients with unresponsive thrombotic microangiopathies.

In pivotal studies and large clinical trials [5, 8], few events have complicated rituximab infusion. Nonetheless, after a decade of use and numerous patients treated, it appears that rituximab may induce a rare but wide panel of potentially serious and even lethal toxicities. This chapter, a systematic review, focuses on these severe adverse events, classified as acute or severe late onset toxicity (Table 2).

To perform the review, we searched the MEDLINE database for all articles concerning rituximab-induced toxicity. We first crossed "rituximab" with "toxicity" as Medical Subject Headings. Then we crossed "Rituximab" with the medical subject heading of any toxicity we found (e.g., "Progressive multifocal leukoencephalopathy"). Any type of manuscript, from 1999 to 2017 was taken into account: case reports, retrospective or prospective series, randomized controlled trials and meta-analyses. Redundant cases were excluded. Only articles written in English or French languages were selected.

Table 2 Major acute and late onset toxicities of rituximab

ACUTE ONSET TOXICITY	SEVERE LATE ONSET TOXICITY
Infusion related reaction	Pneumocystis pneumonia
Tumor lysis syndrome	Viral reactivation (HBV, JC, VZV)
Digestive perforation	Bacterial infection
Thrombocytopenia	Late onset neutropenia
Serum sickness	Hypogammaglobulinemia
Lung toxicity (ARDS)	Organizing pneumonia

ARDS: acute respiratory distress syndrome; *VZV*: Varicella zoster virus; *HBV*: hepatitis B virus

Acute Onset Toxicity

Infusion Reactions

Infusion reaction, also called cytokine release syndrome, is well described in the current literature and has led to the formulation of recommendations for rituximab administration in hematology-oncology patients. It has been reported in 4% [13, 14], 14.6% [15] and 23% [16] of patients depending on the particular study and has especially been encountered during the first infusion of the drug. Usual mild infusion reactions include rash, hot flushes, dyspnea and pruritus [13]. Less common mild reactions may consist of dry throat feeling, palpitations, headaches, restless leg syndrome, chills, hypertension and fever. Severe cytokine release syndrome is infrequent (0.5%) [16] but can be lethal, with anaphylactoid reactions such as bronchospasm, angioedema, shock and hypoxemia [17]. Cardiogenic shock, myocardial infarction and ventricular fibrillation have been reported by the US Food and Drug Administration (FDA). Fatal reactions may occur in 0.04–0.07% of patients [3].

Risk factors identified for a rituximab infusion reaction include: first infusion, large tumor burden or high levels of circulating B lymphocytes [15, 18, 19]. This toxicity has been ascribed to the release of tumor necrosis factor (TNF), interleukin (IL)-6 or other cytokines by B lymphocytes, following the binding of rituximab to CD20 [19]. To prevent these reactions, the FDA recommends slow infusion rates, especially for the first administration of rituximab (initial rate of 50 mg/h with an increase of 50 mg/h every 30 min, to a maximum of 400 mg/h unless signs of infusion reaction occur). Subsequent infusions can be accelerated to 100 mg/h increasing to 400 mg/h by steps of 100 mg/h every 30 min. Recent protocols with 90-minute infusion rates do not seem to increase the incidence of infusion reactions in previously treated patients [13, 15, 19, 20]. Moreover, premedication with antihistamine, steroids and acetaminophen prior to rituximab infusion is often sufficient to prevent infusion reactions [13].

The treatment of infusion reactions consists of infusion interruption and symptomatic treatment. The best-documented case of severe respiratory failure following a first rituximab administration in a case of Asian-variant intravascular lymphoma is shown in Fig. 2.

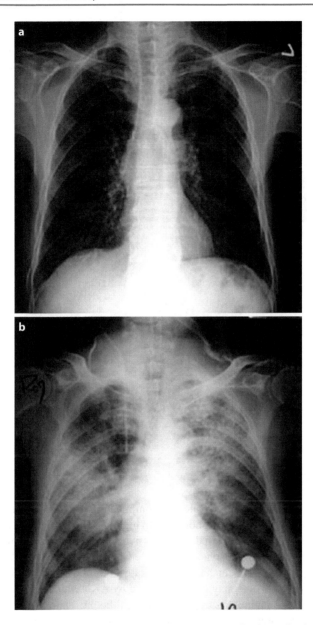

Fig. 2 A very well-documented case of severe pulmonary complications after initial treatment with rituximab for Asian-variant intravascular lymphoma. The chest X-ray before (**a**) and after (**b**) rituximab administration. The post-rituximab chest films showed newly developed infiltrations and consolidation. High-resolution computed tomography of the chest (panel **c**) showed ground-glass opacity and consolidation associated with reticulation in both lungs as well as moderate bilateral pleural effusions. The diagnostic impression was interstitial pneumonitis. Histopathological examination (panel **d**) showed pulmonary hemorrhage with an intra-alveolar proteinaceous exudate containing erythrocytes and necrotic neutrophils suggestive of acute capillaritis. From [84] with permission

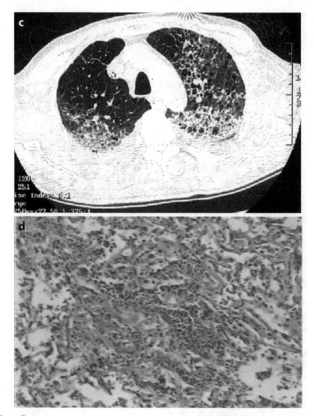

Fig. 2 (Continued)

Tumor Lysis Syndrome

Tumor lysis syndrome is a life-threatening complication of highly aggressive malignancies, described mainly in lymphomas with high tumoral burden and hyperleukocytic leukemias. It is characterized by a massive release of the content of tumoral cells (mainly potassium, phosphate and nucleic acids) into the blood circulation, spontaneously or following cancer chemotherapy, immunotherapy or targeted therapy. Tumor lysis syndrome may be complicated by AKI, which impacts negatively on the prognosis of patients with cancer [21]. Although tumor lysis syndrome is a well-described complication of chemotherapy for aggressive lymphoma, it has not been frequently reported in patients treated with rituximab. Only a few cases have been reported in the literature. In these cases, it is noteworthy that the tumor lysis syndrome occurred in the context of high burden lymphoproliferative disorders (bulky lymphadenopathies or high white blood cell [WBC] count) [22]. Mortality rate was high since 4/8 patients died from the tumor lysis syndrome [23, 24]. However, the lack of case reports of tumor lysis syndrome following rituximab infusion may be linked to a publication bias because only severe or uncommon tumor lysis syndrome cases may have been published.

Digestive Perforation

Digestive tract perforation is a rare but serious complication of rituximab infusion. It was reported in 37 cases/730,000 exposures in a 2006 vigilance report, resulting in 4 deaths [25]. Digestive tract perforation occurred exclusively in the setting of lymphoma, mostly post-transplant lymphoproliferative disorders involving the gut. Although this complication may occur with other chemotherapies, treatment with rituximab increases the risk of digestive perforation from 0.15 to 0.38% [26]. In a series of 46 patients with post-transplant lymphoproliferative disorders receiving rituximab monotherapy, one patient experienced gut perforation [27]. The median time from rituximab infusion to perforation is 6 days (range 1–77) [26]. The small bowel and colon may be involved equally [25, 28–30].

Serum Sickness

Serum sickness is linked to a hypersensitivity reaction (Gell and Coombs classification type III), with immune complex deposits. Indeed, an antigen and its antibody form an immune complex which deposits in vessel walls and tissues and induces complement cascade activation and inflammation. Serum sickness may be a rare complication of rituximab infusion. Clinical signs usually occur between day-7 to day-14 following rituximab infusion, and consist of fever, polyarthritis, purpura, palmar erythema, urticarial rash and AKI. Complement activation is observed as C3, C4 and CH50 rates decrease in the serum [31].

Only 32 cases of rituximab-induced serum sickness have been reported in the literature. This complication occurred mostly in the setting of autoimmune diseases, such as Sjögren syndrome [32] and immune thrombocytopenic purpura [33]. It is less described in the context of non-Hodgkin lymphomas. These different incidences may be explained by the fact that polychemotherapies are often used in non-Hodgkin lymphomas and may reduce the inflammatory reaction; or by the fact that identified risk factors for serum sickness [32], namely polyclonal hypergammaglobulinemia and rheumatoid factor are more frequently reported in autoimmune diseases, especially Sjögren syndrome.

HACAs (human anti-chimeric antibodies) may be observed and could explain part of the physiopathology. HACA and rituximab form immune complex deposits and activate the complement cascade. HACAs were studied in seven cases of serum sickness under rituximab, and were present in five cases [32]. Steroids are often effective to treat this complication [34].

A similar complication may occur when rituximab is used to treat cryoglobulinemic vasculitis. Sène et al. [35] described four cases of severe "flare" and two of serum sickness among 22 patients treated with rituximab for hepatitis C virus

(HCV)-associated mixed cryoglobulinemic vasculitis. The pathophysiology of disease flare is similar to serum sickness as rituximab and cryoglobulin precipitate in vessel walls, inducing vasculitis. This interaction is due to the rheumatoid factor activity of mixed cryoglobulins. Cryoglobulinemia flares with rituximab occurred 1–2 days after rituximab infusion, and were successfully treated by methylprednisolone pulses and plasma exchanges.

Thrombocytopenia

Rituximab-induced acute thrombocytopenia is rare and reported in only 17 case reports in the literature [36, 37]. Identified risk factors included mantle cell lymphoma (70%), splenomegaly and/or bone marrow infiltration by lymphoma. Thrombocytopenia occurred 1–3 days after rituximab infusion and resolved quickly over 7–10 days. It was profound, with a median platelet count of 10,000/mm^3 but benign since no severe hemorrhage was reported. Nonetheless, most patients received platelet transfusion. Thrombocytopenia relapsed in 42% of patients in whom rituximab was reintroduced.

Delayed Onset Toxicity

Lung Toxicity

Rituximab has been involved in several cases of diffuse interstitial pneumonia. Two literature reviews of 45 [38] and 126 [39] cases are available. The overall mortality rate is around 15%. Lung toxicity occurred mostly in the setting of non-Hodgkin lymphoma (93% cases) with an estimated frequency of 0.01–0.03% cases. Three types of diffuse interstitial pneumonia have been described according to their delay of onset:

1. Hyperacute pneumonia (11%), occurring a few hours after rituximab infusion, in the context of infusion reaction. This pneumonia usually evolves to acute respiratory distress syndrome (ARDS) requiring mechanical ventilation. Here, the cytokine release is most likely to be responsible for ARDS as described above and in Fig. 2.
2. Acute/subacute pneumonia (82%), occurring within two weeks following rituximab infusion, after a median of four treatments. Patients describe fever and dyspnea and 27% need mechanical ventilation. Chest computed tomography (CT) usually shows multifocal alveolar densities, associated with ground glass attenuation. Bronchoalveolar lavage (BAL) fluid shows mostly CD4 lymphocyte alveolitis. Organizing pneumonia is the prominent histological pattern at lung biopsy and steroids are effective in most cases. Relapses occur in 80% of cases after rituximab reintroduction.

3. Deferred and chronic pneumonia (7%), occurring in the eight weeks following the final rituximab infusion. Patients have multiple asymptomatic pulmonary macronodules and BAL fluid shows lymphocytic alveolitis. Lung biopsy shows organizing pneumonia and steroids are effective.

Pneumocystis Pneumonia

Pneumocystis jirovecii pneumonia is a dreaded opportunistic infection commonly described in patients with lymphoma, since they exert T cell defects from the lymphoproliferative disease, polychemotherapy and steroid administration. Although *P. jirovecii* pneumonia has been largely attributed to CD4+ lymphocyte immunosuppression, as usually seen in human immunodeficiency virus (HIV) infection, B cells and antibodies seem to be involved in the host defense against this fungal infection [40]. Until recently, it was not clear whether rituximab actually increased the risk for *P. jirovecii* pneumonia or not, because patients on anti-CD20 therapy frequently also receive chemotherapy and steroids (increasing *per se* the risk of *P. jirovecii* pneumonia) and/or co-trimoxazole prophylaxis (decreasing the risk of *P. jirovecii*) [26]. Nonetheless, a recent meta-analysis showed a higher risk of *P. jirovecii* under rituximab therapy in patients treated by polychemotherapy and steroids for lymphoma. The incidence was 28/942 (3%) with rituximab versus 5/977 (0.5%) without rituximab. The relative risk of *P. jirovecii* pneumonia with rituximab is estimated to be 3.65 (IC95% = 0.09–0.94). No case has been described under prophylaxis with co-trimoxazole [41]. In a case series of 30 patients who developed *P. jirovecii* pneumonia under rituximab, 10% had no lymphoma but auto-immune diseases (immune thrombocytopenia, rheumatoid arthritis or granulomatosis with polyangeitis). Moreover, 10% occurred under rituximab alone [40]. *P. jirovecii* pneumonia occurred with a median delay of 77 days after the final rituximab infusion. For the 10 patients with available data, low CD4+ lymphocyte levels were found. The manifestations were serious, as 88.5% of patients had criteria for ARDS and 30% died.

JC Virus Reactivation: Progressive Multifocal Leukoencephalopathy

Progressive multifocal leukoencephalopathy (PML) is a sub-acute/chronic infection of the brain, linked to JC virus (JCV) reactivation, seen in immunocompromised subjects. This opportunistic infection is usually observed in advanced stages of HIV infection, but has also been described in lymphoid neoplasms, and following immunosuppressive drugs, such as rituximab [42]. JCV is a ubiquitous double-stranded DNA virus [43]. Its seroprevalence is estimated at around 80–90% and asymptomatic primary infection occurs in childhood in 75% of the cases. The virus then remains latent in the kidney and mononuclear immune cells [26]. PML is a demyelinating disease of the central nervous system (CNS), occurring when JCV reactivation occurs in the context of lymphoid depletion. The spectrum of clinical manifestations associated with PML includes confusion, motor weakness, ataxia, aphasia, visual symptoms [44]. These manifestations usually progress over weeks to months.

Brain magnetic resonance imaging (MRI) usually shows multifocal areas of subcortical and periventricular white matter demyelination. These lesions typically predominate in the parieto-occipital territory. They are hypointense in T1-weighted sequences, not enhanced after gadolinium injection, and hyperintense in T2-weighted sequences. JCV detection by polymerase chain reaction (PCR) in the cerebrospinal fluid (CSF) has an estimated sensitivity of 92% and a specificity of 92% in patients with acquired immunodeficiency disease (AIDS) [45]. In a series of 57 cases of rituximab-associated PML in non-AIDS patients, JCV was found in the CSF of only 54% of the cases [44]. If there is a high suspicion of PML with a negative PCR, brain biopsy must be performed [42]. No treatment has been shown to be effective except for immune restoration whenever possible. Mortality is high, around 90% over a median of 2 months.

Among 57 patients with PML receiving rituximab therapy [44], 52 had lymphoid malignancy, 2 had systemic lupus erythematosus, 1 had rheumatoid arthritis, and 2 had autoimmune cytopenia. A median of six rituximab doses (1–28) were administered before PML diagnosis (after a median delay of 5.5 months (0.3–66 months) following the last rituximab administration). As PML has largely been described in patients with non-Hodgkin lymphoma, the accountability of rituximab in this context is unclear. Indeed, PML has been associated with non-Hodgkin lymphoma (0.07% cases [44]), resulting from both the disease and the treatment-induced immunosuppression. In a 2005 report of 46 cases of PML occurring after non-Hodgkin lymphoma polychemotherapy, only four patients had received rituximab [46]. Among 307 HIV infected patients treated with rituximab for lymphoproliferative disorders, the incidence of PML was 1.4 cases/1,000 patient-years, which was not higher than what is usually described in AIDS patients (0.5–1.3/1,000 patient years) [43]. Nonetheless, in a monocenter retrospective study, no case of PML was described among 459 patients not exposed to rituximab but five cases were described among 517 exposed patients, making a rate difference of 2.2 (0.1–4.3)/1,000 person-years between the two groups [47].

In patients with connective tissue diseases, PML incidence is much lower. It is estimated to affect 0.4/100,000 patients with rheumatoid arthritis, and 4/100,000 patients with systemic lupus erythematosus [42]. Rituximab is the only disease-modifying drug that is clearly associated with an increased risk of developing PML in patients with rheumatoid arthritis. A 10-fold increased risk is estimated under rituximab therapy for patients with rheumatoid arthritis [42]. For patients with other connective tissue diseases, the risk modification is unknown since the use of rituximab is less common.

Hepatitis B Reactivation

Hepatitis B (HBV) reactivation may occur in patients with occult HBV infection (HbS Ag+, HbCab+, HBV DNA−) treated with anti-cancer polychemotherapy, es-

Table 3 Prevalence of reactivation in hepatitis-B virus (HBV) seroconverted patients receiving rituximab	First author (date, reference)	Prevalence %
	Kim (2013) [81]	2.4%
	Lu (2015) [58]	2.7%
	Matsui (2013) [82]	6.8%
	Hsu (2012) [55]	11.3%
	Huang (2013) [59]	17.9%
	Yeo (2009) [56]	23.8%

pecially when rituximab is added to the regimen. The prevalence of reactivation in these patients is estimated at between 16 and 80% [48]. In a recent meta-analysis, rituximab was a significant risk factor for HBV reactivation in HbSag+ patients treated with polychemotherapy (RR 2.14; 95% CI 1.42–3.22) [49]. Thus, it is recommended that preventive antiviral treatment (lamivudine, entecavir or tenofovir) be given to exposed patients [50–52]. Moreover, rituximab promotes HBV reactivation in patients with 'resolved' (seroconverted) HBV infection (HbSag–, HbCab+, HBV DNA–). Table 3 reports HBV reactivation rates in patients treated with rituximab. The relative risk of HBV reactivation in seroconverted HBV patients under rituximab therapy was estimated to be 5.52 (95%CI: 2.05–14.85) in a recent meta-analysis [49].

In patients with autoimmune diseases, rituximab-induced HBV reactivation in seroconverted patients has been reported as a rare event [53, 54]. The median time from the start of chemotherapy to HBV reactivation is 21 weeks (range, 3–57) [55]. The clinical severity of these reactivations varies from asymptomatic cases to severe hepatitis (2.7%) [55], hepatic failure or death (0.05%) [56]. Moreover, HBV reactivation could be associated with higher mortality rates in non-Hodgkin lymphoma patients, because of the need to discontinue chemotherapy in this context [57]. Identified risk factors for HBV reactivation in HBV seroconverted patients are: undetectable baseline HbSab [56, 58], male sex [56] and elevated International Prognostic Index (IPI) score ≥ 3 [58].

For the prevention of HBV reactivation in HBV-seroconverted patients, two strategies are described in the literature. The first is monthly monitoring of blood HBV DNA, with antiviral treatment only when HBV PCR becomes positive. The second is preventive treatment. Although there seem to be more cases of viral load elevation with the first strategy, both approaches are equally effective to prevent mortality, hepatitis and delayed chemotherapy administration [55, 57–59]. As lamivudine is not effective to reduce mortality in case of HBV reactivation [57], curative treatment with entecavir or tenofovir is recommended.

Varicella-Zoster Virus Reactivation

In several randomized controlled trials (RCTs), varicella-zoster virus (VZV) reactivation was more frequent in groups receiving rituximab [3]. Overall, the incidence of herpes zoster infection increased from 1% (control group) to 4.5% (rituximab group) in elderly patients treated with polychemotherapy for non-Hodgkin lymphoma [5]. In patients with rheumatoid arthritis, rituximab was associated with an incidence of VZV infection of 1.87/100 patient-years. This risk was not higher in the rituximab group than in a group of patients receiving other biotherapies [60] or placebo [16].

Among 64 reported cases of serious viral infections under rituximab, 9.4% were reported to be linked to VZV [61]. For these six patients, there was only cutaneous involvement, but several dermatomes could be involved. There are only three case reports of disseminated VZV infections under rituximab associated with other chemo/immunotherapies, with no clear evidence of rituximab accountability [62]. Despite its severity, with a mortality rate estimated to be 29%, it is most often observed in very immunocompromised patients and the role of rituximab in disseminated VZV infection is controversial [62].

Bacterial Infections

Rituximab does not seem to increase the risk of bacterial infections overall. In the context of polychemotherapy for non-Hodgkin lymphoma, rituximab did not increase the risk of bacterial infections in RCTs or subsequent meta-analyses [3, 63]. In patients with rheumatoid arthritis, the adjunction of rituximab was not associated with a risk of bacterial infection compared to standard treatment alone as published in available RCTs and meta-analyses [16, 64]. Bacterial pneumonias were the most common severe infections (2%). In highly sensitized renal transplant recipients, rituximab did not increase the risk of bacterial infections, compared to other immunosuppressive regimens in a retrospective study [65, 66]. However, when rituximab is used as maintenance monotherapy in indolent non-Hodgkin lymphoma, the risk of severe bacterial infections increases, with one report noting that 19% developed bacterial infections and 1–4% grade III–IV infections [3]. Meta-analyses report a relative risk between 1.67 and 2.85 for the risk of bacterial infections and of 3.55 for grade III–IV infections [8, 67].

Late-Onset Neutropenia

Late-onset neutropenia under rituximab treatment is defined as a leukocyte count $< 1,000/mm^3$, occurring 3–4 weeks after the last injection of the drug and a spontaneous return to a normal neutrophil count thereafter. Overall, late-onset neutropenia is estimated to occur in 14% of patients receiving rituximab therapy [68] and the risk of infection is estimated at 17% in patients with late-onset neutropenia [68]. The incidence of this complication varies according to the indication for rituximab. Neutrophil counts $< 500/mm^3$ were described in 5–13% of patients treated for non-Hodgkin lymphoma, in 42% of patients receiving hematopoietic stem cell transplantation, and in 3% of those treated for autoimmune diseases [68]. Late-onset neutropenia occurred in 42% of kidney transplant recipients receiving rituximab, compared to 28% of patients not receiving rituximab [69].

Late-onset neutropenia has been reported between 46 and 384 days after the first injection of rituximab [26]. Neutrophils return to normal after between 1 to 17 weeks [67, 70, 71]. Late-onset neutropenia resolution can also be obtained using granulocyte colony-stimulating factor (G-CSF) administration [72].

The mechanism of late-onset neutropenia is linked to inhibition of granulopoiesis with a maturation blockade in the bone marrow [70]. The hypothesis that late-onset neutropenia could be due to a defect of granulopoiesis linked to a competition with intra-medullary B lymphopoiesis has been voiced. This hypothesis was sustained by more intense B-cell activating factor (BAFF) elevation in patients with late-onset neutropenia [69, 73]. Other authors have hypothesized that late-onset neutropenia could be due to autoantibody production against neutrophils progenitors [74, 75]. Finally, large granular lymphocyte proliferation was observed in several patients with rituximab-induced late-onset neutropenia [26, 68]. This could explain late-onset neutropenia as large granular lymphocyte oligoclonal proliferation is known to induce neutropenia [76].

Hypogammaglobulinemia

Although rituximab does not target plasmocytes that do not present the CD20 antigen, a decrease in serum immunoglobulin levels has been reported under this treatment [26]. In a series of patients treated with rituximab for indolent non-Hodgkin lymphoma, there was a decrease in IgM levels to 73% of baseline in patients receiving long-term treatment, but not in IgG or IgA levels. These patients did not present more infectious events [77].

In 22.4% of patients with rheumatoid arthritis under rituximab therapy, there was a significant decrease in IgM levels, 3.5% in IgG levels and 1.1% in IgA levels. These patients also had no increased infection rate during follow-up [16]. In a series of 30 children treated with rituximab for immune thrombocytopenia, a slight decrease in IgG, A, and M levels was reported over the year following rituximab therapy, without any case of infection [78]. In a multicenter retrospective study, 3/189 (1.6%) patients receiving rituximab for immune thrombocytopenic purpura developed hypogammaglobulinemia < 5 g/l. They presented chronic sinusitis, recurrent bronchitis, and one case had enteroviral meningoencephalitis. The authors analyzed published data on rituximab use in immune thrombocytopenic purpura and noted that 21/192 (10%) patients had an asymptomatic decrease in gammaglobulins. Moreover, there are only four other cases in the literature of symptomatic hypogammaglobulinemia under rituximab for immune thrombocytopenic purpura. Among them, another case developed enteroviral meningoencephalitis [79].

Conclusion

In summary, rituximab is an effective and widely used treatment for non-Hodgkin lymphoma, autoimmune, inflammatory and orphan diseases, with a good tolerance and safety profile, but rare toxic events. The drug is administered as curative treatment, alone or in combination with chemotherapy, as well as in preventive and maintenance therapy. Therefore, the exposed population is large and increasing, making these toxic events likely to present in our ICUs. Critical care specialists must be aware of the drug's different potentially serious adverse effects, which may occur immediately, or short- or long-term after rituximab infusion, depending on the mechanism of toxicity. The toxicity of more recently released anti-CD20 antibodies is less known. Nonetheless, ofatumumab (used in CLL) or obinutuzumab (used in both CLL and follicular lymphoma) seem to share toxicities with rituximab (e.g., infusion reaction, late cytopenia, progressive multifocal leucoencephalopathy or HBV reactivation [82]), prompting careful surveillance of patients receiving new anti-CD20 antibodies.

References

1. Smith MR (2003) Rituximab (monoclonal anti-CD20 antibody): mechanisms of action and resistance. Oncogene 22:7359–7368
2. Edwards JCW, Cambridge G (2006) B-cell targeting in rheumatoid arthritis and other autoimmune diseases. Nat Rev Immunol 6:394–403
3. Kimby E (2005) Tolerability and safety of rituximab (MabThera). Cancer Treat Rev 31:456–473
4. MacDonald D, Crosbie T, Christofides A et al (2017) A Canadian perspective on the subcutaneous administration of rituximab in non-Hodgkin lymphoma. Curr Oncol Tor Ont 24:33–39
5. Coiffier B, Lepage E, Briere J et al (2002) CHOP chemotherapy plus rituximab compared with CHOP alone in elderly patients with diffuse large-B-cell lymphoma. N Engl J Med 346:235–242
6. Pfreundschuh M, Trümper L, Osterborg A et al (2006) CHOP-like chemotherapy plus rituximab versus CHOP-like chemotherapy alone in young patients with good-prognosis diffuse large-B-cell lymphoma: a randomised controlled trial by the MabThera International Trial (MInT) Group. Lancet Oncol 7:379–391
7. Hallek M, Fischer K, Fingerle-Rowson G et al (2010) Addition of rituximab to fludarabine and cyclophosphamide in patients with chronic lymphocytic leukaemia: a randomised, open-label, phase 3 trial. Lancet 376:1164–1174
8. Vidal L, Gafter-Gvili A, Salles G et al (2011) Rituximab maintenance for the treatment of patients with follicular lymphoma: an updated systematic review and meta-analysis of randomized trials. J Natl Cancer Inst 103:1799–1806
9. Edwards JCW, Szczepanski L, Szechinski J et al (2004) Efficacy of B-cell-targeted therapy with rituximab in patients with rheumatoid arthritis. N Engl J Med 350:2572–2581
10. Stone JH, Merkel PA, Spiera R et al (2010) Rituximab versus cyclophosphamide for ANCA-associated vasculitis. N Engl J Med 363:221–232
11. Guillevin L, Pagnoux C, Karras A et al (2014) Rituximab versus azathioprine for maintenance in ANCA-associated vasculitis. N Engl J Med 371:1771–1780
12. Dumas G, Géri G, Montlahuc C et al (2015) Outcomes in critically ill patients with systemic rheumatic disease: a multicenter study. Chest 148:927–935

13. Arredondo-Garza T, Majluf-Cruz A, Vela-Ojeda J et al (2013) Peri-infusional adverse reactions to rituximab in patients with non-Hodgkin's lymphoma. Arch Med Res 44:549–554

14. Swan JT, Zaghloul HA, Cox JE, Murillo JR (2014) Use of a pharmacy protocol to convert standard rituximab infusions to rapid infusion shortens outpatient infusion clinic visits. Pharmacotherapy 34:686–694

15. Lang DSP, Keefe DMK, Schultz T, Pearson A (2013) Predictors of acute adverse events from rapid rituximab infusion. Support Care Cancer 21:2315–2320

16. van Vollenhoven RF, Emery P, Bingham CO et al (2013) Long-term safety of rituximab in rheumatoid arthritis: 9.5-year follow-up of the global clinical trial programme with a focus on adverse events of interest in RA patients. Ann Rheum Dis 72:1496–1502

17. Plosker GL, Figgitt DP (2003) Rituximab: a review of its use in non-Hodgkin's lymphoma and chronic lymphocytic leukaemia. Drugs 63:803–843

18. Winkler U, Jensen M, Manzke O et al (1999) Cytokine-release syndrome in patients with B-cell chronic lymphocytic leukemia and high lymphocyte counts after treatment with an anti-CD20 monoclonal antibody (rituximab, IDEC-C2B8). Blood 94:2217–2224

19. Sehn LH, Donaldson J, Filewich A et al (2007) Rapid infusion rituximab in combination with corticosteroid-containing chemotherapy or as maintenance therapy is well tolerated and can safely be delivered in the community setting. Blood 109:4171–4173

20. Salar A, Casao D, Cervera M et al (2006) Rapid infusion of rituximab with or without steroid-containing chemotherapy: 1-yr experience in a single institution. Eur J Haematol 77:338–340

21. Canet E, Zafrani L, Lambert J et al (2013) Acute kidney injury in patients with newly diagnosed high-grade hematological malignancies: impact on remission and survival. PLoS One 8:e55870

22. Francescone SA, Murphy B, Fallon JT et al (2009) Tumor lysis syndrome occurring after the administration of rituximab for posttransplant lymphoproliferative disorder. Transplant Proc 41:1946–1948

23. Otrock ZK, Hatoum HA, Salem ZM (2008) Acute tumor lysis syndrome after rituximab administration in Burkitt's lymphoma. Intern Emerg Med 3:161–163

24. Yang B, Lu XC, Yu RL et al (2012) Diagnosis and treatment of rituximab-induced acute tumor lysis syndrome in patients with diffuse large B-cell lymphoma. Am J Med Sci 343:337–341

25. Cornejo A, Bohnenblust M, Harris C, Abrahamian GA (2009) Intestinal perforation associated with rituximab therapy for post-transplant lymphoproliferative disorder after liver transplantation. Cancer Chemother Pharmacol 64:857–860

26. Ram R, Ben-Bassat I, Shpilberg O et al (2009) The late adverse events of rituximab therapy – rare but there! Leuk Lymphoma 50:1083–1095

27. Choquet S, Leblond V, Herbrecht R et al (2006) Efficacy and safety of rituximab in B-cell post-transplantation lymphoproliferative disorders: results of a prospective multicenter phase 2 study. Blood 107:3053–3057

28. Kollmar O, Becker S, Schilling MK, Maurer CA (2002) Intestinal lymphoma perforations as a consequence of highly effective anti-CD20 antibody therapy. Transplantation 73:669–670

29. Kutsch E, Kreiger P, Consolini D, Furuya KN (2013) Colonic perforation after rituximab treatment for posttransplant lymphoproliferative disorder. J Pediatr Gastroenterol Nutr 56:e41

30. Hsu YC, Liao WC, Wang HP et al (2009) Catastrophic gastrointestinal manifestations of posttransplant lymphoproliferative disorder. Dig Liver Dis 41:238–241

31. D'Arcy CA, Mannik M (2001) Serum sickness secondary to treatment with the murine-human chimeric antibody IDEC-C2B8 (rituximab). Arthritis Rheum 44:1717–1718

32. Le Guenno G, Ruivard M, Charra L, Philippe P (2011) Rituximab-induced serum sickness in refractory immune thrombocytopenic purpura. Intern Med J 41:202–205

33. Bennett CM, Rogers ZR, Kinnamon DD et al (2006) Prospective phase 1/2 study of rituximab in childhood and adolescent chronic immune thrombocytopenic purpura. Blood 107:2639–2642

34. Pijpe J, van Imhoff GW, Spijkervet FKL et al (2005) Rituximab treatment in patients with primary Sjögren's syndrome: an open-label phase II study. Arthritis Rheum 52:2740–2750

35. Sène D, Ghillani-Dalbin P, Amoura Z et al (2009) Rituximab may form a complex with IgMkappa mixed cryoglobulin and induce severe systemic reactions in patients with hepatitis C virus-induced vasculitis. Arthritis Rheum 60:3848–3855

36. Sadashiv SK, Rao R, Fazal S, Lister J (2013) Rituximab-induced acute severe thrombocytopenia: a case series in patients with mantle cell lymphoma. Clin Lymphoma Myeloma Leuk 13:602–605

37. El-Osta H, Nair B (2013) Rituximab-induced acute thrombocytopenia: an underappreciated entity. Leuk Lymphoma 54:2736–2737

38. Lioté H, Lioté F, Séroussi B et al (2010) Rituximab-induced lung disease: a systematic literature review. Eur Respir J 35:681–687

39. Hadjinicolaou AV, Nisar MK, Parfrey H et al (2012) Non-infectious pulmonary toxicity of rituximab: a systematic review. Rheumatol Oxf Engl 51:653–662

40. Martin-Garrido I, Carmona EM, Specks U, Limper AH (2013) Pneumocystis pneumonia in patients treated with rituximab. Chest 144:258–265

41. Jiang X, Mei X, Feng D, Wang X (2015) Prophylaxis and treatment of pneumocystis jiroveci pneumonia in lymphoma patients subjected to rituximab-contained therapy: a systemic review and meta-analysis. PLoS One 10:e122171

42. Palazzo E, Yahia SA (2012) Progressive multifocal leukoencephalopathy in autoimmune diseases. Joint Bone Spine 79:351–355

43. Hoffmann C, Gérard L, Wyen C, Oksenhendler E (2012) No evidence for an early excess incidence of progressive multifocal leukencephalopathy in HIV-infected patients treated with rituximab. J Acquir Immune Defic Syndr 60:e121–e122

44. Carson KR, Evens AM, Richey EA et al (2009) Progressive multifocal leukoencephalopathy after rituximab therapy in HIV-negative patients: a report of 57 cases from the Research on Adverse Drug Events and Reports project. Blood 113:4834–4840

45. Cinque P, Scarpellini P, Vago L et al (1997) Diagnosis of central nervous system complications in HIV-infected patients: cerebrospinal fluid analysis by the polymerase chain reaction. AIDS Lond Engl 11:1–17

46. García-Suárez J, de Miguel D, Krsnik I et al (2005) Changes in the natural history of progressive multifocal leukoencephalopathy in HIV-negative lymphoproliferative disorders: impact of novel therapies. Am J Hematol 80:271–281

47. Tuccori M, Focosi D, Blandizzi C et al (2010) Inclusion of rituximab in treatment protocols for non-Hodgkin's lymphomas and risk for progressive multifocal leukoencephalopathy. Oncologist 15:1214–1219

48. Evens AM, Jovanovic BD, Su Y-C et al (2011) Rituximab-associated hepatitis B virus (HBV) reactivation in lymphoproliferative diseases: meta-analysis and examination of FDA safety reports. Ann Oncol 22:1170–1180

49. Dong H-J, Ni L-N, Sheng G-F et al (2013) Risk of hepatitis B virus (HBV) reactivation in non-Hodgkin lymphoma patients receiving rituximab-chemotherapy: a meta-analysis. J Clin Virol 57:209–214

50. Di Bisceglie AM, Lok AS, Martin P et al (2015) Recent US Food and Drug Administration warnings on hepatitis B reactivation with immune-suppressing and anticancer drugs: just the tip of the iceberg? Hepatol Baltim Md 61:703–711

51. European Association For The Study Of The Liver (2012) EASL clinical practice guidelines: management of chronic hepatitis B virus infection. J Hepatol 57:167–185

52. Liaw Y-F, Kao J-H, Piratvisuth T et al (2012) Asian-Pacific consensus statement on the management of chronic hepatitis B: a 2012 update. Hepatol Int 6:531–561

53. Droz N, Gilardin L, Cacoub P et al (2013) Kinetic profiles and management of hepatitis B virus reactivation in patients with immune-mediated inflammatory diseases. Arthritis Care Res 65:1504–1514

54. Ghrénassia E, Mékinian A, Rouaghe S et al (2012) Reactivation of resolved hepatitis B during rituximab therapy for rheumatoid arthritis. Joint Bone Spine 79:100–101

55.

Hsu C, Tsou H-H, Lin S-J et al (2014) Chemotherapy-induced hepatitis B reactivation in lymphoma patients with resolved HBV infection: a prospective study. Hepatol Baltim Md 59:2092–2100

56. Yeo W, Chan TC, Leung NWY et al (2009) Hepatitis B virus reactivation in lymphoma patients with prior resolved hepatitis B undergoing anticancer therapy with or without rituximab. J Clin Oncol 27:605–611

57. Sagnelli E, Pisaturo M, Martini S et al (2014) Clinical impact of occult hepatitis B virus infection in immunosuppressed patients. World J Hepatol 6:384–393

58. Lu S, Xu Y, Mu Q et al (2015) The risk of hepatitis B virus reactivation and the role of antiviral prophylaxis in hepatitis B surface antigen negative/hepatitis B core antibody positive patients with diffuse large B-cell lymphoma receiving rituximab-based chemotherapy. Leuk Lymphoma 56:1027–1032

59. Huang Y-H, Hsiao LT, Hong YC et al (2013) Randomized controlled trial of entecavir prophylaxis for rituximab-associated hepatitis B virus reactivation in patients with lymphoma and resolved hepatitis B. J Clin Oncol 31:2765–2772

60. Yun H, Xie F, Delzell E et al (2015) Risks of herpes zoster in patients with rheumatoid arthritis according to biologic disease-modifying therapy. Arthritis Care Res 67:731–736

61. Aksoy S, Harputluoglu H, Kilickap S et al (2007) Rituximab-related viral infections in lymphoma patients. Leuk Lymphoma 48:1307–1312

62. Tsuji H, Yoshifuji H, Fujii T et al (2017) Visceral disseminated varicella zoster virus infection after rituximab treatment for granulomatosis with polyangiitis. Mod Rheumatol 27:155–161

63. Rafailidis PI, Kakisi OK, Vardakas K, Falagas ME (2007) Infectious complications of monoclonal antibodies used in cancer therapy: a systematic review of the evidence from randomized controlled trials. Cancer 109:2182–2189

64. Salliot C, Dougados M, Gossec L (2009) Risk of serious infections during rituximab, abatacept and anakinra treatments for rheumatoid arthritis: meta-analyses of randomised placebo-controlled trials. Ann Rheum Dis 68:25–32

65. Scemla A, Loupy A, Candon S et al (2010) Incidence of infectious complications in highly sensitized renal transplant recipients treated by rituximab: a case-controlled study. Transplantation 90:1180–1184

66. Kamar N, Milioto O, Puissant-Lubrano B et al (2010) Incidence and predictive factors for infectious disease after rituximab therapy in kidney-transplant patients. Am J Transplant 10:89–98

67. Aksoy S, Dizdar O, Hayran M, Harputluoğlu H (2009) Infectious complications of rituximab in patients with lymphoma during maintenance therapy: a systematic review and meta-analysis. Leuk Lymphoma 50:357–365

68. Wolach O, Bairey O, Lahav M (2010) Late-onset neutropenia after rituximab treatment: case series and comprehensive review of the literature. Medicine (Baltimore) 89:308–318

69. Ishida H, Inui M, Furusawa M, Tanabe K (2013) Late-onset neutropenia (LON) after low-dose rituximab treatment in living related kidney transplantation – single-center study. Transpl Immunol 28:93–99

70. Tesfa D, Gelius T, Sander B et al (2008) Late-onset neutropenia associated with rituximab therapy: evidence for a maturation arrest at the (pro)myelocyte stage of granulopoiesis. Med Oncol 25:374–379

71. Nitta E, Izutsu K, Sato T et al (2007) A high incidence of late-onset neutropenia following rituximab-containing chemotherapy as a primary treatment of CD20-positive B-cell lymphoma: a single-institution study. Ann Oncol 18:364–369

72. Salmon JH, Cacoub P, Combe B et al (2015) Late-onset neutropenia after treatment with rituximab for rheumatoid arthritis and other autoimmune diseases: data from the AutoImmunity and Rituximab registry. RMD Open 1:e34

73. Terrier B, Ittah M, Tourneur L et al (2007) Late-onset neutropenia following rituximab results from a hematopoietic lineage competition due to an excessive BAFF-induced B-cell recovery. Haematologica 92:e20–e23

74. Weissmann-Brenner A, Brenner B, Belyaeva I et al (2011) Rituximab associated neutropenia: description of three cases and an insight into the underlying pathogenesis. Med Sci Monit 17:CS133–CS137
75. Voog E, Morschhauser F, Solal-Céligny P (2003) Neutropenia in patients treated with rituximab. N Engl J Med 348:2691–2694
76. Ghrenassia E, Roulin L, Aline-Fardin A et al (2014) The spectrum of chronic CD8+ T-cell expansions: clinical features in 14 patients. PLoS One 9:e91505
77. Ghielmini M, Rufibach K, Salles G et al (2005) Single agent rituximab in patients with follicular or mantle cell lymphoma: clinical and biological factors that are predictive of response and event-free survival as well as the effect of rituximab on the immune system: a study of the Swiss Group for Clinical Cancer Research (SAKK). Ann Oncol 16:1675–1682
78. Rao A, Kelly M, Musselman M et al (2008) Safety, efficacy, and immune reconstitution after rituximab therapy in pediatric patients with chronic or refractory hematologic autoimmune cytopenias. Pediatr Blood Cancer 50:822–825
79. Levy R, Mahévas M, Galicier L et al (2014) Profound symptomatic hypogammaglobulinemia: a rare late complication after rituximab treatment for immune thrombocytopenia. Report of 3 cases and systematic review of the literature. Autoimmun Rev 13:1055–1063
80. Reagan PM, Friedberg JW (2017) Reassessment of anti-CD20 therapy in lymphoid malignancies: impact, limitations, and new directions. Oncology 31:402–411
81. Kim SJ, Hsu C, Song Y-Q et al (2013) Hepatitis B virus reactivation in B-cell lymphoma patients treated with rituximab: analysis from the Asia Lymphoma Study Group. Eur J Cancer 49:3486–3496
82. Matsui T, Kang J-H, Nojima M et al (2013) Reactivation of hepatitis B virus in patients with undetectable HBsAg undergoing chemotherapy for malignant lymphoma or multiple myeloma. J Med Virol 85:1900–1906
83. Weiner GJ (2010) Rituximab: mechanism of action. Semin Hematol 47:115–123
84. Wu SJ, Chou WC, Ko BS, Tien HF (2007) Severe pulmonary complications after initial treatment with Rituximab for the Asian-variant of intravascular lymphoma. Haematologica 92:141–142

Between Dream and Reality in Nutritional Therapy: How to Fill the Gap

E. De Waele, P. M. Honoré, and M. L. N. G. Malbrain

Introduction

Malnutrition is a robust predictor of mortality and morbidity in patients presenting with critical illness [1]. In specific populations, such as emergency general surgery patients entering an intensive care unit (ICU), 60% were diagnosed with nonspecific malnutrition; a strong correlation with mortality was demonstrated and readmission rates were increased [2]. In adult patients with systemic inflammatory syndrome or sepsis, differential metabolic profiles were associated with malnutrition, and this cohort of patients had a higher 28-day mortality [3]. Nutritional therapy therefore remains of cardinal importance in the treatment of the critically ill.

Interventions to improve quality of care have been implemented at several organizational levels. The European Council formed a resolution in 2003 concerning hospital food and nutritional therapy. Nevertheless, risk assessment varies considerably around the world, and energy goals are frequently not met [4]. The importance of implementation of current guidelines within daily clinical practice has been stressed. 'Nutritionday ICU' is a worldwide prevalence study of nutrition practice in intensive care. Data collected from 2007 to 2013 were analyzed: 9777 patients from 46 countries were included. The conclusion was that most of the patients were underfed while in the ICU. Energy prescription by means of calories did not correlate with patient body weight. Nutritional interventions were slow to start and goals, recommended by international guidelines, were never met. The authors had the impression that nutritional support seemed to be standardized and limited, and concluded that guidelines were poorly observed [5].

In this chapter, we will review the different aspects of nutrition therapy and practical options. The nutrition care process in total should include malnutrition risk screening, nutritional assessment, diagnostic procedures, a nutritional care plan,

E. De Waele (✉) · P. M. Honoré · M. L. N. G. Malbrain
Department of Intensive Care, Universitair Ziekenhuis Brussel, Vrije Universiteit Brussel
Brussels, Belgium
e-mail: elisabeth.dewaele@uzbrussel.be

© Springer International Publishing AG 2018
J.-L. Vincent (ed.), *Annual Update in Intensive Care and Emergency Medicine 2018*,
Annual Update in Intensive Care and Emergency Medicine,
https://doi.org/10.1007/978-3-319-73670-9_44

nutrition therapy, monitoring and documentation to be conform to European guidelines [6]. In analogy to antibiotic stewardship, 'nutrition stewardship' should be adopted. This overview focuses on ownership, screening, assessment, diagnostic procedures and the actual therapy.

Ownership/management

Nutritional therapy is part of the treatment of the critically ill. In a quality management policy, structures concerning nutritional therapy should be developed and tools provided. This includes standardized practice guidelines, interdisciplinary feeding protocols, access to knowledge, clear structures, specific computerized information systems, and dedicated healthcare practitioners. The presence and recommendations of an ICU-based dietician improved nutritional therapy in a Swiss ICU quality improvement program [7]. In a recent Chinese initiative, implementation of an enteral nutrition feeding protocol in 410 patients increased the proportion of patients receiving enteral feeding [8]. Adherence to guideline recommendations is associated with elements of organizational culture, leadership support, shared beliefs on utility and inter-professional collaboration. Strategies on organizational change can positively influence performance of healthcare practitioners and thereby patient outcomes [9]. Since knowledge translation interventions that include protocols with or without education are correlated with the greatest improvements in processes of critical care [10], all the above mentioned tools should be made available in an ICU setting, if one wants to achieve the goal of optimal nutritional therapy. The situation in which nutritional therapy is coordinated solely by the attending physician, with consultation with pharmacists is obsolete. A Nutritional Support Team including physicians from various fields, pharmacists, dieticians and nurses should be initiated and activated. In a neonatal ICU, significant improvements in the delivery of nutrition and a significant reduction in the mean length of ICU stay were observed with this approach [11].

Patient Screening and Assessment

Screening for malnutrition is mandatory for all hospitalized patients, as stated by the European Society for Clinical Nutrition and Metabolism (ESPEN) [12]. The primary aim is to identify patients at risk of malnutrition. Different tools exist for this purpose, with diverging results. The Nutritional Risk Score (NRS) 2002 is validated for a hospital setting [13]. A comparison between the NRS 2002 and the Malnutrition Universal Screening Tool (MUST) in patients on admission to hospital showed that MUST was better correlated with the ESPEN definition of malnutrition [14]. The Nutrition Risk in Critically ill (NUTRIC) score is developed for and can be used in the critically care setting [15]. The NUTRIC score identifies patients who will benefit more from aggressive nutrition. To make it an acceptable clinical tool, a modified version was developed and validated: the modified NUTRIC (mNU-

TRIC). As interleukin-6 (IL-6) is not mandatory in the mNUTRIC, feasibility is high. In critically ill, mechanically ventilated patients, the mNUTRIC score determined a high nutritional risk in 42.5% of patients. This population had increased length of stay and higher mortality [16]. A recent review confirmed a prevalence of malnutrition of up to 78% in ICU patients, and its correlation with increased morbidity and mortality. Assessment tools, such as the Subjective Global Assessment, scored better than screening tools in identifying patients at risk [17]. In an ICU setting, an acute physiology and chronic health evaluation (APACHE) II score > 10 renders the NRS 2002 positive, so that a substantial proportion of patients will be defined nutritionally at risk.

Risk screening should be performed within the first 24–48 h of hospital admission to identify patients at risk. Patients identified as at risk need to be nutritionally assessed conform to the 2017 ESPEN guidelines on definitions and terminology of clinical nutrition [6]. The assessment process should include an evaluation of the risk of developing refeeding syndrome. These metabolic disturbances can be difficult to predict from baseline characteristics. Nevertheless, awareness is important because caloric restriction in these patients is associated with increased survival [18].

Diagnostic Procedures

Objective data should be acquired to complete the nutritional evaluation and guide the management plan. Body weight and length are standard, although body weight measurements are recorded in no more than 13.5 to 55% of patients in hospitals, due to the increased work load and need for equipment [19]. Body mass index (BMI) is important because survival is reduced in patients with BMI values from < 18.5–25 kg/m^2 and > 50 kg/m^2 compared to 25–30 kg/m^2. There is a beneficial role for early enteral nutrition in patients with BMI < 25 kg/m^2, because the mortality disadvantage in this group disappeared when given early enteral nutrition [20]. A more valid evaluation or characterization of a patient's body is his or her body composition. This can reveal important information regarding the background of the patient and be important in predicting clinical outcome. It can also be used for intermediate evaluation of the evolution of the patient, especially in patients with extended ICU stays. There is a large bias between lean body mass measured by computed tomography (CT) and that calculated using existing equations. This is why CT analysis for body composition should be made user-friendly and the development of ICU-specific equations could help fill the gap [21]. A low fat-free mass at ICU admission predicts 28-day mortality. This is also shown with bioelectrical impedance analysis (BIA), more specifically via the phase angle [22]. BIA can be a relevant tool for guiding nutrition but also serves other purposes, such as fluid management [23]. A rising but not yet optimized technique is ultrasonography to measure muscle quality and quantity. This technique is non-invasive, relatively cheap and can be used at the bedside, which is a major advantage. Standardization of measurement procedures and interpretation is mandatory. Nevertheless, in combination with other diagnostic procedures, it can contribute to revealing the metabolic profile of a critically ill patient [24]. In the course of nutritional therapy, feedback information is currently lacking because of insufficient markers of optimal therapy. A 13C-breath test could be used in the setting of feeding optimization [25].

In the broad spectrum of the clinical mapping of the ICU patient, the role of the intestinal microbiome cannot be underestimated. As knowledge improves concerning alterations in the health-promoting gut microbiome during critical illness, the clinical relevance of these changes will soon become obvious. Because of the direct interaction of feeding through the enteral route and gut bacteria, monitoring or assessing the composition of the gut microbiome can be of help, whether to perform baseline evaluation of the critically ill patient or to guide therapy during the course of illness [26].

In the context of muscle strength, hand grip measurements can still be used. A correlation was recently demonstrated between higher amino acid provision by parenteral nutrition and grip strength. These secondary endpoints can be used in research settings but may mirror physical abilities of critically ill patients, who suffer from muscle weakness, especially with extended ICU stay [27]. The possibility of assessing intestinal function, to evaluate enteral tolerance and efficacy of enteral feeding, is a domain with almost no available data. Very recently, methods from other domains of medicine, have been tested in an ICU setting. Assessment of small intestinal function in patients receiving intravenous glutamine using plasma citrulline analysis, obtained by an arterial line, may be of value although no experience with this test has yet been acquired [28]. A non-invasive approach to evaluate intestinal activity, more specifically gastric motility, is modified B-ultrasound. Compared with gastric residual volume measurements, ultrasound-guided enteral nutrition was more successful (shorter ICU and hospital stay and higher levels of serum albumin and pre-albumin) [29]. Albumin and pre-albumin have long been used as nutritional parameters but they correlate strongly with acute inflammation and are therefore non-specific. As a ratio with lactate, albumin is relevant for predicting adverse outcomes in pediatric patients with sepsis, but not useful to assess nutritional status [30]. In cancer patients admitted to the ICU, decreased albumin levels also increase the risk of death. Whether this is a nutrition-related issue has not been proven [31]. More extensive information than that provided by plasma proteins can come from metabolic profiling. Metabolite pathways can be altered in patients admitted with sepsis: a significant correlation between vitamin D status and five metabolites related to glutathione and glutamate was found in a metabolomics study in critically ill patients [32]. A systematic review revealed no improvement of clinical outcome with vitamin D administration, although the authors state that there are not enough data available to draw conclusions on the treatment modalities [33]. Antioxidant micronutrients may play a role in therapy [34]. In the context of evaluating the critically ill patient, the aim is to gather as much information as possible, to be used as baseline knowledge on which to base nutritional therapy, but also as a parameter cloud which can be followed during therapy.

In terms of metabolic activity, the distinction between anabolic and catabolic state can be measured using indirect calorimetry. Because it is the gold standard for measuring energy expenditure, use of indirect calorimetry will increase: continuous metabolic monitoring will be able to provide baseline information but will be a very valuable tool to steer nutritional therapy because it can demonstrate metabolic reactions to feeding regimens [35, 36]. Nitrogen balance should be considered, although the technique is not optimized yet. In the absence of indirect calorimetry, mechanical ventilator information could be used to provide information on energy expenditure. However, because of physiologic and technical issues, this technique remains inferior to indirect calorimetry [37].

Nutritional Care Plan and Nutritional Therapy

A treatment path consists of several aspects. With answers to the relevant questions based on evidence and guidelines, a multidisciplinary care plan can be developed. Experience in cardiac surgery patients has shown a positive effect of a care plan, reducing length of stay in the ICU and hospital and impacting on secondary outcomes [38]. Issues to be addressed are listed in Box 1.

Box 1. Issues to be addressed in a nutritional care plan

Why?	Nutrition therapy will improve outcome
Who?	Which patients will you feed?
What?	What macro and micronutrients will you provide?
Where?	Which access will you use: gastrointestinal? intravenous? subcutaneous?
When?	What will be the time course for your feeding regimen?
How much?	What will be your caloric and protein goals?
How to monitor?	Which data will you collect?

---

a. Why?
   Absence of a clear nutritional plan may increase ICU-related morbidity and mortality, especially in patients with malnutrition and a low BMI.
b. Who?
   In a European setting, it is appropriate to follow the ESPEN guidelines. Users should keep in mind the limitations of insufficient available data, which can undermine the strength of the recommendations, reducing them sometimes to expert opinions. Nevertheless, when implemented in clinical practice, they provide an accepted support and back-up for ICU protocols. Following the guidelines on parenteral nutrition, all patients in the ICU should be fed to avoid starvation and underfeeding, which are correlated with increased mortality and morbidity [12]. In the enteral nutrition recommendations, it is recommended that enteral nutrition be started early in critically ill patients who will likely not be able to eat a full diet by day 3 [39]. Although not considered ideal for ICU use, a posi-

tive NRS can support these interventions as mentioned earlier. It is important to know that the majority of ICU patients will screen positive, because an APACHE score > 10 is one of the criteria for a NRS score of 3 indicating that the patient is nutritionally at-risk. All patients in the ICU should receive an optimal nutrition plan, which can also mean optimization of oral intake. We demonstrated substantial benefit on survival in cardiac surgery patients managed with an optimized nutrition treatment plan, largely composed of dietary adaptations and oral supplements [40].

c. What?

Correct nutritional therapy aims to provide substances necessary to sustain cell function and life. Primarily the aim is to deliver amino acids, glucose, lipids, water, vitamins and trace elements [6]. Variations in medically used nutritional compounds exist, but an overall superiority of, for example, fish oil in parenteral nutrition has not been demonstrated by available data [41].

d. Where?

As the aim is to deliver a correct amount of macro- and micro-nutrients, the route to be used will depend heavily on the patient. A thorough assessment of the patient's clinical condition will guide the prescription of optimal nutritional therapy. The impact of delivering correct amounts of energy and protein, the so called power couple, if necessary in a combined strategy, can optimize clinical outcome [42]. Since data are available on the non-inferiority of the parenteral route in ICU patients, the intravenous route can be used safely to provide a certain amount of nutrients [43]. Promising preliminary data are appearing concerning a less invasive means of delivering nutrients: the subcutaneous route [44]. In the nutritional care plan, all these routes can contribute to provide the necessary feeding regimen to an ICU patient, and this in a continuously evolving and interactive way. Optimization by the use of parenteral nutrition was shown to be cost-saving by reducing nosocomial infections and thereby resource consumption [45]. This renders the argument of cost in the use of parenteral nutrition obsolete.

e. When?

Several studies are being conducted to determine the optimal timing for the initiation of clinical nutrition. Although high impact studies, even with no mortality differences, have influenced medical decision making, in a daily clinical setting it would be appropriate to rely on existing guidelines and initiate feeding within 24 to 48 h of ICU admission [12, 46].

f. How much?

Calorie and protein targeting has proven to be beneficial for critically ill patients. Concerning calories, there is consensus on the use of indirect calorimetry to measure energy expenditure and thereby guide caloric prescriptions [47], using the Weir equation to calculate metabolic rate:

Total heat output in a given time is total kg.cal =

$3.941 \times$ liters of oxygen used $+ 1.106 \times$ liters of CO_2 produced.

With upcoming continuous metabolic monitoring, data on caloric use by the patient's metabolism will be available. Based on big data analysis, a possible approach would be to target 70 to 80% of measured energy expenditure, although prospective randomized data are lacking, as so often encountered in the domain of clinical nutrition [48]. Protein prescriptions will ideally be combined with physical exercise, and may also have an effect on long-term physical abilities of the ICU patient [49]. A calculated dose of 1.5 kg/kg ideal body weight/day is supported by ESPEN guidelines, even though higher doses are currently defended.

g. How to monitor?

Quality control is very important and demands data acquisition and analysis. Computerized systems are widespread in ICUs around the world. These have the main advantage of being able to group relevant nutrition variables, make them visible and provide efficient feedback to the user, i.e., the healthcare practitioner involved in nutrition therapy. In addition, electronic medical files can be stored for prolonged periods, keeping the data available and providing information to oversee the treatment target, mark adjustments to the therapy and facilitate flexible, adaptive, global, optimal nutrition therapy [50].

Conclusion

Nutrition therapy is part of high quality care for critically ill patients. Although primarily the physician's responsibility, it is preeminently a multidisciplinary task. All aspects of the treatment plan should be carefully considered, resulting in a predefined road map. No two road maps will be the same, as to be expected in the era of precision medicine. Moreover, the map will move and change with the patient's journey, in continuous interaction with clinical feedback. Every critically ill patient deserves an optimal nutrition regimen, and all possible tools and interventions should be applied to make this happen. As knowledge, the technical armamentarium and human competence in the field of clinical nutrition grow, the gap between dream and reality will further narrow.

References

1. Mogensen KM, Horkan CM, Purtle SW, Moromizato T, Rawn JD, Robinson MK, Christopher KB (2017) Malnutrition, critical illness survivors, and postdischarge outcomes: a cohort study. JPEN J Parenter Enteral Nutr. https://doi.org/10.1177/0148607117709766 (May 1, Epub ahead of print)
2. Havens JM, Columbus AB, Seshadri AJ et al (2016) Malnutrition at intensive care unit admission predicts mortality in emergency general surgery patients. JPEN J Parenter Enteral Nutr. https://doi.org/10.1177/0148607116676592 (Nov 1, Epub ahead of print)
3. Mogensen KM, Lasky-Su J, Rogers AJ et al (2017) Metabolites associated with malnutrition in the intensive care unit are also associated with 28-day mortality. JPEN J Parenter Enteral Nutr 41:188–197

4. Schindler K, Pernicka E, Laviano A et al (2010) How nutritional risk is assessed and managed in European hospitals: a survey of 21,007 patients findings from the 2007-2008 cross-sectional nutrition Day survey. Clin Nutr 29:552–559

5. Bendavid I, Bendavid I, Singer P et al (2017) NutritionDay ICU: A 7 year worldwide prevalence study of nutrition practice in intensive care. Clin Nutr 36:1122–1129

6. Cederholm T, Barazzoni R, Austin P et al (2017) ESPEN guidelines on definitions and terminology of clinical nutrition. Clin Nutr 36:49–64

7. Soguel L, Revelly JP, Schaller MD, Longchamp C, Berger MM (2012) Energy deficit and length of hospital stay can be reduced by a two-step quality improvement of nutrition therapy: the intensive care unit dietitian can make the difference. Crit Care Med 40:412–419

8. Li Q, Zhang Z, Xie B et al (2017) Effectiveness of enteral feeding protocol on clinical outcomes in critically ill patients: a before and after study. PLoS One 12:e182393

9. Dodek P, Cahill NE, Heyland DK (2010) The relationship between organizational culture and implementation of clinical practice guidelines: a narrative review. JPEN J Parenter Enteral Nutr 34:669–674

10. Sinuff T, Muscedere J, Adhikari NK et al (2013) Knowledge translation interventions for critically ill patients: a systematic review. Crit Care Med 41:2627–2640

11. Eurim J, Young HJ, Seung HS et al (2016) The successful accomplishment of nutritional and clinical outcomes via the implementation of a multidisciplinary nutrition support team in the neonatal intensive care unit. BMC Pediatr 16:113

12. Singer P, Berger MM, Van den Berghe G et al (2009) ESPEN Guidelines on Parenteral Nutrition: intensive care. Clin Nutr 28:387–400

13. Kondrup J, Rasmussen HH, Hamberg O, Stanga Z, ESPEN Working Group (2003) Nutritional risk screening (NRS 2002): a new method based on an analysis of controlled clinical trials. Clin Nutr 22:321–336

14. Poulia KA, Klek S, Doundoulakis I et al (2017) The two most popular malnutrition screening tools in the light of the new ESPEN consensus definition of the diagnostic criteria for malnutrition. Clin Nutr 36:1130–1135

15. Heyland DK, Dhaliwal R, Jiang X, Day AG (2011) Identifying critically ill patients who benefit the most from nutrition therapy: the development and initial validation of a novel risk assessment tool. Crit Care 15:R268

16. Kalaiselvan MS, Renuka MK, Arunkumar AS (2017) Use of Nutrition Risk in Critically ill (NUTRIC) score to assess nutritional risk in mechanically ventilated patients: a prospective observational study. Indian J Crit Care Med 21:253–256

17. Lew CCH, Yandell R, Fraser RJL, Chua AP, Chong MFF, Miller M (2017) Association between malnutrition and clinical outcomes in the intensive care unit: a systematic review. J Parenter Enteral Nutr 41:744–758

18. Olthof LE, Koekkoek W, van Setten C, Kars JCN, van Blokland D, van Zanten ARH (2017) Impact of caloric intake in critically ill patients with, and without, refeeding syndrome: A retrospective study. Clin Nutr. https://doi.org/10.1016/j.clnu.2017.08.001 (Aug 10, Epub ahead of print)

19. Flentje K, Knight C, Stromfeldt I, Chakrabarti A, Friedman ND (2017) Recording patient body weight in hospitals: are we doing well enough? Intern Med J. https://doi.org/10.1111/imj.13519 (Jun 7, Epub ahead of print)

20. Harris K, Zhou J, Liu X, Hassan E, Badawi O (2017) The obesity paradox is not observed in critically ill patients on early enteral nutrition. Crit Care Med 45:828–834

21. Moisey LL, Mourtzakis M, Kozar RA, Compher C, Heyland DK (2017) Existing equations to estimate lean body mass are not accurate in the critically ill: Results of a multicenter observational study. Clin Nutr 36:1701–1706

22. Thibault R, Makhlouf AM, Mulliez A et al (2016) Phase Angle Project Investigators. Fat-free mass at admission predicts 28-day mortality in intensive care unit patients: the international prospective observational study Phase Angle Project. Intensive Care Med 42:1445–1453

23. Malbrain ML, Huygh J, Dabrowski W, De Waele JJ, Staelens A, Wauters J (2014) The use of bio-electrical impedance analysis (BIA) to guide fluid management, resuscitation and dere-suscitation in critically ill patients: a bench-to-bedside review. Anaesthesiol Intensive Ther 46:381–391

24. Mourtzakis M, Parry S, Connolly B, Puthucheary Z (2017) Skeletal muscle ultrasound in critical care: a tool in need of translation. Ann Am Thorac Soc 14:1495–1503

25. Wischmeyer PE, Puthucheary Z, San Millán I, Butz D, Grocott MPW (2017) Muscle mass and physical recovery in ICU: innovations for targeting of nutrition and exercise. Curr Opin Crit Care 23:269–278

26. Krezalek MA, Yeh A, Alverdy JC, Morowitz M (2017) Influence of nutrition therapy on the intestinal microbiome. Curr Opin Clin Nutr Metab Care 20:131–137

27. Ferrie S, Allman-Farinelli M, Daley M, Smith K (2016) Protein requirements in the critically ill: a randomized controlled trial using parenteral nutrition. JPEN J Parenter Enteral Nutr 40:795–805

28. Peters JH, Wierdsma NJ, Beishuizen A, Teerlink T, van Bodegraven AA (2017) Intravenous citrulline generation test to assess intestinal function in intensive care unit patients. Clin Exp Gastroenterol 10:75–81

29. Liu Y, Gao YK, Yao L, Li L (2017) Modified B-ultrasound method for measurement of antral section only to assess gastric function and guide enteral nutrition in critically ill patients. World J Gastroenterol 23:5229–5236

30. Lichtenauer M, Wernly B, Ohnewein B et al (2017) The lactate/albumin ratio: a valuable tool for risk stratification in septic patients admitted to ICU. Int J Mol Sci 18:1893

31. Cheng L, DeJesus AY, Rodriguez MA (2017) Using laboratory test results at hospital admission to predict short-term survival in critically ill patients with metastatic or advanced cancer. J Pain Symptom Manag 53:720–727

32. Lasky-Su J, Dahlin A, Litonjua AA et al (2017) Metabolome alterations in severe critical illness and vitamin D status. Crit Care 21:193

33. Langlois PL, Szwec C, D'Aragon F, Heyland DK, Manzanares W (2017) Vitamin D supplementation in the critically ill: a systematic review and meta-analysis. Clin Nutr. https://doi.org/10.1016/j.clnu.2017.05.006 (May 11, Epub ahead of print)

34. Manzanares W, Dhaliwal R, Jiang X, Murch L, Heyland DK (2012) Antioxidant micronutrients in the critically ill: a systematic review and meta-analysis. Crit Care 16:R66

35. Rogobete AF, Sandesc D, Papurica M et al (2017) The influence of metabolic imbalances and oxidative stress on the outcome of critically ill polytrauma patients: a review. Burn Trauma 5:8

36. Oshima T, Berger MM, De Waele E et al (2017) Indirect calorimetry in nutritional therapy. A position paper by the ICALIC study group. Clin Nutr 36:651–662

37. De Waele E, Honoré PM, Spapen HD (2016) VCO2 calorimetry: stop tossing stones, it's time for building! Crit Care 20:399

38. Kebapçı A, Kanan N (2017) The effects of nurse-led clinical pathway in coronary artery bypass graft surgery: a quasi-experimental study. J Clin Nurs. https://doi.org/10.1111/jocn.14069 (Sep 7, Epub ahead of print)

39. Kreymann KG, Berger MM, Deutz NE et al (2006) ESPEN Guidelines on Enteral Nutrition: intensive care. Clin Nutr 25:210–223

40. De Waele E, Nguyen D, De Bondt K et al (2017) The CoCoS trial: Caloric Control in Cardiac Surgery patients promotes survival, an interventional trial with retrospective control. Clin Nutr. https://doi.org/10.1016/j.clnu.2017.03.007 (Mar 18, Epub ahead of print)

41. Kreymann KG, Heyland DK, de Heer G, Elke G (2017) Intravenous fish oil in critically ill and surgical patients – historical remarks and critical appraisal. Clin Nutr. https://doi.org/10.1016/j.clnu.2017.07.006 (Jul 13, Epub ahead of print)

42. Oshima T, Deutz NE, Doig G, Wischmeyer PE, Pichard C (2016) Protein-energy nutrition in the ICU is the power couple: a hypothesis forming analysis. Clin Nutr 35:968–974

43. Harvey SE, Parrott F, Harrison DA et al (2014) Trial of the route of early nutritional support in critically ill adults. N Engl J Med 371:1673–1684
44. Zaloga GP, Pontes-Arruda A, Dardaine-Giraud V, Constans T, Clinimix Subcutaneous Study Group (2016) Safety and efficacy of subcutaneous parenteral nutrition in older patients: a prospective randomized multicenter clinical trial. JPEN J Parenter Enteral Nutr 41:1222–1227
45. Pradelli L, Graf S, Pichard C, Berger MM (2017) Supplemental parenteral nutrition in intensive care patients: a cost saving strategy. Clin Nutr. https://doi.org/10.1016/j.clnu.2017.01.009 (Jan 25, Epub ahead of print)
46. Casaer MP, Mesotten D, Hermans G et al (2011) Early versus late parenteral nutrition in critically ill adults. N Engl J Med 365:506–517
47. Preiser JC, van Zanten AR, Berger MM et al (2015) Metabolic and nutritional support of critically ill patients: consensus and controversies. Crit Care 19:35
48. Zusman O, Singer P (2017) Resting energy expenditure and optimal nutrition in critical care: how to guide our calorie prescriptions. Crit Care 21:128
49. Weijs PJM (2017) Protein nutrition and exercise survival kit for critically ill. Curr Opin Crit Care 23:279–283
50. Berger MM (2013) How to prescribe nutritional support using computers. World Rev Nutr Diet 105:32–42

Part XIII
Moving the Patient

Inter-hospital Transport on Extracorporeal Membrane Oxygenation

R. S. Stephens, D. Abrams, and D. Brodie

Introduction

Extracorporeal life support, including extracorporeal membrane oxygenation (ECMO) and extracorporeal carbon dioxide removal (ECCO$_2$R), is increasingly used to support patients with severe acute respiratory failure and refractory cardiac failure [1]. With the growth in ECMO utilization, the need to safely transport these severely ill patients to centers where ECMO may be performed is becoming ever more common. Recent experience suggests that cannulating patients for ECMO at the hospital of origin and transporting them to a center with ECMO expertise while the patient is receiving ECMO is an increasingly compelling and generally safe approach [2–7]. Nonetheless, this is a complex endeavor that should be undertaken in a methodical fashion by centers with experience both in ECMO and in the transport of critically ill patients.

Rationale for ECMO Transport Programs

ECMO is a resource-intensive and high-risk support modality which requires substantial institutional commitment and specialized expertise. Additionally, as with many aspects of medical care, outcomes in patients with acute respiratory failure, for example, are generally better at high-volume centers [8, 9]. The same relationship between volumes and outcomes appears to hold true for ECMO [10–12]. Accordingly, a group of experts has suggested that ECMO should ideally be pro-

R. S. Stephens
Division of Pulmonary and Critical Care Medicine, Johns Hopkins University
Baltimore, MD, USA

D. Abrams · D. Brodie (✉)
Division of Pulmonary, Allergy and Critical Care Medicine, Columbia College of Physicians and Surgeons/New York-Presbyterian Hospital
New York, NY, USA
e-mail: hdb5@cumc.columbia.edu

© Springer International Publishing AG 2018
J.-L. Vincent (ed.), *Annual Update in Intensive Care and Emergency Medicine 2018*,
Annual Update in Intensive Care and Emergency Medicine,
https://doi.org/10.1007/978-3-319-73670-9_45

vided at high-volume centers with expertise not only in ECMO, but also in the broader management of acute respiratory failure [13], or by extension, other underlying conditions necessitating the use of ECMO.

Given that ECMO is mostly performed in desperately ill patients, and the difficulty in safely transporting such patients to a center with relevant expertise, it follows that ECMO centers should ideally have the capacity to provide mobile ECMO teams capable of evaluating patients at other medical centers, cannulating and initiating ECMO at those centers, and transporting critically ill patients while receiving ECMO back to the ECMO-capable center. Transport of patients with severe acute respiratory distress syndrome (ARDS) is risky, and death may occur during transport [14]. In some cases, ECMO may be required for the safe transport of patients who could otherwise be managed with prone positioning or other proven therapies which may be impractical or impossible at the center of origin or during routine transport.

Safety and Outcomes

One of the earliest reports of transport during ECMO was in 1977 [15]. As ECMO technology has improved and ECMO use has increased, experience and data regarding transport during ECMO have also expanded. In considering ECMO transport programs, the two most important questions involve safety and efficacy. First, with a complex and high-risk technology such as ECMO, is it safe to initiate ECMO and proceed with transport of patients over considerable distances between two medical facilities? Second, do patients transported while receiving ECMO ultimately have comparable outcomes to similar patients receiving ECMO who did not require transport? There are increasing data available to answer these questions. Several large series (greater than 100 patients) have now been reported, as well as multiple smaller series [2–7, 16].

The earliest large series reporting the transport of patients during ECMO consisted of 100 pediatric and adult patients from the University of Michigan (Ann Arbor, Michigan, USA), published in 2002 [2]. Of these 100 patients, 78 of whom had ARDS, the overall survival to hospital discharge was 66%. Transport-related complications occurred in 17% of patients; electrical power failure was the most common complication. One death occurred during cannulation due to right atrial appendage perforation. An updated report in 2014 reported experience with transporting 221 patients during ECMO, including the initial 100 patients, over a period of more than 20 years (1990–2012) [3]. Again, most patients (81%) had a respiratory indication for ECMO but 52% of patients were placed on venoarterial ECMO. Overall survival to discharge was 62%. One patient died during transport, and four patients (not included in the total survival rate) died after cannulation but prior to transport. Complications during transport were common, including electrical complications (e.g., power loss, 18%) and missing items needed for remote cannulation (10%).

Several other centers, in both the United States and Europe, have published large series of patients transported while receiving ECMO. The University of Arkansas and Arkansas Children's Hospital (Little Rock, Arkansas, USA) published their experience with 112 predominantly pediatric ECMO transports in 2010 [4]. Survival to hospital discharge was 58%, and no major transport complications were reported. In 2015, Columbia University (New York, USA) reported 100 consecutive ECMO transports with a 63% survival to hospital discharge and no major transport complications [5]. Also in 2015, Glenfield Hospital in Leistershire, UK, published their five-year experience with a mobile ECMO service, which included 102 adult patients transported during ECMO from referring centers [6]. Most patients (93%) were transported on venovenous ECMO for severe respiratory failure, with 72% undergoing single-site cannulation, no major transport complications and a survival rate to discharge of 84%.

The largest series of transport during ECMO is from Karolinska University Hospital in Stockholm, Sweden, published in 2015 [7]. This report included 322 adult, pediatric, and neonatal patients over a 4-year period (2010–2013), the vast majority of whom were placed on ECMO for respiratory failure. Overall survival to discharge was 70% for adults with respiratory failure and 92% for pediatric patients with respiratory failure. Of the 300 transports for which documentation was available about the transport, 27% had a complication. These were most commonly patient-related, such as loss of ventilator tidal volume, but also included equipment and vehicle problems.

All of these studies share similar weaknesses: small size, retrospective nature, and single-center design. Two systematic reviews have attempted to compensate for these limitations. The first reviewed 27 case series comprising 643 patients (both pediatric and adult) [3]. This meta-analysis revealed an overall survival of 61% without any major complications or deaths during transfer. Importantly, there was no difference in overall survival rate between these 643 transported patients and the almost 50,000 patients in the Extracorporeal Life Support Organization (ELSO) registry.

A more recent meta-analysis included 38 series with a total of 1481 patients, and reported an overall hospital survival rate of 62% for adults and 68% for pediatric patients (95% CI of 57–68 and 60–75, respectively) [16]. Eighty complications were reported in these 1481 patients, including two deaths during transport; however, 92% of transports had no complications (95% CI 91–94).

An additional paper within the last year reported the rate of adverse events over the course of 514 transports during ECMO [17]. Thirty-two percent involved at least one adverse event, for a total of 206 adverse events. Most of these involved loss of ventilator tidal volume, hypovolemia, hemodynamic instability or bleeding, although equipment failure also occurred.

In summary, the available data suggest that transport of critically patients who are receiving ECMO during transport is safe when conducted by experienced teams. Moreover, outcomes of patients transported during ECMO appear to be similar to those in patients in whom ECMO is initiated at an ECMO center. However, it needs to be emphasized that careful planning, proper staffing and experience are all essential to achieving these good outcomes.

Notification and Initial Evaluation of Patients for Transport

In most cases, deployment of a mobile ECMO team for patient transport begins when a non-ECMO facility contacts an ECMO center to consider the wisdom of ECMO support for a critically ill patient. Many tertiary care centers have a dedicated telephone hotline for referring clinicians and facilities. Once a referring clinician contacts an ECMO center to propose transfer, they are connected to the appropriate ECMO team. Some centers utilize a dedicated nurse or other ECMO specialist to complete a detailed triage assessment before conferencing in the accepting physician [5, 6, 18]; alternatively, the referring clinician may be connected directly to an ECMO attending physician [19–21]. During the telephone conference, an initial evaluation of the patient's candidacy for ECMO support is undertaken. Varying indications and criteria have been reported, but in general, patients should have some form of refractory, but potentially reversible respiratory or cardiac failure [5–7, 19, 22–24]. Irreversible causes of cardiopulmonary failure, severe irreversible brain injury, or any other condition that would limit the potential benefit of ECMO should be viewed as a contraindication to ECMO transport [22]. In all cases, a discussion of the goals of care (including ECMO) should be held, and assurances that the patient or, more commonly, the patient's surrogate, would be amenable to ECMO initiation and transport should be obtained before the ECMO transport team is dispatched.

Transport Team Composition

Once a patient has been determined to be a candidate for ECMO transport, the transport team must be assembled and launched. The composition of such teams differs by institution and geographic locale; various configurations are reported in Table 1. Team composition must balance the need for adequate personnel to manage complex patients and equipment with the logistical need for a team small enough to fit in the confined space of the transport vehicle. Teams typically include (at minimum) a cannulating physician, a critical care nurse or paramedic and an ECMO specialist. European teams are more likely than North American teams to include an anesthesiologist cannulator rather than a surgeon [25]. In all cases, team members should be fully trained on the ECMO device, including cannulation, monitoring, and management of patients during ECMO, device troubleshooting, and response to emergencies. Team member roles and responsibilities must be clearly delineated and understood by all participants, and simulation training is highly recommended.

Table 1 Extracoporeal membrane oxygenation (ECMO) transport team composition

Institution	Team composition (number)	Reference
Arkansas Children's Hospital (Little Rock, USA)	Cardiothoracic surgeon, intensivist, ECMO coordinator, surgical assistant	[4]
Careggi Teaching Hospital (Florence, Italy)	Cardiac surgeon, intensivist, cardiologist, perfusionist, nurse	[20]
Duke University Medical Center (Durham, USA)	Cardiothoracic surgeon or surgical fellow,* critical care nurse (2), perfusionist	[18]
Glenfield Hospital (Leicestershire, UK)	Cannulating physician (cardiothoracic surgeon or intensivist), intensivist^, critical care ECMO specialist nurse, perfusionist	[6]
Heinrich-Heine University (Dusseldorf, Germany)	Cardiovascular surgeon, perfusionist	[23]
Hospital das Clinicas, University of Sao Paulo (Sao Paulo, Brazil)	Intensivists (2), critical care nurse, respiratory therapist	[16]
Karolinska University Hospital (Stockholm, Sweden)	Cardiothoracic surgeon*, ECMO physician (1–2), critical care nurse (1–2)	[7]
New York Presbyterian Hospital/ Columbia University (New York, USA)	Cardiothoracic surgeon, surgical fellow, perfusionists (2), critical care paramedics (2)	[5]
Rikshopitalet University Hospital (Oslo, Norway)	Cardiothoracic surgeon, anesthesiologist, critical care nurse, perfusionist	[27]
University of Michigan Health System (Ann Arbor, USA)	Critical care surgeon, critical care fellow, flight nurses (2), ECMO specialists (2)	[3]
University of Pennsylvania Health System (Philadelphia, USA)	Cardiac surgeon OR cardiac anesthesiologist, critical care nurse, perfusionist, paramedic	[19]
Wilford Hall Medical Center (Lackland Air Force Base, San Antonio, USA)	ECMO director/mission commander, surgeon, intensivist, cardiologist, critical care nurse (2), ECMO coordinator, ECMO specialist (2), respiratory therapist (1–2)	[31]

*If remote cannulation is to be performed
^if cannulating physician is a cardiothoracic surgeon

Transport and Cannulation Equipment

Recent advances in ECMO technology and miniaturization of ECMO machines have greatly facilitated mobile ECMO. Lightweight (10 kg), self-contained ECMO devices with integrated batteries exist, and are well-suited to transport [26]. Other centers deploy a variety of ECMO circuits, often omitting bulkier components such as heat exchangers (Fig. 1) [3, 7, 21]. In addition to the ECMO circuit itself, the transport team requires a variety of specialized equipment. As with team composition, a balance must be struck between space constraints and ensuring the presence and availability of all necessary equipment, including back-up equipment. It is important to recognize that missing essential items is not a rare occurrence and may be very problematic [3, 17]. Equipment checklists are essential to ensure that no critical items are left behind [5, 6]. Many centers pre-package essential equipment

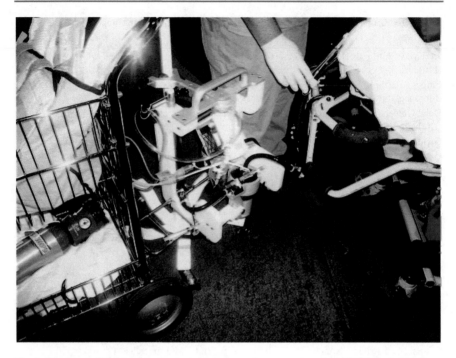

Fig. 1 The streamlined transport extracorporeal membrane oxygenation (ECMO) circuit. From [21] with permission

to facilitate easy assembly for transport [5, 7]. If cannulation is to be performed by the mobile ECMO team prior to transport, requisite surgical equipment, and in some cases, imaging equipment needs to be brought along. Whereas some teams ask the referring hospital to have certain pieces of equipment available (e.g., bedside ultrasound, fluoroscopy, vascular surgical tray) [5], other centers bring all of their own equipment, including portable ultrasounds and transesophageal echocardiography equipment [19]. A variety of different sized cannulas should be available. Similarly, since most cannulations are percutaneous, a variety of guidewires should be available. Site of cannulation is an important consideration. Most venoarterial remote adult cannulations are femoral-femoral, but there is more variability with venovenous cannulation. Whereas some centers utilize single site dual-lumen internal jugular cannulation [6, 21], other centers prefer two site (e.g., femoral-internal jugular) cannulation [7, 16], which may reduce the need for imaging guidance [5], and may be less difficult to position.

Most mobile ECMO teams bring their own cannulating physician to the remote hospital. The legal and administrative logistics are complex, and will vary based on country and region. In the United States, this approach mandates obtaining emergency privileges for that physician at the referring hospital to allow him or her to operate there, and may require an additional medical license if not in the physician's home state. Centers have used varying approaches to obtaining emergency privileges [2, 5, 19].

An alternative approach is to have a physician or surgeon from the referring hospital perform the cannulation procedure if they have the requisite experience with cannulation. In some cases, this approach accounts for the majority of remote cannulations [18]. Although available data are limited regarding this issue, there appears to be no difference in outcomes when cannulation is performed by outside surgeons versus a member of the mobile ECMO team [3, 18]. Regardless of who is performing the cannulation procedure, the team should be prepared to manage cannulation complications, and should recognize that in some situations (e.g., right atrial perforation in a hospital lacking cardiac surgery facilities), cannulation catastrophes may be non-survivable.

Transport Vehicle and Distance

Mobile ECMO transports have utilized ground ambulances, helicopters, and fixed-wing aircraft. Choice of transport modality depends on the distance of the transport, weather conditions, and vehicle availability and suitability (Table 2) [27]. Regardless of the vehicle used, it must be capable of providing adequate power for all equipment (ECMO circuit, ventilator, monitors, infusion pumps, etc.) and should have a redundant power supply in the event of primary generator failure [6]. Adequate oxygen supply must also be available; this may require a careful calculation of worst-case oxygen consumption (e.g., both ventilator and oxygenator receiving 100% oxygen with high minute ventilation and sweep gas flow rates, respectively) plus a safety margin to account for delays, gas leaks and other eventualities. Suction equipment and adequate lighting is essential. The vehicle must have adequate size and weight capacity to accommodate team members, equipment and patient. The mobile ECMO team must be familiar with the vehicle and with the arrangement of equipment within. Consideration must be given to environmental temperature extremes, especially extreme cold, as infusion pumps and lines can freeze [17], and patient hypothermia is a significant consideration. Careful planning is necessary to mitigate the risks inherent in vehicular transport; still, a considerable percentage of transports may be impacted by vehicular or transportation problems [17].

For short-distance transports, ground is typically preferred. To account for all the factors noted above, some centers use a custom-built or dedicated ECMO ambulance [2, 6]. A variety of transport stretchers are available, as are carrying carts for the ECMO equipment, some of which are integrated into the transport stretcher. Before ground transport is commenced, the patient must be adequately stable to leave the referring facility. All equipment, including the transport stretcher, ECMO circuit, transport ventilator, and infusion pumps must be secured in the ambulance before the vehicle is put in motion. The route should be carefully planned, with consideration given to weather, road conditions and traffic. Alternative routes should be planned as needed. Additionally, diversion plans to the nearest emergency room

Table 2 Choice of vehicles for inter-hospital transport of patients on ECMO. Adapted from [27] with permission

Attribute	Ground ambulance	Helicopter	Fixed-wing aircraft
Availability	Excellent	Weather-dependent	Variable
Convenience	Door-to-door	Door-to-door (potentially)	2 airports, 2 ambulances, 4 patient transfers
Safety	Excellent	Good	Good
Space for multiple attendants	Ample	Limited	Variable
Vibration	Little	Severe	Moderate
Noise	Little	Loud	Moderate-loud
Pressurization	Not necessary	Not available	Available and necessary
Distance to referring hospital	0–200 miles (0–320 km)	50–450 miles (80–720 km)	>350 miles (>560 km)
Ability to divert in transport	Excellent	Good	Poor
Cost	Low	High	High
Weight	Virtually unlimited	Limited by aircraft, distance, temperature	Limited by aircraft, distance
Loading	Relatively easy	Limited by aircraft configuration	Varies by aircraft

should be made in the event of an emergency situation beyond the space or equipment capabilities of the transport team [18].

For long distance transports, or if speed is essential, air transport, either helicopter or fixed-wing, may be used. Air transport introduces more regulatory requirements, and equipment often needs to be certified by the appropriate regulatory agency (e.g., the European Aviation Safety Agency or the United States Federal Aviation Administration). Similarly, air logistics are different than ground-based transport, and may be more affected by adverse weather conditions. Air transports may have a higher risk of adverse events than ground transportation, especially if the total duration of the trip (hospital-to-hospital) exceeds 3 h [17]. Helicopters are commonly used for short-duration air transport of ECMO patients. Helicopter transport requires consideration of weight and space limitations, as well as assurance that equipment is compatible with flight. Flight altitude is generally low enough that the effect of cabin pressure on oxygenation is minimal. This may be more of a factor in high-altitude or mountainous environments. Air transport vehicles may be owned by health systems or operated under a standing contract with an aeromedical service. Sometimes, helicopter or fixed-wing support may be provided by governmental or military sources [6, 7, 28].

ECMO transports have been performed over extreme distances, ranging up to more than 13,000 km [5, 17, 29–31]. Distances these great, and indeed any distance greater than the range of a helicopter, requires a fixed-wing aircraft. Unlike helicopters, fixed wing aircraft typically fly at altitudes high enough to require aircraft pressurization, typically to the equivalent of 6,000–8,000 feet of altitude [31, 32]. This is high enough to potentially cause high-altitude physiologic effects, although the real-world consequences for a patient receiving ECMO are unclear. All equipment must be able to tolerate the acceleration, deceleration and vibration inherent in fixed-wing aircraft flight [31].

Whereas many hospitals have on-site landing facilities for helicopters, those that do not and those making use of fixed-wing aircraft require that the patient, ECMO equipment and ECMO team be transported via ambulance to an airport, loaded on the aircraft, and then disembarked at the arrival airport onto a second ambulance for transport to the hospital. This introduces a complex set of logistics: need for two ambulances, access of ambulances to the airport tarmac, and allowance for air-traffic and weather delays [17]. Creative solutions to some of these problems have been developed, including using military cargo aircraft to transport the ambulance (with the patient and ECMO equipment inside the ambulance) [28].

Risks, Safety and Quality Improvement

Transporting the ECMO patient is a highly complex and potentially risky endeavor. Beyond the capital costs of equipping an ECMO transport team, there are personnel costs, especially if a team is kept ready to deploy on short notice at all times. In addition to the resources required for the transport itself, it must be acknowledged that the team (potentially including a physician or perfusionist) will be absent from the hospital for a prolonged period of time, potentially affecting other patients or the performance of surgeries, both elective and emergent. There are medico-legal risks involved in ECMO transport; these vary by country and region, but may be assumed by the ECMO center.

The largest analysis of adverse events during ECMO transport reported adverse events during nearly 32% of transports [17]. Of these, 65% were patient-related (bleeding, hemodynamic instability, loss of tidal volume, etc.), 15% were equipment-related (broken monitoring or lab device, broken heater, hose, power loss, loss of oxygen); 6% were staff flaws (forgotten equipment, failure to secure equipment, unavailable staff), 13% were vehicle- or transportation-related (delay at airport, delayed or wrong ambulance or equipment, ambulance traffic accident, loss of ambulance power), and 2% were environmental (freezing of intravenous lines). Beyond these, there is also the risk of injury to patients and staff due to accidents, lifting heavy equipment (including the stretcher with patient) and slipping during wet or icy conditions. Adverse weather can increase the risk of any type of transport. However, many of these risks can be mitigated or minimized with appropriate planning.

Standardized protocols have been shown to improve quality of care and reduce costs in a number of medical fields [33, 34]. Accordingly, most, if not all, high-volume ECMO transport programs have specific protocols to ensure consistency of performance. Simulation exercises are an important component of preparation, and can be used to practice cannulation, initiation of ECMO, loading of the patient onto the vehicle and response to emergencies [35–38]. Equipment checklists can be useful to make sure that all equipment is available and loaded onto the ECMO transport vehicle [6, 39]. A checklist covering necessary actions to launch the ECMO team and checklists for the outside hospital can ensure that the necessary equipment, power and oxygen supplies are in place. Team safety briefings can be used before deployment of the team, before cannulation and before initiation of transport to ensure that all team members are aware of plans and that anyone with a safety concern speaks up. After-action debriefings and review of outcomes may help ensure the safety of ECMO transport.

Conclusion

In the hands of experienced mobile ECMO teams, remote initiation of ECMO support and transport of patients during ECMO is safe and may allow critically ill patients who would otherwise be too unstable to be safely transported to high-volume centers of excellence. Ground, helicopter and fixed-wing aerial transport are all proven modalities, and ECMO transport is feasible even over extreme distances. To maintain patient and team safety during this complex and high-risk endeavor, meticulous attention to detail, careful planning and extensive training are necessary.

References

1. Karagiannidis C, Brodie D, Strassmann S et al (2016) Extracorporeal membrane oxygenation: evolving epidemiology and mortality. Intensive Care Med 42:889–896
2. Foley DS, Pranikoff T, Younger JG et al (2002) A review of 100 patients transported on extracorporeal life support. ASAIO J 48:612–619
3. Bryner B, Cooley E, Copenhaver W et al (2014) Two decades' experience with interfacility transport on extracorporeal membrane oxygenation. Ann Thorac Surg 98:1363–1370
4. Clement KC, Fiser RT, Fiser WP et al (2010) Single-institution experience with interhospital extracorporeal membrane oxygenation transport: a descriptive study. Pediatr Crit Care Med 11:509–513
5. Biscotti M, Agerstrand C, Abrams D et al (2015) One hundred transports on extracorporeal support to an extracorporeal membrane oxygenation center. Ann Thorac Surg 100:34–39
6. Vaja R, Chauhan I, Joshi V et al (2015) Five-year experience with mobile adult extracorporeal membrane oxygenation in a tertiary referral center. J Crit Care 30:1195–1198
7. Broman LM, Holzgraefe B, Palmer K, Frenckner B (2015) The Stockholm experience: interhospital transports on extracorporeal membrane oxygenation. Crit Care 19:278
8. Kahn JM, Linde-Zwirble WT, Wunsch H et al (2008) Potential value of regionalized intensive care for mechanically ventilated medical patients. Am J Respir Crit Care Med 177:285–291
9. Kahn JM, Goss CH, Heagerty PJ, Kramer AA, O'Brien CR, Rubenfeld GD (2006) Hospital volume and the outcomes of mechanical ventilation. N Engl J Med 355:41–50
10. Noah MA, Peek GJ, Finney SJ et al (2011) Referral to an extracorporeal membrane oxygenation center and mortality among patients with severe 2009 influenza A(H1N1). JAMA 306:1659–1668
11. Barbaro RP, Odetola FO, Kidwell KM et al (2015) Association of hospital-level volume of extracorporeal membrane oxygenation cases and mortality. Analysis of the extracorporeal life support organization registry. Am J Respir Crit Care Med 191:894–901
12. Hayes D Jr., Tobias JD, Tumin D (2016) Center volume and extracorporeal membrane oxygenation support at lung transplantation in the lung allocation score era. Am J Respir Crit Care Med 194:317–326

13. Combes A, Brodie D, Bartlett R et al (2014) Position paper for the organization of extracorporeal membrane oxygenation programs for acute respiratory failure in adult patients. Am J Respir Crit Care Med 190:488–496

14. Peek GJ, Mugford M, Tiruvoipati R et al (2009) Efficacy and economic assessment of conventional ventilatory support versus extracorporeal membrane oxygenation for severe adult respiratory failure (CESAR): a multicentre randomised controlled trial. Lancet 374:1351–1363

15. Bartlett RH, Gazzaniga AB, Fong SW, Jefferies MR, Roohk HV, Haiduc N (1977) Extracorporeal membrane oxygenator support for cardiopulmonary failure. Experience in 28 cases. J Thorac Cardiovasc Surg 73:375–386

16. Mendes PV, de Albuquerque Gallo C, Besen B et al (2017) Transportation of patients on extracorporeal membrane oxygenation: a tertiary medical center experience and systematic review of the literature. Ann Intensive Care 7:14

17. Ericsson A, Frenckner B, Broman LM (2017) Adverse events during inter-hospital transports on extracorporeal membrane oxygenation. Prehosp Emerg Care 21:448–455

18. Ranney DN, Bonadonna D, Yerokun BA et al (2017) Extracorporeal membrane oxygenation and interfacility transfer: a regional referral experience. Ann Thorac Surg 104:1471–1478

19. Gutsche J, Vernick W, Miano TA et al (2017) One-year experience with a mobile extracorporeal life support service. Ann Thorac Surg 104:1509–1515

20. Ciapetti M, Cianchi G, Zagli G et al (2011) Feasibility of inter-hospital transportation using extra-corporeal membrane oxygenation (ECMO) support of patients affected by severe swine-flu(H1N1)-related ARDS. Scand J Trauma Resusc Emerg Med 19:32–38

21. Javidfar J, Brodie D, Takayama H et al (2011) Safe transport of critically ill adult patients on extracorporeal membrane oxygenation support to a regional extracorporeal membrane oxygenation center. ASAIO J 57:421–425

22. Brodie D, Bacchetta M (2011) Extracorporeal membrane oxygenation for ARDS in adults. N Engl J Med 365:1905–1914

23. Aubin H, Petrov G, Dalyanoglu H et al (2016) A suprainstitutional network for remote extracorporeal life support: a retrospective cohort study. JACC Heart Fail 4:698–708

24. Abrams D, Combes A, Brodie D (2014) Extracorporeal membrane oxygenation in cardiopulmonary disease in adults. J Am Coll Cardiol 63:2769–2778

25. Nwozuzu A, Fontes ML, Schonberger RB (2016) Mobile extracorporeal membrane oxygenation teams: The North American versus the European experience. J Cardiothorac Vasc Anesth 30:1441–1448

26. Philipp A, Arlt M, Amann M et al (2011) First experience with the ultra compact mobile extracorporeal membrane oxygenation system Cardiohelp in interhospital transport. Interact Cardiovasc Thorac Surg 12:978–981

27. DiGeronimo RJ, Henderson CL, Grubb PH (2005) Referral and transport of ECMO patients. In: Van Meurs K, Lally KP, Peek G, Zwischenberger JB (eds) ECMO: Extracorporeal Cardiopulmonary Support in Critical Care, 3rd edn. Extracorporeal Life Support Organization, Ann Arbor, pp 157–172

28. Wagner K, Sangolt GK, Risnes I et al (2008) Transportation of critically ill patients on extracorporeal membrane oxygenation. Perfusion 23:101–106

29. Charon C, Allyn J, Bouchet B et al (2017) Ten thousand kilometre transfer of cardiogenic shock patients on venoarterial extracorporeal membrane oxygenation for emergency heart transplantation: Cooperation between Reunion Island and Metropolitan France. Eur Heart J Acute Cardiovasc Care. https://doi.org/10.1177/2048872617719652 (Jun 1, Epub ahead of print)

30. Maillot A, Bussienne F, Braunberger E et al (2016) Long-distance air transfer on commercial long-haul flights for patients on extracorporeal life support. Intensive Care Med 42:949–950

31. Coppola CP, Tyree M, Larry K, DiGeronimo R (2008) A 22-year experience in global transport extracorporeal membrane oxygenation. J Pediatr Surg 43:46–52

32. Aerospace Medical Association, Aviation Safety Committee (2008) Cabin cruising altitudes for regular transport aircraft. Aviat Space Environ Med 79:433–439
33. Fitch ZW, Debesa O, Ohkuma R et al (2014) A protocol-driven approach to early extubation after heart surgery. J Thorac Cardiovasc Surg 147:1344–1350
34. Sinuff T, Muscedere J, Adhikari NK et al (2013) Knowledge translation interventions for critically ill patients: a systematic review. Crit Care Med 41:2627–2640
35. Weems MF, Friedlich PS, Nelson LP et al (2017) The role of extracorporeal membrane oxygenation simulation training at extracorporeal life support organization centers in the United States. Simul Healthc 12:233–239
36. Burkhart HM, Riley JB, Lynch JJ et al (2013) Simulation-based postcardiotomy extracorporeal membrane oxygenation crisis training for thoracic surgery residents. Ann Thorac Surg 95:901–906
37. Grisham LM, Vickers V, Biffar DE et al (2016) Feasibility of air transport simulation training: a case series. Air Med J 35:308–313
38. Alfes CM, Steiner SL, Manacci CF (2015) Critical care transport training: new strides in simulating the austere environment. Air Med J 34:186–187
39. Clark SC, Dunning J, Alfieri OR et al (2012) EACTS guidelines for the use of patient safety checklists. Eur J Cardiothorac Surg 41:993–1004

Early Mobilization of Patients in Intensive Care: Organization, Communication and Safety Factors that Influence Translation into Clinical Practice

C. L. Hodgson, E. Capell, and C. J. Tipping

Introduction

Early mobilization in the intensive care unit (ICU) is currently a hot topic, with more than 15 randomized controlled trials (RCTs) in the past ten years including several high impact publications [1]. However, the largest studies of early mobilization have enrolled 300 patients, and the results of phase II randomized trials, pilot studies and observational studies have been used to encourage practice change [2–5]. There are currently several international practice guidelines available, and early mobilization has consistently been reported as safe and feasible in the ICU setting [6]. There is no doubt that this early intervention in ICU shows exciting potential. The reported benefits of early mobilization, include reduced ICU-acquired weakness, improved functional recovery within hospital, improved walking distance at hospital discharge and reduced hospital length of stay [1]. However, medical research has repeatedly demonstrated that the results of pilot studies and phase II studies may not result in improved patient-centered outcomes when tested in a larger trial [7, 8]. More importantly, it has been difficult to test this complex intervention, with several randomized trials delivering significantly less early mobilization than specified in the study protocol [2, 9] and observational studies reporting very low rates of early mobilization during the ICU stay [10, 11].

This chapter summarizes the considerations for patient safety during early mobilization; including the physiological assessment of the patient, the consideration

C. L. Hodgson (✉) · C. J. Tipping
Australian and New Zealand Intensive Care Research Centre, School of Public Health and Preventive Medicine, Monash University
Melbourne, Victoria, Australia
Department of Physiotherapy, The Alfred Hospital
Melbourne, Victoria, Australia
e-mail: carol.hodgson@monash.edu

E. Capell
Department of Physiotherapy, The Alfred Hospital
Melbourne, Victoria, Australia

© Springer International Publishing AG 2018
J.-L. Vincent (ed.), *Annual Update in Intensive Care and Emergency Medicine 2018*,
Annual Update in Intensive Care and Emergency Medicine,
https://doi.org/10.1007/978-3-319-73670-9_46

of invasive lines and monitoring, the management of sedation, strategies to educate and manage the multidisciplinary team and environmental factors. Importantly, we will consider the long-term effect of early mobilization on patient outcome and the future directions for this important area of work for ICU clinicians.

Safety of Early Mobilization in the ICU: Short-Term Consequences

Early mobilization is a complex intervention that requires careful patient assessment and management, as well as interdisciplinary team cooperation and training [12]. Patient safety is one of the most commonly reported barriers to delivering early mobilization, including respiratory, cardiovascular and neurological stability and the integrity of invasive lines. In a recent systematic review and meta-analysis of patient safety during early mobilization, 48 studies were identified that reported data on safety during early mobilization, including falls, removal of endotracheal tubes (ETT), removal or dysfunction of intravascular catheters, removal of catheters or tubes, cardiac arrest, hemodynamic changes and oxygen desaturation [13]. Five studies were not included as their data were reported in other included publications. The 43 included studies had different descriptions of safety events and, in most, the criteria for ceasing early mobilization were the same criteria used to define a safety event. The most frequently reported safety events were oxygen desaturation and hemodynamic changes, each reported in 33 (69%) of the eligible studies and removal or dysfunction of intravascular catheters reported in 31 (65%) of the eligible studies. Several studies did not report on important safety events, including falls (n = 21, 43%), ETT removal (n = 17, 35%) and cardiac arrest (n = 15, 31%).

Of the 43 included studies, 23 (53%) reported consequences of potential safety events [13]. There were 308 potential safety events from 13,974 mobilization sessions, for an incidence of 2% potential safety events during mobilization. Of these, consequences of the safety event were reported for 78 occasions (0.6%) including 49 debridement or suturing of wounds and 11 tube removals with 4 of these requiring replacement. With regards to adverse events including a high heart rate, low blood pressure or oxygen desaturation, the pooled incidence for each was less than 2 per 1,000 episodes of mobilization. Safety events that resulted in additional care requirements or consequences were very rare.

There have been several publications that recommend criteria for the safe mobilization of patients receiving mechanically ventilated. The first was published approximately 15 years ago, and later adopted as a recommendation by the European Respiratory Society and the European Society of Critical Care Medicine [12, 14]. At this time, the evidence was considered level C and D (observational studies and expert opinions). In particular, these authors recommended identification of patient characteristics that enable treatment to be prescribed and modified on an individual basis, with standardized pathways for clinical decision making. The flow diagram detailing patient assessment prior to early mobilization is a useful tool in clinical practice, and may be used to assist with staff training.

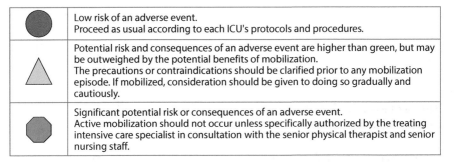

●	Low risk of an adverse event. Proceed as usual according to each ICU's protocols and procedures.
△	Potential risk and consequences of an adverse event are higher than green, but may be outweighed by the potential benefits of mobilization. The precautions or contraindications should be clarified prior to any mobilization episode. If mobilized, consideration should be given to doing so gradually and cautiously.
⬣	Significant potential risk or consequences of an adverse event. Active mobilization should not occur unless specifically authorized by the treating intensive care specialist in consultation with the senior physical therapist and senior nursing staff.

Fig. 1 Expert consensus color coding definitions for safe early mobilization of mechanically ventilated patients [15]

More recently, an international multidisciplinary expert consensus group developed recommendations for consideration prior to mobilization of patients in the ICU during mechanical ventilation [15]. The panel consisted of 23 clinical or research experts from four countries, including 17 physiotherapists, five intensivists and one nurse. Following a modified Delphi process, the group developed a traffic light system for each of the identified safety criteria to determine the risk/benefit of performing early mobilization. Green indicated that there was a low risk of an adverse event, and the benefit outweighed the potential safety consequences of early mobilization. Yellow indicated a potential risk or consequence of adverse event during early mobilization, such that precautions and contraindications should be discussed with the interdisciplinary team prior to mobilization. Red indicated a significant potential risk of an adverse event, where early mobilization should not occur unless it was authorized by the medical team responsible for the overall patient management in ICU.

Importantly, a 'red' sign was not a contraindication to early mobilization, but rather a clear message that the risks may outweigh the benefits in this instance (Fig. 1) [15]. The safety criteria were divided into the categories of respiratory, cardiovascular, neurological and other considerations (e.g., securing intravascular lines). Consensus was achieved on all criteria for safe mobilization with the exception of levels of vasoactive agents, where the panel agreed that more evidence was required to guide the recommendations. At an international meeting, 94 multidisciplinary ICU clinicians concurred with the proposed expert recommendations prior to publication.

The safety criteria developed by the group were intended to be used whenever mobilization was being considered, which might be up to several times per day for an individual patient. In considering the decision to mobilize a patient, the criteria should be assessed based on the status of the patient at the time of planned mobilization, but changes in condition, and direction of trends, in the preceding hours should also be taken into account [15]. The potential consequences of an adverse event in an individual patient should also be considered as part of the overall clinical reasoning process. This group noted that further research was required to validate the traffic light system in centers of clinical expertise and in centers without clinical expertise in early mobilization. They also noted that practice may change and progress in the future, so that areas that were considered a significant potential risk (red) may change to yellow with further investigation, or *vice versa*.

Barriers and Facilitators to Mobilization Reported in Quantitative Studies

Many observational and randomized controlled trials over the past decade have demonstrated that ICU clinicians are reluctant to mobilize mechanically ventilated patients, despite the scarcity of reported adverse events and the potential benefits [11, 16, 17]. The barriers and facilitators to early mobilization can be divided into patient factors, ICU team factors and organizational factors (Table 1). A recent systematic review identified barriers to delivering the Awakening, Breathing Coordination, Delirium and Early mobility/exercise (ABCDE) bundle to minimize adverse outcomes and improve patient care for ICU patients [18]. This study reported 107 barriers, categorized into four classes: patient-related (patient instability); clinician-related (lack of knowledge and staff safety concerns); protocol-related (unclear protocol criteria); and ICU contextual barriers (interdisciplinary team coordination).

Several large, multicenter observational studies have reported barriers to mobilization across regions. For example, a prospective, observational study of mobilization practice in mechanically ventilated patients enrolled 192 patients from 12 ICUs in Australia and New Zealand [11]. The data were collected from 1,288 physiotherapy–patient interactions and no early mobilization occurred in 1,079 (84%) of these episodes during mechanical ventilation. A total of 122 (63.5%) patients did not receive early active mobilization and the main reported barrier to mobilization was sedation, with nearly half of the cohort too sedated for active mobilization on the first two days in the ICU. The study suggests that unit culture, rather than patient-related factors, may be the main barrier to early mobilization in these ICUs. The use of vasopressors was common (n = 127, 66%), however there was no evidence to suggest the appropriate level of vasopressor support to enable safe mobilization. Similarly, a point prevalence study completed across 38 ICUs in Australia and New Zealand showed that no patients mobilized or sat out of bed during mechanical ventilation [16].

Harrold and colleagues compared early mobilization between Australian and Scottish ICUs [10]. This study found that 60.2% (209/347) patients were mobilized in the Australian cohort and 40.1% (68/167) patients were mobilized in the Scottish cohort during the ICU stay. Mobilization in the presence of an ETT was rare in both cohorts (3.4% Scotland and 2.2% in Australia). Physiological instability and the presence of an ETT were frequently reported barriers; however sedation was the most commonly reported barrier to mobilization in both the Australian and Scottish cohorts.

Randomized trials have also had difficulty delivering the planned dose of early mobilization in the intervention group. The TEAM pilot study found that early,

Table 1 Barriers and facilitators to mobilization

Barriers	Facilitators
Patient Factors	
Physiological instability (hemodynamic, respiratory, neurological)	Manage patient physiological instability
	Management of sedation & delirium
Sedation	Sleep
Low Glasgow Coma Scale	Delirium screening/management
Delirium/agitation	Analgesia prior to mobilization
Psychological state	Patient goals
Pain	Family engagement and education
Medical procedures/orders	
Patient refusal/anxiety	
Intensive Care Team Factors	
Poor culture	Develop a positive team culture
Lack of communication	Ward rounds, multidisciplinary team meetings
Lack of leadership	Designated leaders
Disengaged team members	Team planning and communication
Inexperienced staff	Education and up-skilling staff
Lack of planning and coordination	Screening of appropriate patients
Unclear expectations	Flexible and cooperative team members
Risk for mobility providers	Utilization of safety criteria for mobilizing
Femoral lines	mechanically ventilated patients
Early ward transfers	Anticipated benefits
Anticipated risks	
Organizational Factors	
Lack of funding	Business case for additional staff to outline the
Time constraints	economic benefits for the organization
Lack of equipment and resources	Appropriate equipment & resources
Lack of staffing or availability	Dedicated staffing
Busy caseloads	Mobility guidelines/protocol
	Training on appropriate equipment

goal-directed mobility was feasible, safe and resulted in increased duration and level of active exercise [19]. Fifty patients were randomized and the intervention group received a median duration of 20 min/day early goal-directed mobilization, despite the 30–60 min pre-specified goal of the intervention. Although the intervention group did not meet the targeted duration of early mobilization, the proportion of patients that walked in the ICU was almost doubled in the intervention group. Two of the largest randomized trials of early mobilization have also reported difficulties delivering intensive dosage of active mobilization. One study was only able to deliver the intervention on 57% of study days [9], whilst the other was able to complete physical therapy on 55% and progressive resistance exercise on 36% of study days [2]. Sedation management, in particular, limited the number of early mobilization interventions, which may have contributed to the findings that ICU-based physical rehabilitation did not appear to improve physical outcomes at 6 months compared to standard physical rehabilitation.

To address the concern with unit culture and interdisciplinary goals and communication, a multicenter international randomized trial in five university hospitals in

Austria, Germany and the USA was performed where the mobilization goal was defined during daily morning ward rounds and facilitated by interdisciplinary closed-loop communication [4]. The mobilization goal was achieved in 89% of study days in the intervention group. Early goal-directed mobilization improved patient mobilization throughout ICU admission, shortened patient length of stay in both the surgical ICU and hospital, and improved patients' functional mobility at hospital discharge (51% of patients in the intervention group vs 28% of patients in the control group). The current evidence suggests that early mobilization is safe and feasible and may improve functional recovery at hospital discharge; however ICUs are still very conservative in mobilizing mechanically ventilated patients, with some potentially avoidable barriers. Interdisciplinary communication and a clinical lead or champion may reduce barriers to early mobilization [20–22].

Themes that Identify Barriers and Facilitators to Early Mobilization

There have been several studies that have used qualitative methods to establish themes associated with barriers and facilitators to early mobilization in ICU. Barber and colleagues used three discipline-specific focus groups to establish barriers and facilitators to early mobilization amongst 25 ICU staff, including separate focus groups for doctors, nurses and physiotherapists [21]. Three key themes emerged to both barriers and facilitators across all groups. The barriers included: first, culture which included the use of sedation and the reluctance to mobilize patients with an ETT; second, communication which included contacting the appropriate physiotherapist to mobilize a patient, and doctors writing it as a care plan for the day without it being operationalized; and third, a lack of resources, which included staff, training and equipment to safely conduct mobilization in the ICU. The facilitators to early mobilization in the ICU included: organizational change, such as a dedicated mobility team; leadership including a champion who would assist with multidisciplinary team planning, team meetings and daily goal setting; and resources to provide adequate staff, training and equipment for mobilization in this complex area.

Using the theory of planned behavior, Holdsworth and colleagues elicited attitudinal, normative and control beliefs toward early mobilization of mechanically ventilated patients [23]. A nine-item elicitation questionnaire was administered electronically to a convenience sample of 22 staff in the ICU. Respondents wrote the most text about barriers to mobilization, including that it was time consuming, posed a safety risk to patients with line dislodgement or disconnection and unstable patient physiology and that there was a negative workplace culture.

Perhaps the most comprehensive publication in this area is a recent systematic review of quantitative and qualitative studies that identified and evaluated factors influencing physical activity in the ICU setting (and post-ICU setting) [20]. Eighty-nine papers were included with five major themes and 28 sub-themes including: first, patient physical and psychological capability to perform physical activity, including delirium, sedation, motivation, weakness and anxiety; second, safety influences, including physiological stability and invasive lines; third, culture and team influences, including leadership, communication, expertise and administrative buy-in; fourth, motivation and beliefs regarding risks versus benefits; and lastly environmental influences including funding, staffing and equipment. Many of the barriers and enablers to physical activity were consistent across both qualitative and quantitative studies and geographical regions, and they supported themes established from previous research in this area. Barriers and facilitators to physical activity were multidimensional and may be altered by raising general awareness about post-intensive care syndrome and the potential risks versus potential benefits of early mobilization in the ICU.

Drivers of Clinical Decision Making That Are Modifiable

It is possible that several of the drivers of clinical decision making with regards to early mobilization of mechanically ventilated patients are modifiable [20]. In a large prospective cohort study across 12 ICUs, the main reported barrier to early mobilization was sedation [11]. Only one of 12 ICUs in this study routinely used a sedation protocol, including sedation minimization or daily sedation interruption. Implementing a sedation protocol into routine ICU care across regions may facilitate early mobilization by allowing ICU patients to wake and participate in physical activity. These results were also identified in an international study of early mobilization practices in Australia and Scotland [10].

In another observational study, Leditschke and colleagues reported on 327 patient days audited for early mobilization or barriers to early mobilization [22]. Early mobilization did not occur on 151 (46%) of these days and the reasons for inability to deliver early mobilization was potentially avoidable in almost half of these. Potentially avoidable barriers to mobilization included femoral vascular catheters, timing of procedures, sedation management, agitation and early transfer to the hospital ward. Active identification of barriers to early mobilization and strategies to avoid these issues should be included as part of an early mobilization plan.

Early Mobilization and Long-term Consequences

The importance of completing long-term follow-up of patient outcomes after ICU has become well recognized and is now prioritized in research [24, 25]. It is recommended that studies follow up patients for a least six months after ICU admission [26]. Mortality is a commonly reported outcome in critical care research. Due to the complexities of critical care and the interventions provided to patients, it is possible that early mobilization and rehabilitation may have long-term adverse effects on our patients [1]. An updated meta-analysis of controlled and randomized trials of early mobilization and rehabilitation in ICU showed no significant difference in mortal-

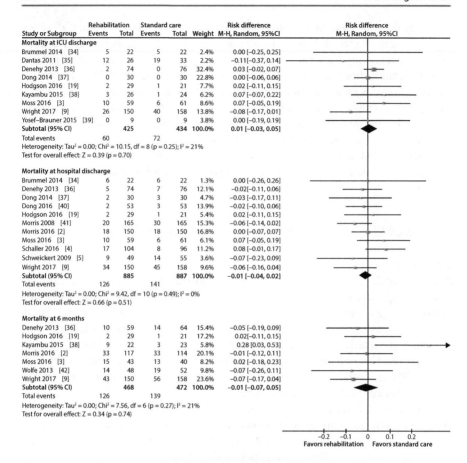

Fig. 2 Forest plot of mortality in ICU, in hospital and at six months comparing early mobilization with standard care in randomized controlled trials

ity at six months between the intervention and control groups (OR –0.01, 95% CI –0.07–0.05, p = 0.74, seven studies, n = 265) (Fig. 2).

Whilst mortality is an important outcome to assess after critical illness, it is long-term physical, psychological and cognitive function that patients and their family members rate as important outcomes post-critical illness [27]. To this end, there are a large number of outcome measures available to assess the key domains after ICU discharge, including physical, cognitive and psychological function [28]. In studies of early mobilization and rehabilitation it is common that different outcome measures are used to assess the same domains across different studies.[1, 20] This makes combining the results in a meta-analysis difficult and makes it challenging to compare the results across studies.

A recent meta-analysis assessed six-month outcomes from randomized and controlled clinical trials of early mobilization and rehabilitation. It reported that there was no significant difference in timed-up-and-go test and the 36 Item Short Form Survey (SF-36) results [1]. It did, however, show significantly higher SF-36 results favoring the intervention group in the role physical and role emotional domains for high-dose rehabilitation compared to low-dose rehabilitation and significantly more days alive and out of hospital favoring the intervention group (mean difference 9.63, 95% CI 1.68–17.57, p = 0.02, five studies, n = 509). There were consistent concerns regarding the high rates of loss to follow up across the studies, making outcomes like the SF-36 and timed-up-and-go difficult to interpret as they do not account for death [1, 29]. There is currently no consistent message regarding the long-term effects of early mobilization in the ICU on physical function or quality of life [30, 31].

Do We Have Consensus on Long-term Outcomes for ICU Survivors?

A two-stage, international Delphi process determined that the following domains are important to assess post-ICU discharge in patients with acute respiratory failure: physical function, cognition, mental health, satisfaction with life and personal enjoyment, survival, pulmonary function, pain and muscle or nerve function [32]. The Delphi process evaluated which outcome measures should be used to assess domains identified as important. Consensus could not be reached on all domains, however the minimal acceptable outcomes to report based on this study are survival, EuroQol-5D (EQ-5D; assessing satisfaction with life and personal enjoyment), hospital anxiety and depression scale and impact of event scale revised (assessing mental health).

Perhaps we can learn some lessons from other acute areas of medicine. A dose-response analysis of early mobilization, completed on the AVERT Study stoke patient data, helps to unravel uncertainties in the dosage, timing and frequency of early mobilization interventions following stroke onset [33]. In the primary analysis, the results demonstrated that very early mobilization in stroke patients resulted in decreased odds of a favorable outcome [7]. The secondary analysis, however, showed a 13% improvement in odds of a favorable outcome with each episode of out-of-bed activity per day, keeping time to mobilization and daily amount constant. Conversely increasing the amount of time doing out-of-bed activity reduced the odds of a favorable outcome. Patients who started mobilizing earlier post-onset of stroke also had more favorable outcomes. The beneficial effect of regular short periods of out-of-bed activity was consistent across most of the analysis. These results may guide further research in the critical care population with regards to the prescription of early mobilization. To date, studies of early mobilization in the ICU have delivered variations in dose, timing and progression of the rehabilitation intervention [1]. This variability has made it challenging to compare the study results and to determine the most appropriate dosage and timing of early mobilization in the ICU.

Conclusion

Currently there is a divide between ICU clinicians who wish to implement early mobilization based on current evidence and clinicians who believe that early mobilization is an intervention that should be tested in a large patient-centered trial to determine long term outcomes (including functional recovery). Despite the publication of safety recommendations and clinical practice guidelines [6, 14, 15], the implementation of early mobilization remains a challenge in the ICU, with limited information on safe levels of vasoactive support, ongoing evidence of over-sedation of mechanically ventilated patients and poor staff resources limiting the ability to deliver early mobilization. Based on current evidence, early mobilization is safe during mechanical ventilation, but the conservative management of ICU patients translates into a culture of bed rest. Some of the drivers of clinical decisions may be modifiable, with better adherence to sedation and mobilization protocols, clinical leadership and increased staff resources and training. However, given our experience in other areas of medicine including stroke and traumatic brain injury, early mobilization should be tested in a patient-centered trial with evaluation of long-term outcomes prior to implementation.

References

1. Tipping CJ, Harrold M, Holland A, Romero L, Nisbet T, Hodgson CL (2017) The effects of active mobilisation and rehabilitation in ICU on mortality and function: a systematic review. Intensive Care Med 43:171–183
2. Morris PE, Berry MJ, Files DC et al (2016) Standardized rehabilitation and hospital length of stay among patients with acute respiratory failure: a randomized clinical trial. JAMA 315:2694–2702
3. Moss M, Nordon-Craft A, Malone D et al (2016) A randomized trial of an intensive physical therapy program for patients with acute respiratory failure. Am J Respir Crit Care Med 193:1101–1110
4. Schaller SJ, Anstey M, Blobner M et al (2016) Early, goal-directed mobilisation in the surgical intensive care unit: a randomised controlled trial. Lancet 388:1377–1388
5. Schweickert WD, Pohlman MC, Pohlman AS et al (2009) Early physical and occupational therapy in mechanically ventilated, critically ill patients: a randomised controlled trial. Lancet 373:1874–1882
6. NICE Guidelines (2009) Rehabilitation after critical illness in adults. https://www.nice.org.uk/guidance/cg83. Accessed 11 January 2018
7. Bernhardt J, Langhorne P, Lindley RI et al (2015) Efficacy and safety of very early mobilisation within 24 h of stroke onset (AVERT): a randomised controlled trial. Lancet 386:46–55
8. Cooper DJ, Rosenfeld JV, Murray L et al (2011) Decompressive craniectomy in diffuse traumatic brain injury. N Engl J Med 364:1493–1502
9. Wright SE, Thomas K, Watson G et al (2017) Intensive versus standard physical rehabilitation therapy in the critically ill (EPICC): a multicentre, parallel-group, randomised controlled trial. Thorax. https://doi.org/10.1136/thoraxjnl-2016-209858 (Aug 5, Epub ahead of print)
10. Harrold ME, Salisbury LG, Webb SA, Allison GT et al (2015) Early mobilisation in intensive care units in Australia and Scotland: a prospective, observational cohort study examining mobilisation practises and barriers. Crit Care 19:336

11. Hodgson C, Bellomo R, Berney S et al (2015) Early mobilization and recovery in mechanically ventilated patients in the ICU: a bi-national, multi-centre, prospective cohort study. Crit Care 19:81

12. Gosselink R, Bott J, Johnson M et al (2008) Physiotherapy for adult patients with critical illness: recommendations of the European Respiratory Society and European Society of Intensive Care Medicine Task Force on Physiotherapy for Critically Ill Patients. Intensive Care Med 34:1188–1199

13. Nydahl P, Sricharoenchai T, Chandra S et al (2017) Safety of patient mobilization and rehabilitation in the intensive care unit. systematic review with meta-analysis. Ann Am Thorac Soc 14:766–777

14. Stiller K, Phillips A (2003) Safety aspects of mobilising acutely ill inpatients. Physiother Theory Pract 19:239–257

15. Hodgson CL, Stiller K, Needham DM et al (2014) Expert consensus and recommendations on safety criteria for active mobilization of mechanically ventilated critically ill adults. Crit Care 18:658

16. Berney S, Harrold M, Webb S et al (2013) Intensive care unit mobility practices in Australia and New Zealand: a point prevalence study. Crit Care Resus 15:260–265

17. Nydahl P, Ruhl AP, Bartoszek G et al (2014) Early mobilization of mechanically ventilated patients: a 1-day point-prevalence study in Germany. Crit Care Med 42:1178–1186

18. Costa DK, White MR, Ginier E et al (2017) Identifying barriers to delivering the awakening and breathing coordination, delirium, and early exercise/mobility bundle to minimize adverse outcomes for mechanically ventilated patients: a systematic review. Chest 152:304–311

19. Hodgson CL, Bailey M, Bellomo R et al (2016) A binational multicenter pilot feasibility randomized controlled trial of early goal-directed mobilization in the ICU. Crit Care Med 44:1145–1152

20. Parry SM, Knight LD, Connolly B et al (2017) Factors influencing physical activity and rehabilitation in survivors of critical illness: a systematic review of quantitative and qualitative studies. Intensive Care Med 43:531–542

21. Barber EA, Everard T, Holland AE, Tipping C, Bradley SJ, Hodgson CL (2015) Barriers and facilitators to early mobilisation in intensive care: a qualitative study. Aust Crit Care 28:177–182

22. Leditschke IA, Green M, Irvine J, Bissett B, Mitchell IA (2012) What are the barriers to mobilizing intensive care patients? Cardiopulm Phys Ther J 23:26–29

23. Holdsworth C, Haines KJ, Francis JJ, Marshall A, O'Connor D, Skinner EH (2015) Mobilization of ventilated patients in the intensive care unit: an elicitation study using the theory of planned behavior. J Crit Care 30:1243–1250

24. Iwashyna TJ, Ely EW, Smith DM, Langa KM (2010) Long-term cognitive impairment and functional disability among survivors of severe sepsis. JAMA 304:1787–1794

25. Needham DM, Davidson J, Cohen H et al (2012) Improving long-term outcomes after discharge from intensive care unit: report from a stakeholders' conference. Crit Care Med 40:502–509

26. Blackwood B, Marshall J, Rose L (2015) Progress on core outcome sets for critical care research. Curr Opin Crit Care 21:439–444

27. Angus DC, Carlet J (2003) Surviving intensive care: a report from the 2002 Brussels Roundtable. Intensive Care Med 29:368–377

28. Turnbull AE, Rabiee A, Davis WE et al (2016) Outcome measurement in ICU survivorship research from 1970 to 2013: a scoping review of 425 publications. Crit Care Med 44:1267–1277

29. Hodgson C, Cuthbertson BH (2016) Improving outcomes after critical illness: harder than we thought! Intensive Care Med 42:1772–1774

30. Hodgson CL, Iwashyna TJ, Schweickert WD (2016) All that work and no gain – what should we do to restore physical function in our survivors? Am J Respir Crit Care Med 15:1071–1072

31. Hodgson CL, Fan E (2016) Better measures, better trials, better outcomes in survivors of critical illness? Crit Care Med 44:1254–1255
32. Needham DM, Sepulveda KA, Dinglas VD et al (2017) Core outcome measures for clinical research in acute respiratory failure survivors: an international modified delphi consensus study. Am J Respir Crit Care Med 196:1122–1130
33. Bernhardt J, Churilov L, Ellery F et al (2016) Prespecified dose-response analysis for A Very Early Rehabilitation Trial (AVERT). Neurology 86:2138–2145
34. Brummel NE, Girard TD, Ely EW et al (2014) Feasibility and safety of early combined cognitive and physical therapy for critically ill medical and surgical patients: the activity and cognitive therapy in ICU (ACT-ICU) trial. Intensive Care Med 40:370–379
35. Dantas CM, Silva PF, Siqueira FH et al (2012) Influence of early mobilization on respiratory and peripheral muscle strength in critically ill patients. Rev Bras Ter Intensiva 24:173–178
36. Denehy L, Skinner EH, Edbrooke L et al (2013) Exercise rehabilitation for patients with critical illness: a randomized controlled trial with 12 months of follow-up. Crit Care 17:R156
37. Dong ZH, Yu BX, Sun YB, Fang W, Li L (2014) Effects of early rehabilitation therapy on patients with mechanical ventilation. World J Emerg Med 5:48–52
38. Kayambu G, Boots R, Paratz J (2015) Early physical rehabilitation in intensive care patients with sepsis syndromes: a pilot randomised controlled trial. Intensive Care Med 41:865–874
39. Yosef-Brauner O, Adi N, Shahar BT, Yehezkel E, Carmeli E (2015) Effect of physical therapy on muscle strength, respiratory muscles and functional parameters in patients with intensive care unit-acquired weakness. Clin Respir J 9:1–6
40. Dong Z, Yu B, Zhang Q et al (2016) Early rehabilitation therapy is beneficial for patients with prolonged mechanical ventilation after coronary artery bypass surgery. Int Heart J 57:241–246
41. Morris PE, Goad A, Thompson C et al (2008) Early intensive care unit mobility therapy in the treatment of acute respiratory failure. Crit Care Med 36:2238–2243
42. Wolfe KS, Wendlandt BN, Patel SB et al (2013) Long-term survival and health care utilization of mechanically ventilated patients in a randomized controlled trial of early mobilization. Am J Respir Crit Care Med 187:A5235 (abst)

Part XIV
The Future

The Emerging Role of the Microbiota in the ICU

N. S. Wolff, F. Hugenholtz, and W. J. Wiersinga

Introduction

In recent years, the surge of culture-independent methods to study bacterial populations has led to an increasing body of evidence pointing towards the microbiome as an important player in the pathophysiology of a whole spectrum of diseases that affect the critically ill, including trauma and sepsis [1–4]. Techniques such as 16S rRNA and shotgun metagenomic sequencing have opened up a new area of research, enabling detailed investigations of complex populations of bacteria and their effects on health and disease [5, 6]. Some have even called the microbiome a separate organ given its numerous roles in metabolism, development of the immune system and host defense against pathogens [7].

Microbiota is an overarching term for all the microbes in a population, consisting of bacteria, archaea and eukarya [8]. Most studies that have been performed look at the bacterial microbiota because of its high abundance and high diversity. The collective of microbes in a population is referred to as the microbiota and the genetic content as the microbiome.

The real value of all this novel knowledge for the clinical care of patients on the intensive care unit (ICU) still has to be established. Nonetheless, data are accumulating that underscore the potential importance of the microbiome for intensive care

N. S. Wolff · F. Hugenholtz
Center for Experimental and Molecular Medicine, Academic Medical Center, University of Amsterdam
Amsterdam, Netherlands

W. J. Wiersinga (✉)
Center for Experimental and Molecular Medicine, Academic Medical Center, University of Amsterdam
Amsterdam, Netherlands
Department of Medicine, Division of Infectious Diseases, Academic Medical Center, University of Amsterdam
Amsterdam, Netherlands
e-mail: w.j.wiersinga@amc.uva.nl

© Springer International Publishing AG 2018
J.-L. Vincent (ed.), *Annual Update in Intensive Care and Emergency Medicine 2018*,
Annual Update in Intensive Care and Emergency Medicine,
https://doi.org/10.1007/978-3-319-73670-9_47

medicine. On any given day, three-fourths of all patients on the ICU are treated with antibiotics, which are known to cause severe collateral damage to the microbiome [9]. Besides antibiotics, there are multiple external modulators of the gut microbiota applied during the clinical care of patients on the ICU, such as gastric acid inhibition, the route of feeding, sedatives and opioids [3, 10]. Novel strategies are being designed to intervene on the microbiome to prevent or treat trauma and sepsis. Excitingly, a very recent randomized, placebo-controlled trial among 4556 healthy infants in India showed that the oral administration of *Lactobacillus plantarum* in combination with fructooligosaccharide in the first week of life could reduce the occurrence of sepsis in the first 60 days of life [4]. Other evidence points towards the use of synbiotics as an adjunctive therapy to prevent postoperative complications, such as surgical site infections and sepsis among adult surgical patients [11]. Most research in this field has focused on the intestinal microbiome; however, current research is also starting to show the importance of the lung microbiome for ICU patients [1]. For example, enrichment of the lung microbiome with gut bacteria seems to play a role in the pathogenesis of acute respiratory distress syndrome (ARDS) [12].

In this chapter, we will discuss the emerging role of the bacterial microbiotas in the gut and the lung in the critically ill. First, we will discuss the techniques available to study the bacterial microbiome, then we will continue into the gut and lung microbiome and end with some key questions for future research in the field of microbiota-targeted therapies on the ICU.

Microbiota Analyses

The composition of the microbiota in the gut has been studied extensively using 16S ribosomal RNA (rRNA) gene-targeted approaches. The use of this single genetic marker has revolutionized microbial ecology [13, 14]. It has become relatively easy to amplify the 16S rRNA encoding genes from environmental DNA. Nowadays, with next-generation sequencing techniques, many microbial environments can be studied in depth and at high resolution in space and time, using relatively straightforward procedures.

To address not only microbiota composition, but rather focus on the metabolic potential and actual activity of the intestinal microbiota, "meta'omic" approaches have emerged during the last decade and are now widely used [15–17]. Each of the meta'omic approaches provides different information about the functional potential or activity profiles of a microbial community.

Metagenomics is used to determine the collective genomes of members present in a microbial community as well as their functional capacity. Metagenomics was used in the Meta HIT (Metagenomics of the Human Intestinal Tract) project and provided a human microbiome-derived gene catalogue with over 3 million genes, indicating a community of over 150 species in an individual and a 100-fold larger non-redundant gene set compared to the human gene complement [16].

Metatranscriptomics and metaproteomics are able to provide information about the functions expressed by the members of the community. For example, metaproteomics analysis in healthy humans revealed a difference in the amount of proteins expressed and the proteins predicted by metagenomics. Moreover, metaproteomics in fecal material not only gives information on the bacterial proteins, but also on the major human proteins, giving insights into the main host responses [18]. However, it is difficult and sometimes not possible to use conserved proteins to distinguish between species or even higher taxonomic levels (e.g., genus or family). Consequently, by using this technique, you lose some of the taxonomic information otherwise gained by using metagenomics, metatranscriptomics or targeted 16S rRNA sequencing.

Metatranscriptome analysis of the gastrointestinal tract microbiota enables elucidation of the specific functional roles microbes have in this complex community. Although initial studies on the human large intestine revealed that different functions are expressed among individuals, core functions of the microbiota appear to be consistently expressed in different individuals [19, 20]. Moreover, metatranscriptome analyses of the small intestinal microbiota underpinned the cross-feeding between two dominant members of the small intestinal microbiota, i.e., *Streptococcus* spp. and *Veilonella* spp., in which the lactate produced by *Streptococcus* spp. is used as a carbon and energy source by the *Veillonella* spp. [17]. Metatranscriptome analysis of the microbiota in humanized mice revealed that mice colonized with the microbiota obtained from a lean human donor had greater expression of genes involved in polysaccharide breakdown and in propionate and butyrate production as compared to those colonized with the microbiota of an obese human donor [21]. These findings imply that metatranscriptomics can provide insight into the differential activity profiles in the intestinal microbiota, and enables reconstruction of the metabolic activity profile of microbial communities.

Metabolomic approaches are used to detect and quantify the metabolites that are produced by the microbial community. This approach has been suggested to be applicable as a diagnostic tool in diseases that involve aberrations of the intestinal microbiota composition and activity [22]. However, as with metaproteomics, you also lose information on the specific bacteria producing these metabolites. To overcome the loss of taxonomic information in metaproteomics and metabolomics, these techniques are often combined with 16S rRNA sequencing, metagenomics or metatranscriptomics.

These tools often generate very complex datasets with many different measurements (e.g., species or function) under various conditions. Therefore, these multivariate meta'omics datasets need tools to simplify the datasets and focus on correlations between points of interest, such as dietary interventions and the bacterial community or the bacterial community and host responses. Multivariate statistics are used to handle these large datasets and enable a relatively quick focus on data of importance [23]. An overview of available techniques to analyze the microbiome is provided in Fig. 1.

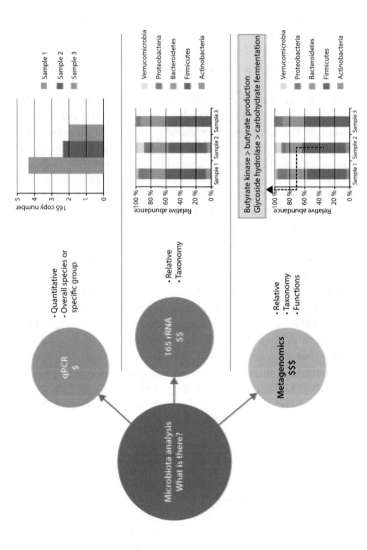

Fig. 1 Overview of techniques to detect bacterial microbiota. To detect which bacterial species there are in a sample, there are three options: 1) use quantitative polymerase chain reaction (qPCR) to detect total bacterial 16S rRNA gene and/or in combination with a specific qPCR for a bacterial group or species; 2) use 16S rRNA gene for amplicon multiplex sequencing to get information on the taxonomic distribution in a sample; 3) use total DNA of a sample for shot-gun sequencing of the metagenomics content to get information on taxonomic distribution and functions, examples of which are indicated in the box, to show that you have functional information within a taxonomic group, in this case butyrate kinase and glycoside hydrolase. The dollar sign below the different techniques is an indicator of the price: depending on the sample type and information depth, prices are variable, but, roughly, a one-dollar sign is around 5–10 dollars per sample; the two-dollar sign is 50–150 dollars per sample, and the three-dollar sign is 300–1000 dollars per sample

The Gut Microbiota

Human individuals can harbor over 150 different microbial species in their gut, which collectively encode more than 100-fold more non-redundant genes than there are in the human genome [16, 24]. More recent data, however, has challenged this number, suggesting that the ratio between bacteria and human cells is closer to 1:1 [25]. In healthy humans, the intestinal microbiota consists of members of all three domains of life: bacteria, archaea and eukarya, of which the bacterial community is the most abundant and diverse [8]. Nine different bacterial phyla have been recorded in humans so far, of which the bacteroidetes and firmicutes dominate [8, 16, 24]. Many of these bacteria in the gut have not been cultivated. Recent breakthroughs in the successful culture of the previously 'unculturable' human microbiota have revealed a whole spectrum of novel bacterial species and taxa [26]. The application of novel sequencing techniques provides an opportunity to understand this complex ecosystem much better [8, 13].

The intestinal microbiota plays a critical role in priming the host's immune system, gut maturation and gut functions, such as nutrient uptake and metabolism, mucosal barrier function, enteric nervous system and motility [27–29]. Numerous host genes seem to be specifically altered in response to various members of the microbiota, showing the importance of the microbial composition to the body's response [30, 31].

Modulators of the Microbiota on the ICU

The healthy intestinal microbiota is affected primarily by the host and the diet. In critically ill patients, these two factors both play an important role. However, in the critically ill it is also important to note that pathogens are able to outcompete other members of the intestinal microbiota more easily than in healthy humans, also changing the microbial composition. These pathogens benefit from a changed environment in critically ill patients, which are (though not *per se* all at the same time) decreased transit time, lack of 'normal' nutrition, oxygen levels and antibiotic usage [1]. Most of these opportunistic pathogens, except for *Clostridium difficile* infections, are Gram-negative aerobic species belonging to the proteobacteria, which thrive under the changed environment in critically ill patients. The universal use of antibiotics is probably the main cause of the severe bacterial dysbiosis seen in patients admitted to the ICU [32–36]. In addition, because of no or limited nutritional intake by patients on the ICU, nutrition for the microbiota in the intestine also decreases, affecting the microbiota composition. For example, in the large intestine, the microbiota ferments non-digested dietary fibers and dietary and host-derived proteins. The fermentation of fibers is necessary for the production of butyrate by the microbiota, which epithelial cells use as an energy source. The study of the clinical relevance of these effects in critically ill patients is, however, still in its infancy.

The Potential Clinical Relevance of the Gut Microbiota on the ICU

An imbalance in the homeostasis or 'dysbiosis' of the gut microbiota has been associated with a range of different diseases, including diabetes, obesity, inflammatory
bowel disease and rheumatoid arthritis [5, 6]. This association with disease has led
to investigations into the gut microbiota's involvement at the systemic level. In the
critically ill, the intestinal microbiota has been analyzed in a couple of studies so far.
In general, we can state that critically ill patients admitted to the ICU have a state of
dysbiosis of the intestinal microbiota [32–34]. Fig. 2 shows a schematic representation of the composition of the intestinal microbiota in the critically ill in comparison
to a healthy human. Overall, the intestinal microbiota of critically ill patients admitted to the ICU with sepsis is characterized by lower diversity, lower abundance of
key commensal genera (such as *Faecalibacterium, Blautia, Ruminococcus*), and in
some cases overgrowth (over 50% relative abundance) by one genera, such as *Es-
cherichia/Shigella, Salmonella, Enterococcus, C. difficile* or *Staphylococcus* [32–
36].

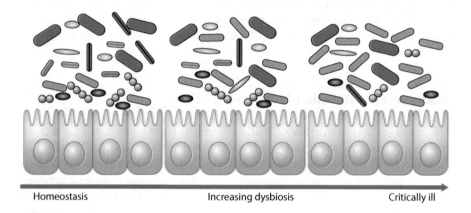

| Homeostasis | Increasing dysbiosis | Critically ill |

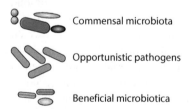

Commensal microbiota

Opportunistic pathogens

Beneficial microbiotica

Fig. 2 Intestinal microbiota in health and critical illness. The microbiota in a healthy individual
is a diverse ecosystem with beneficial and commensal bacteria and low abundances of opportunistic pathogens, which are not harmful in small numbers. As a result of certain therapies, such as
antibiotics, the microbial composition can be disrupted. The intestinal microbiota of critically ill
patients is less diverse and contains more opportunistic pathogens and less beneficial and commensal bacteria

A normal, healthy intestinal microbiota protects against an invasion of pathogens like *Enterococcus faecium, Escherichia coli* and *C. difficile*. It comes as no surprise that severe infections caused by these pathogens often occur in patients with a recent history of antibiotic use. The microbiota of these patients is therefore probably disrupted, which allows for the overgrowth of antibiotic-resistant pathogenic and opportunistic bacteria that are frequently encountered in hospital settings [37].

In sepsis, the focus often lies on the identification of a single pathogen as the causative agent. However, there is an increasing realization that most pathogens do not act in isolation and that infections have 'polymicrobial' phenotypes and are thus linked to the status of the microbiota in the patient. The initial state of the microbiota can influence susceptibility to infection [38] and severity of infection [39]. Recent preclinical data derived from animal models suggest that the gut microbiome plays a protective role in the host defense against sepsis [39–41]. As an example, antibiotic induced disruption of the gut microbiome leads to increased inflammation and bacterial dissemination in murine models of both Gram-positive and Gram-negative pneumosepsis [39, 40]. ICU patient data have suggested that the loss of microbiome diversity could predict the length of stay of patients on the ICU further underscoring the potential clinical relevance of the gut microbiome for intensive care medicine [33].

The Evolving Role of the Lung Microbiota in Critical Illness

Healthy lungs were long thought to be sterile, until recent studies showed that bacteria can be cultured from healthy lungs [42]. The lung environment is less advantageous for bacteria to grow and flourish when compared to the intestine, leading to a less dense bacterial community compared to the gut. A lack of nutrients, the bidirectional movement of the lung, the aerobic environment, and the coating of alveoli with a lipid-rich surfactant that has bacteriostatic effects all contribute to this harsh environment for bacteria [42, 43]. Furthermore, obtaining a sample from the lung is far more invasive than obtaining a stool sample to study the microbiome. Contamination from the sampling device or from the upper respiratory tract is another point to take into consideration.

In a healthy lung, the microbiota is delicately balanced by the reproduction rate of present bacteria and the immigration and elimination rate of bacteria. Under normal circumstances, the reproduction rate of bacteria remains low and the immigration and elimination high. However, in critical illness, sedatives and endotracheal intubation can decrease the mucociliary clearance and cough reflex, leading to decreased microbial elimination. Furthermore, mechanical ventilation can cause an increase in alveolar edema, which can lead to an increase in available nutrients in the lung and areas where the oxygen levels are lower, allowing bacteria to thrive [1].

In healthy lungs, it is thought that most of the bacteria come from the oral microbiota. The lung microbiota most closely resembles the microbiota of the oropharynx, more so than that of the nasopharynx, gastrointestinal tract or inhaled air [42]. The healthy oropharynx contains benign *Veillonella* spp. and *Prevotella* spp, and, therefore, these are also found in healthy lungs. During critical illness, the oropharynx can become overpopulated with pathogenic proteobacteria, such as *Pseudomonas aeruginosa* and *Klebsiella pneumoniae*. Furthermore, in critical illness the stomach and small intestine can become the primary source of bacterial migration to the lung [1, 42].

ARDS and pneumonia are thought to cause alveolar injury and as a consequence induce changes in the microbiome. The alveoli become covered with protein-rich fluids and the bactericidal surfactant from the alveoli becomes inactivated, making the alveoli a more hospitable environment for bacteria [1]. Furthermore, Dickson et al. [44] proposed a theory regarding the existence of a positive feedback loop between the growth of certain bacterial species in the lung and the local inflammatory response; as the bacterial population grows, it starts to limit itself due to nutrient shortage while it also provokes an increased inflammatory response. This inflammatory response can consequently lead to endothelial and epithelial injury, releasing fluids that are rich in proteins and nutrients, thus stimulating bacterial growth. Further bacterial growth will increase the local inflammation, thus creating a positive feedback loop. This suggests that in some cases the body's inflammatory response may be making the infection worse.

The Link between the Microbiota and the Gut-lung Axis

The intestinal microbiota has emerged as a key component of both local and systemic immunity. Epithelial and immune cells gain information directly from bacteria and local cytokine responses and subsequently adjust inflammatory responses. Microbiome research combining the gut and lung has started to show an association between the composition of the intestinal microbiota and lung health [45, 46]. Experimental germ-free and antibiotic murine models have shown that the body's microbiota is important in the defense against influenza and several types of bacterial pneumonia [46]. Moreover, probiotics containing *Lactobacillus* spp. and *Bifidobacterium* spp. have been shown to improve incidence and outcome of respiratory infections. Additionally, exposure to Toll-like receptor (TLR) agonists and nucleotide-binding oligomerization domain (NOD)-like receptors in the intestine, by substances such as lipopolysaccharide (LPS), peptidoglycan and lipoteichoic acid, has been shown to increase the lungs' ability to clear bacteria [45]. These studies suggest that the intestinal microbiota is important for airway defenses. Moreover, human and murine studies have shown that the lungs can contain gut-associated bacteria during sepsis and ARDS. However, this gut-lung axis does not seem to be a one-way street. Pulmonary infection with tuberculosis, influenza and *Burkholderia pseudomallei* have all been shown to have a significant effect on the composition of the gut microbiome in murine models [40, 47, 48]. Fig. 3 shows a schematic overview of the potential consequences of microbial dysbiosis in the critically ill in both the lung and intestine.

Healthy | Critically ill

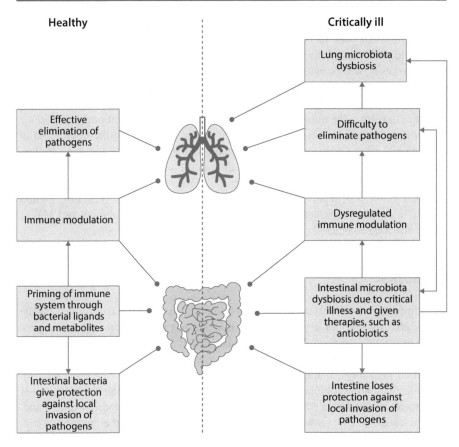

Fig. 3 The gut and lung microbiota in critical illness. A healthy gut microbiome plays a protective role in host defense against local and pulmonary pathogen invasion. In the critically ill, there is often dysbiosis in the lung and intestinal microbiotas, which can contribute to diseases like pneumonia and acute respiratory distress syndrome (ARDS)

The Road Ahead

Hospital-acquired infections are a huge problem in patients on the ICU. Antibiotic administration is the usual form of treatment or prevention of these infections and is lifesaving. However, as a side-effect, it severely affects the microbiota, risks induction of antibiotic resistant pathogens and potentially even the new onset of severe infection. Restoring the microbiota after antibiotic treatment has the potential to reduce infections [10, 23]. Different approaches can be utilized: probiotics, prebiotics (a dietary ingredient that promotes beneficial microbiota) and synbiotics (a combination of a probiotic with a prebiotic) have all been tested in various patient groups on the ICU with mixed results [4, 49]. Probiotics will not reestablish a complete microbiota. This can be achieved to a larger extent by performing a fecal microbiota transfer (FMT). FMT has been used successfully to restore re-occurring *C. difficile* infections in patients on the ICU. The first case reports on the successful use of FMT in patients with therapy-refractory sepsis have been published [10]. A key factor, however, will be establishing the exact mechanism by which certain components of the gut and/or lung microbiome play their presumed protective effects on the health of patients admitted to the ICU. This could enable us to develop targeted therapies to restore the microbiome in this very vulnerable patient population.

At the present time, we lack information on the dynamics of the microbiota in the critically ill in order to develop targeted therapies to restore the microbiome. There is a need for information on how the microbiota restores with and without interference or therapies in the critically ill. Moreover, these patients should be followed for long-term periods to monitor re-occurring infections. This information will aid in developing targeted approaches, such as the use of probiotics or FMT, to restore the microbiota and prevent infections during a patient's recovery.

Conclusion

The importance of the intestinal and lung microbiotas is often overlooked on the ICU. Currently, we can explore the microbiome using a vast array of techniques, giving us 'meta' libraries of data, which has allowed researchers to show the potential crucial role of the microbiota for ICU patients. During a patient's stay on the ICU, their microbiota is influenced by both their illness and the care provided. For example, the gut microbiota of critically ill patients admitted to the ICU with sepsis is characterized by lower diversity, lower abundance of key commensal genera and, in some cases, an overgrowth by one genera. These changes in the microbiota can, in turn, affect patient outcome and susceptibility to infection. Furthermore, the lung microbiota has only recently been shown to be important in the critically ill. Intriguingly, recent evidence also points to a bi-directional microbiota-mediated role between the gut and the lung, the so called gut-lung axis. The importance of these microbiotas is pushing us towards new types of treatments, in which we also start to treat the microbiota.

Acknowledgements

This work was supported by the Netherlands Organization for Scientific Research (NWO), the Horizon2020 Marie Skłodowska-Curie International Training Network "the European Sepsis Academy" and The Netherlands Organization for Health Research development (ZonMw).

References

1. Dickson RP (2016) The microbiome and critical illness. Lancet Respir Med 4:59–72
2. Baumler AJ, Sperandio V (2016) Interactions between the microbiota and pathogenic bacteria in the gut. Nature 535:85–93
3. Haak BW, Wiersinga WJ (2017) The role of the gut microbiota in sepsis. Lancet Gastroenterol Hepatol 2:135–143
4. Panigrahi P, Parida S, Nanda NC et al (2017) A randomized synbiotic trial to prevent sepsis among infants in rural India. Nature 548:407–412
5. Blaut M, Clavel T (2007) Metabolic diversity of the intestinal microbiota: implications for health and disease. J Nutr 137(3 Suppl 2):751S–755S
6. Guarner F (2006) Enteric flora in health and disease. Digestion 73(Suppl 1):5–12
7. Baquero F, Nombela C (2012) The microbiome as a human organ. Clin Microbiol Infect 18(Suppl 4):2–4
8. Rajilic-Stojanovic M, de Vos WM (2014) The first 1000 cultured species of the human gastrointestinal microbiota. FEMS Microbiol Rev 38:996–1047
9. Vincent J-L, Rello J, Marshall J et al (2009) International study of the prevalence and outcomes of infection in intensive care units. JAMA 302:2323–2329
10. Haak BW, Levi M, Wiersinga WJ (2017) Microbiota-targeted therapies on the intensive care unit. Curr Opin Crit Care 23:167–174
11. Kasatpibal N, Whitney JD, Saokaew S, Kengkla K, Heitkemper MM, Apisarnthanarak A (2017) Effectiveness of Probiotic, prebiotic, and synbiotic therapies in reducing postoperative complications: a systematic review and network meta-analysis. Clin Infect Dis 64(suppl 2):S153–S160
12. Dickson RP, Singer BH, Newstead MW et al (2016) Enrichment of the lung microbiome with gut bacteria in sepsis and the acute respiratory distress syndrome. Nat Microbiol 1:16113
13. Tringe SG, Hugenholtz P (2008) A renaissance for the pioneering 16S rRNA gene. Curr Opin Microbiol 11:442–446
14. Pace NR, Sapp J, Goldenfeld N (2012) Phylogeny and beyond: scientific, historical, and conceptual significance of the first tree of life. Proc Natl Acad Sci U S A 109:1011–1018
15. Fritz JV, Desai MS, Shah P, Schneider JG, Wilmes P (2013) From meta-omics to causality: experimental models for human microbiome research. Microbiome 1:14
16. Qin J, Li R, Raes J et al (2010) A human gut microbial gene catalogue established by metagenomic sequencing. Nature 464:59–65
17. Zoetendal EG, Raes J, van den Bogert B et al (2012) The human small intestinal microbiota is driven by rapid uptake and conversion of simple carbohydrates. ISME J 6:1415–1426
18. Verberkmoes NC, Russell AL, Shah M et al (2009) Shotgun metaproteomics of the human distal gut microbiota. ISME J 3:179–189
19. Franzosa EA, Morgan XC, Segata N et al (2014) Relating the metatranscriptome and metagenome of the human gut. Proc Natl Acad Sci U S A 111:E2329–E2338
20. Gosalbes MJ, Durban A, Pignatelli M et al (2011) Metatranscriptomic approach to analyze the functional human gut microbiota. PLoS One 6:e17447
21. Ridaura VK, Faith JJ, Rey FE et al (2013) Gut microbiota from twins discordant for obesity modulate metabolism in mice. Science 341:1241214
22. De Preter V, Verbeke K (2013) Metabolomics as a diagnostic tool in gastroenterology. World J Gastrointest Pharmacol Ther 4:97–107
23. Martin FP, Wang Y, Sprenger N et al (2008) Top-down systems biology integration of conditional prebiotic modulated transgenomic interactions in a humanized microbiome mouse model. Mol Syst Biol 4:205
24. Backhed F, Ley RE, Sonnenburg JL, Peterson DA, Gordon JI (2005) Host-bacterial mutualism in the human intestine. Science 307:1915–1920

25. Sender R, Fuchs S, Milo R (2016) Are we really vastly outnumbered? revisiting the ratio of bacterial to host cells in humans. Cell 164:337–340

26. Browne HP, Forster SC, Anonye BO et al (2016) Culturing of 'unculturable' human microbiota reveals novel taxa and extensive sporulation. Nature 533:543–546

27. Ciccia F, Guggino G, Rizzo A et al (2017) Dysbiosis and zonulin upregulation alter gut epithelial and vascular barriers in patients with ankylosing spondylitis. Ann Rheum Dis 76:1123–1132

28. Nicholson JK, Holmes E, Kinross J et al (2012) Host-gut microbiota metabolic interactions. Science 336:1262–1267

29. Backhed F, Roswall J, Peng Y et al (2015) Dynamics and stabilization of the human gut microbiome during the first year of life. Cell Host Microbe 17:690–703

30. Hooper LV, Wong MH, Thelin A, Hansson L, Falk PG, Gordon JI (2001) Molecular analysis of commensal host-microbial relationships in the intestine. Science 291:881–884

31. Leser TD, Molbak L (2009) Better living through microbial action: the benefits of the mammalian gastrointestinal microbiota on the host. Environ Microbiol 11:2194–2206

32. Lankelma JM, van Vught LA, Belzer C et al (2017) Critically ill patients demonstrate large interpersonal variation in intestinal microbiota dysregulation: a pilot study. Intensive Care Med 43:59–68

33. McDonald D, Ackermann G, Khailova L et al (2016) Extreme dysbiosis of the microbiome in critical illness. Msphere 1:e00199–16

34. Wischmeyer PE, McDonald D, Knight R (2016) Role of the microbiome, probiotics, and 'dysbiosis therapy' in critical illness. Curr Opin Crit Care 22:347–353

35. Zaborin A, Smith D, Garfield K et al (2014) Membership and behavior of ultra-low-diversity pathogen communities present in the gut of humans during prolonged critical illness. MBio 5:e1361–14

36. Ojima M, Motooka D, Shimizu K et al (2016) Metagenomic analysis reveals dynamic changes of whole gut microbiota in the acute phase of intensive care unit patients. Dig Dis Sci 61:1628–1634

37. Pamer EG (2016) Resurrecting the intestinal microbiota to combat antibiotic-resistant pathogens. Science 352:535–538

38. Yooseph S, Kirkness EF, Tran TM et al (2015) Stool microbiota composition is associated with the prospective risk of Plasmodium falciparum infection. BMC Genomics 16:631

39. Schuijt TJ, Lankelma JM, Scicluna BP et al (2016) The gut microbiota plays a protective role in the host defence against pneumococcal pneumonia. Gut 65:575–583

40. Lankelma JM, Birnie E, Weehuizen TAF et al (2017) The gut microbiota as a modulator of innate immunity during melioidosis. PloS Negl Trop Dis 11:e5548

41. Deshmukh HS, Liu Y, Menkiti OR et al (2014) The microbiota regulates neutrophil homeostasis and host resistance to Escherichia coli K1 sepsis in neonatal mice. Nat Med 20:524–530

42. Huffnagle GB, Dickson RP, Lukacs NW (2017) The respiratory tract microbiome and lung inflammation: a two-way street. Mucosal Immunol 10:299–306

43. Dickson RP, Huffnagle GB (2015) The lung microbiome: new principles for respiratory bacteriology in health and disease. PloS Pathog 11:e1004923

44. Dickson RP, Erb-Downward JR, Huffnagle GB (2014) Towards an ecology of the lung: new conceptual models of pulmonary microbiology and pneumonia pathogenesis. Lancet Respir Med 2:238–246

45. Budden KF, Gellatly SL, Wood DL (2017) Emerging pathogenic links between microbiota and the gut-lung axis. Nat Rev Microbiol 15:55–63

46. Marsland BJ, Trompette A, Gollwitzer ES (2015) The gut-lung axis in respiratory disease. Ann Am Thorac Soc 12(Suppl 2):S150–S156

47. Winglee K, Eloe-Fadrosh E, Gupta S, Guo H, Fraser C, Bishai W (2014) Aerosol Mycobacterium tuberculosis infection causes rapid loss of diversity in gut microbiota. PLoS One 9:e97048
48. Deriu E, Boxx GM, He X et al (2016) Influenza virus affects intestinal microbiota and secondary salmonella infection in the gut through type i interferons. PloS Pathog 12:e1005572
49. Manzanares W, Lemieux M, Langlois PL, Wischmeyer PE (2016) Probiotic and synbiotic therapy in critical illness: a systematic review and meta-analysis. Crit Care 19:262

In Pursuit of Precision Medicine in the Critically Ill

M. Shankar-Hari, C. Summers, and K. Baillie

Introduction

> For it is not enough to recognize that all our knowledge is, in a greater or less degree, uncertain and vague; it is necessary, at the same time, to learn to act upon the best hypothesis without dogmatically believing it (From 'Philosophy for Laymen' by Bertrand Russell).

Critical care medicine is, at present, a specialty of broad syndromes. This reflects the similarity in therapeutic approach required for the final common physiology that follows from many different pathological processes. Since their original definitions and descriptions, sepsis and acute respiratory distress syndrome (ARDS) are the two clinical conditions that have shaped health policy and dominated the research agenda in critical care [1, 2]. It is a truism to state that these are conglomerates of numerous different sub-syndromes; to make this observation is simply to restate the definition of sepsis and ARDS as common patterns arising from numerous different injuries. But it is also clear that, if we take the simple example of organ failure arising from a sterile versus an infectious insult, there is a very high likelihood that patients will respond differently to treatment with antibiotics. Or to take a more ambitious example, if we could diagnose, at presentation, the infectious agent caus-

M. Shankar-Hari (✉)
Guy's and St Thomas' NHS Foundation Trust, St Thomas' Hospital
London, UK
Division of Infection, Immunity and Inflammation, Kings College London
London, UK
e-mail: manu.shankar-hari@kcl.ac.uk

C. Summers
Department of Medicine, University of Cambridge School of Clinical Medicine
Cambridge, UK

K. Baillie
Intensive Care Unit, Royal Infirmary of Edinburgh
Edinburgh, UK
Roslin Institute, University of Edinburgh
Easter Bush, Midlothian, UK

© Springer International Publishing AG 2018
J.-L. Vincent (ed.), *Annual Update in Intensive Care and Emergency Medicine 2018*,
Annual Update in Intensive Care and Emergency Medicine,
https://doi.org/10.1007/978-3-319-73670-9_48

ing sepsis, we could then confidently treat with narrow spectrum antibiotics. In this way, sub-classifications of critical illness are almost certainly directly applicable to clinical practice.

With numerous statistically negative randomized controlled trials (RCTs) reported in both sepsis and ARDS, and strong conceptual arguments that patients presenting with these two conditions are heterogeneous, the idea of providing clinical care based on some patient level characteristic, along similar lines highlighted in cancer medicine is very appealing. Thus, critical care is contemplating approaches that are considered useful in cancer medicine and other clinical fields such as respiratory medicine, to inform clinical trials in sepsis and ARDS. However, the challenges with precision medicine in the critically ill could be related to the classic paper by Geoffrey Rose; "Sick Individuals and Sick Populations" [3]. The key principle is that individual and population approaches to improving health achieve different aims: the individual approach aims to protect susceptible (high-risk) patients, whereas the population approach aims to reduce the group level incidence of or outcome from diseases. In this short perspective, after discussing the rationale for current definitions, we discuss whether the heterogeneity and precision medicine concepts could inform future studies in sepsis and/or ARDS.

Rationale for ARDS and Sepsis Definitions with Predictive Validity

The latest ARDS [2] and sepsis definitions [1] and the corresponding clinical criteria [4–6] were derived to identify patient populations with predictive validity, by combining the consensus conference discussions with empirical evaluation of clinical data, resulting in valid and reliable critical illness syndromic definitions. ARDS is defined as acute onset hypoxemic respiratory failure despite a positive end-expiratory pressure (PEEP) of $5\,cmH_2O$ or greater, with non-cardiogenic pulmonary edema evidenced by bilateral chest opacities. With this definition, stages of mild, moderate, and severe ARDS based on severity of hypoxemia, were associated with significantly higher mortality and increased median duration of mechanical ventilation in survivors [2]. Sepsis is defined as life-threatening organ dysfunction caused by a dysregulated host response to infection, with organ dysfunction defined as an increase in the sequential organ failure assessment (SOFA) score of 2 points or more [4]. Septic shock was defined as a subset of sepsis in which profound circulatory, cellular, and metabolic abnormalities are associated with a greater risk of mortality than with sepsis alone. Patients with septic shock can be clinically identified by a vasopressor requirement to maintain a mean arterial pressure (MAP) of 65 mmHg or greater and serum lactate level greater than 2 mmol/l in the absence of hypovolemia [5]. With this definition, sepsis and septic shock were associated with significantly higher mortality, compared to uncomplicated infection [1]. The predictive validity for mortality categories could potentially inform clinical care and trial design. For example, worsening ARDS severity has been aligned with treatment options, with severe ARDS aligned with need for neuromuscular blockade, prone position and extracorporeal support [6].

Heterogeneity

Heterogeneity is the interindividual variation in susceptibility to either the illness or the outcome from illness or both. When risk factors for the illness or outcome are reported, the unstated (and likely incorrect) assumption is that these risk factors confer similar risk to individuals in a population, which is often overlooked during design, conduct and interpretation of studies [7]. Variation in the risk of illness or outcome is generated either as a random phenomenon, or due to measurable differences in biological characteristics in patients [8, 9], resulting from genetic and/or environmental influences. It is challenging to discern the relative contribution of each of these influences on outcomes in a critically ill patient with ARDS or sepsis. For contextualization to ARDS and sepsis patients, heterogeneity could be categorized into patient, illness biology and treatment response level differences.

Patient-level Heterogeneity

Patient-level heterogeneity contemplates broadly two questions – (a) why did this patient get this disease at this time [3]?; and (b) why did this patient have a different outcome, compared to another patient who appeared similar in many aspects of illness? The answers to these questions rely on understanding the determinants of susceptibility amongst individuals to the illness (risk of illness) and the illness-related outcomes (risk of outcome). For example, as sepsis is infection-related organ dysfunction, the risk factors for sepsis would include risk factors for infection and risk factors for developing organ dysfunction in the context of infection. The risk factors for developing organ dysfunction in the context of infection are poorly understood. The risk factors for infection include age with an inverted parabolic distribution with highest risk at extremes of age; male sex; ethnicity with black race and Asians having a greater risk; and presence of one or more comorbidity [10].

Genetic predisposition to infectious diseases is strongly heritable [11, 12], presumably because of the strong selective pressure exerted by pathogens on our ancestors. Identifying – and understanding – the genetic factors underlying predisposition may lead directly to tractable therapeutic targets in the host [13]. Several strong associations with susceptibility to infections have been discovered (e.g., human immunodeficiency virus [HIV], West Nile virus [WNV], tuberculosis, malaria, influenza, meningococcus) [14–16], but these tend to be highly pathogen-specific. Whether there is general genetic susceptibility to sepsis, or even more broadly to a deleterious response to sterile injury, remains an open question. However, several lines of evidence suggest that responses to critical illness are likely to exhibit heritable variation in human populations. First, the consensus in critical care medicine, supported by many years of clinical and animal model research, is that organ failure seen during critical illness is complex, driven by immune-mediated injury and alterations in bioenergetics [17, 18], alongside individual predisposition discussed as patient heterogeneity. Second, immune phenotypes tend to be strongly heritable, and numerous genetic associations for both autoimmune and infectious diseases have been discovered. Importantly, many of these disease associations are pleiotropic [19]. Hence, variation in the host responses to severe systemic injury is likely to be in part genetically-determined. Finally, and most directly, the results of the Genomic Advances in Sepsis (GAinS) and GenoSept studies have discovered some genetic associations with outcome in sepsis [20], which will be important candidates for further biological investigation.

Similarity within Sepsis and ARDS Biological Heterogeneity

Acute immune changes in sepsis, studied using whole blood transcriptomics, identifies a complex set of pro- and anti-inflammatory abnormalities in the innate and adaptive immune systems and alteration in genes highlighting mitochondrial dysfunction [21]. Antigen presenting cells, such as dendritic cells, monocyte-macrophage system, follicular dendritic cells, are impaired and there is accelerated depletion of B- and T-lymphocytes. When the same biology is studied by looking for unsupervised clustering algorithms, between 2 and 4 different sub-phenotypes within sepsis have been observed [18, 22–25]. At a clinical characteristic level, site of infection, numbers of organ dysfunctions, types of organ dysfunction and combination of organ dysfunctions also influence outcome from sepsis and add to this heterogeneity [26]. In ARDS, structural and functional disruption of the alveolar endothelial and epithelial barrier occur as a result of the generation of inflammasome and signalosome complexes, by leukocyte sensing of danger signals [27, 28]. The endothelial abnormalities and inflammatory responses observed in ARDS are also seen in sepsis and trauma [23, 29]. Furthermore, patients with ARDS could also be grouped into hyperinflammatory and non-reactive ARDS subphenotypes based on biomarkers and/or clinical variables [30–34] (Table 1).

Heterogeneity in Treatment Responses

For any treatment, the essential drivers arguing for a precision medicine approach, in the clinical or trial setting, include between-patient differences in treatment responses, patient-level interaction with treatment due to individual heterogeneity and the variation in treatment response determined by stage of illness due to variability in the lag time between onset of illness to treatment [35]. A simple example for the impact of time on treatment effect is the relationship between time to antibiotic treatment and outcome. In a cohort study, Seymour et al. highlighted that in patients who had the 3-hour Surviving Sepsis Campaign Bundle (blood culture, antibiotic therapy and measurement of lactate) completed within a 12-hour period, every extra hour taken to complete the bundle was associated with a significant increase in mortality [36]. Similarly, the treatment effect of drugs has been shown to vary with illness severity, using activated protein C trials in sepsis and effect of PEEP in ARDS [37] as examples. A related concept in this context is heterogeneity in treatment response, which is a crude omnibus test for differences in responses to

Table 1 Recent studies describing acute respiratory distress syndrome (ARDS) and sepsis sub-phenotypes

First author [reference] (population)	Sub-phenotypes	Comment
Calfee [33] (ARDS)	Hyperinflammatory phenotype versus phenotype-1	Latent class analysis-based grouping based on clinical and biomarker data. The discriminant markers between phenotypes were IL-6, sTNFR1, vasopressor use, IL-8, bicarbonate
Famous [32] (ARDS)	Hyperinflammatory phenotype versus pPhenotype-1	Latent class analysis-based grouping based on clinical and biomarker data. The discriminant markers between phenotypes were IL-8, sTNFR1, vasopressor use, bicarbonate, minute ventilation
Bos [30] (ARDS)	Reactive phenotype versus uninflamed phenotype	Agglomerative hierarchical cluster analyses based only on biomarker data. The discriminant markers between phenotypes were IL-6, IFNγ, ANG1/2, PAI-1
Davenport [23] (Sepsis)	Sepsis response signature-1 versus sepsis response signature-2	Agglomerative hierarchical clustering based on Ward's method using pan-leukocyte transcriptome using microarray. The discriminant markers between two phenotypes were seven genes – *DYRK2, CCNB1IP1, TDRD9, ZAP70, ARL14EP, MDC1*, and *ADGRE3*
Scicluna [25] (Sepsis)	Four molecular endotypes named as Mars1 to Mars4	Agglomerative hierarchical clustering based on Ward's method using pan-leukocyte transcriptome using microarray. The study showed that a 140-gene expression signature reliably stratified patients with sepsis to the four endotypes. The study also reported biomarkers for each endotype to facilitate clinical use: Mars1 = BPGM and TAP2; Mars2 = GADD45A and PCGF5; Mars3 = AHNAK and PDCD10; Mars4 = IFIT5, NOP53

IL: interleukin; *sTNFR1*: soluble tumor necrosis factor receptor; *IFNγ*: interferon gamma; *ANG1/2*: angiotensin; *PAI-1*: plasminogen activator inhibitor-1; *DYRK2*: dual specificity tyrosine phosphorylation regulated kinase 2; *CCNB1IP1*: cyclin B1 interacting protein 1; *TDRD9*: tudor domain containing 9; *ZAP70*: zeta chain of T-cell receptor associated protein kinase 70; *ARL14EP*: ADP ribosylation factor like GTPase 14 effector protein; *MDC1*: mediator of DNA damage checkpoint 1; *ADGRE3*: adhesion G protein-coupled receptor; *E3BPGM*: bisphosphoglycerate mutase; *TAP2*: ATP binding cassette subfamily B member transporter 2; *GADD45A*: growth arrest and DNA damage inducible alpha; *PCGF5*: polycomb group ring finger 5; *AHNAK*: AHNAK nucleoprotein; *PDCD10*: programmed cell death 10; *NOP53*: ribosome biogenesis factor

treatment and illness-related outcomes arising from all factors contributing to heterogeneity and stochasticity of risk. This has been illustrated using simulation of sepsis and ARDS RCTs [38] and by using completed RCT data from intravenous immunoglobulin trials in sepsis [39]. As the risk of death changes in a trial population, the differences in mortality between the intervention arm and the usual arm also changes. This could potentially highlight a risk of outcome-specific subgroups within ARDS and sepsis who are likely to benefit the most from the intervention.

Stratified Medicine and Enrichment

Stratified medicine refers to identifying groups of patients based on either characteristics of disease or likely treatment response at a population level. Enrichment markers are biomarkers that help identify treatment responders and/or patients with higher risk of certain outcomes [40]. Thus, in the context of sepsis and ARDS, stratified medicine (enrichment) of clinical trial populations is a potentially viable strategy, as differential biological mechanisms and the technical ability to prospectively identify patient subsets exist. For example, in children with septic shock, using a 100-gene profile and serum protein biomarkers, it is possible to identify two patient subsets, with different outcomes, and differential responses to corticosteroid treatment [41]. Similarly, in adults with septic shock, corticosteroid responders can be identified using a three-biomarker panel [42]. Similarly, ARDS subsets, which respond differently to ventilator and fluid management, have been identified using data from completed ARDS trials [32, 33].

In 2007, Trusheim et al. [40] proposed three necessary conditions required for effective stratified medicine for a disease: (a) differential biological mechanisms; (b) multiple treatment options; and (c) a clinical biomarker that links patient subsets to treatment responses. Sadly, in critical care medicine, we are a long way from meeting the second criterion: multiple treatment options.

However, as efforts have progressed to achieve these goals, both in critical care medicine and beyond, it has become clear that a necessary first step is the identification of a pattern, or subgroup, within heterogeneous patient populations. In itself, this is purely an exercise of academic interest, but where a common biological mechanism can be found, there is a reasonable chance that some current or future therapy might have a different effect in patients belonging to a given subgroup – this essentially is the definition of a disease endotype [43]. The process of identifying endotypes is conceptually identical to the approach taken by our medical forebears: a syndrome becomes a disease when the underlying mechanism is thought to be known. Given the interplay of multiple mechanisms, two or more endotypes are likely in ARDS and sepsis.

The identification of a disease endotype has immediate clinical relevance, since it is likely that patients with a given endotype will respond differently to some therapies when compared with patients having other patterns of disease. Once an endotype is convincingly discovered, considerable academic and commercial investment is applied to identifying treatments and viable biomarkers with which to make the diagnosis [44]. It is therefore important to consider carefully what criteria must be met for this enterprise to proceed. Differential response to therapy is probably too high a bar in critical care medicine, because in many cases the fundamental problem is that we lack specific diseases and therapies for those diseases. Thus, a major aspiration of this field is that, by better understanding the underlying biology, we may be able to create or repurpose drug treatments to modulate the host response to injury. At present, however, efforts to achieve this goal have failed. Aside from heterogeneity, this is not necessarily because of lack of understanding of the molecular mechanisms involved, but due to the complex interplay of many mechanisms contributing to the final outcome; targeting one particular mechanism may not yield the desired treatment benefit. Progress in identifying distinct disease processes in critical illness should not be held back by this limitation.

We therefore propose the following, permissive criteria to conclude that valid and reliable endotypes exist in critically ill populations. Subgroups should be:

1. Consistency
2. Biological plausibility
3. Clinical plausibility
4. Feasibility of implementation in clinical care and/or trials

Consistency can be measured using standard criteria for generalizability to other populations of similar patients. Where, as is often the case, expensive new technologies have been used to observe patterns in a group of patients, consistency must necessarily be determined within the original population, using a bootstrapping approach or similar.

Plausibility is a vague and subjective concept but we contend that most investigators know it when they see it. Biological plausibility can – in some cases – be determined by statistical tests applied to the biological signature that defines membership of a subgroup. Such signatures may depend on systematic collections of known biology, for example for pathway enrichment, or genome-wide methods [45], such as co-expression module enrichment [46]. If the number of tests performed is faithfully reported, these approaches can provide convincing evidence that a given grouping is biologically real. Clinical plausibility is an extension of this concept. Biological plausibility has obvious limitations: there are many real subgroupings of any population of patients. Hence, if there is not a predictable mechanism by which a given subgrouping could turn out to have a differential treatment effect, or at least a differential effect on prognosis, then the risk of failure is expected to be high.

Finally, feasibility represents a compromise between the truth of detection (validity) and reliability of measurements to identify subgroups. For example, a cytokine profile for identifying corticosteroid responders in septic shock [42] could be considered to have greater feasibility compared to a 100-gene expression panel [41], but with different reliability and validity. Importantly, it is possible, but not necessary, for clinical outcome to be different between endotypes: patients with different diagnoses can have identical statistical probabilities for a given outcome. A focus on outcome runs the risk of detecting severity markers, rather than distinct biological processes.

Precision Medicine

Fundamentally, precision medicine represents a scenario where detecting one or more biological abnormalities in patients helps pair them to treatment(s), based on the individuals' favorable treatment response–adverse effect profiles. Most precision medicine advances have been in oncology, although consistent success is limited. For example, super-responders to everolimus treatment considered as exemplar for precision oncology [47] have not been consistently replicated. Furthermore, the cancer-free survival amongst patients with relapse and/or refractory tumors is not impressive and super-responders to targeted chemotherapy may be a much smaller cancer population than previously considered [48]. For example, a recently published phase II multicenter RCT enrolled 741 adult patients with any kind of metastatic solid tumour refractory to standard of care. From this population, 40% of patients had at least one molecular alteration that matched with one of the 10 treatment regimens and 195 patients were randomized to receive experimental treatment specific for pathway mutations or standard of care. There were no differences in efficacy or adverse event endpoints between the intervention and control arms [49]. These lessons from precision oncology approaches must be seriously considered [50], when testing precision medicine in critically ill patients with heterogeneous syndromes such as sepsis or ARDS.

Conclusion

ARDS and sepsis often occur in older patients with comorbidity, resulting in critical illness. Heritable characteristics and environmental factors influence the incidence and outcomes from ARDS and sepsis. We have begun to group ARDS and sepsis patients with similar biological characteristics and consider stratified or precision medicine as the solution for overcoming statistically negative clinical trials. Key biological and clinical plausibility challenges need to be addressed to achieve major breakthroughs in future trials and in the clinical care of sepsis and ARDS patients.

References

1. Singer M, Deutschman CS, Seymour CW et al (2016) The Third International Consensus Definitions for Sepsis and Septic Shock (Sepsis-3). JAMA 315:801–810
2. Force ADT, Ranieri VM, Rubenfeld GD et al (2012) Acute respiratory distress syndrome: the Berlin definition. JAMA 307:2526–2533
3. Rose G (2001) Sick individuals and sick populations. Int J Epidemiol 30:427–432
4. Seymour CW, Liu VX, Iwashyna TJ et al (2016) Assessment of clinical criteria for sepsis: for the third international consensus definitions for sepsis and septic shock (Sepsis-3). JAMA 315:762–774
5. Shankar-Hari M, Phillips GS, Levy ML et al (2016) Developing a new definition and assessing new clinical criteria for septic shock: for the third international consensus definitions for sepsis and septic shock (Sepsis-3). JAMA 315:775–787
6. Ferguson ND, Fan E, Camporota L et al (2012) The Berlin definition of ARDS: an expanded rationale, justification, and supplementary material. Intensive Care Med 38:1573–1582
7. Aalen OO, Valberg M, Grotmol T, Tretli S (2015) Understanding variation in disease risk: the elusive concept of frailty. Int J Epidemiol 44:1408–1421
8. Smith GD (2011) Epidemiology, epigenetics and the 'Gloomy Prospect': embracing randomness in population health research and practice. Int J Epidemiol 40:537–562
9. Pearson H (2011) Epidemiology: study of a lifetime. Nature 471:20–24
10. Mayr FB, Yende S, Angus DC (2014) Epidemiology of severe sepsis. Virulence 5:4–11

11. Petersen L, Sorensen TI, Andersen PK (2010) A shared frailty model for case-cohort samples: parent and offspring relations in an adoption study. Stat Med 29:924–931

12. Sorensen TI, Nielsen GG, Andersen PK, Teasdale TW (1988) Genetic and environmental influences on premature death in adult adoptees. N Engl J Med 318:727–732

13. Baillie JK (2014) Translational genomics. Targeting the host immune response to fight infection. Science 344:807–808

14. Hill AV (2012) Evolution, revolution and heresy in the genetics of infectious disease susceptibility. Philos Trans R Soc Lond B Biol Sci 367:840–849

15. Everitt AR, Clare S, Pertel T et al (2012) IFITM3 restricts the morbidity and mortality associated with influenza. Nature 484:519–523

16. Glass WG, McDermott DH, Lim JK et al (2006) CCR5 deficiency increases risk of symptomatic West Nile virus infection. J Exp Med 203:35–40

17. Singer M (2014) The role of mitochondrial dysfunction in sepsis-induced multi-organ failure. Virulence 5:66–72

18. van der Poll T, van de Veerdonk FL, Scicluna BP, Netea MG (2017) The immunopathology of sepsis and potential therapeutic targets. Nat Rev Immunol 17:407–420

19. Sivakumaran S, Agakov F, Theodoratou E (2011) Abundant pleiotropy in human complex diseases and traits. Am J Hum Genet 89:607–618

20. Rautanen A, Mills TC, Gordon AC et al (2015) Genome-wide association study of survival from sepsis due to pneumonia: an observational cohort study. Lancet Respir Med 3:53–60

21. Sweeney TE, Shidham A, Wong HR, Khatri P (2015) A comprehensive time-course-based multicohort analysis of sepsis and sterile inflammation reveals a robust diagnostic gene set. Sci Transl Med 7:287ra271

22. Burnham KL, Davenport EE, Radhakrishnan J et al (2017) Shared and distinct aspects of the sepsis transcriptomic response to fecal peritonitis and pneumonia. Am J Respir Crit Care Med 196:328–339

23. Davenport EE, Burnham KL, Radhakrishnan J et al (2016) Genomic landscape of the individual host response and outcomes in sepsis: a prospective cohort study. Lancet Respir Med 4:259–271

24. Rautanen A, Mills TC, Gordon AC et al (2015) Genome-wide association study of survival from sepsis due to pneumonia: an observational cohort study. Lancet Respir Med 3(1):53–60

25. Scicluna BP, van Vught LA, Zwinderman AH et al (2017) Classification of patients with sepsis according to blood genomic endotype: a prospective cohort study. Lancet Respir Med 5:816–826

26. Shankar-Hari M, Harrison DA, Rowan KM (2016) Differences in impact of definitional elements on mortality precludes international comparisons of sepsis epidemiology—a cohort study illustrating the need for standardized reporting. Crit Care Med 44:2223–2230

27. Dolinay T, Kim YS, Howrylak J et al (2012) Inflammasome-regulated cytokines are critical mediators of acute lung injury. Am J Respir Crit Care Med 185:1225–1234

28. Matthay MA, Ware LB, Zimmerman GA (2012) The acute respiratory distress syndrome. J Clin Invest 122:2731–2740

29. Xiao W, Mindrinos MN, Seok J et al (2011) A genomic storm in critically injured humans. J Exp Med 208:2581–2590

30. Bos LD, Schouten LR, van Vught LA et al (2017) Identification and validation of distinct biological phenotypes in patients with acute respiratory distress syndrome by cluster analysis. Thorax 72:876–883

31. Calfee CS, Janz DR, Bernard GR et al (2015) Distinct molecular phenotypes of direct vs indirect ARDS in single-center and multicenter studies. Chest 147:1539–1548

32. Famous KR, Delucchi K, Ware LB et al (2017) Acute respiratory distress syndrome subphenotypes respond differently to randomized fluid management strategy. Am J Respir Crit Care Med 195:331–338

33. Calfee CS, Delucchi K, Parsons PE et al (2014) Subphenotypes in acute respiratory distress syndrome: latent class analysis of data from two randomised controlled trials. Lancet Respir Med 2:611–620
34. Calfee C, Matthay M (2010) Clinical immunology: culprits with evolutionary ties. Nature 464:41–42
35. Senn S (2016) Mastering variation: variance components and personalised medicine. Stat Med 35:966–977
36. Seymour CW, Gesten F, Prescott HC et al (2017) Time to treatment and mortality during mandated emergency care for sepsis. N Engl J Med 376:2235–2244
37. Shankar-Hari M, Rubenfeld GD (2017) The use of enrichment to reduce statistically indeterminate or negative trials in critical care. Anaesthesia 72:560–565
38. Iwashyna TJ, Burke JF, Sussman JB, Prescott HC, Hayward RA, Angus DC (2015) Implications of heterogeneity of treatment effect for reporting and analysis of randomized trials in critical care. Am J Respir Crit Care Med 192:1045–1051
39. Welton NJ, Soares MO, Palmer S et al (2015) Accounting for heterogeneity in relative treatment effects for use in cost-effectiveness models and value-of-information analyses. Med Decis Making 35:608–621
40. Trusheim MR, Berndt ER, Douglas FL (2007) Stratified medicine: strategic and economic implications of combining drugs and clinical biomarkers. Nat Rev Drug Discov 6:287–293
41. Wong HR, Atkinson SJ, Cvijanovich NZ et al (2016) Combining prognostic and predictive enrichment strategies to identify children with septic shock responsive to corticosteroids. Crit Care Med 44:e1000–e1003
42. Bentzer P, Fjell C, Walley KR, Boyd J, Russell JA (2016) Plasma cytokine levels predict response to corticosteroids in septic shock. Intensive Care Med 42:1970–1979
43. Russell CD, Baillie J (2017) Treatable traits and therapeutic targets. Curr Opin Syst Biol 2:140–146
44. Lotvall J, Akdis CA, Bacharier LB et al (2011) Asthma endotypes: a new approach to classification of disease entities within the asthma syndrome. J Allergy Clin Immunol 127:355–360
45. Khatri P, Sirota M, Butte AJ (2012) Ten years of pathway analysis: current approaches and outstanding challenges. PloS Comput Biol 8:e1002375
46. Forrest AR, Kawaji H, Rehli M et al (2014) A promoter-level mammalian expression atlas. Nature 507:462–470
47. Iyer G, Hanrahan AJ, Milowsky MI et al (2012) Genome sequencing identifies a basis for everolimus sensitivity. Science 338:221
48. Prasad V (2016) Perspective: the precision-oncology illusion. Nature 537:S63–S63
49. Le Tourneau C, Delord JP, Goncalves A et al (2015) Molecularly targeted therapy based on tumour molecular profiling versus conventional therapy for advanced cancer (SHIVA): a multicentre, open-label, proof-of-concept, randomised, controlled phase 2 trial. Lancet Oncol 16:1324–1334
50. Stewart DJ, Kurzrock R (2013) Fool's gold, lost treasures, and the randomized clinical trial. BMC Cancer 13:193

Future Roles for Xenon in Emergency Medicine and Critical Care

T. Laitio and M. Maze

Introduction

We are at an auspicious juncture regarding the clinical use of xenon, the rarest of the noble gases, present at only 89 parts/billion in the earth's atmosphere. A half-century after xenon's discovery by Sir William Ramsay and Dr. Morris Travers in 1898, Lawrence reported on its anesthetic properties in preclinical studies [1]. Shortly thereafter, Cullen and Gross published on xenon's administration (50%) to volunteers in which its analgesic and subjective effects were compared to nitrous oxide; the authors also self-administered xenon (70%) and described rapid onset of loss and return of consciousness [2]. These two intrepid investigators also provided the first documented cases of general anesthesia in two adult surgical patients and again reported on its rapid onset and offset [2]. After a further 50 years, xenon received market authorization for its clinical use as an anesthetic, first in Russia and subsequently in Western Europe where it received a label for use in general anesthesia for American Society of Anaesthesiologists physical classification (ASA) I–II patients in 2005.

At the turn of the century, work from Nick Franks' laboratory addressed the molecular sites of anesthetic action; their findings of xenon's antagonist action at the N-methyl-d-aspartate (NMDA) subtype of the glutamate receptor ushered in an intense period of preclinical investigations that identified several organ protective effects [3]. Recently, these investigations have culminated in clinical trials testing

T. Laitio
Division of Perioperative Services, Intensive Care Medicine and Pain Management, Turku University Hospital
Turku, Finland

M. Maze (✉)
Center for Cerebrovascular Research, Department of Anesthesia and Perioperative Care, University of California
San Francisco, CA, USA
e-mail: Mervyn.maze@ucsf.edu

© Springer International Publishing AG 2018

J.-L. Vincent (ed.), *Annual Update in Intensive Care and Emergency Medicine 2018*,
Annual Update in Intensive Care and Emergency Medicine,
https://doi.org/10.1007/978-3-319-73670-9_49

the efficacy and safety of xenon for brain and other organ protection in the acute care settings.

In this chapter, we will provide the scientific basis for the various medical applications of xenon, ranging from anesthesia/sedation, imaging, through to acute ongoing neurological injury. Thereafter, we will discuss in some detail the conduct and results of recently completed clinical trials and finally consider the future uses of xenon.

Molecular Basis for Xenon's Medical Uses

Anesthesia

According to the Meyer-Overton hypothesis of anesthetic action, xenon was predicted to exert a narcotizing effect based upon its high solubility in olive oil. Xenon's Ostwald coefficient, the ratio of the concentration in solvent to the concentration in the gas in contact with the solvent, is 1.8 for oil/gas. More remarkable is how insoluble xenon is in blood with a blood/gas solubility of 0.115, which provides the physico-chemical basis for the extremely fast onset and offset of xenon [4].

The lipid theory of anesthetic action, based on the Meyer-Overton hypothesis, has now been discredited [5] leading to a concerted effort to discover specific protein sites for anesthetic action. For xenon, this is particularly intriguing because of its chemical non-reactivity, a feature shared with the other noble gases. With an octet of tightly-bound electrons in its outer orbital, xenon exists in an extremely stable and minimum energy configuration. Therefore, xenon is unable to form covalent bonds and remains in its mono-atomic form and cannot form adducts, as electrons cannot be added or subtracted from its outermost orbital. Yet xenon can interact with other molecules because the arrangement of the electrons can be induced to form dipoles that line up to match the charges of adjacent molecules, thereby attracting xenon through London dispersion forces, part of the Van Der Waals interaction. These weak forces exist over a very short distance and therefore xenon has to 'fit' into a pre-formed space quite snugly in order to perturb a neighboring molecular species.

A plethora of protein candidates has been advanced as molecular targets for general anesthetic action, none more so than the gamma amino butyric acid (GABA) receptor [6]. Unlike most other general anesthetics, xenon has no activity at the $GABA_A$ receptors as shown initially by *in vitro* studies [7] and subsequently confirmed by positron-emission tomography (PET) scanning studies in human volunteers [8]. As there are more than 250 structures containing xenon in the Research Collaboratory for Structural Bioinformatics (RCSB) protein data bank (http://www.rcsb.org) there have been exhaustive studies to identify the precise molecular species for xenon's anesthetic action. We now focus on the likeliest of the possible candidates.

NMDA Subtype of the Glutamate Receptor

Franks' group showed an important interaction with NMDA receptors, a pivotal protein thought to be involved in the anesthetic action of compounds such as ketamine and nitrous oxide. In their demonstration, xenon inhibited NMDA-evoked currents in cultured hippocampal neurons by ~60% at a xenon concentration (80% of one atmosphere) that was close to minimum anesthetic concentration [3]. Unlike most NMDA antagonists that have an ion-pore blocking action, xenon competes with glycine for the NMDA receptor's co-activation site [9]. *In vivo* confirmation for the NMDA receptor as a site for xenon's anesthetic effect is lacking.

α-Amino-3-hydroxy-5-methyl-4-isoxazolepropionic Aide (AMPA)/Kainate Subtype of the Glutamate Receptor

While Franks' group found little evidence for xenon's actions at the AMPA receptor when glutamate was the applied agonist [6], there was a significant inhibitory effect when kainate was the agonist [10]. Others have now confirmed with patch-clamping of brain slices that AMPA transmission is inhibited by xenon under physiological conditions [11]. Thus far there has been no *in vivo* confirmation for the AMPA/kainate receptor being the site of xenon's anesthetic action.

Hyperpolarization-activated Cyclic Nucleotide-gated (HCN)-1 Channel

HCN-1 channels are highly-expressed in regions of the brain that are most affected by general anesthetics and are considered to be the site for the hypnotic action of ketamine [12]. Using an impressive array of both *in vitro* and *in vivo* techniques, Mattusch and colleagues showed a significant inhibition of this channel in thalamocortical tracts and the absence of xenon's sedative effect when tested in mice lacking this channel [13].

Neuroprotection

NMDA Subtype of the Glutamate Receptor

As we have alluded to in the section on possible targets for xenon's anesthetic action the NMDA receptor is inhibited by xenon [3]. While it is not known whether this effect is the mechanism for xenon's anesthetic action, it is likely that the NMDA subtype is a target for xenon's neuroprotective properties because of the key mediating role of glutamate-induced excitotoxicity in acute ongoing neurologic injury. Therefore, the finding that an over-abundance of glycine overcomes both xenon's NMDA-induced inhibition as well as its protective effect in a traumatic brain slice injury model is quite compelling [14].

Two-pore-domain Potassium Channels

These channels provide a background "leak" current that attenuates neuronal excitability and confers neuroprotection [15] including that produced by sevoflurane preconditioning [16]. Therefore, the finding that xenon potently activates TREK-

1 channels provides another possible mechanism for its neuroprotective properties [17].

Plasmalemmal Adenosine Triphosphate-sensitive Potassium Channels (K$_{ATP}$ Channels)

In an *in vitro* neuronal-glial co-culture model, xenon protected against oxygen-glucose deprivation injury through activation of the K$_{ATP}$ channels in the plasmalemma [18]

Organ Protective Effects

Perhaps the most unique property of xenon is its ability to increase translation and expression of the transcription factor hypoxia-inducible factor-1α (HIF-1α) under normoxic conditions [19]. HIF-1α binds to hypoxia-responsive elements on a number of genes resulting in upregulation of cytoprotective factors, such as erythropoietin and vascular endothelial growth factor (VEGF) that are known to be protective in several organ injury models.

Myocardial Protection

In myocardial models of ischemia/reperfusion injury, xenon preconditioning limits injury through phosphorylation and hence activation of protein kinase Cε as well as P38 mitogen-activated protein kinase (MAPK) [20].

Lung Protection

In a transplant model of acute lung injury, xenon conferred protection by mitigating the translocation of high-mobility group box 1 protein (HMGB1) from cell nuclei thereby limiting activity in the Toll-like receptor-4-nuclear factor-kappa B (TLR4-NF-κB) inflammatory pathway [21].

Kidney Protection

Xenon protects against kidney injury in several different models including (i) gentamycin-induced nephrotoxicity through an antioxidant effect [22]; (ii) transplantation with cold ischemia/reperfusion by enhanced expression of the anti-apoptotic factor, BCl-2, and heat shock protein (HSP) 70 [23]; and (iii) with prolonged hypothermic storage of allografts through increased expression of HSP 70 and heme oxygenase-1 [24].

Imaging

Xenon has many different isotopes, eight of which are stable, and more than 30 are radioactive. Several of these isotopes have been investigated for their use in imaging brain, heart and lung using three different technical approaches. First, stable isotopes can be used as contrast agents because they are radiopaque and have been used with computed tomography (CT) imaging of cerebral blood flow [25]. The stable isotope ^{131}Xe has been widely used to determine regional ventilation and perfusion in the lung and has been explored for diagnostic imaging in pancreatic and hepatic disease [26]. Second, trace amounts of radioactive isotopes, usually ^{133}Xe, can be used in single photon emission CT (SPECT). Finally, some xenon isotopes, especially ^{129}Xe, can be spin-polarized as a method for enhancing contrast [27].

Foundation Preclinical Studies for Present and Future Medical Uses of Xenon

Anesthesia/Sedation

Lawrence and colleagues exposed six mice to one atmosphere of xenon-oxygen gas containing no less than 20% oxygen and noted a rapid onset of a narcotizing effect in 5 of the 6 mice [1].

Neuroprotection

Hypoxic-ischemic encephalopathy
The combination of xenon with modest hypothermia provided a synergistic neuroprotective effect (by morphological and functional endpoints) in the Rice-Vannucci model of neonatal asphyxia in rats [28]. Similarly, in neonatal piglets, xenon augmented the neuroprotective effect of hypothermia assessed by magnetic resonance spectroscopy (MRS) [29]. Thoresen's group showed significant improvement in outcome at 10 weeks when the combination of xenon and hypothermia was administered in the Rice-Vannucci injury model [30].

Out-of-hospital Cardiac Arrest
In an adult model of cardiac arrest in pigs, prior administration of xenon was associated with reduced levels of a neurochemical biomarker of brain injury [31]. Xenon exposure, beginning 1 h after cardiac arrest in adult pigs, improved brain morphological outcome [32]. A combination of mild hypothermia and xenon after 10 min of cardiac arrest in pigs also improved functional outcome within the first 5 days [33].

Stroke
Using different rodent stroke models, Warner's group demonstrated a dose-dependent improvement in both functional and histologic outcomes following xenon exposure in transient middle cerebral artery occlusion [34] and, either alone or with hypothermia, xenon showed an enduring benefit following either an ischemic or hemorrhagic stroke-type injury [35].

Traumatic Brain Injury

In a brain slice model of traumatic injury, xenon reduced morphologic changes even when administered up to 3 h post-injury [36]. Similarly, xenon improved both functional and morphological outcomes when exposure occurred after a controlled cortical impact in mice [37].

Cardiopulmonary Bypass

In a rat model of cardiopulmonary bypass (CPB)-induced brain injury, exposure to xenon during CPB provided functional and morphological improvement in outcome [38].

Postoperative Cognitive Decline

Postoperative cognitive decline is thought to be due to an inflammatory response to surgical trauma through the engagement of the innate immune system by HMGB1 that is released by tissue injury [39]. Neuroinflammation has also been documented in patients with postoperative cognitive decline [40]. Xenon has been shown to retain HMGB1 in the nuclear compartment thereby preventing its release and consequent inflammation, which may benefit postoperative cognitive decline [21].

Myocardial Protection

When rats were pretreated with three pulses of xenon prior to coronary artery occlusion-reperfusion, the size of myocardial infarction was diminished [20]

Renal Protection

Xenon pre-conditioning limited morphological and functional damage in ischemic-reperfusion kidney injury in mice [19]. In a syngeneic rat model of kidney transplantation, xenon exposure to either the donor or the recipient improved post-transplant kidney function [23]. In a prolonged hypothermic renal graft injury, xenon administered to either the donor or the recipient improved post-transplant graft survival [24]. When the solution containing a renal graft was supplemented with xenon, both functional and morphological outcomes were improved post-transplant [41].

Clinical Experience with Xenon in Critical Care and Emergency Medicine

Neuroprotection

Following the compelling preclinical evidence establishing xenon's neuroprotective properties, several groups have conducted clinical trials to investigate xenon's efficacy and safety in patients suffering from acute ongoing neurological injury [42–46].

Xe-HypotheCA Trial (NCT00879892)

A randomized, single blinded, phase II clinical drug trial investigated the effects of xenon on the extent of brain white matter damage assessed by diffusion tensor imaging sequence (DTI) of magnetic resonance imaging (MRI) scan in comatose survivors from out-of-hospital cardiac arrest (OHCA) [43]. Patients were randomized to receive either therapeutic hypothermia treatment at 33 °C alone for 24 h (defined as the control group) or inhaled xenon (~ 40–50%) with hypothermia (33 °C) for 24 h (xenon group). The main inclusion criteria were witnessed OHCA from shockable initial rhythm and restoration of spontaneous circulation (ROSC) within 45 min. Further details of inclusion and exclusion criteria are listed in Laitio et al. [43]. Xenon inhalation was initiated in the ICU within 4 h after arrival to hospital and was continued until completion of the 24-hour cooling period.

After re-warming was completed, MRI was performed with a 3 T scanner with tract-based spatial statistical analysis (TBSS) [47]. Lower fractional anisotropy values reflect more extensive white matter damage [48]. One hundred and ten patients were enrolled and randomly assigned to xenon and control groups (n = 55/group). There were 34 non-survivors of whom 29 (85.3%) had a neurological mode of death. DTI-MRI data for TBSS analysis were obtained from 48 patients in the xenon group and from 49 patients in the control group. The age, sex and site-adjusted mean global fractional anisotropy (GFA) value was 3.8% higher in the xenon group (adjusted mean difference 0.016 [95% CI 0.005–0.027], p = 0.006). The 3.8% magnitude of change needs to be considered in the context of a 6.4% difference in GFA values between survivors and non-survivors. Each 0.01 unit increase in GFA decreased the risk of death by 19%; age, sex, group and site-adjusted hazard ratio (HR) 0.81 (95% CI 0.69–0.94, p = 0.006). These results indicate that there had been more severe damage of white matter in the control group (Fig. 1). Regarding clinical outcome (for which the study was not powered) 6-month mortality was 15/55 (27.7%) in the xenon group and 19/55 (34.5%) in the control group (adjusted HR 0.49 [95% CI 0.23–1.01], p = 0.053). The neurological outcome at six months was similar between the groups.

CoolXenon Trial (NCT02071394)

In a single arm dose-escalation feasibility study, xenon (50%) was administered to 14 infants who received therapeutic hypothermia for hypoxic-ischemic encephalopathy [44]. Primary outcome (cardiorespiratory stability, electroencephalography [EEG] parameters and feasibility) was compared to 42 case-matched neonates that received only therapeutic hypothermia. At 18 months, 7 of 14 patients survived with a good clinical outcome; 3 died while in hospital and 4 survivors had disability at 18 months. Therefore, death and disability occurred in 50% of patients; historically this number is 75%. The ongoing CoolXenon trial involves randomization to either therapeutic hypothermia alone or xenon (50% for 18 h) plus therapeutic hypothermia. The co-primary outcomes are death and disability

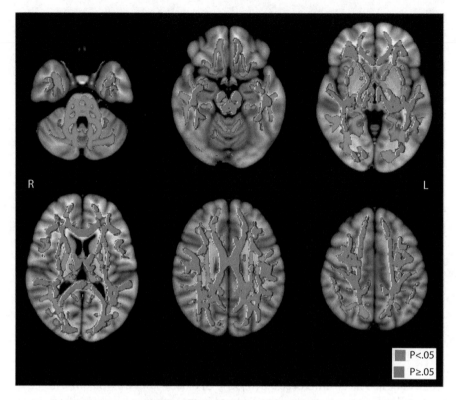

Fig. 1 The visualization presents the results of the voxel-wise tract-based spatial statistics analysis of fractional anisotropy values between the xenon group and the control group. Voxels with significantly (p < 0.05, family-wise error corrected for multiple comparisons) higher fractional anisotropy values in the xenon group were identified and are shown in *red* in the statistical visualization (i.e., 41.7% of all 119,013 analyzed voxels), whereas areas in which there were no significant differences in fractional anisotropy values between the groups are shown in *green* (i.e., 58.3% of all analyzed voxels). Reproduced from [43] with permission

at 18 months. Secondary endpoints include MRI brain scan within 2 weeks of birth. At the time of writing, a further 9 patients are required to achieve their target enrollment of 52 patients (Personal Communication – Dr. John Dingley).

TOBY-Xe Trial (NCT00934700)
A randomized open label clinical trial assessed whether the combination of cooling (33°C for 72 h beginning within 6 h of birth) with inhaled xenon (30% beginning within 12 h of birth) could improve neurological outcomes after hypoxic ischemic encephalopathy [46]. Full details of the inclusion and exclusion criteria were reported in an earlier feasibility and safety report at which time fewer seizures were noted in the xenon group [45]. Pre-enrolment, it was estimated that a sample size of 138 would have 80% power to detect a difference (2-sided 5% significance level) in the geometric mean lactate to N-acetyl aspartate ratio between groups. Only 92

of the targeted 138 patients were enrolled with 46 in each group and scans were obtained in 37 (80%) of 46 infants in the cooling group and 41 (89%) in the cooling plus xenon group. There was no difference observed in either of the two co-primary outcomes namely, a reduction in lactate to N-acetyl aspartate ratio in the thalamus detected by MRS or better preservation of fractional anisotropy in the posterior limb of the internal capsule assessed by TBSS. Nine (20%) infants in the cooling group and 11 (24%) in the cooling plus xenon group died (relative risk 1.22, 99% CI 0.44–3.41). Neither event rates of adverse outcomes nor other clinical measures examined before discharge from hospital nor the distribution of MRI scores between groups differed significantly. These data are consistent with preclinical studies in which xenon only provided a neuroprotective effect if the delay to treatment was less than 5 h.

HIPELD Trial (NCT01199276)

Coburn and colleagues evaluated the safety of xenon and its effects on the incidence of postoperative delirium in elderly ($\geq$ 75 years old) hip fracture surgery patients who are at high risk for postoperative complications [49]. In a phase II, multicenter, randomized, double-blind, parallel-group, controlled clinical trial, 260 hip fracture patients were randomized to receive either xenon (n = 124) or sevoflurane-based (n = 132) general anaesthesia during surgery. Patients in the xenon group received $60 \pm 5\%$ xenon (approximately 1 MAC) and patients in the sevoflurane group received 1 MAC of sevoflurane with titration of anaesthetic supplements using depth of anaesthesia monitoring with the bispectral index (40–60). The sample size was based on an expected postoperative delirium event rate of 30% within 4 days after surgery with sevoflurane anaesthesia and a 50% reduction by xenon. Xenon (9.7%, 95% CI 4.5–14.9) was associated with a non-statistically lower incidence of postoperative delirium than sevoflurane (13.6%, 95% CI: 7.8–19.5). Sequential organ failure assessment (SOFA) scores were significantly (p = 0.017) lower with xenon as was the incidence of serious adverse events (SAEs). Mortality rate trended lower in the xenon group (0% vs 3.8%; p = 0.06). The lower-than-expected incidence of postoperative delirium in the sevoflurane group (expected rate of 30% and observed rate of 13.6%) resulted in an underpowered study that precluded a type 2 error for the primary endpoint. The exploratory observations concerning postoperative SOFA scores, SAEs, and deaths warrant further study of the potential benefits of xenon in this surgical population.

Feasibility and Safety of Receiving Xenon During CPB

A Phase I open-label dose-escalation study (0, 20, 35, 50% xenon in oxygen and air) investigated the safety and feasibility of administering xenon to sixteen patients undergoing coronary artery bypass grafting (CABG) while on hypothermic cardiopulmonary bypass [50]. Middle cerebral artery Doppler showed no evidence of increased emboli with xenon. Patients receiving xenon had no major organ dysfunction: Troponin I and S100 levels tended to be lower in patients receiving xenon. Further studies are warranted to investigate xenon's clinical benefit in patients undergoing cardiac surgery.

Planned Phase III Trial of Xenon for Neuroprotection for OHCA (NCT03176186)

Following the demonstration of both safety and efficacy in the Imaging Biomarker phase II (Xe-Hypotheca) study, NeuroproteXeon will launch a pivotal phase III trial entitled XePOHCAS, Xenon for Post Out-of-Hospital Cardiac Arrest Syndrome. In 1436 successfully resuscitated adult survivors following an OHCA, standard-of-care for post-cardiac arrest intensive care (including 24 h targeted temperature management [TTM]) will be compared to the same treatment with the addition of 50% xenon for 24 h by inhalation. The primary objective is to evaluate, at 30-days and 90-days post-OHCA, whether there is a difference in good functional outcome (modified Rankin Scale score of ≤ 2) in comatose subjects after OHCA who were treated during TTM with xenon 50% + oxygen vs. those receiving similar oxygen treatment during TTM, but without supplementary xenon. Among the secondary objectives, the trial will evaluate whether there is a difference in survival to day 30 and day 90. The inclusion criteria will be similar to those of Xe-Hypotheca but inclusion is not limited to patients with an initial shockable rhythm [43]; new exclusion criteria include a ROSC of > 30 min and hypoxemia (oxygen saturation of < 90%) with a fraction of inspired oxygen (FiO_2) of $\geq 50\%$. There will be an interim and final analysis; the same primary and secondary endpoint analyses will be performed in each. The analyses will use an O'Brien-Fleming sequential design and stopping rules.

Myocardial Protection

Xe-HypotheCA Trial (NCT00879892)

In the Xe-HypotheCA Trial, an *a priori* defined analysis for the effect of xenon on myocardial injury revealed that the xenon-exposed TTM patients had significantly less troponin T release than the patients who received TTM alone [51]. Furthermore, in the setting of CABG surgery, xenon-exposed patients had significantly less myocardial injury, as reflected by troponin I release than those who were randomized to receive propofol and a non-inferior impact compared to sevoflurane-receiving CABG patients [52].

Conclusion

Xenon has an enviable safety record in acute care settings and is arguably the safest general anesthetic in use today. Because of its scarcity, the costs of xenon are quite high and sophisticated delivery systems are needed to mitigate the expense. Although there are suitable alternatives for general anesthesia, xenon's future entry into clinical practice will be for intensive care and emergency medicine conditions in which there are no appropriate alternatives. Foremost amongst these is the use of xenon to prevent acute ongoing neurological injury, also termed neuroprotection. Studies have now progressed to a pivotal phase III randomized clinical trial for comatose victims at risk of further neurologic injury from the post-cardiac arrest syndrome, a global type of ischemia/reperfusion injury. For this hospital-based intervention, xenon 50% will be delivered for the 24-hour period that the patient receives TTM. The primary endpoint will be survival with good functional outcome measured at both 30 and 90 days. If the pivotal trial is successful then xenon should be further considered for other settings in which neuroprotection may be beneficial including stroke and traumatic brain injury. However, for these clinical indications, pre-hospital xenon administration will be required, necessitating the development of a delivery system that can be used in the field by emergency medical services.

References

1. Lawrence JH, Loomis WF, Tobias CA, Turpin FH (1946) Preliminary observations on the narcotic effect of xenon with a review of values for solubilities of gases in water and oils. J Physiol 105:197–204
2. Cullen SC, Gross EG (1951) The anesthetic properties of xenon in animals and human beings, with additional observations on krypton. Science 113:580–582
3. Franks NP, Dickinson R, de Sousa SL, Hall AC, Lieb WR (1998) How does xenon produce anaesthesia? Nature 396:324
4. Goto T, Suwa K, Uezono S, Ichinose F, Uchiyama M, Morita S (1998) The blood-gas partition coefficient of xenon may be lower than generally accepted. Br J Anaesth 80:255–256
5. Franks NP, Lieb WR (1984) Do general anaesthetics act by competitive binding to specific receptors? Nature 310:599–601
6. Forman SA, Miller KW (2016) Mapping general anesthetic sites in heteromeric gamma-aminobutyric acid type a receptors reveals a potential for targeting receptor subtypes. Anesth Analg 123:1263–1273
7. de Sousa SL, Dickinson R, Lieb WR, Franks NP (2000) Contrasting synaptic actions of the inhalational general anesthetics isoflurane and xenon. Anesthesiology 92:1055–1066
8. Westkaemper RB, Glennon RA (1991) Approaches to molecular modeling studies and specific application to serotonin ligands and receptors. Pharmacol Biochem Behav 40:1019–1031
9. Banks P, Franks NP, Dickinson R (2010) Competitive inhibition at the glycine site of the N-methyl-D-aspartate receptor mediates xenon neuroprotection against hypoxia-ischemia. Anesthesiology 112:614–622
10. Plested AJ, Wildman SS, Lieb WR, Franks NP (2004) Determinants of the sensitivity of AMPA receptors to xenon. Anesthesiology 100:347–358
11. Haseneder R, Kratzer S, Kochs E, Mattusch C, Eder M, Rammes G (2009) Xenon attenuates excitatory synaptic transmission in the rodent prefrontal cortex and spinal cord dorsal horn. Anesthesiology 111:1297–1307
12. Zhou C, Douglas JE, Kumar NN, Shu S, Bayliss DA, Chen X (2013) Forebrain HCN1 channels contribute to hypnotic actions of ketamine. Anesthesiology 118:785–795
13. Mattusch C, Kratzer S, Buerge M et al (2015) Impact of hyperpolarization-activated, cyclic nucleotide-gated cation channel type 2 for the xenon-mediated anesthetic effect: evidence from in vitro and in vivo experiments. Anesthesiology 122:1047–1059
14. Harris K, Armstrong SP, Campos-Pires R, Kiru L, Franks NP, Dickinson R (2013) Neuroprotection against traumatic brain injury by xenon, but not argon, is mediated by inhibition at the N-methyl-D-aspartate receptor glycine site. Anesthesiology 119:1137–1148
15. Feliciangeli S, Chatelain FC, Bichet D, Lesage F (2015) The family of K2P channels: salient structural and functional properties. J Physiol 593:2587–2603
16. Tong L, Cai M, Huang Y, Zhang H, Su B, Li Z, Dong H (2014) Activation of K(2)P channel-TREK1 mediates the neuroprotection induced by sevoflurane preconditioning. Br J Anaesth 113:157–167

17. Gruss M, Bushell TJ, Bright DP, Lieb WR, Mathie A, Franks NP (2004) Two-pore-domain K+ channels are a novel target for the anesthetic gases xenon, nitrous oxide, and cyclopropane. Mol Pharmacol 65:443–452

18. Bantel C, Maze M, Trapp S (2009) Neuronal preconditioning by inhalational anesthetics: evidence for the role of plasmalemmal adenosine triphosphate-sensitive potassium channels. Anesthesiology 110:986–995

19. Ma D, Lim T, Xu J et al (2009) Xenon preconditioning protects against renal ischemic-reperfusion injury via HIF-1alpha activation. J Am Soc Nephrol 20:713–720

20. Weber NC, Toma O, Wolter JI et al (2005) The noble gas xenon induces pharmacological preconditioning in the rat heart in vivo via induction of PKC-epsilon and p38 MAPK. Br J Pharmacol 144:123–132

21. Zhao H, Huang H, Ologunde R et al (2015) Xenon treatment protects against remote lung injury after kidney transplantation in rats. Anesthesiology 122:1312–1326

22. Jia P, Teng J, Zou J et al (2013) Intermittent exposure to xenon protects against gentamicin-induced nephrotoxicity. PLoS One 8:e64329

23. Zhao H, Watts HR, Chong M et al (2013) Xenon treatment protects against cold ischemia associated delayed graft function and prolongs graft survival in rats. Am J Transplant 13:2006–2018

24. Zhao H, Yoshida A, Xiao W et al (2013) Xenon treatment attenuates early renal allograft injury associated with prolonged hypothermic storage in rats. FASEB J 27:4076–4088

25. Yonas H, Wolfson SK Jr et al (1984) Clinical experience with the use of xenon-enhanced CT blood flow mapping in cerebral vascular disease. Stroke 15:443–450

26. Lusic H, Grinstaff MW (2013) X-ray-computed tomography contrast agents. Chem Rev 113:1641–1666

27. Kauczor H, Surkau R, Roberts T (1998) MRI using hyperpolarized noble gases. Eur Radiol 8:820–827

28. Ma D, Hossain M, Chow A et al (2005) Xenon and hypothermia combine to provide neuro-protection from neonatal asphyxia. Ann Neurol 58:182–193

29. Faulkner S, Bainbridge A, Kato T et al (2011) Xenon augmented hypothermia reduces early lactate/N-acetylaspartate and cell death in perinatal asphyxia. Ann Neurol 70:133–150

30. Hobbs C, Thoresen M, Tucker A, Aquilina K, Chakkarapani E, Dingley J (2008) Xenon and hypothermia combine additively, offering long-term functional and histopathologic neuroprotection after neonatal hypoxia/ischemia. Stroke 39:1307–1313

31. Schmidt M, Marx T, Gloggl E, Reinelt H, Schirmer U (2005) Xenon attenuates cerebral damage after ischemia in pigs. Anesthesiology 102:929–936

32. Fries M, Nolte KW, Coburn M et al (2008) Xenon reduces neurohistopathological damage and improves the early neurological deficit after cardiac arrest in pigs. Crit Care Med 36:2420–2426

33. Fries M, Brucken A, Cizen A et al (2012) Combining xenon and mild therapeutic hypothermia preserves neurological function after prolonged cardiac arrest in pigs. Crit Care Med 40:1297–1303

34. Homi HM, Yokoo N, Ma D et al (2003) The neuroprotective effect of xenon administration during transient middle cerebral artery occlusion in mice. Anesthesiology 99:876–881

35. Sheng SP, Lei B, James ML et al (2012) Xenon neuroprotection in experimental stroke: interactions with hypothermia and intracerebral hemorrhage. Anesthesiology 117:1262–1275

36. Coburn M, Maze M, Franks NP (2008) The neuroprotective effects of xenon and helium in an in vitro model of traumatic brain injury. Crit Care Med 36:588–595

37. Campos-Pires R, Armstrong SP, Sebastiani A et al (2015) Xenon improves neurologic outcome and reduces secondary injury following trauma in an in vivo model of traumatic brain injury. Crit Care Med 43:149–158

38. Ma D, Yang H, Lynch J, Franks NP, Maze M, Grocott HP (2003) Xenon attenuates cardiopulmonary bypass-induced neurologic and neurocognitive dysfunction in the rat. Anesthesiology 98:690–698

39. Vacas S, Degos V, Tracey KJ, Maze M (2014) High-mobility group box 1 protein initiates postoperative cognitive decline by engaging bone marrow-derived macrophages. Anesthesiology 120:1160–1167
40. Forsberg A, Cervenka S, Jonsson Fagerlund M et al (2017) The immune response of the human brain to abdominal surgery. Ann Neurol 81:572–582
41. Zhao H, Ning J, Savage S et al (2013) A novel strategy for preserving renal grafts in an ex vivo setting: potential for enhancing the marginal donor pool. FASEB J 27:4822–4833
42. Arola OJ, Laitio RM, Roine RO et al (2013) Feasibility and cardiac safety of inhaled xenon in combination with therapeutic hypothermia following out-of-hospital cardiac arrest. Crit Care Med 41:2116–2124
43. Laitio R, Hynninen M, Arola O et al (2016) Effect of inhaled xenon on cerebral white matter damage in comatose survivors of out-of-hospital cardiac arrest: a randomized clinical trial. JAMA 315:1120–1128
44. Dingley J, Tooley J, Liu X et al (2014) Xenon ventilation during therapeutic hypothermia in neonatal encephalopathy: a feasibility study. Pediatrics 133:809–818
45. Azzopardi D, Robertson NJ, Kapetanakis A et al (2013) Anticonvulsant effect of xenon on neonatal asphyxial seizures. Arch Dis Child Fetal Neonatal Ed 98:F437–F439
46. Azzopardi D, Robertson NJ, Bainbridge A et al (2016) Moderate hypothermia within 6 h of birth plus inhaled xenon versus moderate hypothermia alone after birth asphyxia (TOBY-Xe): a proof-of-concept, open-label, randomised controlled trial. Lancet Neurol 15:145–153
47. Smith SM, Nichols TE (2009) Threshold-free cluster enhancement: addressing problems of smoothing, threshold dependence and localisation in cluster inference. Neuroimage 44:83–98
48. Le Bihan D (2003) Looking into the functional architecture of the brain with diffusion MRI. Nat Rev Neurosci 4:469–480
49. Coburn M, Sanders RD, Maze M et al (2018) The hip fracture surgery in elderly patients (HIPELD) study to evaluate xenon anaesthesia for the prevention of postoperative delirium: a multicenter, randomised, controlled clinical trial. Br J Anaesth 120:127–137
50. Lockwood GG, Franks NP, Downie NA, Taylor KM, Maze M (2006) Feasibility and safety of delivering xenon to patients undergoing coronary artery bypass graft surgery while on cardiopulmonary bypass: phase I study. Anesthesiology 104:458–465
51. Arola O, Saraste A, Laitio R et al (2017) Inhaled xenon attenuates myocardial damage in comatose survivors of out-of-hospital cardiac arrest: the Xe-Hypotheca trial. J Am Coll Cardiol 70:2652–2660
52. Hofland J, Ouattara A, Fellahi JL et al (2017) Effect of xenon anesthesia compared to sevoflurane and total intravenous anesthesia for coronary artery bypass graft surgery on postoperative cardiac troponin release: an international, multicenter, phase 3, single-blinded, randomized noninferiority trial. Anesthesiology 127:918–933

Electronic Health Record Research in Critical Care: The End of the Randomized Controlled Trial?

S. Harris, N. MacCallum, and D. Brealey

Introduction

We believe it is the duty of every hospital to establish a follow-up system, so that as far as possible the result of every case will be available at all times for investigation by members of the staff, the trustees, or administration, or by other authorized investigators or statisticians (Ernest Amory Codman).

Codman was a surgeon from Boston, practicing at the beginning of the 20th century. He instituted the practice of morbidity and mortality conferences, and personally tracked all his patients using 'End Result Cards'. Upon these he recorded demographics, diagnosis, treatment and outcomes. He argued that we should follow-up all cases to improve the quality of care. We wish to argue here that we should capture all healthcare information to benefit the science of clinical medicine. This is indeed the promise of the electronic health record (EHR) – healthcare's own 'big data'[1].

However, big data alone will not be a panacea. It has all the same fallibilities that we have learned to be wary of in observational studies. In this chapter, we will provide a brief history of big data starting with the triumph of measurement over diktat in the scientific revolution. We will review the state of big data in critical care with particular reference to the Critical Care Health Informatics Collaborative (CCHIC), a partnership between the UK's National Institute of Health Research (NIHR) and five leading NHS hospital trusts. CCHIC is a nascent multicenter, scalable and linkable repository of the full EHR with the explicit purpose of enabling and facilitating research for patient benefit.

Finally, we will discuss why the randomized controlled trial (RCT) is not an adequate solution to scientific progress. It might however be ably supported in this

---

[1] Big data is often characterized by the 4 'V's: volume, variety, velocity, and veracity.

S. Harris (✉) · N. MacCallum · D. Brealey
Critical Care Department, University College London Hospitals NHS Foundation Trust
London, UK
e-mail: doc@steveharris.me

© Springer International Publishing AG 2018
J.-L. Vincent (ed.), *Annual Update in Intensive Care and Emergency Medicine 2018*,
Annual Update in Intensive Care and Emergency Medicine,
https://doi.org/10.1007/978-3-319-73670-9_50

endeavour by the opportunities created by big data when combined with the rigor of the new field of causal inference. Despite the provocative title, we are not arguing that the RCT is in danger, but are proposing that its podium position in the hierarchy of evidence might soon need to be shared.

A Brief History of Measurement

One Measure

The Paris meridian, long term rival to the Greenwich meridian as the prime meridian, sits on the north-south line of longitude running from Dunkirk to Barcelona. This represents one-quarter of the arc connecting the North Pole to the Equator. Its measurement in 1798 defined the meter as one ten-millionth of the full arc. It also proved Newton's hypothesis that the earth was an oblate spheroid with flattening equal to 1/230.

That the resolution of the argument as to the shape of the earth was through observation and measurement was the triumph of empiricism and the scientific revolution. However, the revolution was incomplete, and the instinct that there was one true, even divine, measurement lingered. In fact, simultaneous measures of the meridian arc were conducted by the French Academy of Sciences in Peru (1735–1739) and in Lapland (1735–1739), by a papal mission in Rome (1750–52), and by the Portuguese in Brazil (1743). Unsurprisingly, the true measure was still a relative judgement depending on whether you harkened from Paris, Lisbon, or Rome.

Many Measures

The resolution of the problem can be attributed to a Croatian astronomer and mathematician, Roger Boscovich, who radically judged each measure equally regardless of the measurer. Each vote counted, and a better version of the truth could be approached by combining all measures rather than choosing one. The best measure, the arithmetic mean, was that which minimized the distance between all measures [1]. Replacing the one divine measure with a democracy of measures mirrored the contemporaneous French and American political revolutions. This was the *vox populi*, the wisdom of the crowd.[2]

The key is that the best answer is derived from all opinions, or, in science, from all measurements. Each measurement is a vote, a single piece of information but one that carries a degree of error. Since errors can be in either direction, then aggregated they will cancel each other out, and the average will move closer to the truth.

---

[2] A hundred years later, Francis Galton, of regression and eugenics fame, observed the efficacy of a crowd of 800, in guessing the weight of a slaughtered bull at a country fair: the median response was within 1% of the true value [2].

All Measures: Big Data

Big data is the final step in the empirical revolution. Until the computer age, measurement was expensive. The original expedition to measure the meridian arc purportedly cost more than the large hadron collider at the European Council for Nuclear Research (CERN). At such cost, it is little wonder that the democratization of measurement took so long. Digitalization has changed this. In our own lifetimes, new prefixes for quantities of data enter the vernacular every few years: kilo, mega, giga, tera and now peta. Exabytes, a billion billion bytes, can only be a few years away. The democracy of measures has not been satisfied with universal suffrage but is relentlessly extending its plebiscite to every aspect of our lives. The EHR is simply shorthand for clinical big data.

This revolution faces two principle challenges: one social and one scientific. First, such pervasive observation must not become surveillance. We, the public, are rightly suspicious of both governments and commercial organizations handling our data. Neither have as yet proven themselves as worthy guardians of this public good.

Second, measurement alone does not advance science. Just because I can count every rain drop in a cloud does not automatically allow me to recommend carrying an umbrella. Boscovich's method of the means was the start of the statistical revolution that has taken us from one to many measures. The democracy of statistics allows us to see that there is error in every measurement. We use probability to quantify the error, and demarcate the signal from the noise. However, statistics has always had an Achilles heel. If the measurement machine is badly calibrated, the result will always be inaccurate even if it eventually becomes precise. In clinical medicine this means if there is bias or confounding, our knowledge will not improve with many, or even millions of measures. It is to this second theme that we will return after a brief tour of big data in critical care.

Big Data in Critical Care

By the very nature of our speciality, we will be at the forefront of the big data revolution in medicine. There is no other environment where patients are monitored more closely, or with such a broad range of measures. Uniquely this multi-parameter data stream is actually a panel of correlated time-series measures that are sampled as often as 300 times per second (e.g., heart rate and blood pressure recordings).

Since 2001, such data has been hosted as the Medical Information Mart for Intensive Care (MIMIC) database at the Lab for Computational Physiology at the Massachusetts Institute of Technology (Boston, USA) [3]. This database now contains more than 40,000 patient records from a single center in North America. Despite the risks, both the funders and the MIMIC development team have prioritized making the data open access. This has enabled research in complementary disciplines including engineering, physiology and computer science. Making available some of the most important data we hold, human physiology and health outcome data, to a very wide range of researchers is a laudable achievement.

Critical care also leads with some of the largest healthcare audit programs in the world. The UK's Intensive Care National Audit and Research Centre Case Mix Programme Database (ICNARC CMPD) has been running since 1994 and currently contains around 2 million records. Similarly, the Australia and New Zealand Intensive Care Society's Adult Patient Database (ANZICS APD) has been reporting since 1992 and contains more than 1.5 million records.

Critical Care Health Informatics Collaborative (CCHIC)

Building on these two traditions, the UK NIHR founded the Health Informatics Collaborative (HIC) in 2013. This project aims to make available routinely collected healthcare data to researchers within the National Health Service (NHS) with a number of clear ambitions:

- make available the phenotypical description of disease characterized in the clinical record such that it could complement the emerging 'omics' (genomics, transcriptomics, etc) data sets
- make clinical data available to epidemiologists, health services researchers, and improvement scientists to improve the delivery of care to existing patients
- make clinical data available to trialists and other researchers who normally have to employ dedicated researchers to transcribe clinical data into dedicated case report forms

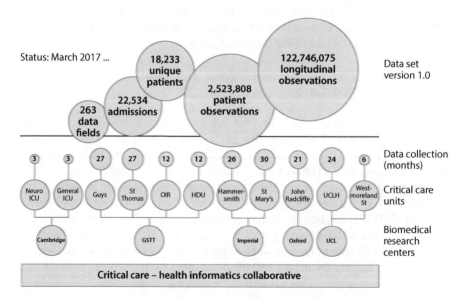

Fig. 1 Summary of data within the Critical Care Health Informatics Collaborative (CCHIC) as of March 2017

Critical care was one of the five founding clinical themes alongside renal transplant, acute coronary syndromes, ovarian cancer and viral hepatitis (and now joined by infection and breast, colorectal, lung and prostate cancers). Each theme contributes a catalog of the domain specific data which is made available to researchers.

Critical care has taken the additional important step of agreeing *a priori* to curate the data itself. At the time of writing, the database holds the records of more than 25,000 critical care admissions with more than 250 data items per record (Fig. 1). This amounts to around 2.5 million time-invariant (e.g., age, sex) and 120 million time-varying observations (e.g., heart rate, norepinephrine dose).

CCHIC Design Principles

The design of CCHIC has been based on the following principles

1. to protect the privacy of the patients from whom data has been recorded
2. to support research for patient benefit, specifically excluding commercial exploitation
3. to facilitate that research by building a scalable pipeline for extracting, processing and sharing the data

Principle 1: Patient Privacy

Being able to protect patient privacy with confidence is the first and foremost consideration for this data resource. Extensive patient and public engagement work has been performed to ensure that this resource is seen as a public good by a broad cross-section of constituents. The particular problem with critical care research is that the patients themselves are either temporarily or permanently incapacitated and therefore unable to offer explicit permission. In the UK, this triggers the need for an application to the Secretary of State for Health to hold these data without consent (as per Section 251 of the NHS Act 2006). Permission is only granted when the physical security of the data can be guaranteed, and when the justification for holding the data is in the public interest (hence principle 2).

The data are encrypted before leaving each hospital, and then moved to the data safe haven at University College London. Access to the identifiable data is strictly controlled, but an anonymization step in the data pipeline makes an extract of the data ready for the end-researcher (principle 3).

Principle 2: Research for Patient Benefit

Even after privacy is protected, there a widely reported distinction in the public perception of rights to use data. The furore over the partnership between the Royal Free NHS Foundation Trust and Google DeepMind in 2016 was not just because of the transfer of identifiable patient records. The public have a deep suspicion of the motives of commercial organizations, especially those with the pervasive reach of Google.

In the DeepMind case, the purported use of the data was to simply develop an alerting system for patients with acute kidney injury (AKI). However calculating the AKI class from a laboratory creatinine is so simple that it is hard to believe this was Google's end game. In fact the Information Sharing Agreement that was signed in 2015 placed no restrictions on the data to be analyzed, or the technologies that might be used [4].

In contrast, for CCHIC the data cannot be used for commercial purposes, the research question must be explicitly for patient benefit, and even anonymized data releases must be proportional to the researcher's need.

Principle 3: Research Ready

Principle 1 protects the patient, and Principle 2 justifies the risks, however small, of making health care data available. Principle 3 enables the researcher to deliver on the promise of their research. Most data analysis requires a huge amount of preparation.

We therefore developed an automated data processing pipeline to process and curate data submitted by individual ICUs (Fig. 2). In brief,

1. A centrally agreed data dictionary defines a specification for each data item, and is used to validate an XML export from individual hospitals.
2. We extract physiological EHR data using a combination of manual, semi-automatic or entirely automatic methods adapted to local ICU clinical information systems.
3. Uniquely, the patient identifier is retained with the record to permit linkage to external health and social care data sets to better understand the antecedents of critical illness, and its long-term consequences.
4. The identifiable data are uploaded and processed within the UCL Data Safe Haven – a secure data processing platform that operates under the ISO/IEC 27001:2013 information security standard.
5. We quality control the data following a philosophy of reproducing accurately the local EHR rather than curating a 'corrected' data set for audit, benchmarking or quality control.[3] An audit trail is created to identify the provenance of each data item.

Having created a central data repository, we must make the data safely available to authorized researchers without compromising the privacy of the patients who have contributed data.

---

[3] For example, aberrant invasive blood pressure readings of 300 mmHg occur when the transducer system is flushed, and exposed to the attached pressure bag instead of the patient. For benchmarking, it is important to identify and exclude these values before using them to adjust for patient outcomes. However, it is exactly this sort of artefact that must be handled by the designer of a clinical monitoring system. Such use cases are very much part of the justification for CCHIC. Similarly, missing data might need imputation to allow between-patient comparison for audit, but the pattern of missingness has turned out to be an important input for computer scientists trying to predict patient outcomes [5].

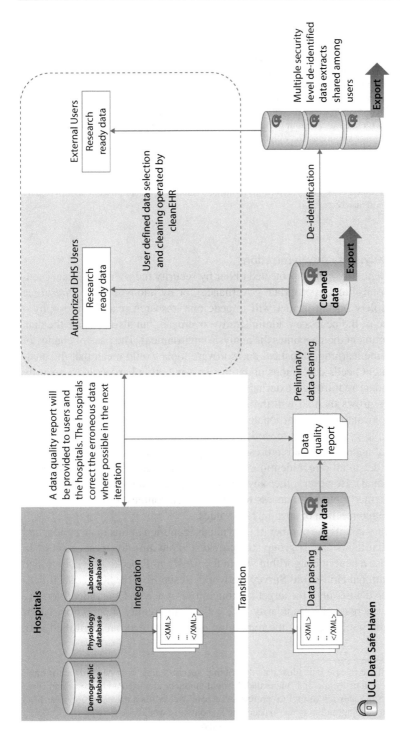

Fig. 2 Data processing pipeline. Data moves from the hospital electronic health record (EHR) to the University College London (UCL) Data Safe Haven as an XML file, and is validated before appending to the central database. A data quality report is then returned to the submitting site. Preliminary cleaning removes out-of-range and invalid entries. The database can then be queried in its identifiable form by authorized users within the safe haven, or a separate anonymizer can produce extracts for external collaborators

Fig. 3 Flow diagram for data anonymization. A summary of the anonymization process applied before any data release. 1. Removal of direct identifiers: all unique identifiers including NHS number and hospital number will be removed from the data before release. 2. Remove high-risk individuals and specific opt-outs. 3. Date and time metadata: all timestamps are converted to data and time differences from the instant of critical care admission. 4. Aggregate continuous and date-time key variables: Because we cannot group patients by a continuous measure, the concept of k-anonymity only applies to categorical variables (e.g., we can group patients by eye color, but not hair length). Where a key variable is continuous then we will run an initial conversion to a categorical version by aggregating. The unit of aggregation will be the natural unit of the measurement (e.g., years for age or kilograms for weight), and the initial aggregation will be some multiple of that unit (e.g., 2 years and 5 kg, respectively). Thus multiples will be initially small in order to minimize information loss, but will be increased during the iterative specific anonymization step until the necessary k-anonymity and l-diversity is reached. 5. Remove living subjects (where possible: the Data Protection Act only applies to living individuals so where possible data will only be released for non-survivors) ▶

Research Ready: Data Anonymization

Patient confidentiality can be protected either by security measures (physical security, access control and appropriate governance), or by anonymization. We argue that relying solely on the former will impede our 'research ready' philosophy – partly because of the necessary administrative overhead, but also because the data storage environment then becomes the analysis environment. The pace of change of modern machine learning, statistical and software tools would mean that the analysis environment needs continuous updating. This is both a burden and a security risk (each update requires an external ingest of code). Moreover, as the number of researchers grows then so will the number of tools and risk of external exposure. Making available a proportionate anonymized extract of the data solves this problem and allows researchers to work with their own tools (Fig. 3). The new compromise is that anonymization requires data suppression and therefore information loss. We first delete all direct identifiers (e.g., NHS numbers which uniquely identify an individual). However, other key variables can be combined by a motivated intruder, particularly one with access to external data sources, to re-identify individuals by the intersection of specific rare values.

K-anonymity counts the number of individuals identified at this intersection, and we set k so that this smallest group still provides anonymity for its members.[4] In practice, we use a heuristic algorithm within the *sdcMicro* R package [6] developed by the International Household Survey Network[5] to suppress (remove) quasi-identifiers from the dataset until the target k-anonymity is reached. Quasi-identifiers are aggregated to increase the granularity before the k-anonymity suppression. Additionally, for the public release, the remaining quasi-identifiers are perturbed with noise.

---

[4] For example, if we release individual data describing 'species', and 'favorite sandwich filling', then the intersection of 'bears' and 'marmalade' would uniquely identify Paddington Bear. If we generalize 'favorite sandwich filling' to 'prefers sweet sandwiches' then because Pooh Bear likes honey as well as Paddington liking marmalade, the k-anonymity would rise to two.

[5] http://www.ihsn.org/software/disclosure-control-toolbox.

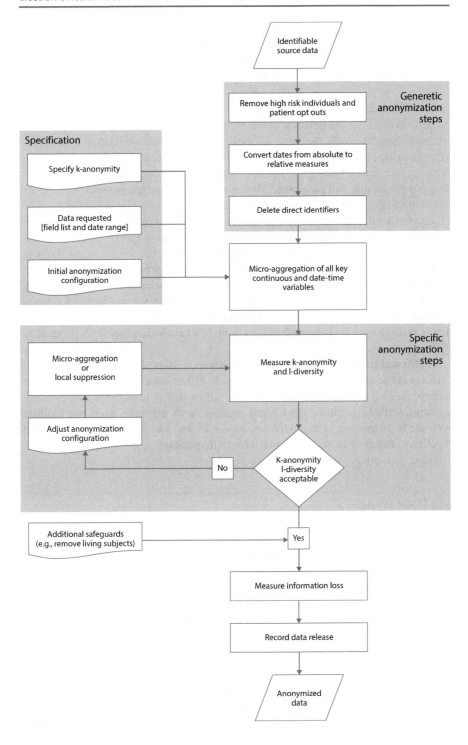

In addition, we prospectively identify sensitive data items such as those recording (alcoholic) cirrhosis or human immunodeficiency virus (HIV) status. These are either suppressed if homogeneous, or released if heterogeneous. In this way, the disease status of the members of even the smallest (k) group remains uncertain.[6]

Research Ready: The cleanEHR Toolkit

As described above, the data that is released is a 'warts and all' version of the EHR record integrated across the sites. Although being faithful to the original record is a design principle, it leaves most researchers with the huge task of cleaning the data. We therefore provide alongside the data a set of tools covering the most common data pre-processing and post-processing operations. These are provided as an open source package, cleanEHR, for the R statistical programming language.

The most important of these operations is a function that converts the various asynchronous lists of time-dependent measurements into a table of measurements with a customizable cadence. For example, if the researcher wishes to use the data every hour then a skeleton table is built with one row per critical care admission per hour from the time of admission to the time of discharge. For time-invariant data, the data items are repeated across all rows. For time-varying items, a value is inserted if a value has been recorded in that hour.[7] The end result is a data frame that is ready for analysis in applications from Microsoft Excel to SPSS, from R to Python.

Additional functionality includes the ability to re-label the data fields at will, to perform range and consistency checks, and to either impute missing values or to remove episodes with excess missingness. All of this is performed by providing a simple text file[8] with the configuration requests so that even users not familiar with the R programming language can configure the data processing and cleaning pipeline to match their requirements. The entire package is provided with tutorials and documentation.

Big Data Hype

The CCHIC program, like those before it, is implicitly assuming that this effort to bring healthcare data to researchers is justified. Yet since the beginning of the evidence-based medicine (EBM) movement, we have been taught that "observational studies [are] low quality evidence" [7]. Making an observational study 'big' does not solve that problem. In fact it just creates more opportunities for the cliché that 'correlation is not causation'.

---

[6] This is known as *l-diversity* and guarantees that even if an individual can be identified as belonging to a small group (cell) there is sufficient variability of these sensitive items within that group that uncertainty remains as to a specific individual's status.

[7] Where more than one item is available in that time period, the most recent measurement is used by default although other selection algorithms are possible.

[8] The text file is specified using the human readable and writeable version of XML called YAML. Learning the formatting rules for this should take no more than ten minutes.

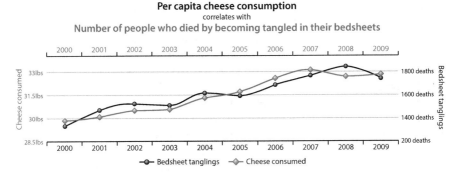

Fig. 4 Correlation is not causation. From [8]

The Spurious Correlations project [8] is a humorous example of this very problem. Here an automated script searches the internet for publicly available time-series datasets, checks for correlations and posts the best to a website. The current number 3 in the hit list shows a 95% correlation between death by bed sheet tangling (Centres for Disease Control & Prevention) and per capita cheese consumption (US Department of Agriculture) (Fig. 4).

We are only in danger of accepting this relationship if we forget the data generating mechanism (a random, never-ending computer search). The data are not experimental. We have neither control of US cheese consumption, nor do we have a theory of cheese and bedsheets that would lead us to test this relationship. The correlation is spurious in the same way that a lottery winner is lucky.

The error is in thinking that there is an equivalence between the strength of the correlation and its plausibility. The proper application of statistics, given the information about the lottery of relations that were examined, has no difficulty in reminding us that if we search in the noise for long enough we can always find a pattern. The deeper problem is that correlation is also a feature of confounding. Confounding has, to date, always been managed by resorting to randomization but this is not an option for big data.

Using Randomization to Learn

Confounding is not a new problem. In medicine, the RCT has been seen as the antidote to poorly conducted observational research. This is the synthesis of two streams of thinking. The first is the clinical trial which is often attributed to James Lind's investigation of treatments for scurvy[9] (although the old testament recounts a similar approach when the Israelite Daniel was offered food by the Babylonian King Nebuchadnezzar) [9].

---

[9] Demonstrating the success of the treatment was made easier by the choice of the controls, which included sulphuric acid, vinegar, and brine.

The second is Ronald Fisher's solution to the problem that controlling such comparisons becomes increasingly difficult as the number of factors to be controlled increases. In fact, the 'curse of dimensionality' states that the required sample size increases exponentially. A two-by-two table summarizes a treatment comparison with one control. The table becomes a cube for two controls, and an $n+1$ dimensional hypercube for n controls. The population must be divided between cells in the cube, and, very quickly, the number of cells exceeds the available population.

This was the exact problem faced by Fisher in the 1920s at the Rothamsted Experimental agricultural station where he was required to analyze crop yields after controlling for the field location, the time of the year, the preceding crop, the crop preceding that, the weather and more. Fisher realised that rather than trying to control for everything, you could instead control for nothing if the treatment assignment was itself deliberately random.

There is a genius in the symmetry of Fisher's solution to this problem. The desire is to ensure that the confounders are randomly allocated and so do not upset the treatment-control comparison. In other words, there is no other systematic bias or difference between the groups. Since this is impossible to achieve because the confounders are numerous and uncontrollable, Fisher inverted the process to achieve the same result. He randomly allocated the treatment. If a treatment is allocated on the basis of a coin flip, then the only confounder that remains is the coin itself. Randomize patients with pneumonia to penicillin or placebo, and if survival improves either the coin has divine properties or the penicillin is effective. Science was happy to discard the divine effect of the coin, and embrace the result of the trial.

Fisher was not alone in this approach. Charles Peirce, a lecturer in logic at Johns Hopkins University, came to the same conclusion in his 1887 publication "Illustrations of the Logic of Science". Nonetheless, the insight that measurement alone is insufficient to advance knowledge is a clear bookend to the Scientific Revolution from three centuries previously. The implicit suggestion is that we cannot learn by just observing, in Paul Holland's words, "there is no causation without manipulation" [10].

Experimental Design and Statistics

The pairing of randomization and statistics creates an enormously powerful tool for learning from data. Randomization means we have only one relationship to examine, and statistics allows us to discuss the plausibility of that relationship. However, RCTs are expensive juggernauts more akin to measuring the meridian line in terms of cost, time and effort.[10]

---

[10] There are new strategies that aim to make the clinical trial more agile including platform trials, and now REMAP (Randomized Embedded Multifactorial Adaptive Platform). Here, new treatment options are continuously added and removed, as they are discovered and assessed, and the randomization is embedded in health care delivery. The EHR can even provide the realtime data collection and feedback loop [11].

We have had to rely on the design of the experiment [12] because while statistics allows us to quantify the plausibility of a result, it has no language to handle confounding. Statistics can quantify the relationship between a disease and symptoms, but it cannot evaluate whether the disease causes the symptoms, or the symptoms cause the disease. The equation in a regression model is symmetrical, and can be written in either direction. It is only with external knowledge (the experiment) that we know one thing preceded the other, and that we can attribute cause and effect.

Big data without the experiment will fall short of being the powerful tool promised. No amount of machine learning would help if we have no theory to manage causality in general, and in particular confounding. Fortunately, we now do in something called a graphical model.

Graphical Models

Graphical models are simply graphical representations of the world. They are made up of nodes (or vertices) connected by arrows (or edges). The nodes are symbols representing observable or unobservable entities (sometimes drawn as boxes and circles respectively). The arrows then indicate a possible causal link between the nodes. We say possible here because the lack of an arrow between two nodes is a statement that there is no causal relationship. Taking the classic example of smoking, lung cancer and carrying matches then we would draw just two arrows: one from smoking to carrying matches, and one from smoking to lung cancer (Fig. 5). The lack of an arrow between carrying matches and lung cancer is an implicit assumption that we do not believe that carrying matches causes cancer. Conversely, the presence of an arrow does not require there to be a relationship. It just says that one may exist, and we wish to estimate its magnitude (which may be zero).

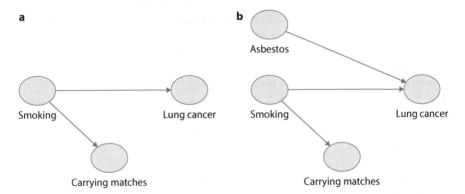

Fig. 5 Graphical models (or directed acyclic graphs [DAG]). Bias from confounding is seen in (**a**) where a backdoor path exists from lung cancer to carrying matches via smoking. Bias is induced by selection in (**b**) where lung cancer is a collider for smoking and asbestos exposure

The power of these models is in how they easily capture relationships, and then provide a theoretical basis for handling confounding, selection bias and other issues in epidemiology that have only had a narrative description hitherto.

Confounders and Backdoor Paths

For example, the definition of a confounder is immediately clear from the diagram. Smoking confounds the relationship between carrying matches and lung cancer because it is a common cause. In the literature, this is known as a backdoor path because we proceed against the flow of causality from lung cancer to smoking to make the journey to matches. By measuring, and controlling, a node on each backdoor path between the exposure and the outcome, we can get at the true, unconfounded relationship. The graphical model identifies the minimum set of controls that we need, and makes explicit the assumptions in any estimate we produce. Sometimes we cannot block each backdoor path because we cannot measure one or more of the nodes (or because there is a circular relationship between exposure and outcome). In which case, we say that the solution is not identifiable. Where a relationship is identifiable, then we can set about gathering the data, and using the machinery of statistics to estimate the magnitude of the relationship.

Colliders and Berkson's Paradox

The power of graphical models can be demonstrated by how they clearly handle a more subtle form of bias known as Berkson's paradox. This states that false relationships may be created when we limit our enquiries to a population that is defined as a consequence of the outcome being studied.

Consider an attempt to study the relationship between asbestos exposure, smoking and lung cancer. Assume that both smoking and asbestos exposure do cause lung cancer. If we study patients with lung cancer, we will almost certainly discover these factors are inversely related: the more you smoke, the lower your asbestos exposure. This is because controlling for a common effect of two exposures is akin to not controlling for a common cause. Lung cancer in patients who never smoked must be driven by a strong history of asbestos exposure, and lung cancer in those never exposed to asbestos must be the consequence of a heavier smoking history.

The graphical representation is much simpler: we draw arrows from smoking to lung cancer, from asbestos to lung cancer, and between asbestos and smoking (Fig. 5). The arrows downstream from smoking and asbestos collide on lung cancer. Including a collider in your model, either a control or by selecting on that factor, induces a false relationship. The corollary is that just as we must control for backdoor paths, we must exclude colliders.

Experimental and Natural Randomization

The graphical representation of experimental randomization is the simplest of all. The first node is the coin, the second the treatment, and the third the outcome with a single path made up of two arrows, from coin to treatment, from treatment to outcome. The treatment is determined by the coin with no other ancestors so there is no confounding hence relationship between the treatment, and the outcome is identifiable, and we can then lean on the probability theory underpinning statistics to determine the strength and the plausibility of that relationship.

Beyond experimental randomization, the graphical model also allows us to encode the assumptions of natural experiments. Famous examples range from the near experimental to the truly opportunistic. The Oregon Experiment, where the extension of Medicaid was assigned by lottery, is an example of the former [13]. In critical care, the latter strategy has been used to evaluate the effect of delayed admission to critical care on outcome using the 'lottery' of bed availability in a healthcare system where critical care bed supply is constrained [14].

These are usually termed instrumental variable analyses where we assert that the instrument operates only on the treatment [15]. Just like in the RCT, we draw an arrow from the instrument to the treatment, but no arrow from the instrument to the outcome. If accept that ICU occupancy cannot affect ward outcomes other than through the arrow connecting delayed admission to outcome, then the effect of delay is identifiable. There is no backdoor connection, and no confounding.

Other similar natural experimental opportunities exist. Physician prescribing preference studies exploit Dr A's preference for drug X, and the randomness of a patient falling ill when Dr A is on-call [16]. Anesthesia techniques for hip surgery have been explored based on the variation in practice between hospitals rather than physicians. Patients living halfway between a hospital that prefers general anesthesia and a hospital that prefers regional (neuraxial) techniques are effectively randomized by the ambulance choosing to turn left or right [17].

Another opportunity is created by rule-based behavior based on a continuous measures: these are known as regression discontinuity designs [18]. Take, for example, a rule that mandates medical review when urine output drops below 0.5 ml/kg/h. A patient with a urine output of 0.49 ml/kg/h will be treated differently to one with a urine output of 0.51 ml/kg/h, yet the difference in urine output between the two is clinically negligible. With enough data, the arbitrary threshold allows comparison of different treatment strategies in otherwise similar patients.

Conclusion: Big Data and Graphical Models

Just as a century ago the pairing of randomization and statistics created a new tool for learning, we can now combine big data with the modern tools of causal inference. There is now theory to untangle not just the spurious correlations that arise by chance, but also the much thornier problems of confounding. The theory of graphical models [19] won its creator, Judea Pearl, the Turing Award, the 'Nobel Prize of Computing'.[11] However, graphical models are part of a larger field of causal inference that includes potential-outcome frameworks and structural equation models [20].

---

[11] Other recipients include Tim Berners-Lee who won the 2016 Turing Award for inventing the world wide web.

The field allows the researcher to move from the narrative description taught on public health programs to a testable framework of relationships. They permit encoding of external knowledge about systems and then provide guidance as to which relationships can be evaluated. Moreover, they provide very explicit guidance as to how these relationships should be evaluated to get at the true effect. They define which factors to control (common causes) and which to exclude from control (common effects). Although they lay no claim on the thorny Rumsfeldian problem of unknown unknowns they at least make explicit our current state of knowledge [21].

Those of us who practice critical care will find ourselves in the midst of the big data revolution sooner than most. MIMIC, ICNARC, ANZICS and now CCHIC and others provide an exciting opportunity. The RCT may seem like the end of this history.[12] However, in critical care we are more aware than most that this would be a poor ending. Clinical trials have been notoriously fruitless in our field, especially in the field of sepsis research [22].

EHR research will not replace the RCT, but we can allow ourselves to be excited by the possibilities. For once, it's not all hype.

References

1. Stigler SM (1986) The history of statistics. Harvard University Press, Cambridge
2. Galton F (1907) Vox populi. Nature 75:450–451
3. Johnson AEW, Pollard TJ, Shen L et al (2016) MIMIC-III, a freely accessible critical care database. Sci Data 3:160035
4. Powles J, Hodson H (2017) Google DeepMind and healthcare in an age of algorithms. Health Technol 29:1–17
5. Alaa AM, Yoon J, Hu S, van der Schaar M (2017) Personalized risk scoring for critical care prognosis using mixtures of Gaussian processes. Ieee Trans Biomed Eng 65:207–218
6. Templ M, Kowarik A, Meindl B (2015) Statistical disclosure control for micro-data using the r package sdcMicro. J Stat Softw 67:1–36
7. Guyatt GH, Oxman AD, Kunz R, Vist GE, Falck-Ytter Y, Schünemann HJ, Working Group (2008) What is "quality of evidence" and why is it important to clinicians? BMJ 336:995–998
8. Vigen T. Spurious Correlations Project. www.tylervigen.com/spurious-correlations. Accessed 10 January 2018
9. Lewis EJ (2003) Ancient clinical trials. N Engl J Med 348:83–84
10. Holland PW (1986) Statistics and causal inference. J Am Stat Assoc 81:945–960
11. Angus DC (2015) Fusing randomized trials with big data: the key to self-learning health care systems? JAMA 314:767–768
12. Fisher R (1935) The design of experiments. Macmillan, London
13. Baicker K, Taubman SL, Allen HL et al (2013) The Oregon experiment – effects of medicaid on clinical outcomes. N Engl J Med 368:1713–1722
14. Harris S, Singer M, Rowan K, Sanderson C (2015) Delay to admission to critical care and mortality among deteriorating ward patients in UK hospitals: a multicentre, prospective, ob- servational cohort study. Lancet 385:S40

---

[12] The End of History is a 1992 essay by Francis Fukuyama that argued that Western liberal democ- racy would be the final endpoint for social and political development. A quarter of a century later this claim seems rather premature.

15. Hernan MA, Robins JM (2006) Instruments for causal inference: an epidemiologist's dream? Epidemiology 17:360–372
16. Rassen JA, Schneeweiss S, Glynn RJ, Mittleman MA, Brookhart MA (2009) Instrumental variable analysis for estimation of treatment effects with dichotomous outcomes. Am J Epidemiol 169:273–284
17. Neuman MD, Rosenbaum PR, Ludwig JM, Zubizarreta JR, Silber JH (2014) Anesthesia technique, mortality, and length of stay after hip fracture surgery. JAMA 311:2508–2510
18. Geneletti S, O'Keeffe AG, Sharples LD, Richardson S, Baio G (2014) Bayesian regression discontinuity designs: incorporating clinical knowledge in the causal analysis of primary care data. Stat Med 34:2334–2352
19. Pearl J (1988) Probabilistic Reasoning in Intelligent Systems: Networks of Plausible Inference. Morgan Kaufmann Publishers, San Francisco
20. Greenland S, Brumback B (2002) An overview of relations among causal modelling methods. Int J Epidemiol 31:1030–1037
21. Rumsfeld DH (2002) DoD news briefing – secretary Rumsfeld and gen. Myers. http://archive.defense.gov/Transcripts/Transcript.aspx?TranscriptID=2636. Accessed 4 January 2018
22. Riedemann NC, Guo RF, Ward PA (2003) The enigma of sepsis. J Clin Invest 112:460–467

Using Telemedicine in the ICU Setting

P. R. Menon, T. D. Rabinowitz, and R. D. Stapleton

Introduction

Each year, approximately 6 million people in the US are admitted to an intensive care unit (ICU), accounting for roughly 30% ($67 billion) of total hospital costs [1]. Patients admitted to the ICU have an extremely high risk of morbidity and mortality, with mortality approaching 10% or 540,000 deaths annually [1, 2]. In the face of a shortage of intensivists and an aging population, ICU telemedicine has grown dramatically over the past decade. Currently, telemedicine programs support more than 11% of all critically ill patients admitted to private US ICUs [3].

Telemedicine is defined as the delivery of healthcare services or the transmission of healthcare information using telecommunications technology [4]. The US National Aeronautics and Space Administration (NASA) first introduced telemedicine in the 1960s to gather physiologic data from astronauts in space [5, 6]. Telemedicine has since evolved to provide both general medical care from a distance to underserved areas and subspecialty services to smaller hospitals. The use of telemedicine in rural and underserved areas has been shown to effectively address specific issues that rural physicians often encounter, including isolation, poor interprofessional communication, lack of onsite specialists and limited access to current medical information and continuing medical education. In addition, utilization of telemedicine has been shown to improve patients' perceptions of the quality of care received and to decrease the financial impact of illness because it often obviates the need for travel to another facility to receive subspecialty services [7, 8]. In addition to providing patient care, telemedicine has been studied in other settings as a mode of communicating and connecting with rural providers, patients and families. Telemedicine may be a useful critical care tool to provide effective early communication with family members of patients who transfer from rural hospitals to tertiary care centers. In

P. R. Menon (✉) · T. D. Rabinowitz · R. D. Stapleton
University of Vermont College of Medicine
Burlington, VT, USA
e-mail: Prema.menon@uvmhealth.org

© Springer International Publishing AG 2018   691
J.-L. Vincent (ed.), *Annual Update in Intensive Care and Emergency Medicine 2018*,
Annual Update in Intensive Care and Emergency Medicine,
https://doi.org/10.1007/978-3-319-73670-9_51

this chapter, we describe the current roles that telemedicine plays within critical care and propose future areas where telemedicine may be highly impactful.

Current Uses of Telemedicine in the Intensive Care Unit

Over the past several decades, there has been a rapid growth of telemedicine implementation across many healthcare fields. Increased use of telemedicine in critical illness has been particularly notable and may substantially impact processes of care.

Telemedicine was first implemented in the ICU in response to two major areas of concern: heterogeneous critical care delivery and workforce shortage. High variability in critical care delivery due to varying organizational structures within the healthcare system may be responsible for more than 100,000 preventable annual deaths in the US, primarily due to lack of implementation of best practices [9]. As the US population continues to age, the need for ICU providers has risen significantly, leading to a shortage of critical care providers. According to a 2006 Health Resources and Services Administration study, the US will need 4,300 critical care physicians by 2020 with a predicted shortfall of 1,500 intensivists nationally [10]. Thus, telemedicine in the ICU began in an effort to improve overall standardization of ICU care in compliance with guidelines and as a potential solution for provider shortages.

Tele-ICU or e-ICU is the provision of critical care by a critical care provider(s) via a computer and audiovisual or telecommunication system. In its most common form, ICU telemedicine involves remote monitoring of ICU patients using fixed installations. Monitoring occurs either continuously or only during nighttime hours, when physicians may not be present at the bedside but can monitor critically ill patients remotely. Tele-ICU care has been shown to decrease overall length of stay (LOS) in the ICU, with several studies demonstrating a reduction in ICU LOS from 1–2 days [2, 11–15]. Studies investigating the association of telemedicine utilization to ICU mortality have demonstrated mixed results, with some studies finding a significant improvement and others finding no change in mortality [2, 11–14, 16–20]. In addition, use of tele-ICU is associated with improved overall ICU quality metrics due in large part to better adherence to best practices such as protocol based management of sepsis, low tidal volume ventilation strategies, and prevention of ventilator associated complications in the ICU [16, 21–23].

At present, tele-ICU is the most commonly used application of telemedicine within critical care. Beyond remote monitoring of patients, telemedicine can provide educational opportunities to rural hospital providers (e.g. teaching case conferences and discussions). Additionally, telemedicine is also used for 'virtual' consultations. In these instances, telemedicine is used to discuss cases among providers with subsequent recommendations for care without actively involving nurses or patients [24]. Within pediatric ICUs, telemedicine is used to connect children with their family members who are unable to be present due to long distances or who need to continue to go to work. Telemedicine with videoconferencing has provided a practical solution to these barriers that limit family presence and participation in care [25].

Barriers and Facilitators to Telemedicine in the ICU

Although telemedicine has been in existence in various forms since the 1970s, it was not introduced widely in the ICU until 2000 and meaningful adoption did not begin until 2003, with subsequent rapid growth [2, 26]. The overall number of US ICU beds covered by telemedicine increased from 0.4 to 7.9% between 2003 and 2010. Most of that growth occurred between 2003 and 2007 (annual rate of growth of 101.1% per year) compared to 2008–2010 where the average rate of growth was 8.1% per year [27]. This slowing growth is likely not explained by the technology reaching its saturation point, but rather by the fact that the majority of hospitals to implement ICU telemedicine capabilities to date are large teaching hospitals in metropolitan areas, without much adoption in smaller rural hospitals [27, 28]. The reasons for the lag in adoption remain unclear but may include barriers to implementation such as high cost, lack of staffing capabilities, and negative perceptions of telemedicine. The recent slower growth in utilization of telemedicine has made investigating user acceptance an increasingly critical technology implementation and management issue. Previous investigations have studied the utilization and efficiency of telemedicine through the technology assessment model (TAM), an information systems theory that models how users come to accept and use a technology [29]. This model incorporates perceived usefulness, perceived ease of use, attitude toward use, behavioral intention to use and other external variables to evaluate actual system use. One study applying the TAM model specifically towards telemedicine found that perceived usefulness was the most significant factor affecting acceptance. Attitude towards telemedicine was also considered an important factor, but has not been elucidated in its entirety. Interestingly, perceived ease of use was considered significantly less important [30]. Additional studies, discussed below, have examined costs, perceptions, and other barriers independent of the TAM model.

Costs of Tele-ICU

It has been estimated that full implementation of a tele-ICU system in community hospitals nationwide could prevent between 5,400 and 13,400 deaths and potentially save $5.4 billion annually in the US. However, one of the primary barriers to disseminated adoption has been the cost of implementation. These costs, at a minimum, include construction, installation and training. The average cost of implementing a tele-ICU system is $50,000–$100,000 per bed (approximately $2–$3 million per institution) in addition to annual operating costs of about $300,000–$1 million. Several studies have suggested that the initial set up and annual operating costs are offset by approximately $1–2 million saved annually through overall decreased ICU LOS, and adherence to best practices such as avoidance of iatrogenic complications, stewardship of antibiotics, and decreased blood transfusions [31, 32].

A recent simulation cost-effectiveness analysis comparing ICUs with and without telemedicine showed an incremental cost-effectiveness ratio (the difference in costs divided by the difference in their effect) of \$50,265 to \$375,870 [33]. These economic evaluations, coupled with further experience, will help individual hospitals determine the impact of telemedicine in the ICU.

Perceptions

The interpersonal dynamics of ICU staff are influenced by the use of tele-ICU for monitoring and intervention by specialists. Understanding impact on staff is imperative as perceptions and perceived benefits of tele-ICU coverage are important for implementing, operating and maintaining a tele-ICU system. Many studies have evaluated pre- and post-implementation acceptance of tele-ICU coverage, and overall general acceptance is favorable. One study evaluating nurses' pre-implementation perceptions found that on a five-point Likert scale (1 = not favorable and 5 = favorable), nurses' perceived tele-ICU usefulness and overall attitude toward tele-ICU was average (2.8 and 3.3 respectively) [34]. However, post implementation, mean satisfaction with tele-ICU coverage ranged from 4.2 to 4.5 [35]. Another study found that prior to implementation, 67% of ICU physicians and nurses believed that tele-ICU coverage could enhance ICU quality of care, and post-implementation 82.3% reported increased quality [36–38]. An additional investigation demonstrated that 67% of ICU staff believed tele-ICU coverage would improve communication between ICU nurses and intensivists before implementation; post-implementation, 94% found that collaboration was facilitated by tele-ICU and overall communication between intensivists improved [39].

There are also data suggesting that tele-ICU decreases provider burden of caring for patients in the ICU, is encouraged and facilitated by hospital administration, and helps with recruitment and retention of healthcare professionals at smaller hospitals [40]. One small study assessed patients' and families' perceptions of care in 10 ICUs supported by tele-ICU coverage. Items with which patients and family members were most satisfied included feeling that patients were treated as individual people and comforted that they were being monitored. They felt that they received appropriate explanations of care and that their needs were responded to in a timely manner, suggesting that tele-ICU may also enhance patient and family experience in the ICU [41].

In addition to the perceived benefits of tele-ICU, several barriers to tele-ICU acceptance beyond costs have been identified. Although there is considerable improvement in post-implementation perceptions, the attitudes of physicians and nurses who have not used telemedicine is a significant barrier. Moreover, there is widespread concern about privacy issues, as well as nurse and physician perceptions that tele-ICU may decrease the ability to personally know and establish a relationship with the tele-ICU staff. There are also concerns about disruptions to workflow, confusion about how to use tele-ICU software and hardware, and uneasiness with unmet expectations such as how telemedicine will be rolled out, how responsibilities might change, etc. [42]. Physicians remain concerned that positive cost savings are not guaranteed and may not meaningfully affect a hospital's financial security. Moreover, although physician reimbursement is increasingly common, very few payers, including Medicare (the most common payer for US ICU patients), reimburse for critical care services provided via telemedicine [43].

Telemedicine for Communication

Although interventions, such as establishing best practices and implementation of novel technologies within ICUs, have led to improvement in survival rates, overall ICU mortality remains high. Many studies have demonstrated that the majority of deaths in the ICU involve withholding or withdrawing life-sustaining therapies [44]. Therefore, the ICU represents a setting where, in addition to decisions about acute life-sustaining therapies, decisions about managing death and dying are frequently made. Studies have found that family members rate communication with health-care providers as one of the most important factors of care, often equal to or more important than clinical skills [46]. Effective communication is therefore crucial for excellent ICU care, and research demonstrates that high quality early communication in the ICU improves family satisfaction, perceived quality of death and dying among family members whose loved ones died in an ICU, reduces symptoms of depression and decreases costs [47, 48].

Despite the robust evidence supporting high quality communication, most ICU physicians do not conduct family conferences until shortly before the decision is made to withhold/withdraw life sustaining therapies, and many physicians remain uncomfortable beginning these discussions early in an ICU stay [46]. In addition, there is an even larger communication gap among family members of patients who are transferring from a rural hospital to a larger tertiary care center ICU. Long distances, financial restrictions, and other responsibilities often impair the ability of family members to travel to a tertiary care center to participate in ICU family conferences, and thus communication with families of patients who transfer very rarely occurs early in these patients' care. Telemedicine may therefore positively impact communication with families of critically ill patients in smaller rural hospitals.

Telemedicine has been used in the non-ICU setting for teleconsultations in a variety of medical specialties including radiology, dermatology, surgery, pediatrics and psychiatry. In most of these consultative processes, communication through telemedicine is most often physician-centered. In telepsychiatry and telepsychology, however, an emphasis is placed on increasing patient communication and improving physician awareness and response to verbal and non-verbal cues. Some studies have evaluated the efficacy of telemedicine to assist in both communication with patients and the development of an effective therapeutic alliance between patient and a healthcare professional [48]. These studies have found that effective communication and development of a therapeutic alliance rely heavily on the experiences of the patient during their first telemedicine encounters. Patients who felt they had adequate time to talk and ask questions, were not rushed, and when heard had higher rates of satisfaction with the telemedicine experience. Likewise, patients who received interventions via telemedicine did not report any difference in the experience compared to in-person communication interventions. Although these studies were performed in the outpatient specialty setting (psychology and pulmonary), these data demonstrate that communication through telemedicine, when performed optimally, is feasible and acceptable to patients. In spite of the importance of communication in the ICU, there are few studies of tele-ICU for improving communication with family members of patients who cannot be present for an early family conference.

Early Communication in the ICU Using Telemedicine

Because communication with patients who transfer from rural hospitals to larger tertiary care center ICUs is often delayed, their families may benefit from early communication to discuss diagnosis, prognosis, goals of care and treatment plans via telemedicine. We have been investigating telemedicine as a tool for early family conferences and palliative care consultations for critically ill patients being transferred from rural health centers to a tertiary care center (Fig. 1). Our work thus far demonstrates that physicians and nurses are responding positively to this use of telemedicine and that these consultations lead to high quality patient goal-oriented end of life care. In fact, we have found that often times patients/family members choose not to transfer to a tertiary care center if not consistent with overall goals of care [49, 50].

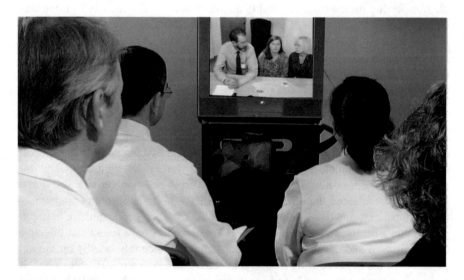

Fig. 1 Photograph of telemedicine videoconference (obtained during simulated conference with simulated patients for a video we recorded to demonstrate telemedicine capabilities to small rural hospitals)

Conclusion

Telemedicine in the ICU may reduce ICU mortality, hospital mortality and ICU LOS. However, tele-ICU programs are not associated with overall decreased lengths of hospital stay and the long-term cost effectiveness of the programs requires further exploration. Additional uses of telemedicine programs in the ICU setting should be considered, including providing early and effective communication for patients in rural settings considering transfer to a tertiary care ICU. Further detailed studies that address both barriers and facilitators of using telemedicine to communicate with families are needed. These studies should incorporate the concepts of the technology acceptance model to provide the most comprehensive review of barriers and facilitators.

Understanding these issues will be the key to designing, implementing and analyzing a successful and sustainable telemedicine practice.

References

1. Halpern NA, Pastores SM (2010) Critical care medicine in the United States 2000–2005: an analysis of bed numbers, occupancy rates, payer mix, and costs. Crit Care Med 38:65–71
2. Breslow MJ, Rosenfeld BA, Doerfler M et al (2004) Effect of a multiple-site intensive care unit telemedicine program on clinical and economic outcomes: an alternative paradigm for intensivist staffing. Crit Care Med 32:31–38
3. Lilly CM, McLaughlin J, Zhao M et al (2014) Critical care telemedicine: evolution and state of the art. Crit Care Med 42:2429–2436
4. Yeo W, Ahrens SL, Wright T (2012) A new era in the ICU: the case for telemedicine. Crit Care Nurs Q 35:316–321
5. Pitts JAS (1985) The human factor: biomedicine in the manned space program to 1980. The NASA History Series. https://history.nasa.gov/SP-4213.pdf. Accessed 10 January 2018
6. Vakoch DA (2011) Psychology of space exploration: contemporary research in historical perspective. NASA history series. https://www.nasa.gov/pdf/607107main_PsychologySpaceExploration-ebook.pdf. Accessed 10 January 2018
7. Hicks LL, Boles KE, Hudson ST et al (2001) Using telemedicine to avoid transfer of rural emergency department patients. J Rural Health 17:220–228
8. Nesbitt TS, Marcin JP, Daschbach MM et al (2005) Perceptions of local health care quality in 7 rural communities with telemedicine. J Rural Health 21:79–85
9. Pronovost PJ, Rinke ML, Emery K et al (2004) Interventions to reduce mortality among patients treated in intensive care units. J Crit Care 19:158–164
10. Duke EM (2006) The critical care workforce: a study of the supply and demand for critical care physicians. Health Resources and Services Administration. http://www.mc.vanderbilt.edu/documents/CAPNAH/files/criticalcare.pdf. Accessed 10 January 2018
11. Lilly CM, Cody S, Zhao H et al (2011) Hospital mortality, length of stay, and preventable complications among critically ill patients before and after tele-ICU reengineering of critical care processes. JAMA 305:2175–2183
12. Sadaka F, Palagirl A, Trottier S et al (2013) Telemedicine intervention improves ICU outcomes. Crit Care Res Pract 2013:456389
13. Willmitch B, Golembeski S, Kim SS et al (2012) Clinical outcomes after telemedicine intensive care unit implementation. Crit Care Med 40:450–454
14. Rosenfeld BA, Dorman T, Breslow MJ et al (2000) Intensive care unit telemedicine: alternate paradigm for providing continuous intensivist care. Crit Care Med 28:3925–3931

15. Vespa PM, Miller C, Hu X et al (2007) Intensive care unit robotic telepresence facilitates rapid physician response to unstable patients and decreased cost in neurointensive care. Surg Neurol 67:331–337
16. McCambridge M, Jones K, Paxton H et al (2010) Association of health information technology and teleintensivist coverage with decreased mortality and ventilator use in critically ill patients. Arch Intern Med 170:648–653
17. Morrison JL, Cai Q, Davis N et al (2010) Clinical and economic outcomes of the electronic intensive care unit: results from two community hospitals. Crit Care Med 38:2–8
18. Nassar BS, Vaughan-Sarrazin MS, Jiang L et al (2014) Impact of an intensive care unit telemedicine program on patient outcomes in an integrated health care system. JAMA Intern Med 174:1160–1167
19. Thomas EJ, Lucke JF, Wueste L et al (2009) Association of telemedicine for remote monitoring of intensive care patients with mortality, complications, and length of stay. JAMA 302:2671–2678
20. Young LB, Chan PS, Lu X et al (2011) Impact of telemedicine intensive care unit coverage on patient outcomes: a systematic review and meta-analysis. Arch Intern Med 171:498–506
21. Kalb T, Raikhelkar J, Meyer S et al (2014) A multicenter population-based effectiveness study of teleintensive care unit-directed ventilator rounds demonstrating improved adherence to a protective lung strategy, decreased ventilator duration, and decreased intensive care unit mortality. J Crit Care 29:691.e7–691.e14
22. Lilly CM, McLaughlin JM, Zhao H et al (2014) A multicenter study of ICU telemedicine reengineering of adult critical care. Chest 145:500–507
23. Scales DC, Dainty K, Hales B et al (2009) An innovative telemedicine knowledge translation program to improve quality of care in intensive care units: protocol for a cluster randomized pragmatic trial. Implement Sci 4:5
24. Meyers L, Gibbs D, Thacker M et al (2012) Building a telehealth network through collaboration: the story of the nebraska statewide telehealth network. Crit Care Nurs Q 35:346–352
25. Parsapour K, Kon AA, Dharmar M et al (2011) Connecting hospitalized patients with their families: case series and commentary. Int J Telemed Appl 2011:804254
26. Grundy BL, Crawford P, Jones PK et al (1977) Telemedicine in critical care: an experiment in health care delivery. JACEP 6:439–444
27. Kahn JM, Cicero BD, Wallace DJ et al (2014) Adoption of ICU telemedicine in the United States. Crit Care Med 42:362–368
28. Angus DC, Shorr AF, White A et al (2006) Critical care delivery in the United States: distribution of services and compliance with Leapfrog recommendations. Crit Care Med 34:1016–1024
29. Holden RJ, Karash B (2010) The technology acceptance model: its past and its future in health care. J Biomed Inform 43:159–172
30. Chau PYK, Hu PJH (2002) Investigating healthcare professionals' decisions to accept telemedicine technology: an empirical test of competing theories. Inf Manag 39:297–311
31. Coustasse A, Deslich S, Bailey D et al (2014) A business case for tele-intensive care units. Perm J 18:76–84
32. Fortis S, Weinert C, Bushinski R et al (2014) A health system-based critical care program with a novel tele-ICU: implementation, cost, and structure details. J Am Coll Surg 219:676–683
33. Yoo BK, Kim M, Sasaki T et al (2016) Economic evaluation of telemedicine for patients in ICUs. Crit Care Med 44:265–274
34. Kowitlawakul Y (2011) The technology acceptance model: predicting nurses' intention to use telemedicine technology (eICU). Comput Inform Nurs 29:411–418
35. Marttos A, Wilson K, Krauthamer S et al (2008) Telerounds in a trauma ICU dept. Crit Care Med 36:A120 (abst)
36. Faiz SA, Zachria A, Weavind L, Patel B (2006) Fellowship education in remote telemonitoring units. Chest 130(Suppl):113S (abst)

37. Heath B, Salerno R, Hopkins A et al (2009) Pediatric critical care telemedicine in rural under-served emergency departments. Pediatr Crit Care Med 10:588–591

38. Mora A, Faiz S, Kelly T et al (2007) Resident perception of the educational and patient care value from remote telemonitoring in a medical intensive care unit. Chest 132:443a (abst)

39. Chung KK, Poropatich RK (2009) Bedside nurse perceptions of intensive care unit telemedicine. Crit Care Med 37:A441 (abst)

40. Ward MM, Ullrich F, Potter AJ et al (2015) Factors affecting staff perceptions of tele-ICU service in rural hospitals. Telemed J E Health 21:459–466

41. Golembeski S, Willmitch B, Kim SS (2012) Perceptions of the care experience in critical care units enhanced by a tele-ICU. AACN Adv Crit Care 23:323–329

42. Moeckli J, Cram P, Cunningham C et al (2013) Staff acceptance of a telemedicine intensive care unit program: a qualitative study. J Crit Care 28:890–901

43. McCambridge MM, Tracy JA, Sample GA (2011) Point: Should tele-ICU services be eligible for professional fee billing? Yes. Tele-ICUs and the triple aim. Chest 140:847–849

44. Vincent J-L, Parquier JN, Presier JC et al (1989) Terminal events in the intensive care unit: review of 258 fatal cases in one year. Crit Care Med 17:530–533

45. Hickey M (1990) What are the needs of families of critically ill patients? A review of the literature since 1976. Heart Lung 19:401–415

46. Lautrette A, Darmon M, Megarbane B et al (2007) A communication strategy and brochure for relatives of patients dying in the ICU. N Engl J Med 356:469–478

47. Curtis JR, Treece PD, Nielsen EL et al (2016) Randomized trial of communication facilitators to reduce family distress and intensity of end-of-life care. Am J Respir Crit Care Med 193:154–162

48. Wootton R, Liu J, Bonnardot L (2015) Relationship between the quality of service provided through store-and-forward telemedicine consultations and the difficulty of the cases – implications for long-term quality assurance. Front Public Health 3:217

49. Menon PR, Stapleton RD, McVeigh U et al (2015) Telemedicine as a tool to provide family conferences and palliative care consultations in critically ill patients at rural health care institutions: a pilot study. Am J Hosp Palliat Care 32:448–453

50. Menon PR, Prelock P, Rose GL et al (2016) Clinicians' perceptions of telemedicine for conducting family conferences prior to transfer to a tertiary care center intensive care unit. J Int Soc Telemed eHealth 4:20–24

Index

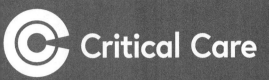
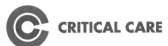
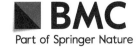